Nursing Care
of Older Adults

Theory and Practice

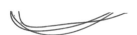

Third Edition

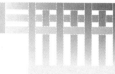

Nursing Care of Older Adults

Theory and Practice

Carol A. Miller, M.S.N., R.N., C.

Gerontological Clinical Nurse Specialist
Care & Counseling, Miller/Wetzler Associates
Cleveland, Ohio

Clinical Faculty
Frances Payne Bolton School of Nursing
Case Western Reserve University
Cleveland, Ohio

Nursing Consultant
Western Reserve Geriatric Education Center
Case Western Reserve University
Cleveland, Ohio

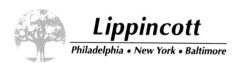

Lippincott

Philadelphia • New York • Baltimore

Acquisitions Editor: Susan M. Keneally
Production Editor: Virginia Barishek
Senior Production Manager: Helen Ewan
Production Service: P. M. Gordon Associates, Inc.
Compositor: The PRD Group
Printer/Binder: R. R. Donnelley & Sons/Crawfordsville
Cover Designer: Joan Wendt
Cover Printer: Lehigh Press

Third Edition

9 8 7 6 5 4 3 2 1

Library of Congress Cataloging-in-Publication Data

Miller, Carol A.
   Nursing care of older adults : theory and practice / Carol A. Miller. — 3rd ed.
      p.   cm.
   Includes bibliographical references and index.
   ISBN 0-7817-1623-3
   1. Geriatric nursing.   I. Title.
   [DNLM: 1. Geriatric Nursing.   WY 152 M563n 1999]
   RC954.M55   1999
   610.73'65—dc21
   DNLM/DLC   98-45982
   for Library of Congress   CIP

*This book is dedicated, with love,
to my parents, Margaret and Bob Miller,
who are inspiring examples of continued growth
throughout adulthood.*

*I also dedicate this work to the many older adults
and their families who have been a source of inspiration
in the past decade as I have been privileged to share
in the most challenging years of their lives
through my private practice.*

Reviewers

Lorraine Elliott Boyd, MSN, RN, C
Assistant Professor
Columbus State Community College
Columbus, OH

Katharine Kolcaba, PhD, RN, C
Assistant Professor
College of Nursing
The University of Akron
Akron, OH

Rosanna Marinpetro, MSN, RN
Teaching Specialist
School of Nursing
Shadyside Hospital
Pittsburgh, PA

Terri T. Small, MSN, RN, C
Assistant Professor of Nursing
Waynesburg College
Waynesburg, PA

Sharon Staib, MS, RN, CS
Nursing Instructor
Ohio University–Zanesville
Zanesville, OH

Foreword

Although older adults have always been a focus of nursing care, only in recent decades has gerontological nursing grown as a specialty within the nursing profession. Today, nurses are seeking answers to crucial questions such as, What is unique about nursing care needs of older adults? and How can nurses effectively care for older adults? *Nursing Care of Older Adults: Theory and Practice* answers such questions. A product of Carol A. Miller's twenty-eight years of experience and expertise in caring for older adults, this text reflects her high degree of sensitivity to the unique nursing needs of older adults. Moreover, Miller provides a theoretical base for the practice of gerontological nursing, thereby making a unique and valuable contribution to the field.

In contrast to the many nursing texts that focus on the illness aspects of aging, this text is wellness oriented and focuses on the quality of life of older adults. Miller uses her *functional consequences theory of gerontological nursing* throughout this text to examine normal aging processes and risk factors that affect the health and functional level of older adults. Then she extends far beyond simply *assessing* function and presents nursing interventions directed toward *improving* the functional level of older adults. In this third edition, Miller has addressed the increasing need to provide culturally sensitive nursing care to a population of older adults that is rapidly growing in diversity. As in the previous editions, the framework of Miller's functional consequences theory provides a practical approach that nurses can use to facilitate positive functional consequences, such as improved quality of life, for older adults.

Nursing Care of Older Adults: Theory and Practice challenges the "What-do-you-expect-you're-old" attitude and provides a theoretical base from which nurses can assist older adults in realizing their tremendous potential for continued growth and better health. Gerontological nurses and older adults for whom they care will benefit greatly from this far-reaching, well-grounded, and sensitively written text. Nurses and nursing students will find that this text is truly a positive life-affirming approach to care of older adults.

May L. Wykle, Ph.D., R.N., F.A.A.N.
Florence Cellar Professor of Gerontological Nursing and
Associate Dean for Community Affairs
Frances Payne Bolton School of Nursing
Case Western Reserve University

Director, University Center on Aging and Health
Case Western Reserve University

Preface

With the exception of nurses who work solely with young people, most nurses realize at some point in their career that at least half of the people for whom they provide care could be defined chronologically as "old." Along with this recognition often comes an uncomfortable awareness of their lack of information about distinctive aspects of nursing care of older adults. *Nursing Care of Older Adults: Theory and Practice* has been written for nursing students and nurses who are knowledgeable about nursing care of adults and desire to enhance their knowledge about the unique responses of *older* adults to actual or potential health problems. This text covers all aspects of physical and psychosocial function that distinguish gerontological nursing from other types of nursing. It is unique in focusing on age-related changes and risk factors that affect the level of function and quality of life of older adults. Assessment guidelines identify risk factors and functional consequences that can be addressed through nursing care, and interventions are applicable not only in acute care settings but also in home, community, and long-term care settings.

Chapters are organized around the *functional consequences theory of gerontological nursing*. Each facet of physiologic or psychosocial function is discussed as follows: age-related changes, risk factors, functional consequences, nursing assessment, nursing diagnosis, nursing goals, nursing interventions, and evaluation of nursing care. Also, each chapter has learning objectives, a chapter summary, critical thinking exercises, and a case example and nursing care plan. The case examples address day-to-day nursing situations that reflect the diversity of settings in which nurses care for ill and healthy older adults.

Special features of this text include tables and illustrations that summarize age-related changes, risk factors, and functional consequences. Designated and shaded displays summarize guidelines for nursing assessment and highlight nursing interventions for each topic. Nursing interventions focus on teaching older adults and their caregivers how to improve functional abilities, and some of the intervention displays are written in a format that can be used for health education. At the end of each chapter is a list of educational resources that provide free or low-cost health education materials pertinent to the topic of the chapter. Nurses and nursing students are encouraged to obtain these educational materials and to give the names of these organizations to older adults and their caregivers. The Appendix provides an additional review of age-related changes, risk factors, negative functional consequences, nursing assessment, nursing interventions, and positive functional consequences for each area of physiologic function.

A special feature of the third edition is the attention to cultural considerations of aging and older adults. Thirty-five specially designated Culture Boxes address cultural differences in specific aspects such as dietary habits, expressions of symptoms, family caregiving expectations, and health and socioeconomic characteristics. A cultural self-assessment tool is included, and many cultural aspects of psychosocial assessment, such as the use of interpreters, also are addressed. Another special feature of the third edition is the inclusion of 15 displays that summarize alternative and preventive health care practices for specific health concerns. A third new feature of this edition is the addition of Internet connections for the educational resources that are listed at the end of every chapter. Critical Thinking Exercises also have been added in this edition.

The text is divided into five parts and twenty-two chapters. Part I provides an overview of gerontological nursing and a perspective on older adults and older adulthood. Particular attention is paid to cultural aspects of aging in Chapter 1. Also, this part reviews theories regarding aging and explains the functional consequences framework underpinning the text. Part II discusses cognitive and psychosocial function of older adults and includes a comprehensive nursing assessment of mental status and other components of psychosocial function. The chapter on psychosocial assessment has been updated significantly to address multicultural aspects of assessment. Parts III and IV cover the following areas of physiologic function: hearing, vision, digestion and nutrition, urinary elimination, cardiovascular function, respiratory function, mobility and safety, skin, sleep, thermoregulation, and sexual function.

Part V addresses multidimensional aspects of care and includes the following topics: functional assessment, medications, dementia, depression, elder abuse and neglect, and health care for older adults. The chapter on dementia is updated to include the latest developments in the causes of and treatments for Alzheimer's disease. The chapter on health care for older adults addresses nursing implications of legal and ethical issues. This chapter also includes information about the recent changes and developments in health insurance and the increasingly diverse settings for the practice of gerontological nursing.

Gerontological nursing provides an opportunity to share in the stage of life that can be approached with either fear and anxiety or a sense of challenge. The goal of *Nursing Care of Older Adults: Theory and Practice* is to provide nurses with the knowledge base needed to help older adults function at their highest level, despite the presence of age-related changes and risk factors. Using this text, nurses and nursing students can assist older adults in meeting the many challenges of older adulthood in a positive and creative way.

Carol A. Miller, M.S.N., R.N., C.

Acknowledgments

I am deeply grateful to my many friends and colleagues who have supported me on my journey as this book has grown from a dream to a reality and now into its third edition. Pat Rehm, in particular, has been a constant source of encouragement on my journey as an author. My family has always encouraged me to believe in my dreams, and my sister, Kathleen Unetic, enjoys with me the rewards of our nursing profession. Many older adults and their families have taught me valuable lessons that contribute to the strength of this text. These experiences, which cannot be learned in books, have taught me to care deeply about and to care sensitively for older adults. I thank these older adults and their families and I appreciate their contributions to my life and my writings.

I appreciate and acknowledge the many people who assisted me in developing my original text and the revisions. Margaret Andrews contributed significantly to Chapter 5 of this edition and has been a challenging source of inspiration regarding cultural aspects of aging and older adulthood. Georgia Anetzberger co-authored Chapter 21, and Betsy Todd contributed to Chapter 18. Katharine Kolcaba contributed to Chapters 1, 2, and 22 and helped me clarify and articulate my theory of gerontological nursing. June Allen and her colleagues at Lorain Community College contributed a wealth of ideas for the resource materials that accompany this text.

I appreciate the thoughtful comments and suggestions offered by the reviewers. I am grateful to Susan Keneally and the many other people in the nursing division of Lippincott Williams & Wilkins who have led the way and guided me on my text-writing journey. Debby Stuart and the capable people at P. M. Gordon Associates did a wonderful job of copyediting and were most helpful during the final phases of book development.

I thank all of you, and many unnamed people, for the advice, guidance, support, and encouragement on my journey through the first, second, and third editions of *Nursing Care of Older Adults: Theory and Practice*.

Carol A. Miller

Credits

Diagrams pages 9, 13, 54, 75, 113, 188, 212, 246, 273, 304, 331, 360, 386, 408, 428, 456, 482–483, 508, 586, and 603, Asterisk Group; interior photographs pages 1 (group—Part I), 67 (seniors group—Part II), 477 (group—Part V), 113 (Fig. 4-1), Paul Beck; pages 1 (man and dog—Part I), 67 (boy and man—Part II), 75 (Fig. 3-1), 456 (Fig. 16-1), Father James F. Flood; page 375 (grandson and grandmother—Part IV), Danielle DiPalma; pages 177 (Part III), 375 (guitar player—Part IV), 477 (woman and baby—Part V), Kathy Sloane

Contents

Part III
Changes, Consequences, and Care Related to Physiologic Function   177

Part IV

Changes, Consequences, and Care Related to Comfort and Pleasure   375

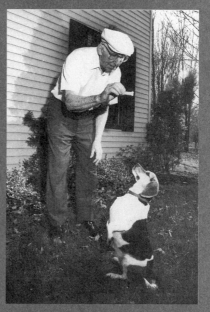

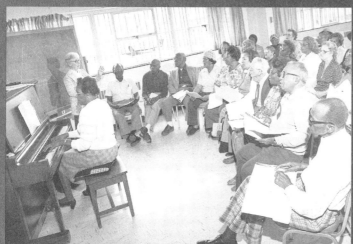

*Introduction to Nursing
Care of Older Adults*

Perspectives on Older Adults and Gerontological Nursing

Chapter

1

Learning Objectives	1. *Discuss the concepts of geriatrics and gerontology.*
	2. *Describe the health and social characteristics of older adults, emphasizing the diversity and cultural aspects of these characteristics.*
	3. *Discuss the implications of changing demographic patterns for the provision of health care in our society.*
	4. *Examine definitions of aging.*
	5. *Recognize attitudes, stereotypes, and sociocultural factors that influence perspectives on aging, older adulthood, and nursing care of older adults.*
	6. *Delineate myths and realities about aging.*
	7. *State at least five factors that contribute to the complexity of providing health care to older adults.*
	8. *Discuss recent challenges related to multiculturalism and alternative health care practices.*
	9. *Describe the scope of gerontological nursing practice.*

Gerontology, Geriatrics, and Gerontological Nursing

Gerontology is the branch of science that deals with aging and the problems of aging people. Gerontology is multidisciplinary and is a specialized area within various disciplines, such as nursing, psychology, social work, and certain allied health professions. The term "geriatrics" usually is associated with the realm of medicine because it encompasses the disease and disabilities of old people. Geriatrics is a subspecialty of internal medicine or family practice that has as its focus the medical aspects of older people. Since 1976, the American Nurses Association (ANA) has advocated using the term "gerontological nursing," rather than "geriatric nursing," because the former more accurately reflects the scope of nursing. If nurses practiced geriatric nursing, their care would focus primarily on the disease conditions of older people, which, for the most part, are much the same as those that affect all adults. However, there are several factors that make the care of this older population unique, among them the response of older people to disease, the manifestations of various disease states in this population, and the functional consequences of these illnesses. Therefore, because nurses focus on the response of individuals to actual or potential health problems, it is more appropriate to say that they practice gerontological nursing.

Demographic changes have had significant implications for our society in general, for the health care industry, and for the nursing profession. For example, in the early 1900s, life expectancy in the United States was only 47 years, and older people constituted only 4% of the population. Very few people were cared for in hospitals, and the field of geriatrics had not yet been developed. In 1996, life expectancy was

76 years, and people aged 65 years or older constituted almost 13% of the population in the United States. Yet another recent demographic phenomenon that has affected health care is the disproportionate increase in the number of "oldest old" in the United States and in other industrialized societies. In 1996, the number of people aged 85 years and older was 31 times greater than in 1900, whereas the number of people aged 65 to 74 years was only 8 times greater. Major demographic changes also are occurring in terms of the cultural diversity of older adults. In 1996, minority groups constituted about 15% of older adults, of which approximately 8% were Black, 5% were Hispanic origin, 2% were Asian or Pacific Islander, and about 1% were Native Alaskan or American Indian (American Association of Retired Persons [AARP] and Administration on Aging, 1997).

Because of demographic trends such as those just cited, the specialties of geriatric medicine and gerontological nursing have become increasingly accepted, integral components of the medical and nursing professions. Also, there has been a growing recognition of the need to address the health care needs of special populations, such as older women, rural elders, older adults of various cultural backgrounds, older adults with mental health problems, and older adults with long-term care needs (Buckwalter et al., 1997). Despite the fact that nurses have cared for older adults for centuries, gerontological nursing has only recently "come of age" as a specialty.

Characteristics of Older Adults in the United States

Two major demographic trends that affect gerontological nursing and the health care system are the rapid growth of the old-old subgroup of older adults and the increasing diversity, including increasing cultural diversity, of the older adult population. The chief implication of the rapid growth of the old-old population is that this group is most likely to have significant functional impairments and, therefore, is most likely to need gerontological nursing care. An implication of the increasing diversity of the older adult population is that the nursing care of these older adults must take into account the unique needs of each individual receiving care. The following sections discuss some of the characteristics of older adults that are most pertinent to the provision of culturally sensitive gerotological nursing care. In reviewing these characteristics, the reader should keep in mind that older adults are a highly diverse group of individuals, and that these characteristics are generalizations that may not apply to a specific older adult. As one well-known gerontologist who was describing the psychosocial profile of older adults noted:

> One feature of late life that promises to endure is that of diversity. In ethnic origin, language, health, family relations, intelligence, life style, educational background, and socioeconomic status, it is difficult to pinpoint an average older person. The profile of today's and tomorrow's older people can only be reduced to a series of prototypes drawn with the broadest of strokes that touch on some common denominators. With every broad stroke that is made, it must be assumed there are many exceptions to the rule. (Silverstone, 1996, p. 27)

Diversity

In the early decades of gerontology, all people aged 65 years or older were grouped together as the population of old people. In the past several decades, however, gerontologists have recognized the need to identify the characteristics of subgroups, such as people who are older than 75 or 85 years. It is now quite common for the subgroup of people 85 years or older to be referred to as the oldest old. Another gerontological trend is to differentiate members of this population according to their functional abilities, distinguishing between "frail elderly" and those who can be classified as "able elderly," or those experiencing "robust aging" or "successful aging." The frail elderly tend to belong to the oldest-old group, whereas able elderly persons usually belong to the young-old or middle-old groups. Frail elderly is a term applied to older adults who are medically ill or incapacitated most of the time and who, therefore, have the greatest health care needs. This subgroup is the opposite extreme of the majority of older adults who are able to function in the community with little assistance. The medically frail older person typically is 85 years or older, is functionally disabled, takes several medications, and has few social supports. What is of concern to health care planners and providers is that the group of people older than 85 years of age has become the fastest growing population group. Because not all people aged 85 years or older are frail and dependent, gerontologists are trying to identify characteristics that determine robust aging and successful aging. A recent study of characteristics of robust aging in people aged 60 years and older revealed that the most robustly aging people reported high levels of social contact, good health and vision, and few major life events occurring in the past 3 years (Garfein and Herzog, 1995). Three components of successful aging that have been identified are active engagement with life, high cognitive and physical function, and low probability of disease and disability (Rowe and Kahn, 1997).

The concept of cultural diversity generally is used in reference to groups of people who share a common heritage. By the year 2050, it is projected that culturally diverse groups in the United States will constitute 25% of the older adult population, compared to 15% in 1996 (AARP and Administration on Aging, 1997). Between 1995 and 2050, the percentage increase in people aged 65 years and older, grouped by categories, is as follows: White, 114%; Black, 217%; other (Aleuts, Asians, Eskimos, Pacific Islanders, and American Indians), 657%, and Hispanic origin, 815% (National Aging Infor-

mation Center, 1997). Projections for the year 2050 indicate that the greatest increases in the minority elderly population will be among Hispanics, who will constitute 15.5% of the older adult population, and Asians and Pacific Islanders, who will account for 7.4% of the older adult population. The disproportionate increase in these minority groups is partly attributable to their past and future immigration patterns (U.S. Bureau of the Census and National Institute on Aging, 1993). Moreover, one must be mindful that data about cultural groups of older adults in the United States were not available until recently, and that the information that is available is limited by the factors described in the accompanying Culture Box.

Life Expectancy, Morbidity, and Mortality

In 1996, approximately 2 million people in the United States were classified as having reached "old age" by virtue of turning 65 years of age. By contrast, only 1.7 million people exited this old age category by dying, resulting in a net increase of 890 old persons per day (AARP and Administration on Aging, 1997). By the middle of the next century, 5% of all Americans and 25% of the people older than 65 years of age will be classified as belonging to the category of oldest old (i.e., 85 years or older). Although the proportion of old to young people in the United States is partially influenced by diminishing birthrates, the principal reasons for the recent upsurge in the growth of the older population are a rising life expectancy and a declining mortality rate. Among the factors contributing to this increased life expectancy in industrialized societies are improved control of infectious diseases, increased emphasis on health promotion, heightened efforts in the prevention and treatment of cardiovascular diseases, and improvements in maternal-infant-child care. In addition to increased life expectancy in industrialized societies, there has been a steady decrease in birth-

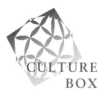

CULTURE
BOX

Gerontological Research Regarding Cultural Aspects of Aging and Older Adulthood

Primary Focus of Research: A Timeline

1960s   African Americans

1970s   Hispanic Americans, primarily Mexican Americans

1980s   Native Americans, Asian and Pacific Islanders, and older adults of European origin

Limitations

- Many subgroups are clustered together: some groupings are inconsistent (see below).
- Most of the emphasis is on morbidity, mortality, risk of disease, and negative aspects of aging; little attention is paid to the multicultural aspects of successful aging.
- Little or no distinction is made between immigrants and nonimmigrants of the same cultural group, or between the first American-born generation, the second American-born generation, and so on.
- Little or no attention is paid to diversity and variations within cultural groups.
- Much of the research compares one or two racial or ethnic groups with White Americans; few studies include more than two or three groups.
- Little attention has been paid to gender differences.
- Until recently, there has been no effort to distinguish the effects of ethnicity from the effects of other factors, such as socioeconomic status.
- Official census data do not yet provide specific information about the numerous "other" cultural groups comprising an increasing percentage of the U.S. population.

Common Cultural Groupings

- African Americans or Blacks, including Africans, West Indians, and Caribbean Islanders
- Asian Americans and Pacific Islanders, including Chinese, Japanese, Filipinos, Koreans, Asian Indians, and Native Hawaiians (according to the U.S. Census Bureau)
- Hispanics, including Cubans, Spaniards, Mexicans, Puerto Ricans, and Central or South Americans
- Japanese Americans, classified according to the following groups:
  - *Issei:* First-generation immigrants to the United States
  - *Nisei:* Second generation (first American-born generation)
  - *Sansei:* Third generation
  - *Yonsei:* Fourth generation
- Native Americans, including Aleuts, Eskimos, Native Hawaiians (according to the Older Americans Act), and more than 500 tribes of American Indians

rate, causing a reversal in the ratio of young to old people in the United States.

Tremendous changes are taking place in life expectancy. Consider, for example, the fact that, in 1940, about 7% of people who reached the age of 65 years could expect to survive to 90 years. In 2000, that percentage will rise to 26%; by 2050, that percentage is expected to increase to 42%. Projections for 2050 estimate that life expectancy will be 82 years, and that people aged 65 years and older will represent about 20% of the population. There are, however, significant racial and gender variations in the rates. In 1991, White men and women reaching the age of 65 years could expect to live an additional 15 or 19 years, respectively, whereas Black men and women could expect to live an additional 13 or 17 years, respectively (U.S. Bureau of the Census, 1996). The gap in life expectancy between Blacks and Whites narrows with increasing age until, around the age of 80 years, the life expectancy of Blacks begins to exceed that of Whites. At the age of 85 years, White and Black women are likely to live an additional 6.3 and 6.5 years, respectively. For White and Black men, life expectancy at the age of 85 years is 5.1 and 5.3 years, respectively (U.S. Bureau of the Census, 1996). Although some questions have been raised about the accuracy of mortality estimates for Hispanics and Native Americans, current estimates suggest that the life expectancy disadvantage of these groups is diminishing (Markides and Rudkin, 1996). The life expectancy of Asians and Pacific Islanders is higher than that of any other group in the United States.

Mortality rates are graphically represented in a survivorship curve, which illustrates the changes occurring in death rates over a period of time. In Figure 1-1, the vertical axis designates the percentage of survivors, ranging from a theoretical 0% at the bottom to 100% at the top, whereas the horizontal axis represents the age of survivorship. As is evident from this graph, the curves are becoming increasingly elongated—nearly rectangular, in fact—owing to

changes caused by various factors occurring at different points in time. For example, the first major change in survival resulted from improved housing and sanitation practices, whereas the second major change was brought about by the advent of immunization programs and other advances in public health practices. The major change occurring between 1960 and 1980 is attributable to biomedical breakthroughs, such as organ transplants, heart-lung machines, and increasingly effective cancer treatments. More recent increases in adult life expectancy can be attributed to declines in stroke and heart disease mortality (Manton et al., 1993). Between 1982 and 1989, disability and morbidity rates both declined, resulting in increased life expectancy at late ages. These recent declines are at least partly attributable to preventive measures, such as increased exercise levels, nutritional changes, reductions in smoking, improvements in antioxidant intake, and use of exogenous estrogens for women (Manton et al., 1995).

The squaring, or rectangularization, of the curve signifies that, for people who reach the age of 75 or 80 years, longevity is not increased, and life expectancy is not prolonged significantly. Despite advances in health care and medical technology, this trend is not expected to change owing to the inherent teleology of human beings. That is, we seem to be programmed genetically to live for about 100 years, even under the best of circumstances. People today are surviving illnesses that led to early deaths in previous decades, but they still tend to suffer from chronic illnesses that do not lead to death. As a consequence, people today spend a relatively greater proportion of their lives in a state of some level of dependency. This has prompted geriatricians and gerontologists to begin to address the concept of "active life expectancy" as an indicator of quality of life during older adulthood. This concept is based on the number of years spent at a high functional level. Function may be evaluated on a continuum of four

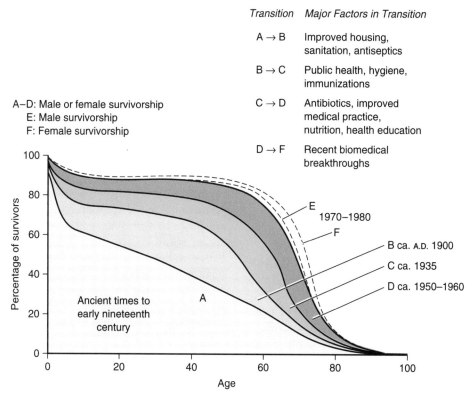

FIGURE 1-1. Human survivorship curve. *Source:* Adapted from B. L. Strehler, (1975), "Implications of aging research for society," *Federation Proceedings* (Federation of American Societies for Experimental Biology), *34,* 6. Used with permission.

states, ranging from inability to perform activities of daily living to full ability to perform activities and instrumental activities of daily living (Crimmins et al., 1996).

This "rectangularization of the curve" has been traced back to the 1920s, and it was first applied to gerontology as a concept in the 1960s. In the early 1980s, interest in this concept was stimulated by the growing awareness of an increasing number of older people. In 1980, James Fries, a physician, stirred much controversy with the publication of an article about the "compression of morbidity" in the *New England Journal of Medicine* (Fries, 1980). Fries argued that the onset of significant illness could be postponed, but that one's life span could not be extended to the same extent. Fries and a colleague emphasized that efforts must be directed toward postponing the onset of chronic illnesses through preventive approaches (Fries and Crapo, 1981). Support for this perspective has been increasing steadily during the past 2 decades, and gerontologists and health care practitioners now consistently emphasize the role of lifestyle, environment, and other factors as determinants of aging. Although these factors are independent of aging, they nevertheless strongly influence the way in which a person ages (Finch and Tanzi, 1997; Lamberts et al., 1997; Rowe and Kahn, 1997).

Cultural Aspects

As noted previously, information about the cultural diversity of groups in the United States has only recently become available, and there are many problems with this information. Of particular concern is the clustering of multiple subgroups. Gerontologists today are keenly aware of the need for information that helps us understand within-group diversity, especially for Hispanics, Native Americans, and Asians and Pacific Islanders (Markides and Rudkin, 1996). Most gerontologists also recognize the fact that, until recently, the study of aging in the United States has essentially been a study of the aging of White Americans.

Gerontological nurses can begin to provide culturally sensitive nursing care by learning about the backgrounds of the many ethnic groups that have immigrated to the United States. The accompanying Culture Box provides a very brief overview of a few of the major cultural groups living in the United States today. Nurses are encouraged to supplement this information by reading journals and other references, and by obtaining information from the Internet and other sources listed in the Educational Resources section of this chapter. Additionally, all health care professionals are encouraged to obtain culturally specific information about groups that reside in their locale. For example, nursing journals frequently publish articles about specific groups, such as the Amish (Yoder, 1997) or South Asians (Narayan and Rea, 1997). One pocket guide, entitled *Culture and Nursing Care* (listed in the Educational Resources section), provides an excellent and practical overview of information that may be helpful in providing culturally competent health care to 24 different groups of people in the United States.

Economic Characteristics

Although the overall economic status of older adults has improved significantly during the past 2 decades, there are tremendous variations in these income gains and, as always, income discrepancies exist among different groups. The Culture Box on page 13 illustrates the changes and differences in rates of poverty for 1979 and 1989 among groups of older adults classified by sex, race, and Hispanic origin. As is clear from this illustration, women, Blacks, and Hispanics, as well as American Indians, Eskimos, and Aleuts, are the groups of older adults that are most likely to be poor. Other factors that increase the likelihood of an older adult living in poverty are widowhood, advanced old age, low educational level, low occupational status, and residence in a rural area or a southern state. A recent study has revealed that the association between low socioeconomic status and poor health continues into old age, and among older adults of varying cultural backgrounds, it is associated with a relatively lower level of function (Berkman and Gurland, 1998).

Social Characteristics

Although gerontologists have been studying the social characteristics of older adults for several decades, only in recent years has a distinction been made between young-old and old-old individuals with regard to social and health characteristics. The social characteristics of culturally diverse groups of older adults in the United States have only begun to be delineated, and little of the available information addresses the differences between young-old and old-old members of culturally diverse groups. Because of the great diversity of the older adult population and the limitations of the information currently available about social characteristics, it is difficult to present a composite picture of typical older adults. Currently, there is no concise information about the social characteristics of all five major population groups that are clustered together in the U.S. census (i.e., White, Black, Hispanic, American Indian, Asian/Pacific Islander). There is some information available about the social characteristics of older adults grouped by

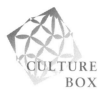

CULTURE
BOX

Brief Overview of Some of the Culturally Diverse Groups of Older Adults in the United States

African Americans

History in America
- African Americans came to America as indentured servants beginning in 1619: about 8 million Africans were sold as slaves in the United States during the 18th and 19th centuries.

Language
- Most African Americans speak English, although some traditional dialects are spoken in the southern states. Black English (ebonics) may be spoken as a second language in urban areas.

Dominant Values and Beliefs
- Good health indicates harmony in life; illness may be a natural event with spiritual influences (i.e., it may be divine punishment for sinful behavior).

American Indians

History in America
- American Indians are the only minority group indigenous to the United States; they were the original settlers in North America. Currently, there are more than 500 federally recognized tribes and an additional 100 to 200 native societies (unrecognized tribes).

Language
- Most American Indians speak English, but there are more than 150 indigenous languages that continue to be spoken.

Dominant Values and Beliefs
- Harmony, thanks, sharing, hospitality, appreciation; close family bonds; respect for all life; reverence for the Great Creator.

Hispanic Americans

History in America
- Mexican Americans came to the Southwest in the late 1800s to build railroads; others arriving during the "bracero" period (1940s to 1960s) became agricultural laborers. Recent immigration patterns involve younger generations, including many people who are undocumented immigrants.
- Cubans initially immigrated in the late 1800s to work in the tobacco industry. A second influx occurred between 1940 and 1950 when Cubans came to help with the war industry. The largest number of Cuban immigrants came to the United States between 1959 and 1979 when many middle- and upper-class citizens were fleeing the country for political reasons.
- Currently, more than 50% of older Hispanics are Mexican Americans; Cubans, Puerto Ricans, and Central and South Americans are the other large groups within this category.

Language
- Most Hispanics speak Spanish, English, or both.

(continued)

Brief Overview (continued)

Dominant Values and Beliefs
- Respect for people by virtue of age, service, or experience (*respeto*); emphasis on the needs of the group or family over the needs of the individual.

Asian Americans

History in America
- The Chinese immigrated as laborers between 1840 and 1882, after which time immigration to America was suspended until 1924 when annual quotas were established. In 1965, the Quota Act was abolished.
- Filipinos initially immigrated in the early 1700s to New Orleans; in the early 1900s, they came as agricultural workers. In 1934, they were limited to an annual immigration quota of 50. From 1946 to 1965, they could become United States citizens by joining the armed services or coming as students, professionals, or war brides. In 1965, the quotas were relaxed.
- Japanese people began immigrating to America in 1885, and immigration peaked between 1900 and 1910. In 1924, they were barred from entering the United States, and in 1942, all Japanese people living in the United States were relocated to internment camps. Immigration resumed in the 1950s.
- Koreans immigrated, particularly to Hawaii, in the early 1900s seeking plantation work. Between 1950 and 1965, a second major wave of Koreans came, many of whom became war brides of American servicemen. After the Immigration Act of 1965 was enacted, many middle-class and college-educated Koreans (particularly health care professionals) came to the United States.
- Vietnamese people and Cambodians came to America as political refugees after 1965.

Language
- Most American-born Asians speak English. Some Asian immigrants speak only their native language or are bilingual.

Dominant Values and Beliefs
- Health is a state of spiritual and physical harmony; illness occurs when the *yin* and *yang* are out of balance.
- Koreans and, to a lesser extent, Japanese people, may be especially concerned about *che-myun*, or face-saving; this may interfere with acceptance of services or acknowledgment of problems.

ages (i.e., 65–74 years, 75–84 years, and 85 years of age and older), but even this information is not presented consistently using the same age groups. Table 1-1 summarizes a few of the social characteristics of older adults that have been identified. Because most of this information is derived from data pertaining to the U.S. older adult population in general, a summary of the social characteristics of specific cultural groups is presented separately in a Culture Box. As this information is only a brief synopsis, the reader is encouraged to seek out supplemental

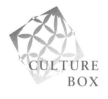

CULTURE
BOX

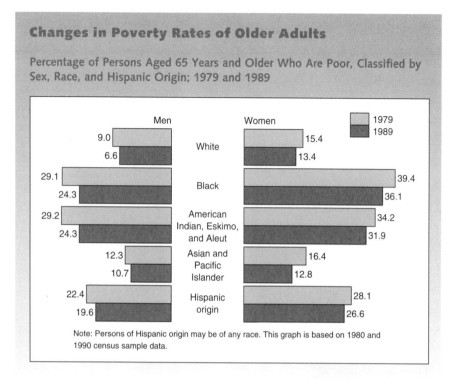

Changes in Poverty Rates of Older Adults

Percentage of Persons Aged 65 Years and Older Who Are Poor, Classified by Sex, Race, and Hispanic Origin; 1979 and 1989

Note: Persons of Hispanic origin may be of any race. This graph is based on 1980 and 1990 census sample data.

information from other resources, such as those listed in the Educational Resources at the end of this chapter.

Family Caregiving Trends

One of the most significant recent population trends in the United States is the increased number of multigenerational families, a phenomenon that is a direct result of the increasing number of people living into advanced old age. Consider these statistics: 25% of people aged 58 to 59 years have at least one living parent; 10% of older people have at least one offspring who is also older than 65 years of age. Moreover, of the people aged 65 years or older who have children, 94% are grandparents and 46% are great-grandparents. These statis-

tics represent a dramatic change in the ratio of old-old parents to old children. This "parent support ratio" is defined as the number of persons aged 85 years and older per 100 persons aged 50 to 64 years. The parent support ratio tripled from 1950 to 1993, and it is expected to triple again by the year 2050 (U.S. Bureau of the Census, 1996). Demographics such as these have influenced patterns of family caregiving, particularly for women. For example, the mid-1980s marked the beginning of an era in which the average woman in the United States spent more time caring for her parents than for her children. The term "sandwich generation" was coined to describe the many middle-aged women who must simultaneously juggle the demands of caring for older and younger generations.

TABLE 1-1
Social Characteristics of Older Adults

Characteristic	65–74 Years of Age	85+ Years of Age
Marital Status		
Married with spouse present		
Men	78%	54%
Women	52%	10%
Widowed		
Men	9%	39%
Women	35%	79%
Living Arrangements		
Living alone		
Men	13%	28%
Women	33%	57%
Living in nursing home	1%	23%
Number of Men Alive per 100 Women	80	39
	65+ Years	
Completing High School or Higher Level of Education		
White	66.7%	
Black	37%	
Hispanic (of any race)	30%	
Participating in Labor Force		
Men	15%	
Women	9%	

This recent increase in the number of multigenerational families has implications not only in terms of caregiving for older adults, but also in terms of older adults who assume responsibilities for other family members. Of particular interest is the dramatic 44% increase during the past decade in the number of children living with grandparents and other relatives. Articles are appearing more and more frequently in nursing and gerontological journals about issues involving older adults who assume long-term caregiving responsibilities for grandchildren (e.g., Emick and Hayslip, 1996; Kelley et al., 1997). The phrase "downward extension of households" is being used to refer to households in which grandchildren or adult children live with and are in some way dependent upon grandparents and older parents. This family configuration contrasts with the more customary "upward extension" of intergenerational households in the United States. In the latter case, older adults reside with adult children or grandchildren so as to receive care. Again, though, the importance of diversity must be emphasized, as the stereotype of dependent older people is being replaced by multiple scenarios in which older adults assume roles as caregivers as well as care receivers, involved in complex relationships with peers and younger and older generations (Silverstone, 1996). The current trend is toward a continuing prevalence of upwardly extended households

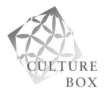

Socioeconomic Conditions of Some Cultural Groups in the United States

African Americans

- *Typical Black elder*: Poor; female; widowed, divorced, separated from spouse; shares a home with a grown child, usually a daughter; previously held an unskilled job (Wykle and Kaskel, 1994).
- *Geographic locations*: Highest concentrations in New York, California, Texas, the southeastern states, and large metropolitan areas.

American Indians

- *Typical American Indian elder*: Poor; has less than a high school education; lives in a rural area with family or alone.
- *Geographic locations*: 45% of older American Indians live in four states: Arizona, California, New Mexico, and Oklahoma.

Asian Americans

- *Characteristics of Asian elderly*: In contrast to all other groups, there is a disproportionately greater number of older Asian men than women; this is due to immigration policies that restricted the immigration of women.
- *Characteristics of Korean elderly*: Although Korean families enjoy a higher income than the average American family, Korean elderly have a higher-than-average rate of poverty.
- *Geographic locations*: Highest concentrations in major cities in the following states: California, Illinois, Hawaii, and New York.

Hispanic Americans

- *Typical Hispanic American elder*: Increased rate of poverty, especially among older Puerto Ricans, as compared with the general United States population.
- *Geographic locations*: Concentrated in major cities in the following states: Arizona, California, Florida, New Jersey, New Mexico, New York, and Texas.

among Whites and downwardly extended households among Blacks (Szinovacz, 1998). One recent study has indicated that caregiving by grandparents is becoming a more common phenomenon and that, although this trend cuts across class, ethnic, and gender lines, single women, African Americans, and low-income people are disproportionately represented (Fuller-Thomson et al., 1997). Diversity also is evident in the wide variety of family relation-

ships and caregiving expectations that characterize different cultural groups in the United States, as summarized in the Culture Box.

Health Characteristics

Health characteristics of older adults are of importance to gerontological nurses for several reasons. First, the subgroup of older adults is the population in the United States that receives

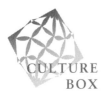

Family Caregiving Expectations of Some Cultural Groups in the United States

African Americans
- Strong family and kinship networks usually exist, with elder care provided in extended family homes.

American Indians
- Children and grandchildren may provide care for elders.

Chinese Americans
- Elder care is provided by the family with the expectation that the wife becomes part of the husband's family.

Filipinos
- Female family members are expected to provide care at home, and admission of an older person to a nursing home may be viewed as disrespectful.

Japanese Americans
- The family is expected to care for dependent elders.

Koreans
- Elders often live in multigenerational families, with the expectation that the oldest son provides elder care in return for the family inheritance.

Mexican Americans
- Women are expected to care for elders.

Puerto Ricans
- Men and women share responsibilities for elder care in the family.

South Asians
- Elders usually live with a married son and grandchildren; female family members are expected to give care at home.

Source: J. G. Lipson, S. L. Dibble, and P. A. Minarik, (1996), *Culture and nursing care: A pocket guide* (San Francisco: UCSF Nursing Press).

the most health care services. Although older people constitute 13% of the population, they occupy about half of the available adult hospital beds, use more than two thirds of the available health care services, and spend 3 times as many days in hospitals and 30 times as many days in long-term care settings than younger people. Therefore, with the exception of those nurses who work exclusively with pediatric or young adult populations, nurses focus more of their care on older adults than on any other age group. Second, the health care system is currently attempting to address the escalating costs of care, and services to older adults are being targeted for cost-cutting measures. Much of this cost-cutting has been focused on the high cost of caring for people with chronic illnesses and impaired function. Because of this emphasis, increased attention has been directed toward preventive care and improved function, and there are increasing opportunities for nurses to assist in the development and implementation of health promotion programs for older adults. Identifying the health characteristics of older adults provides a basis for planning these programs. Finally, because the emphasis of gerontological nursing is on improving the functional status of older adults, the various functional patterns of this population must be identified. This is especially important in light of the growing recognition that much of the health care that is provided to older people involves chronic care related to functional impairments. This contrasts with the emphasis of health care services in younger populations, which tends to be acute rather than chronic in nature.

Because the focus of health care for older adults is primarily on maintaining and improving function, gerontologists and health planners have been particularly interested in statistics about impaired function in daily life. Functional abilities are related to types of chronic illness, chronologic age, and the quantity and quality of social supports, including financial assets. The degree of disability characteristically varies according to the factors just mentioned, and the following chronic conditions have been correlated most consistently with the development of physical disability in older adults: stroke, depression, diabetes, claudication, heart disease, hip fracture, visual impairment, cognitive impairment, knee osteoarthritis, and chronic obstructive pulmonary disease (Fried and Guralnik, 1997). One noted gerontologist used data from a National Center for Health Statistics survey from the years 1961–1962 and 1980–1981 to address the question of whether increased life expectancy had resulted in improved health or increased disability (Palmore, 1986). Palmore used the following indicators to compare the health and function of older adults over a 20-year period: injuries, acute conditions, hearing impairments, visual impairments, severe visual impairments, days of bed disability, and days of restricted activity. He concluded that although disabilities increase with age, "there has been a consistent and substantial trend to-

ward better relative health among the aged between 1961 and 1981" (p. 301). Included in his findings were three possible explanations for this trend. First, cohorts moving into the category of old age are increasingly healthier than previous cohorts because of improved health practices throughout life, as well as higher income and higher levels of education. Second, Medicare and Medicaid have improved health care for older people. Third, the increasing availability of social, economic, nutritional, and psychological programs for older adults has had indirect, beneficial effects on their health status. A recent study supports the conclusion that the underlying reasons for the improved health of older adults are increasingly healthy lifestyles and a decrease in the prevalence of chronic conditions (Fries et al., 1992).

Gerontologists currently are addressing differences in health and function among various subgroups of older adults. For example, information is now available regarding chronologic subgroups (i.e., young-old, middle-old, old-old, and oldest-old populations), and some information about ethnic populations, particularly Black and Hispanic older adults, is becoming available. Data on both health and functional status consistently indicate that older ethnic minority groups have more chronic illnesses, lower functional levels, and poorer self-health ratings compared to White Americans. One recent study indicated that cultural factors, rather than socioeconomic factors, were responsible for between-group differences in disability (Tennstedt and Chang, 1998). However, another recent study revealed that income and education were the most significant predictors of a decline in health for older African Americans when compared with older White Americans (Peek et al., 1997).

Rural and nonmetropolitan elderly are other subgroups that have been the subject of gerontological studies in the 1990s. This attention is warranted by the fact that about 25% of the elderly in the United States live in nonmetropoli-

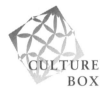

Health Characteristics of Some Cultural Groups in the United States

African Americans

- Worse self-perceptions of health compared to Whites
- Increased impairments in performing daily activities compared to Whites
- Excess prevalence of stroke, cancer, arthritis, diabetes, glaucoma, hypertension, heart disease, alcoholism, and cerebrovascular disease
- Lower rate of osteoporosis than other groups

American Indians

- Higher rates of impaired functional status compared to Whites
- Highest prevalence of diabetes of any group
- Excess prevalence of cancer, obesity, arthritis, cataracts, alcoholism, tuberculosis, kidney disease, rheumatoid diseases, liver and gallbladder disease
- Lowest cancer survival rate of any group
- Higher-than-average risk of dying from accidents (motor vehicle accidents, falls, and fires)

Asian and Pacific Islanders

- Excess prevalence of hypertension, diabetes, certain cancers, thalassemias (anemia), hepatitis B and other liver diseases, and tuberculosis (including multiple-drug–resistant strains),
- Lower rate of osteoporosis than Whites

Hispanic Americans

- Excess prevalence of diabetes, obesity, malnutrition, tuberculosis, and cancer of the cervix, uterus, trachea, and lungs
- Higher rates of functional impairment than Whites
- Lower rate of osteoporosis than Whites

tan areas. People aged 65 years and older constitute 15% of the population in nonmetropolitan areas, and this percentage is increasing because of the in-migration of retired persons and the out-migration of younger adults. In contrast to older adults living in metropolitan areas, a greater percentage of the elderly in nonmetropolitan areas assess their health as fair or poor, but no significant differences have been found in the percentage of elderly who limit their activities because of illness (Van Nostrand, 1993). Display 1-1 presents a health profile of older adults, and the Culture Box above summarizes some of the health characteristics of older adults in a few of the various cultural groups in the United States.

Aging

Much of the previous discussion has centered on characteristics of older adults that influence their health care needs. There is one other concept, however, that is important for gerontological practitioners to understand: aging is a process that has many definitions and many

DISPLAY 1-1
A Brief Profile of the Health Status of Older Adults in the United States

- Seventy-two percent of people aged 64 to 74 years and 66% of people aged 75 years or older rate their health as good, very good, or excellent.
- Eighty percent of older adults have at least one chronic condition.
- Nine percent of people aged 64 to 69 years and nearly 50% of the people aged 85 years and older need assistance with daily activities.

- The most prevalent chronic conditions affecting older Americans are arthritis, hypertension, heart disease, hearing impairments, vision impairments, cancer, diabetes, and orthopedic impairments.
- Restrictions in daily activities increase with increasing age.
- Seventy-five percent of all deaths in the elderly population are caused by heart disease, cancer, and stroke.

consequences. Because our society—and, in fact, the older population itself—views older adults in so many different ways, it is helpful to examine some of the definitions of aging and resulting behaviors, along with their implications for professional nursing practice.

Definitions of Aging

Any discussion of definitions of aging must first underscore the great degree of variation that exists in the way individuals age. Gerontologists are of one accord in their conclusion that aging includes a number of processes that are highly variable and individualized. Two recently evolving trends with regard to aging must be emphasized: (1) there are significant cross-cultural as well as intragroup variations in aging, and (2) lifestyle factors and social factors, such as meaningful relationships, have an important bearing on successful aging. An example of cross-cultural variation in definitions of aging can be found in the age criterion of the Older Americans Act (OAA) that is applied to American Indians and Native Americans. In Montana, American Indians and Native Americans qualify for OAA-funded programs at the age of 45 years, whereas in other states, they qualify for OAA-funded nutritional programs at the age of 55 years.

Aging has been defined both objectively and subjectively by gerontologists and lay people alike. Although aging is defined objectively as a universal process that begins at birth, aging is associated subjectively with old age or older adulthood. Subjectively, people define aging in terms of personal meaning and experience. Children generally do not view themselves as aging, but they delight in announcing how old they are. They usually view birthdays as positive experiences that will permit them to enjoy additional opportunities and responsibilities. Adolescents, likewise, perceive aging as the mechanism that allows them to participate legally in coveted activities, such as driving. In adulthood, however, aging is negatively associated with being old, and "old age" is often arbitrarily defined as an age that is several years or a decade beyond a person's current age. This perspective is evident in the fact that many people whose chronologic age is 70 years, 75 years, or older refer to "old people" as if they were a group distinct from themselves.

Gerontologists have defined "subjective age" from a number of perspectives. Some of the categories of age identified in the gerontological literature include feel-age, identity age, cognitive age, stereotype age, comparative age, and perceived or self-perceived age. The concept of age identification has been the focus of many studies, and it is widely perceived as a continuum of subjective wellness. At one end of the age identification continuum is old age, characterized by feelings of ineffectiveness, whereas at the other end is the perception or sense of being young, with corresponding feelings of control and vital purpose (Baum, 1983–1984). Studies of subjective age suggest that between the ages of 30 and 80 years, people report themselves to be younger than their chronologic age. This finding may be at least partially attributable to the youth bias of modern society, which, beginning in the 4th decade, influences the perceived and reported feel-age of adults (Goldsmith and Heiens, 1992).

Objectively, people define age as the length of time that has passed since one's birth. North American culture is particularly fascinated by numbers, quantities, and relative values that can be measured. Among the questions frequently asked and answered are: How much? How far? How often? How old? Our fascination with age is particularly evident in newspaper articles, which invariably state the age of the subjects, regardless of the relevance of age to the topic. In addition to being easily measured, an advantage of chronologic age is that it serves as an objective basis for social organization. For example, societies establish chronologic age criteria for certain activities, such as education, driving, marriage, employment, alcohol consumption, military service, and the collection of retirement benefits. To participate legally in these activities, people must provide documentation of a certain chronologic age.

With the passage of the 1935 Social Security Act and the 1965 amendment that created Medicare, the age of 65 years was established as the standard age criterion for eligibility for retirement and health care benefits in the United States. Thus, in America, 65 years of age is accepted as the designated age for becoming a senior citizen and enjoying the benefits of the so-called Golden Age. Until recently, gerontologists also viewed 65 years of age as an acceptable chronologic criterion for aging processes. This criterion, however, has now been widely challenged by gerontologists, most of whom have come to recognize the tremendous diversity among people who are defined chronologically as old. As one of the first gerontologists to challenge this categorization stated:

> We have used sixty-five as the economic marker, then as the social and psychological marker, of old age. A set of stereotypes has grown up that older persons are sick, poor, enfeebled, isolated, and desolated. While these stereotypes have been greatly overdrawn even for the old-old, they have become uncritically attached to the whole group over sixty-five. (Neugarten, 1978, pp. 47–48)

The recent trend in gerontology to divide old age into chronologic categories of young-, middle-, and old-old is an improvement over the categorization of all people older than 65 years of age as one homogeneous group, but it has the disadvantage of creating additional age biases. For example, if a chronologically old-old person needs a complicated or expensive medical treatment to maintain or potentially improve their health status, such treatment may be denied or withheld because of the person's advanced age.

Although chronologic age has the advantages of being easily measured, widely accepted, and readily understood, it has many disadvantages, especially in gerontology. From both scientific and humanistic perspectives, a person's age is relatively insignificant. For gerontological practitioners, the important indicators of a person's age are physiologic health, psychological well-being, socioeconomic factors, and the ability to function and socialize to the extent that one desires. For several decades now, the concept of functional age has been used by gerontologists as an alternative to chronologic age. This concept is associated with a shift in emphasis from external factors, such as the passage of time, to factors such as whether individuals can contribute to society and benefit others and themselves. Functional age is a concept that has been used worldwide, but its definition has varied according to the specific cultural context. For example, industrialized societies may associate functional age with self-sufficiency and physiologic function, whereas other cultures might associate it more closely with social or psychological function than with physiologic function. Older adults themselves tend to associate being old with being less functional, both physically and psychologically. Indeed, a recent study revealed that community-living older adults attributed 15% to 30% of their functional decline in performing various daily tasks to "old age" (Williamson and Fried, 1996). One advantage of functional definitions of age over chronologic definitions is that the former are associated with higher levels of well-being and more positive attitudes about aging. Because nursing addresses the response of people to actual or potential health problems, the concept of functional age provides a more rational basis for care than the measurement of how many years have passed since the person was born. Thus, the question How functional? becomes more relevant than How old? For gerontological nurses, the concept of chronologic age is of minimal importance. The more important questions are How well do you feel? and Is there anything that you would like to do that you cannot do?

Ageism and Stereotypes

Although old age has not always been viewed as something to look forward to, until recently it was at least viewed as something to be respected. Fischer (1977) has analyzed trends in attitudes toward old people in the United States from the early 1600s to the present. Data from this analysis indicate that the first period—extending from 1607 to 1820—was characterized by gerontocratic attitudes, or a veneration of old people. Fischer has emphasized, however, that the median age in 1790 was barely 16 years old, and that respect for age was at least partly attributable to its relative rarity. In early America, then, old age was sometimes hated and feared, but more often, it was honored and obeyed. Fischer cites evidence of a subsequent revolution in attitudes, occurring between 1770 and 1820, which sparked a long period of gerontophobia characterized by an idealization of youth. According to Fischer, the "cult of youth . . . became most extreme in the 1960s, when mature men and women followed fashions in books, music, and clothing which were set by their adolescent children. . . . But always, old was out and youth was in" (pp. 132–133). At the same time that youth was being idealized, old age was being identified as a medical problem and labeled as a social problem. Although Fischer did not use the term "ageism" in his book, he discussed the importance of efforts "to oppose the age prejudice which has grown so strong in America" (p. 195).

The term ageism was coined by Robert Butler in 1968 and was first used in a publication (*The Gerontologist*) 1 year later (Butler, 1969). With the publication of Butler's Pulitzer Prize–winning book *Why Survive? Being Old in America* (1975), ageism became an accepted new word in the English language. Butler defines ageism as "the prejudices and stereotypes that are applied to older people sheerly on the basis of their age. . . . Ageism, like racism and sexism, is a way of pigeonholing people and not allowing them to be individuals with unique ways of living their lives" (Butler et al., 1991, p. 243). Some historians and gerontologists view ageism as an outcome of modernization. It is likely that the increased emphasis on the negative and debilitative aspects of old age correlates with the change in perception of the usefulness of older people brought about by urbanization and industrialization (Covey, 1988). Gerontologists continue to advocate addressing ageism as a form of oppression that affects everyone who lives long enough (Laws, 1995). However, one gerontologist has proposed that, rather than affecting all old people, ageism affects only those who are disabled (Cohen, 1988). Cohen further suggests that discrimination against older disabled people arises from the societal perception of them as "biologically inferior and hence incapable of levels of self-fulfillment and self-realization comparable to those of the dominant reference group" (p. 25). Cohen asserts that older disabled people who are the target of ageism share similarities with other groups who have fought against prejudices.

As a consequence of ageism, many stereotypes about older adults have arisen. Although the concept of "old" is not inherently positive or negative, when it is used in reference to people, it seldom applies to a healthy and active person (Cornman and Kingson, 1996). Although the effects of negative stereotypes are hard to measure, Butler repeatedly emphasizes the detrimental impact of negative stereotypes on the self-esteem of older people (Butler, 1975; Butler et al., 1991). He states that "This reaction of the victims of discrimination has been called 'self-hatred' and takes the form of depression, with passive giving up or active self-denigration. These elderly people see themselves as so many younger people see them and thus do not like what they see" (Butler et al., 1991, p. 452). Thus, the consequences of ageism can be quite serious for those older people who believe in the stereotype, as it can become a self-fulfilling prophecy. Caution must be used, however, in applying this conclusion to all older people. A study of the self-perceptions of older Anglo-Americans, Chinese Americans, and Chinese in Taiwan explored cross-cultural differences and similarities in self-perceptions of aging (Tien-Hyatt, 1986–1987). The results of this study indicate that all three groups held positive views of aging, and that the group that represented the highest degree of industrialization and modernization held the most positive view of aging.

Studies of ageism have focused considerable attention on negative attitudes toward older people. A recent summary of the results of such studies has indicated that (1) negative attitudes about older adults are widespread; (2) older adults often hold negative attitudes about themselves as well as about young people; and (3) in some cases, providing accurate information to young adults can change their attitudes toward older adults (McGowan, 1996). Other researchers have looked at the impact of ageism and negative attitudes on nurses and other gerontological health care practitioners. One such study concluded that "As currently conceptualized and measured, negative attitudes toward the aged exist among health care workers. . . . In turn, positive attitudes toward the aged are related to an increased number of positive interactions between nurses and patients as well as a rehabilitative versus a custodial orientation" (Wright, 1988, pp. 813–814). Cohen (1988) has suggested that disabled elderly are victims of low goal formulation, underestimated potential for self-realization, and less than full participation in society. If this supposition is true, gerontological nurses have tremendous opportunities for positively affecting the self-realization of older adults, particularly those who are most disabled. Nurses cannot exert a positive influence, however, until they have identified and addressed their own attitudes about aging, many of which may be based on myths rather than realities. Table 1-2 identifies some of the myths about aging that are commonly accepted as truths, as well as some of the realities of aging. Each of the myths is addressed in a chapter of this text, and a reference to the appropriate chapter is given for each reality. Nurses can address their own attitudes toward older adults through experiential educational activities. For example, *Into Aging* is a simulation game that has been developed by nurses to challenge the myths of aging (see the Educational Resources section of this chapter). This game has been used successfully in a variety of settings to improve attitudes toward aging and to change staff behaviors (e.g., Samter and Voss, 1992).

TABLE 1-2
Myths and Realities of Aging

Myth	Reality
People consider themselves to be old at the age of 65 years.	People usually feel old based on their health and function, rather than on their chronologic age. (*Chapter 1*)
Gerontologists have discovered that, by the age of 75 years, people are quite homogeneous as a group.	The more gerontologists learn about aging, the more they realize that, with increased age, people become more diverse, and individuals become less like their age-peers. (*Chapter 1*)
Ageism is endemic in all societies.	Ageism is much more common in industrialized societies and is highly influenced by stereotypes and cultural values. (*Chapter 1*)
Gerontologists have recently discovered a theory that explains biologic aging.	Theories about biologic aging continue to evolve, and there is little agreement on any one theory. (*Chapter 2*)
In today's society, families no longer care for older people.	In the U.S., 80% of the care of older adults is provided by their families. (*Chapter 22*)
As people grow older, it is natural for them to want to withdraw from society.	Because older people are unique individuals, each of them responds differently to society. (*Chapter 2*)
By the age of 70 years, an individual's psychological growth is complete.	People never lose their capacity for psychological growth. (*Chapters 2 & 4*)
Increased disability in older people is attributable to age-related changes alone.	Although age-related changes increase one's vulnerability to functional impairments, the disabilities are attributable to risk factors, such as diseases and adverse medication effects. (*Chapter 2*)
Widowhood and other specific life events have been found to have a consistently negative impact on older people.	No one life event affects all old people negatively. The most important consideration governing the impact of an event is its unique meaning for the individual. (*Chapter 3*)
In old age, there is an inevitable decline in all intellectual abilities.	A few areas of cognitive ability decline in older adulthood, but other areas show improvement. (*Chapter 4*)
Older adults cannot learn complex new skills.	Older adults are capable of learning new things, but the speed with which they process information slows with age. (*Chapter 4*)
Constipation develops primarily because of age-related changes.	Constipation is attributable primarily to risk factors, such as restricted activity and poor dietary habits. (*Chapter 8*)
Urinary incontinence is best managed by using an indwelling catheter or incontinence products.	In most cases, urinary incontinence can be alleviated by addressing its cause. (*Chapter 9*)
Skin wrinkles can be prevented by using oils and lotions.	The best way to prevent skin wrinkles is to avoid exposure to ultraviolet light. (*Chapter 13*)
Older people decrease the level of their sexual activity because they are less able to perform sexually.	If sexual activity in older people declines, it is because of social reasons (e.g., loss of partner) or risk factors, such as diseases and adverse medication effects. (*Chapter 16*)
Older people experience the same adverse medication effects as younger people.	Older people are more likely to experience mental changes as an adverse medication effect. (*Chapter 18*)
Some degree of "senility" is normal in very old people.	"Senility" is an inaccurate term used to refer to dementing conditions, which are always caused by pathologic changes. (*Chapter 19*)
Most old people are depressed and should be allowed to withdraw from society.	About one third of older people exhibit depressive symptoms; however, depression is a very treatable condition at any age. (*Chapter 20*)

Cultural Perspectives on Aging in the United States

Ageism is a phenomenon that does not exist in all cultures. In the United States, ageism has developed and grown as a result of dominant cultural beliefs and trends, such as the glorification of youth, the ideal of socioeconomic competition, the perception of the individual as autonomous, and the equating of human worth with economic worth. "These values create a cultural environment in which the drawbacks of aging are emphasized, the benefits of aging are ignored, and individual elders are blamed for problems they have not created (for example, being unemployed due to job discrimination)" (McGowan, 1996, p. 71). A potentially positive outcome of the increasing cultural diversity in the United States is that the dominant cultural values that foster ageism may be challenged by cultural values of other groups. The Culture Box on page 25 presents a summary of various cultural perspectives on aging, elders, and ageism.

As the so-called baby boom generation, one of the most diverse generations in American history, reaches older adulthood, some of the long-held American values that have promoted ageism may be challenged and perhaps even replaced with different values that do not foster ageism. The questions that follow are among those that need to be addressed by gerontologists and others in the United States as planning for the aging of the baby boom cohort proceeds.

> Should society automatically marginalize one-fifth of its population because of a chronological age? . . . What roles and responsibilities ought older people to have as individuals to families and to society? . . . Should society care about the quality of life of older persons? . . . Ought society to be concerned if significant numbers of older people are economically poor and/or experience significant health problems? . . . How might we best support the efforts of family members to provide care to persons with significant functional disabilities? (Cornman and Kingson, 1996, p. 24)

The Challenge for Gerontological Nurses

What emerges from the overview of characteristics of older adults is a picture of a diverse group of men and women with various sociocultural backgrounds who are more heterogeneous than homogeneous. Stereotypes of older adults are becoming increasingly fallacious as the diversity within this population grows. What is becoming clear to all people in the field of gerontology, regardless of their specific discipline, is that, as people age, they become less and less like others of the same age. Indeed, the most universal characteristic of increasing age is increasing uniqueness. As was stated in a recent article, "The complexity and elusiveness of the concepts of 'aging' and 'aged' can be summed up in one word: 'diversity'" (Cornman and Kingson, 1996, p. 21). The increasing heterogeneity of older people has implications for health care practitioners, as discussed in the following sections.

Complexity of Health Care for Older Adults

At the same time that gerontologists have become more aware of the increasing diversity among older people, health care providers have become more aware of the increasing complexity of caring for older individuals. Not only are the manifestations of illness less predictable in the elderly, but the causes of illness are more variable and the consequences are more far reaching. Symptoms of illness, even acute illness, in older adults tend to be more subtle and less predictable than in other segments of the population. For example, an older person with a myocardial infarction may not feel any pain or experience any other "typical" manifestation. Similarly, older adults are much more likely than their younger counterparts to experience mental changes or functional declines, rather than

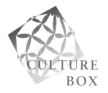

CULTURE
BOX

Cultural Perspectives on Aging, Elders, and Ageism

African Americans, Asian Americans, and Many Other Groups

- Elders are respected and honored and are viewed as a source of wisdom.
- Elders often assume responsibility for the care of younger generations in the immediate and extended family.

American Indians

- Elder status is determined not by age but by the assumption of new social roles, such as teaching, counseling, or grandparenting.
- Expectations of elders include self-control, self-discipline, and positive attitude toward the living.

Gypsies

- Elders are highly respected for their ability to survive hardship and their superior knowledge of Gypsy culture and history.
- Elders are feared for their power within the group.

Mexican Americans

- Elders are treated with respect and reverance, and in a formal manner.
- Elders are involved in the care and education of children.

Puerto Ricans

- *La abuela*(o) (elders or grandparents) are figures of respect, wisdom, and admiration.

South Asians

- The presence of an elder in a family is considered a blessing; elders are very highly respected.
- Elders usually live with their children; they provide child care and teach religion and cultural values to their grandchildren.

White Americans (Dominant Culture in the United States)

- Aging is viewed as a socioeconomic problem. Stereotypes of older people continue to include images of declining health, social isolation, diminished capabilities, and financial problems (AARP, 1995).
- Ageism is fostered by values that emphasize individualism, economic competition, glorification of youth, and reduction of human worth to economic use (McGowan, 1996).

Source: J. G. Lipson, S. L. Dibble, and P. A. Minarik, (1996), *Culture and nursing care: A pocket guide* (San Francisco: UCSF Nursing Press).

physical complaints, in response to medications and physiologic disturbances. Another example of such differences is that older adults with infections may have little or no temperature elevation. Furthermore, by the time illnesses in older adults are noted and attended to, the underlying physiologic disturbance may be in an advanced stage, and additional complications may have developed. A recent article has suggested that any of the following may be possible causes of atypical manifestations of disease in older adults: underreporting of symptoms, complex interactions of several disease conditions, age-related loss of functional and physiologic reserve, and age-related changes that blunt the response to illness (Emmett, 1998).

Another complicating factor is that, for any one manifestation of illness in an older adult, there are usually at least three possible explanations. Changes in function usually are related to a combination of the following: (1) acute illness, (2) psychosocial factors, (3) environmental conditions, (4) age-related changes, (5) a new chronic illness, (6) an existing chronic illness, or (7) an adverse effect of medication(s) or other treatments. When older people are depressed, cognitively impaired, or otherwise psychosocially compromised, accurate assessment of a physiologic illness becomes even more difficult. Cognitively impaired people may not be able to describe their symptoms accurately, and depressed people may either ignore or exaggerate symptoms of physical illness.

The consequences of illness are likely to have an increased impact on the older adult, and they may combine with other factors to compromise the person's functional status and quality of life. An older person who has a fractured hip, for example, is much more likely than a younger person to become permanently impaired. If the older person had previously lived alone and managed independently, if marginally, any functional impairment secondary to the fracture might result in a permanent move to a setting where dependency needs can be met. In addition

to the functional consequences of illness in this population, there are often serious psychosocial consequences for older adults. For example, older people who have experienced a fall may develop an exaggerated fear about falling, and they may limit their mobility as a safety precaution. In the United States, fear of being "put away" in a nursing home is a common anxiety among older people. Because of this anxiety, older people may deny symptoms of illness for fear that the "solution" will result in a loss of independence. Because of such fears, which often are unfounded, people may avoid the health care system and may experience unnecessary anxiety about minor or treatable illnesses.

Care of older people is further complicated by a lack of knowledge on the part of health care practitioners regarding the unique manifestations of aging and disease and the relationships between disease and age-related changes. Although this knowledge deficit is diminishing, many nurses, primary care providers, and other health care practitioners still lack the necessary skills to assess and treat common geriatric conditions accurately and effectively. Indeed, one recent study revealed that family practice residents could correctly differentiate between signs of normal and pathologic aging only 75% of the time (Beall et al., 1996).

Because of all the factors just discussed, the assessment of illness in older adults may require a detective-like approach, rather than the usual diagnostic process. In a health care system in which patients and providers have become accustomed to quick answers based on readily available diagnostic measures, such a time-consuming, puzzle-solving process often ends up being shortened, to the detriment of the older person. Moreover, our current health care system does not provide compensation for time spent listening to lengthy explanations or exploring multiple causes, so the complex health care needs of the older person may be given short shrift. Accordingly, it is often the gerontological nurse who is in a position to ensure that the assessment approach addresses the complexity of the older individual's situation. As every chapter of this text underscores, the more that is learned about any one aspect of gerontological health care, the more questions that are raised. Indeed, it seems that the more that is known, the greater the realization of how little is known! As more is learned about the physiologic and psychosocial function of older adults, it becomes less likely that conditions will be attributed inaccurately to old age, and more likely that the "what-do-you-expect-you're-old" explanation will be relegated to history.

As gerontologists struggle to differentiate between age-related and disease-related factors, they often conclude that very few functional consequences are attributable to age-related changes alone, or to any other single factor. As one's age increases, the number of plausible explanations for a functional change also increases. Thus, the more we learn about the complexity and diversity of older people, the more we realize that it is impossible to classify their health problems in clear and simple categories. This is one reason that gerontological care, by its very nature, is interdisciplinary. No one profession has all the answers to the questions about older people and older adulthood. The challenge of gerontological nursing, therefore, is to work with other professionals to care for people who bring to old age all the complex and unique characteristics of their 70, 80, or more years of living.

Recent Challenges: Multiculturalism and Alternative Health Care Practices

The decade of the 1990s has been characterized by an increasing awareness of the growing cultural diversity of American society and an increasing acceptance and use of alternative or complementary health care practices. These trends must be addressed in all areas of health care practice, including gerontological nursing.

As discussed earlier in this chapter, the proportion of non-Hispanic Whites in the United States is decreasing, whereas the number of older adults in other cultural groups is increasing dramatically. Current projections indicate that this trend will continue at an accelerated rate during the next few decades. Thus, each chapter in this text attempts to include information that is relevant to different cultural groups. Readers must recognize, however, that pertinent multicultural information about older adults in the United States has only recently become available and is limited in scope. Nurses who care for people of diverse cultural groups often can obtain additional information from local resources, particularly in geographic areas where large numbers of ethnic groups live. Also, information is available from the organizations listed in the Educational Resources at the end of this chapter. Because this is a rapidly evolving area of gerontology, nurses are encouraged to access Internet sites that can provide relevant information. Many Internet sites provide health information about particular conditions that is written in several languages. For example, the Alzheimer's Association provides information written in both Spanish and English.

In recognition of the increasing role that alternative or complementary health care practices have assumed in the health care of older adults, this text provides information about these practices that is relevant to specific aspects of physiologic function. The term "alternative," as opposed to "complementary," is used to underscore the wide range of healing and treatment choices available in the United States today. It is important to recognize, however, that people may consult more than one type of health care practitioner or may follow more than one course of treatment. In such cases, they are choosing "complementary" health care practices/practitioners. For most people, this approach is appropriate, especially if they take care to inform all health care practitioners of the full range of modalities being used.

Many people, especially those from non-Western cultural backgrounds, choose a health care approach or practitioner that is not considered to be part of the dominant biomedical model of Western medicine. Indeed, not all people who live in the United States accept the biomedical model of health care. In these situations, the person is not using complementary practices, but is using alternative practices. Currently, in the United States, the broad concept of alternative practices includes all therapies and healing modalities that might be used to address a particular health care concern and that have not been part of the traditional biomedical model of care. (In some countries, prescription medications may be viewed as alternative therapies.)

When considering alternative health care practices, it is important to keep in mind that the relative importance of different health care practices/practitioners varies depending on the person's circumstances. For example, predominantly healthy people may be well served by a nurse practitioner or, if they have a non-Western cultural background, by healers of their own culture. People with treatable medical conditions generally are best served by primary care providers and other health care practitioners trained in biomedical practices. Anyone with symptoms of disease should seek appropriate diagnosis before initiating self-treatment. People with complicated conditions may best be served by a team of practitioners who communicate with each other about different health care options and approaches. The role of the gerontological nurse is to identify sources of health care, as well as self-care practices, and to assess the need for additional or alternative health care practices/practitioners. In some cases, it may be appropriate for the gerontological nurse to encourage an older person to consult a primary care provider; in other cases, the nurse may advise the person to consult another type of health care practitioner. If there has been a major change in the older person's functional or mental status, the nurse may suggest a multidisciplinary geriatric assessment. In all situations, the nurse must seek to ensure that all practitioners involved with the person's care know about the full range of health care practices/practitioners the person is using. In this text, information about alternative and preventive health care practices is included to give the reader an overview of some of the common practices used to promote various aspects of function; it is not to be interpreted as an endorsement of any particular alternative practice. Anyone using alternative health care practices should become knowledgeable about the benefits and risks of those practices. Chapter 18 presents guidelines for the use of herbs and homeopathy and discusses the role of gerontological nurses with regard to assessment of and education about these alternative practices. Nurses are encouraged to use the Internet to gather up-to-date information about alternative health care practices. However, caution must be exercised because much of the information on the Internet is provided by groups that stand to benefit from the use of those alternative health care products and practices. The Office of Alternative Medicine, which is part of the National Institutes of Health, is a good resource for such information (see the Educational Resources listed at the end of this chapter).

Gerontological Nursing Today and Tomorrow

Increasing numbers of nurses are assuming leadership roles in the development of innovative and cost-effective methods for delivering health care to older adults. The ANA states that "gerontological nursing is one of the profession's most challenging practice areas" (1995, p. 6). The ANA statement regarding the scope of gerontological nursing is as follows:

Gerontological nursing practice involves assessing the health and functional status of aging adults, planning and providing appropriate nursing and other health care services, and evaluating the effectiveness of such care. Emphasis is placed on maximizing functional ability in ADLs [activities of daily living]; promoting, maintaining, and restoring health, including mental health; preventing and minimizing the disabilities of acute and chronic illness; and maintaining life in dignity and comfort until death. Gerontological nursing, which focuses on the client and family (both family members and significant others), may be practiced in any setting: the nursing facility, the hospital, the aging person's own home, the clinic, and the community. (ANA, 1995, p. 7)

In addition to traditional nursing care responsibilities, some current roles of gerontological nurses include consultant, nurse practitioner, case or care manager, individual/group counselor, and multidisciplinary team member/leader. Because of recent changes in nursing home regulations, new roles are evolving for nurses. For example, nurses can develop innovative programs in any of the following areas: health promotion, quality assurance, staff and consumer education, prevention of hospitalization, prevention and early detection of acute illnesses, and consultation to Licensed Practical Nurses in the absence of full-time registered nurse coverage (Brandriet, 1992). The development of special care units for people with Alzheimer's disease, along with recent advances in genetic research, has led to newly evolving roles for gerontological nurses as genetic counselors (Schutte et al., 1998). In addition to traditional settings, such as hospitals, private homes, and nursing facilities, any of the following also may be settings for gerontological nursing: senior centers, respite care programs, congregate housing, geropsychiatric programs, rehabilitation programs, geriatric assessment programs, assisted living facilities, group meal programs, protective service agencies, geriatric care management practices, adult day care centers, and community offices on aging.

Increasingly, innovative roles are being developed for gerontological nurses involved in the care or counseling of older adults living in the community, dependent older adults in various institutional settings, and caregivers of dependent older adults. Indeed, there is growing concern about the needs of caregivers of dependent older adults, and gerontological nurses have many opportunities for expanding their roles to address those needs. Geriatric care management services and caregiver counseling and education are rapidly becoming essential components of gerontological nursing. Nurses are involved in formally assessing not only the needs of older adults, but also the needs of their caregivers, who may or may not be older adults themselves. As evidence, terms, such as "respite" and "caregiver stress," have become part of the daily vocabulary of gerontological nurses. Interventions are directed as much toward the caregivers of dependent older people as toward the older people themselves. It has become increasingly common for gerontological nurses to work in collegial relationships with other members of a multidisciplinary team, including primary care providers, psychiatrists, social workers, physical therapists, and other health care providers. The American Nurses Credentialing Center offers certification in any of the following areas specific to gerontological nursing: Gerontological Nurse, Clinical Specialist in Gerontological Nursing, and Gerontological Nurse Practitioner. Home Health Nurse and Nursing Case Manager are two additional certification areas that may be relevant to gerontological nurses. The range of opportunities is limited only by the number of innovative approaches developed for the care of older adults, which has finally "come of age" as a specialty.

Research Imperatives

The rationale for the seventh Standard of Professional Gerontological Nursing Performance states that "Gerontological nurses are responsible for improving nursing practice and the future health care for aging persons by participating in research" (ANA, 1995, p. 25). This standard mandates that nurses ask questions about the care of older adults, participate in designing and conducting studies to address these questions, and submit articles for publication to disseminate the results of their research. In 1993, the 7-year-old National Center for Nursing Research was elevated to the status of a national institute within the National Institutes of Health. The National Institute of Nursing Research (NINR) supports multidisciplinary studies on innovative approaches to promoting health and preventing disease, minimizing the effects of acute and chronic illness and disability, and speeding recovery from disease. Current NINR initiatives that are pertinent to gerontological nursing include the following: examination of preventive measures for people at risk for cognitive impairment; development and testing of biobehavioral and environmental interventions for cognitive impairment; testing of interventions that increase individual and family adaptation to chronic illness; and examination of community-based nursing models, particularly among rural, underserved, and minority populations. In the late 1990s, NINR-funded studies addressed such issues as prevention of pressure sores, decisions about hormonal replacement therapy, the use of hip pads to prevent fractures, and quality of life for Alzheimer's patients and their caregivers. Nurses are encouraged to contact the NINR or visit their Internet site, listed in the Educational Resources at the end of this chapter, for information about these important areas of nursing research.

A recent survey of The National Gerontological Nursing Association (NGNA) identified the following priorities for gerontological nursing research: to identify methods of promoting and maintaining the health and independence of older adults; to measure the efficacy of interventions; and to discern nursing actions to motivate older adults to change lifestyles and behaviors (Luggen, 1997). A prominent leader in geronto-

logical nursing has emphasized that the care of older adults requires an understanding of the complex relationships that exist between the following factors: normal aging, lifestyle, life stresses, acute and chronic illnesses, and the environment (Wells, 1992). Wells has further stated that the bottom line, in terms of the care of older adults, is function in areas such as mobility, cognition, and urinary control, for "function is the pulse beat of gerontological nursing" (Wells, 1992, p. 22). The functional consequences theory of gerontological nursing, presented in the next chapter, provides a framework for such research.

Chapter Summary

The specialties of geriatrics, gerontology, and gerontological nursing have evolved in the past few decades because of rapidly changing demographics in industrialized societies. The older adult population in the United States is characterized by increasing numbers and proportions of old-old people, and by a marked growth in diversity. This chapter reviews the health and social characteristics of older adults in the United States, with emphasis on the diversity and cultural aspects of these characteristics. Because attitudes and stereotypes can influence the way a society views and treats its members, as well as the way individuals perceive and care for themselves, it is important to recognize and address ageist attitudes and stereotypes as they relate to the care of older adults. Nurses can challenge ageist attitudes by questioning some of the dominant values in American society that foster ageism, as well as by debunking the myths and reinforcing the realities of aging as they care for older adults. Because people become more heterogeneous as they age, the care of older adults is very complex and must be provided with cultural sensitivity and within a multidisciplinary context. Nurses must also be prepared to address issues related to the increasing use of alternative and complementary therapies. Numerous roles and opportunities are available for the practice of gerontological nursing today and in the future. The challenge for gerontological nurses is to base their care on a model that identifies and addresses the complexity of interactions between age-related changes and the multiple factors that influence function in older adults. The functional consequences theory of gerontological nursing, discussed in the next chapter, provides such a model.

Critical Thinking Exercises

1. You are asked to staff a booth at a career-day exposition for first-year college students. What information would you give with regard to the following questions?
   a. Why is there an increasing need for people to be educated in areas of gerontology?
   b. What trends in the United States today will make it interesting and challenging to provide health care to older people in the coming years?
   c. What additional areas of study would you recommend (i.e., elective courses) for a nursing student who wants to specialize in the care of older adults?
   d. What activities would you suggest a student pursue if he or she is considering a career in gerontoloigcal nursing?
2. Define aging from each of the following perspectives: chronologic aging, subjective aging, functional aging. How would you define old age?
3. From your cultural perspective, how would you define alternative health care practices? Have you in the past, or do you currently use any alternative health care practices? Choose a cultural perspective other than your own and then define alternative health care practices.

Educational Resources

American Nurses Credentialing Center
600 Maryland Avenue SW, Suite 100W, Washington, DC 20024-2571
(800) 284-2378
www.nursingworld.org

Culture and Nursing Care: A Pocket Guide
UCSF Nursing Press
521 Parnassus Avenue, San Francisco, CA 94143
(415) 476-4992

Into Aging—Understanding Issues Affecting the Later Stages of Life
Boxed Simulation Game, SLACK Inc., 6900 Grove Road, Thorofare, NJ 08086
(800) 257-8290
www.slackinc.com

National Asian Pacific Center on Aging
1511 3rd Avenue, Suite 914, Seattle, WA 98101
(206) 624-1221

National Association for Hispanic Elderly
3325 Wilshire Boulevard, Suite 800, Los Angeles, CA 90010
(800) 953-8553

National Association for Spanish Speaking Elderly
2025 I Street NW, Suite 219, Washington, DC 20006
(202) 293-9329

National Caucus and Center on Black Aged, Inc.
1424 K Street NW, Suite 500, Washington, DC 20005
(202) 637-8400

National Hispanic Council on Aging
2713 Ontario Road NW, Washington, DC 20009
(202) 265-1288

National Indian Council on Aging
6400 Uptown Boulevard NE, Suite 510W, Albuquerque, NM 87110
(505) 888-3276

National Institute of Nursing Research
Building 31, Room 5B13, Bethesda, MD 20892
(301) 496-0207
www.nih.gov/ninr

National Resource Center on Native American Aging
P.O. Box 7090, Grand Forks, ND 58202-7090
(800) 896-7628
www.und.nodak.edu/dept/nrcnaa

Native Elder Health Care Resource Center
University of Colorado Health Sciences Center
4455 East 12th Avenue, Room 329, Denver, CO
80220
(303) 372-3250

Office of Alternative Medicine, National Institutes of Health
P. O. Box 8218, Silver Spring, MD 20907-8218
(888) 644-6226
htpp://altmed.od.nih.gov

Organization of Chinese Americans
1001 Connecticut Avenue NW, Washington, DC
20036
(202) 223-5500

References

American Association of Retired Persons (AARP). (1995). *Images of aging in America.* Washington, DC: AARP.

American Association of Retired Persons (AARP) & Administration on Aging, U.S. Department of Health and Human Services. (1997). *A profile of older Americans: 1997.* Washington, DC: AARP.

American Nurses Association (ANA). (1995). *Scope and standards of gerontological nursing practice.* Washington, DC: ANA.

Baum, S. K. (1983–1984). Age identification in the elderly: Some theoretical considerations. *International Journal of Aging and Human Development, 18*(1), 25–30.

Beall, S. C., Baumhover, L. A., Maxwell, A. J., & Pieroni, R. E. (1996). Normal versus pathological aging: Knowledge of family practice residents. *The Gerontologist, 36,* 113–117.

Berkman, C. S., & Gurland, B. J. (1998). The relationship among income, other socioeconomic indicators, and functional level in older persons. *Journal of Aging and Health, 10*(1), 81–98.

Brandriet, L. M. (1992). Intrapreneurial/entrepreneurial roles for nurses in long-term care. *Journal of Gerontological Nursing, 18*(12), 9–14.

Buckwalter, K., Ebersole, P., Fulmer, T. T., McDowell, J. B., Wall, A. L., & Wykle, M. L. (1997). Nursing. In S. M. Klein (Ed.), *A national agenda for geriatric education* (pp. 1–26). New York: Springer.

Butler, R. N. (1969). Ageism: Another form of bigotry. *The Gerontologist, 9,* 243–246.

Butler, R. N. (1975). *Why survive? Being old in America.* New York: Harper & Row.

Butler, R. N., Lewis, M. I., & Sunderland, T. (1991). *Aging and mental health* (4th ed.). New York: Merrill/Macmillan.

Cohen, E. S. (1988). The elderly mystique: Constraints on the autonomy of the elderly with disabilities. *The Gerontologist, 28* (Suppl.), 24–31.

Cornman, J. M., & Kingson, E. R. (1996). Trends, issues, perspectives, and values for the aging of the baby boom cohorts. *The Gerontologist, 36,* 15–26.

Covey, H. C. (1988). Historical terminology used to represent older people. *The Gerontologist, 28,* 291–297.

Crimmins, E. M., Hayward, M. D., & Saito, Y. (1996). Differentials in active life expectancy in the older population of the United States. *Journal of Gerontology: Social Sciences, 51B,* S111–S120.

Emick, M. A., & Hayslip, B. (1996). Custodial grandparenting: New roles for middle-aged and older adults. *International Journal of Aging and Human Development, 43*(2), 135–154.

Emmett, K. R. (1998). Nonspecific and atypical presentation of disease in the older patient. *Geriatrics, 53*(2), 50–60.

Finch, C. E., & Tanzi, R. E. (1997). Genetics of aging. *Science, 278,* 407–411.

Fischer, D. H. (1977). *Growing old in America.* New York: Oxford University Press.

Fried, L. P., & Guralnik, J. M. (1997). Disability in older adults: Evidence regarding significance, etiology, and risk. *Journal of the American Geriatrics Society, 45,* 92–100.

Fries, J. F. (1980). Aging, natural death, and the compression of morbidity. *New England Journal of Medicine, 303,* 130–135.

Fries, J. F., & Crapo, L. M. (1981). *Vitality and aging: Implications of the rectangularization of the curve.* San Francisco: W. H. Freeman.

Fries, J. F., Williams, C. A., & Morfeld, D. (1992). Improvement in intergenerational health. *American Journal of Public Health, 82,* 109–112.

Fuller-Thomson, E., Minkler, M., & Driver, D. (1997). A profile of grandparents raising grandchildren in the United States. *The Gerontologist, 37,* 406–411.

Garfein, A. J., & Herzog, A. J. (1995). Robust aging among the young-old, old-old, and oldest-old. *Journal of Gerontology: Social Sciences, 50B,* S77–S87.

Goldsmith, R. E., & Heiens, R. A. (1992). Subjective age: A test of five hypotheses. *The Gerontologist, 32,* 312–317.

Kelley, S. J., Yorker, B. C., & Whitley, D. (1997). To grandmother's house we go . . . and stay: Children raised in intergenerational families. *Journal of Gerontological Nursing, 23*(9), 12–20.

Lamberts, S. W. J., Beld, A. W., van den, & Lely, A-J. van der. (1997). The endocrinology of aging. *Science, 278,* 419–424.

Laws, G. (1995). Understanding ageism: Lessons from feminism and postmodernism. *The Gerontologist, 35,* 112–118.

Luggen, A. S. (1997). NGNA's strategic plan. *Geriatric Nursing, 18,* 33–37.

Manton, K. G., Corder, L. S., & Stallard, E. (1993). Estimates of change in chronic disability and institutional incidence and prevalence rates in the U.S. elderly population from the 1982, 1984, and 1989 National Long Term Care Survey. *Journal of Gerontology: Social Sciences, 48,* S153–S166.

Manton, K. G., Stallard, E., & Corder, L. S. (1995). Changes in morbidity and chronic disability in the U.S. elderly population: Evidence from the 1982, 1984, and 1989 National Long Term Care Surveys. *Journal of Gerontology: Social Sciences, 50B,* S194–S204.

Markides, K. S., & Rudkin, L. (1996). Racial and ethnic diversity. In J. E. Birren (Ed.), *Encyclopedia of gerontology: Age, aging, and the aged: Vol. 2* (pp. 371–376). San Diego: Academic Press.

McGowan, T. G. (1996). Ageism and discrimination: In J. E. Birren (Ed.), *Encyclopedia of gerontology: Age, aging, and the aged: Vol. 1* (pp. 71–80). San Diego: Academic Press.

Narayan, M. C., and Rea, H. (1997). Nursing across cultures: The South Asian client. *Home Healthcare Nurse, 15,* 461–469.

National Aging Information Center. (1997). Aging into the 21st century. Washington, DC: Administration on Aging.

Neugarten, B. L. (1978). The rise of the young-old. In R. Gross, B. Gross, & S. Seidman (Eds.), *The new old: Struggling for decent aging* (pp. 47–49). Garden City, NY: Anchor Press/Doubleday.

Palmore, E. B. (1986). Trends in the health of the aged. *The Gerontologist, 26,* 298–302.

Peek, C. W., Coward, R. T., Henretta, J. C., Duncan, R. P., & Dougherty, M. C. (1997). Differences by race in the decline of health over time. *Journal of Gerontology: Social Sciences, 52B,* S336–S344.

Rowe, J. W., & Kahn, R. L. (1997). Successful aging. *The Gerontologist, 37,* 433–440.

Samter, J., & Voss, B. J. (1992). Challenging the myths of aging. *Geriatric Nursing, 13,* 17–21.

Schutte, D. L., Williams, J., Schutte, B. C., & Maas, M. (1998). Alzheimer's disease genetics: Practice and education implications for special care unit nurses. *Journal of Gerontological Nursing, 24*(1), 40–48.

Silverstone, B. (1996). Older people of tomorrow: A psychosocial profile. *The Gerontologist, 36,* 27–32.

Szinovacz, M. E. (1998). Grandparents today: A demographic profile. *The Gerontologist, 38,* 37–52.

Tennstedt, S., & Chang, B-H. (1998). The relative contribution of ethnicity versus socioeconomic status in explaining differences in disability and receipt of informal care. *Journal of Gerontology: Social Sciences, 53B,* S61–S70.

Tien-Hyatt, J. L. (1986–1987). Self-perceptions of aging across cultures: Myth or reality? *International Journal of Aging and Human Development, 24*(2), 129–148.

U.S. Bureau of the Census. (1996). Sixty-five plus in the United States. *Current population reports, special studies* (Series P23–190). Washington, DC: U.S. Government Printing Office.

U.S. Bureau of the Census & National Institute on Aging. (1993, November). Racial and ethnic diversity of America's elderly population. *Profiles of America's elderly* (No. 3). Washington, DC: U.S. Government Printing Office.

Van Nostrand, J. F. (Ed.). (1993). Common beliefs about the rural elderly: What do national data tell us? *Vital and health statistics* (Series 3, No. 28). Hyattsville, MD: U.S. Department of Health and Human Services.

Wells, T. J. (1992). Managing falls, incontinence, and cognitive impairment: Nursing research. In S. G. Funk & E. M. Tornquist (Eds.), *Key aspects of elder care* (pp. 20–27). New York: Springer.

Williamson, J. D., & Fried, L. P. (1996). Characterization of older adults who attribute functional decrements to "old age." *Journal of the American Geriatrics Society, 44,* 1429–1434.

Wright, L. K. (1988). A reconceptualization of the "negative staff attitudes and poor care in nursing homes" assumption. *The Gerontologist, 28,* 813–820.

Wykle, M., & Kaskel, B. (1994). Increasing the longevity of minority older adults through improved health status. In J. S. Jackson (Ed.), *Minority elders: Five goals toward building a public policy base* (pp. 32–39). Washington, DC: The Gerontological Society of America.

Yoder, K. K. (1997). Nursing intervention considerations among Amish older persons. *The Journal of Multicultural Nursing & Health, 3*(2), 48–52, 60.

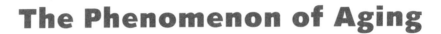

The Phenomenon of Aging

Chapter

2

Learning Objectives

1. *Explain the role of theory in understanding aging.*
2. *Discuss biologic theories of aging and their relevance to gerontological nursing.*
3. *Discuss sociologic theories of aging and their relevance to gerontological nursing.*
4. *Discuss psychological theories of aging and their relevance to gerontological nursing.*
5. *Explain the role of theory in the nursing care of older adults.*
6. *Explicate the functional consequences theory of gerontological nursing.*
7. *Identify cultural considerations with regard to the concepts of person, nursing, health, and environment.*

*S*ince early times, scientists have theorized about the universal human phenomenon of aging, with most of the early theories being limited to biologic aging. For example, Aristotle, Hippocrates, Galen, and other early philosopher-scientists associated aging with a decrease in body heat and fluid. As scientists expanded their knowledge, improved their research methods, and discovered more about aging, it became clear that aging, in fact, was extremely complex and variable. During the 20th century, biologists, sociologists, and psychologists developed theories to explain the phenomenon of aging from their three perspectives. This led to the suggestion that aging could be defined in the following ways: (1) biologic age, encompassing measures of functional capacities of vital or life-limiting organ systems; (2) social age, involving the roles and age-graded behaviors of people in response to the society of which they are a part; and (3) psychological age, referring to the behavioral capacities of people to adapt to changing environmental demands.

Contemporary gerontologists have begun to recognize the importance and value of non-Western perspectives on philosophy and aging.

For example, Native North American traditions and the views held by followers of Confucianism and Buddhism are now being seriously considered by gerontologists who have predominantly Western, traditional perspectives (Kenyon, 1996). In addition to exploring aging from a multicultural perspective, gerontologists have come to recognize the importance of exploring aging across various disciplines. Aging is now viewed as a highly complex phenomenon that must be addressed from a multidisciplinary and multicultural perspective. In addition, disciplines that include subspecialties in gerontology, such as geriatric medicine and gerontological nursing, are now proposing theories about phenomena relating to the unique aspects of care of older adults.

In the next sections, some of the biologic, sociologic, and psychological theories of aging are reviewed, and their relevance to gerontological nursing is discussed. Because of the inherent multidisciplinary nature of gerontology, knowledge of these theories is helpful to gerontological nurses in their care of older adults. Furthermore, because nursing views the health of the whole person in relation to his or her environment, theories from other disciplines contribute to an understanding of the inherent complexity of the older adults for whom nurses care. Despite their relevance to nursing, however, these theories cannot explain the unique relationship between the nurse and the older person. Thus, in the last section of this chapter, a theory for gerontological nursing is proposed. Before the discussion of discipline-based theories, however, the role of theory in understanding aging is briefly discussed.

The Role of Theory in Understanding Aging

Theories make sense of phenomena; they give order and a perspective from which to view the facts. With regard to theories of aging, for instance, gerontologists are trying to use theories to answer certain philosophical questions (Kenyon, 1996). For example, as we extend physical life, what is the purpose of that longer life? What are the elements of a meaningful or worthwhile life (e.g., work, health, companionship, and meaning itself)? For many generations, philosophers of science have thought about the value of, and the criteria for, evaluating theory. Nurses, also, have examined criteria for evaluating theories. Hardy (1978, p. 44) has proposed the following set of questions to evaluate the relevance of a theory to clinical practice:

1. Is it internally consistent or logically adequate?
2. How sound is its empirical support?
3. Does the theory present concepts and conditions that can actually be modified by the nurse?
4. Can the theory be used in bringing about a major, favorable change?

Because nursing is a practice discipline, the last criterion is an especially important one for evaluating nursing theories.

In addition to considering these criteria, it is important to consider how a question is posed, because this directs its possible solutions. For example, if a problem, such as discrimination against older people, exists in the larger societal framework, solutions may be found in sociology. As discussed in Chapter 1, phenomena related to aging, older adults, and older adulthood are highly complex, and the answers to questions about these phenomena are rooted in several disciplines. Improved function in older adults, for instance, often depends on a number of influences, including physiologic, psychosocial, and environmental factors. Gerontological nurses and other gerontological practitioners, therefore, must draw on many perspectives to synthesize particular theories on which they can base their care of older adults.

Although all gerontological practitioners draw from many of the same theories, each discipline has a unique approach to assessing situations, planning care, and solving problems. Over the past few decades, geriatric medicine has relied heavily on biologic theories to explain how biologic changes associated with the aging process affect the physiologic function of the human body. Other disciplines, such as nursing, psychiatry, and sociology, have integrated many theories of aging with the unique perspective of their own discipline. Nurses focus on autonomous people who have nursing problems, psychiatrists try to identify and cure psychopathologic conditions, and sociologists inquire about cohorts of older people who share specific characteristics. Each discipline has a prescribed realm of practice, but each is enriched by knowledge from other disciplines.

Biologic Theories of Aging

Biologic theories of aging address questions about the basic aging processes that affect all living organisms. These theories answer questions, such as How do cells age? and What triggers the process of aging? In addition, biologic aging theories attempt to identify those physiologic processes that occur independently of external or pathologic influences. Leonard Hayflick, one of the first gerontologists to propose a theory of biologic aging, emphasized that a theory of aging or longevity must explain several types of age-related changes, including changes that are: (1) *deleterious,* resulting in reduced function; (2) *progressive,* occurring gradually; (3) *intrinsic,* not attributable to modifiable environmental agents; and (4) *universal,* affecting all members of a species if given the opportunity by virtue of age (Hayflick, 1988). The continuing proliferation of biologic theories of aging is important for conceptualizing the process of aging from a broad perspective. The process of biologic aging is obviously a complex one, and no single theory will suffice to explain the many variations in rates of aging and specific vulnerabilities in each human system. There is much scientific support for the widespread belief that there is a great deal of biologic variability among people.

All biologic theories attempt to explain the characteristics of age-related changes, but each theory is developed from a different perspective. Some of the major biologic theories are considered in this chapter, but readers must keep in mind that these theories are only a sampling of the various perspectives that have been proposed and that continue to evolve. As one commentary on theories of aging has emphasized, biologic aging is not a single mechanism, but should be viewed as processes, mechanisms, and complex phenomena (Evans, 1993). Similarly, the author of a recent review of biologic theories has pointed out that "no single, overarching, predictive theory of senescence will ever be found for humans, because aging human beings undergo changes in all domains of their lives: genetic, biochemical, metabolic, physiological, psychological, social, and for some, even spiritual" (Yates, 1996, p. 547). Thus, there are numerous biologic theories, each one attempting

to explain a particular aspect of aging from one particular perspective. The following discussion of biologic theories of aging presents some of the theories that address questions about biologic human aging, as well as the theories that address questions about the relationships among aging, disease, and function. The discussion also covers the relevance of a particular theory to gerontological nursing.

Genetic Theories

Genetic theories emphasize the role of genes in the development of age-related changes. One of the most popular of the genetic theories is the "program theory of aging," proposed by Hayflick in the 1960s. This theory states that the life span of animals is predetermined by a genetic program, or a so-called biologic clock (Hayflick, 1965). In humans, for instance, the program allows for a maximum of about 110 years. Hayflick (1974) estimates that normal human cells divide 50 times in this number of years. Moreover, according to Hayflick, cells are genetically programmed to stop dividing after achieving 50 cell divisions, at which time they begin to deteriorate. The number of times cell division takes place is different for each species of animal, and the longer a species' life expectancy, the more cell divisions that animal has in its genetic program. Abnormal cells, however, are not subject to this predictable program, and can proliferate an indefinite number of times. Some genetic theories, called mutation theories, suggest that aging is the result of mutations of somatic cells or alterations in DNA repair mechanisms.

Genetic theories of aging are supported by studies that indicate that life expectancy is genetically preprogrammed within a species-specific range. For example, Lints (1978) looked at the similarities in the life expectancies of family members. He found that children of parents who died before the age of 60 years had a life expectancy that was 20 years shorter than that of children of parents who lived more than 80 years. Moreover, in studies comparing identical twins to fraternal twins, Lints demonstrated that the former had more similar life expectancies and more similar causes of death than the latter.

Genetic theories of aging continue to evolve. Currently there is much interest in studying the failures of aging tissues that are likely to result from both genetic changes and environmental insults (Baker and Martin, 1997; Cristofalo, 1996).

Wear-and-Tear Theories

The first wear-and-tear theory was based on a 19th century theory that attempted to explain the difference between immortal germ plasm and mortal soma. In 1891, August Weismann theorized that normal somatic cells were limited in their ability to replicate and function. Weismann postulated that death occurred because worn-out tissues could not forever renew themselves (Hayflick, 1988a). Simply stated, the wear-and-tear theory suggests that organisms have fixed amounts of energy available, and that they will wear out on a scheduled basis. When enough cells wear out, the body does not function well. The wearing-out process is aggravated by harmful stress factors, such as smoking, poor diet, muscular strain, or an excessive intake of alcohol. This theory of aging is supported by microscopic signs of wear and tear in the cells of striated skeletal tissue, heart muscle, and all nerve cells. According to the wear-and-tear theory, the body can be likened to a machine that is expected to function well during the period of its warranty, but that will wear out at a fairly predictable time. Parts can be fixed or replaced, but eventually, the machine no longer functions because of the extensive accumulation of wear and tear. Like the machine, the longevity of the human body will be affected by the care it receives, as well as by its genetic components. Unlike the machine, however, the human body can repair many of its own parts well into old age.

Immunity Theories

Immunity theories are based on the knowledge that immune system components—particularly the thymus and immunocompetent cells in the bone marrow—are affected by the aging process. Because of the age-related, diminished function of the immune system, called immunosenescence, the older person has fewer defenses against foreign organisms and thus has increased susceptibility to cancer, infections, and autoimmune diseases, such as lupus or rheumatoid arthritis. According to immunity theories, diminished immune functioning can lead to an increase in the body's autoimmune responses. When autoimmunity occurs, the body reacts against itself and produces antibodies in response to its own constituents. Autoimmunity theory could explain the fact that older adults often manifest allergies to food and environmental conditions that they previously never experienced. Despite the common occurrence of autoimmunity in old age, however, it is not necessarily the sole or primary cause of autoimmune disease, and many healthy older people test positive for autoantibodies. Rather, it is thought that genetic errors may account for autoimmune diseases and the low-grade autoimmunity in older people (Heidrick, 1987).

Cross-Linkage Theory

The cross-linkage theory proposes that molecular structures that normally are separated may be bound together through chemical reactions. According to this theory, a cross-linking agent attaches itself to a single strand of a DNA molecule and damages that strand. Under normal circumstances, natural defense mechanisms are marshalled to repair the damage. With increasing age, however, the defense mechanisms are weakened, and the cross-linking process continues until irreparable damage occurs. The end result is an accumulation of cross-linking compounds that causes mutations in cells, inability to eliminate wastes and transport ions, and a protein system that is inelastic and ineffective. It is thought that the irreversible aging of proteins, such as collagen, eventually leads to tissue and organ failure (Rockstein and Sussman, 1979). This theory would explain arteriosclerosis and age-related skin changes.

Lipofuscin and Free Radical Theories

The free radical theory, first proposed in the mid-1950s, provides the basis for much of the current research on aging (Harman, 1956). Free radicals are highly unstable and reactive molecules (particularly true of oxygen molecules) that are formed when an electron pair is separated. Free radicals can be produced by normal metabolism, reactions to irradiation, chain reactions with other free radicals, and oxidation of certain environmental pollutants, such as ozone, pesticides, and air pollutants. Free radicals and their conjugated compounds are capable of attacking other molecules because they possess an extra electric charge, or free electron. Free radicals do not contain DNA; therefore, they can cause genetic disorder and produce waste products that accumulate in the nucleus and cytoplasm. The human body has natural protective mechanisms, or antioxidants, that slow the rate of oxidation or counteract the effects of free radicals. Beta-carotene and vitamins C and E are examples of antioxidants that are thought to play a protective role against free radicals.

The free radical theory postulates that protective mechanisms decrease, or free radical formation increases, with advancing age. When free radicals attack molecules, they damage the cell membranes; aging is thought to occur because of accumulative cell damage that eventually interferes with function. Support for this theory is found in lipofuscin, a pigmented waste material that is rich in lipids and proteins. Lipofuscin, which causes age spots, is a by-product of oxidation and therefore seems to be related to free radicals. The key role of lipofuscin in aging may be its ability to interfere with cell transport and

DNA replication (Gordon, 1974). The role of lipofuscin in causing cell damage has been questioned recently, but the role of lipofuscin as an indicator of the aging process remains unquestioned (Brody, 1987).

Neuroendocrine Theories

Neuroendocrine and neurochemical theories are in the early stage of development, but they are the focus of intense interest. These theories postulate that changes in the brain and endocrine glands cause aging. One such theory—the neurotransmitter theory—proposes that an imbalance of thought-transmitting chemicals in the brain interferes with cell division throughout the body. Neuroendocrine theories attribute aging to anterior pituitary hormones that are thought to accelerate aging. Finally, viral theories of aging have been the focus of recent scientific attention. Some of these theories are based on the belief that, at any time, a virus may enter the body and, after an incubation period of several decades, begin to affect any system of the body.

The Single-Organ Theory

The single-organ theory views aging as a disease-related failure of a vital body organ. Based on this theory, people do not die of old age. Rather, they die because a disease, or routine wear and tear, causes a vital part of the body to cease function while the rest of the body is still capable of living. In many such cases, organ transplants or artificial mechanisms have been successful in prolonging life. This theory is similar to the competing risk factor model, which assumes that if a person does not die from one health risk, he or she will die from another risk. These theories assume that if there were no disease and no accidents, death would not occur.

Longevity and Senescence Theories

A discussion of biologic theories of aging would be incomplete without an exploration of theories that address the question of why people live as long as they do. This question is particularly important to gerontological practitioners, who are concerned not only with prolonging life, but also with improving the quality of life. By studying long-lived people who are healthy and functional, we may find answers to the most important question of all: How can we live a life that is not only long, but also functional, productive, and satisfying? Possible answers to this question are found in studies of centenarians.

Alexander Leaf observed three groups of people who were both healthy and long-lived (1973a, 1973b, 1973c). Although his observations are not entirely scientific, they provide some information about factors that contribute to healthy aging. A summary of findings regarding long-lived healthy people throughout the world and in the United States identified the following significant influences: (1) genetic factors; (2) physical environment; (3) physical activity throughout life; (4) consumption of moderate amounts of alcohol; (5) sexual activity persisting into advanced years; (6) dietary factors, such as low animal fat intake; and (7) factors relating to social environment, such as an acquired status of wisdom and dignity (Pelletier, 1986). Gerontologists (e.g., Smith, 1997) consistently point to heredity as one of the strongest predictors of life span. A review of several studies of centenarians identified the following additional factors that were thought to contribute to longevity: laughter; low ambitions; a daily routine; belief in God; close family ties; freedom and independence; organized, purposeful behavior; and a positive view of life (Palmore, 1987).

Kohn (1982) proposed the senescence theory, which is based on postmortem studies of 200 people who died at the age of 85 years or older. Of that group, at least 26% had no acceptable cause of death listed on the death certificate. Kohn determined this by comparing findings from extensive postmortem examinations with the listed cause of death. When decisions about

the accuracy of the cause of death were questionable, the evaluations were weighted in favor of the listed cause. Based on the results of these autopsies, Kohn concluded that, if the same degree of disease occurred in middle-aged people, the condition would not have been fatal. Thus, aging itself was thought to be the actual cause of death in a large fraction of the aged population (Kohn, 1982). Kohn further suggested that, when death in older people cannot be ascribed to a disease process that would cause death in middle-aged people, the cause of death should be listed on the death certificate as senescence. According to Kohn (1982), the relationship between aging and disease is very clear: "The aging syndrome should be viewed as a universal, progressive, and ultimately fatal disease" (p. 2797).

A variation of the senescence theory has been proposed to explain the relationships among aging, health beliefs, and health behaviors (Newquist, 1987). According to Newquist, there are three models for viewing these relationships. In the *siege model*, illness is viewed as a necessary concomitant of being old. The attitude of people with this perspective is "Get ready to be sick, you're old." In the *senescence model*, illness and aging represent the same entity. Illnesses are viewed as age-induced changes ("just old age") and are not seen as pathologic conditions. In the *vanquished model*, sickness is viewed as pathologic, but it is seen as something to be accepted if one is old. According to this model, not only does sickness invariably accompany old age, it is untreatable because of old age (Newquist, 1987).

Active Life Expectancy and Functional Health Theories

Spurred partly by the compression of morbidity theory (discussed in Chapter 1), gerontologists have been trying to predict the probable "active life expectancy" for people. This issue is of particular interest to health planners and policy makers because the cost of medical care is significantly related to the degree of an individual's disability. Health care providers are also interested in this issue because quality of life depends significantly on the level of function. Using life-table methods and the activities of daily living index as a measure of health, Katz and co-workers (1983) analyzed data for noninstitutionalized older people in an attempt to predict active life expectancy. The results showed that people entering the age category of 65 to 69 years had 10 years of "functional well-being" remaining, whereas those in older groups had progressively fewer years. For people 85 years of age or older, the active life expectancy was 2.5 years.

An article that appeared in 1983 in the *Journal of the American Medical Association* (Kennie, 1983) might be viewed as an early attempt to articulate the functional approach to geriatric medical care. The Scottish geriatrician who wrote it stated that the "most important and distinguishing aspect of good health care for the elderly is the switch in emphasis away from dealing strictly with pathology and organ-specific disease [and] toward restoring the patient's resultant loss of function" (Kennie, 1983, p. 770). During the following year, an article appearing in the *Journal of the American Geriatrics Society* proposed a conceptual framework for a "functional approach to the care of the elderly" (Becker and Cohen, 1984). It emphasized the complex relationships between the social, biologic, and psychological variables that influence a person's functional abilities and well-being. Moreover, it emphasized that age-related, as well as disease-related, changes can interfere with functional status. Accordingly, the "ultimate goal of the clinician is to orchestrate compensatory responses in an effort to restore, maximize, and maintain a person's functional status and independence for as long as possible" (p. 928). In the late 1980s, the American College of Physicians and the American Geriatrics Society cited the importance of incorporating a functional assessment into routine clinical geriatrics as a major component of quality of life and as a critical component of appropriate health care. In Chapter 17, additional concepts pertinent to functional assessment are discussed, and a nursing model for functional assessment is presented, along with guidelines for its use.

Medical Theories

Geriatric medical theories try to explain how biologic changes associated with the aging process affect the physiologic function of the human body. Biogerontology is a recent subspecialization, the aim of which is to determine the connections between specific diseases and aging processes (Miller, 1997). These theories address specific questions, such as How are aging and disease processes related, as well as distinguished? and What is different about the medical care of older people? In recent years, many questions have been raised about conclusions drawn from cross-sectional studies, which shed light on age differences rather than age-related changes. As more sophisticated research methods have been used and more data have been collected from healthy subjects in longitudinal studies, some of the conclusions drawn from these cross-sectional studies have been challenged. For example, the popular belief that renal function declines with increased age has recently been called into question by data derived from the Baltimore Longitudinal Study of Aging (Williams, 1987).

As knowledge about aging and disease increases, more questions are being raised about the relationship between these processes. For example, if aging and disease are interdependent processes, then longitudinal studies must attempt to describe the natural history of diseases and their underlying processes as part of the overall aging process (Fozard et al., 1990). Increasing emphasis is also being placed on individual variability. These are especially important considerations in light of the many times health and medical practitioners say or hear such statements as "What do you expect? You're old!" in reference to older people's complaints about changes in their abilities.

Throughout this text, theoretical explanations of specific functional aspects of aging are discussed in the sections on age-related changes. The reader will undoubtedly notice that opposing conclusions and controversial findings are sometimes cited as explanations for age-related or disease-related changes. Whenever possible, theories and conclusions that have generated the greatest concordance are summarized. In all cases, an attempt is made to reflect accurately the current theoretical base. Readers must keep in mind, however, that all theories of aging are in a state of intense flux and growth. As knowledge of this population continues to expand at a rapid pace, current theories may be challenged or supplanted by other theories.

The early medical theories of aging were limited in scope to questions about the relationship between disease and aging. In recent years, however, medical theories of aging have increasingly focused on assessing and improving the functional health of older people (e.g., Crimmins and Saito, 1993; Siu et al., 1993). During the 1990s, geriatric research and practice have undergone a revolution in thinking, with the result that less attention is now being focused on disease processes per se, and more attention is being directed toward the functional losses that are of key importance to older people (e.g., Burns et al., 1997). Evolving theories about functional health are particularly important because they are the underpinnings for the functional consequences theory of gerontological nursing, a theory that is developed in the following sections and that provides a framework for this text. In addition to the theories discussed here, the theory of the compression of morbidity, discussed

in Chapter 1, can be viewed as a theory explaining the relationship between disease and life expectancy.

Relevance for Gerontological Nursing

The relevant question for gerontological nursing that is addressed in biologic theories of aging is How does aging affect physiologic function? The answers to this question provide a basis for identifying ways to improve the physiologic function of older adults, which is the focus of this gerontological nursing text. Conclusions that can be drawn from biologic theories of aging include:

1. Biologic aging affects all living organisms.
2. Biologic aging is natural, inevitable, irreversible, and progressive with time.
3. The course of aging varies from individual to individual.
4. The rate of aging for different organs and tissues varies within individuals.
5. Biologic aging is influenced by nonbiologic factors.
6. Biologic aging processes are different from pathologic processes.
7. Biologic aging increases one's vulnerability to disease.

With this knowledge of the aging process, gerontological nurses can begin to understand the differences between age-related changes and the risk factors that affect the functional status of older adults. For example, it is important to distinguish between biologic aging changes and pathologic processes that commonly affect older adults. This knowledge can be used in teaching older adults that certain conditions are not inevitable just because the person has reached a certain age. Concepts from specific theories are also useful to gerontological nurses. For example, the knowledge that the immune system is affected by aging may explain the altered response to infections among older adults. Applying this knowledge, gerontological nurses can be increasingly vigilant about preventing infections and observing for subtle signs of infections in older adults. Concepts gleaned from wear-and-tear theories provide a rationale for gerontological nurses to plan interventions aimed at reducing the effects of psychological and physiologic stress.

In contrast to the studies that treat aging as strictly a biologic phenomenon, the studies of healthy and long-lived people offer a more holistic perspective on older people. Gerontological nurses must be as concerned about improving the quality of life in later adulthood as they are about extending the quantity of life. Many of the factors that contribute to a healthy, long life fall within the realm of health behaviors. Therefore, the importance of health-promotion activities is significant. For example, education about nutrition and physical exercise can be provided, with emphasis on their role in improving function in later adulthood. Psychosocial interventions, such as efforts directed toward increasing the quality of social supports, are particularly important for older adults. Gerontological nurses often work with older adults and their caregivers in addressing many quality-of-life issues. Theories about longevity can be used, along with sociologic and psychological theories, to provide a framework for addressing challenging questions about choices involving quality of life or prolongation of life. By identifying factors that contribute to longevity as well as to quality of life, older adults and their caregivers can make informed choices about lifestyles, health practices, and medical interventions.

Like nurses, primary care providers are asking questions that address the uniqueness of caring for older people. In addition, both nurses and primary care providers are asking other questions, such as How can the functional abilities of older adults be improved? Unlike nurses,

however, primary care providers focus primarily on disease processes. When function is diminished in an older person, these practitioners attempt to identify a pathologic cause of the problem and then initiate appropriate medical interventions. Theories about disease and aging, therefore, provide a basis for addressing the disease-related factors that influence functional abilities. As will be discussed in the next section and emphasized throughout this text, gerontological nursing considers not only the pathologic factors involved, but also the many additional risk factors that may significantly influence the functional status of older adults.

Although the functional assessment theories provide the most rational approach to the care of older people, many primary care providers base their practice on different theoretical perspectives. It is helpful, therefore, for nurses to be familiar with some of the other medical approaches. If medical care is based on the "what-do-you-expect-you're-old" theory, for example, primary care providers might ignore treatable disease conditions. Similarly, if primary care providers subscribe to the theory that "aging is an ultimately fatal disease," their attitude may reflect a hopelessness that prevades their approach to caring for older patients. In these situations, nurses may have to focus their assessments specifically on the identification of treatable, disease-related factors.

Because nurses generally spend more time with patients than do primary care providers, nurses are a vital communication link between older adults and their care providers. In this role, nurses have many opportunities to inform older adults of the alternative, more rational, functional approach to health care when other, more disease-focused, approaches are being applied. In this role, too, gerontological nurses can act as advocates for older adults whose care might be based on outdated approaches. Using the functional consequences theory of gerontological nursing, which is explicated in this chapter, nurses can encourage all health care providers to apply the functional approach to their care of older adults.

If the biologic theories were the only theories of aging, there would be reason to be pessimistic or even fatalistic about aging. After all, these theories point to unalterable and detrimental physiologic changes that eventually lead to death. If only these theories were applied, there would be a tendency to adhere to ageist attitudes and to use denial of the aging process as a defense mechanism against inevitable decline. These theories do not consider the influence of social, nursing, and medical interventions that can improve one's functional status and life expectancy. Biologic theories, however, do highlight the need for good health care to minimize damage that can be caused by disease. For example, much of the recent emphasis on the use of antioxidants is based on the free radical theory. From a broader perspective, aging is more than an unrelenting progression of cellular deterioration. Survival to old age is an accomplishment that denotes strong will and the ability to adapt. Older adulthood can be a rewarding part of the life cycle, during which one experiences personal growth and self-understanding, fulfillment of potential, and the ability to establish clear priorities. These aspects of aging are addressed in the sociologic and psychological theories of aging that are discussed in the following sections.

Sociologic Theories of Aging

Sociologic theories of aging attempt to explain questions such as How does a society influence its old people? and How do old people influence a society? Early sociologic theories of aging, developed during the 1960s, focused on adjustments of old people to losses within the context of roles and reference groups. Disengagement, activity, subculture, and continuity theories are some of the theories based on this theme. Beginning in the 1970s, social gerontologists broadened their perspective to focus on larger societal and structural factors that influence aging. Age stratification is one theory in which this larger focus is dominant. More recently, social gerontologists have begun to explore in depth the complex interrelationship between old people and their physical, political, and socioeconomic environments. Another recent emphasis is on life-course approaches, which are discussed in the section Psychological Theories of Aging. Some of the principles that social gerontologists agree on in terms of life-course perspectives are: (1) aging is a lifelong process, (2) aging influences and is influenced by social processes, and (3) the age structure changes over time and is experienced differently by different cohorts (Marshall, 1996). Another current focus of social gerontologists is the application of feminist perspectives to sociologic theories of aging. These perspectives focus on critiquing the dominant male-centered view of aging, which bases most sociologic theories on the experiences of White, middle-class men (Lynott and Lynott, 1996). The following sections present a sampling of the more well-developed sociologic theories of aging.

Disengagement Theory

In 1961, Cumming and Henry published the first sociologic theory of aging in their book, *Growing Old: The Process of Disengagement* (Cumming and Henry, 1961). According to this theory, the maintenance of social equilibrium is achieved by a mutually beneficial process of reciprocal withdrawal between society and older people. The process occurs systematically and inevitably and is governed by society's needs, which override individual needs. This theory further states that older people desire this withdrawal and are happy when disengagement occurs. As the number, nature, and diversity of the older person's social contacts diminish, disengagement becomes a circular process that further limits opportunities for interaction. The original theory was later amended to reflect the complexity and diversity of older people. The usefulness of this theory lies in the controversies it has inspired, challenging traditional beliefs about the relationship between a person and society. For instance, considerable controversy has arisen regarding whether the disengagement process is, in fact, universal, inevitable, and beneficial to the person. Controversy also has focused on the fact that this theory ignores the nature of people and their unique responses to aging and society. The disengagement theory is now viewed as a flawed theory that served as a milestone in the systemic study of aging (Achenbaum and Bengston, 1994).

Activity Theory

The widespread belief that the way to age successfully is to keep active was first proposed in the early days of social gerontology. Havighurst and Albrecht (1953) are credited with the first explicit statement about the importance of social role participation in positive adjustment to old age. Ten years later, Havighurst and colleagues (1963) coined the term "activity theory" to reflect this point of view. It was almost another decade, however, before Lemon and colleagues (1972) formalized this theory.

The activity theory is based on the supposition that older people remain psychologically and socially fit if they remain active. This theory reflects the belief that one's self-concept is affirmed through activities associated with various roles. Loss of roles in old age negatively affects life satisfaction. Lemon and colleagues (1972) tested this theory and found a significant relationship between informal activity and life satisfaction. They concluded that the quality or type of interaction was more important than the quantity of activity. A replication of this study revealed that informal activities promoted wellbeing; formal, structured activities led to lowered life satisfaction, and solitary activities had little or no effect on life satisfaction (Longino

and Kart, 1982). Busywork, for example, did not promote self-esteem, but meaningful interaction with one or more people did.

Continuity Theory

Continuity theory was first advanced by Neugarten and colleagues (1968) because neither the activity theory nor the disengagement theory adequately explained successful aging. These social gerontologists believed that what was missing in these theories was the relationship of personality to successful aging. Thus, they proposed a personality-continuity, or developmental, theory of aging (Neugarten et al., 1968). According to this theory, a person's characteristic coping strategies are in place long before old age; however, personality features are also dynamic and continually evolving. Applying this theory, the best way to predict how a person will adjust to being old is to examine how that person has adjusted to changes throughout life. Recent longitudinal studies support this theory and confirm that stability of personality is the rule rather than the exception. These studies further suggest that some of the personality traits that are sometimes attributed to age-related changes may instead reflect generational trends that are the result of early socialization of cohorts (Field, 1991; Field and Millsap, 1991; Hagberg et al., 1991; Schaie and Willis, 1991).

Subculture Theory

The subculture theory, first proposed by Rose in the early 1960s, states that old people, as a group, have their own norms, expectations, beliefs, and habits; therefore, they have their own subculture (Rose, 1965). Moreover, the theory maintains that older people are less well integrated into the larger society and interact more among themselves compared to people from other age groups. Moreover, the theory holds that the aged subculture is primarily a response to loss of status, which is so negatively defined in the United States that people do not want to be viewed as old. In the aged subculture, individual status is based on health and mobility, rather than on the occupational, educational, or economic achievements that were previously important. Rose envisioned that one outcome of the aged subculture would be the development of an "aging group consciousness" that would serve to improve the self-image of older people and change the negative cultural definition of aging (1965).

Because the aged subculture has millions of members in this country, it constitutes a minority group that can organize as such and make public demands. The growth of groups, such as the American Association of Retired Persons (AARP), whose membership exceeds 34 million people, is evidence of the social importance of the aged subgroup. When considered along with the activity theory, the subculture theory supports the social gerontological view that there is a strong relationship between peer group participation and the adjustment process of aging.

Age Stratification Theory

The age stratification theory, first proposed by Riley and colleagues (1972), addresses the interdependencies between age as an element of the social structure and the aging of people and cohorts as a social process. This theory emphasizes the following concepts: (1) people pass through society in cohorts that are aging socially, biologically, and psychologically; (2) new cohorts are continually being born and each experiences a unique sense of history; (3) a society can be divided into various strata according to age and roles; (4) society itself is continually changing, as are the people and their roles in each age strata; and (5) a dynamic interplay exists between individual aging and social change. Thus, aging people and the larger society are constantly influencing each other and changing both the cohorts and the society. Today, this theory provides a useful tool for understanding the place, problems, and potential of older adults in their families, societies, workplaces, communities, and other social institutions (Riley, 1996).

Person-Environment Fit Theory

The person-environment fit theory considers the interrelationships between personal competence and the environment (Lawton, 1982). According to this theory, personal competence includes the following processes that collectively describe the person's functional ability: ego strength, motor skills, biologic health, cognitive capacity, and sensory-perceptual capacity. The environment is viewed in terms of its potential for eliciting a behavioral response from the person. Lawton asserts that, for each person's level of competence, there is a level of environmental demand, or "environmental press," that is most advantageous to that person's function. People who function at relatively lower levels of competence can tolerate only low levels of environmental press, whereas people who function at higher levels of competence can tolerate increased environmental demands. An often-quoted correlate is that the more impaired the person, the greater the impact of the environment. This theory is often used in planning appropriate environments for older adults with disabilities. Today, the person-environment fit theory, in conjunction with the life span development models, is applied by ergonomics professionals who recognize that aging cannot be defined as an entity independent of environment when function is being considered (Vercruyssen et al., 1996). This theory is also used to assess the environmental qualities that are essential components for quality of life among older people (Lawton et al., 1997).

Relevance for Gerontological Nursing

Sociologic theories of aging help nurses view older adults as people who function in relation to their environments and who are influenced by the society in which they live. Some of the influences that are addressed in theories of social gerontology are culture, family, education, community, ascribed roles, home and living setting, and personal and political economics. Although there are patterns of similar responses among cohorts in specific cultures, the theories remind health care workers that, within those larger patterns, each person is unique. Some may achieve their identity in an elderly subculture, others may define successful aging in relation to their activities, and still others may find new roles in society. Sociologic theories of aging can shed light on the unique ways that older people cope with stress, respond to illness, and achieve healthy aging.

Gerontological nurses can apply concepts from the activity, disengagement, and continuity theories, particularly when they assess coping mechanisms and plan interventions to facilitate healthy adjustments. For example, it is helpful to understand that the way in which people respond to changes in older adulthood is probably an extension of the way they learned to cope throughout their lifetimes. By identifying usual activity patterns and coping mechanisms from the past, nurses can help older adults find new activities that will contribute to self-fulfillment and effective coping. An article by Onega and Tripp-Reimer (1997) discusses the application of the continuity theory to gerontological nursing practice and includes an excellent case example. Using concepts from the person-environment fit theory, gerontological nurses can come to appreciate the importance of environmental adaptations as interventions to improve functional status, especially when working with dependent older adults. In addition, these theories emphasize the importance of assessing both environmental and psychosocial factors that influence the function of an older person. Lawton's theory also suggests that, when an older person has difficulty coping, interventions can be directed toward improving personal competency or decreasing environmental demands, or both.

Psychological Theories of Aging

Psychological theories of aging address questions about the behavioral and developmental aspects of later adulthood, such as How is behavior affected by aging? and Do patterns of behavior change over time in any identifiable way? These theories are broad in their scope because psychological aging is influenced by biologic and social factors, and it also involves the use of adaptive capacities for exercising behavioral control or self-regulation. These adaptive capacities include learning, memory, feelings, intelligence, and motivations. In recent years, gerontologists also have addressed questions about why people age differently, with attention being focused on the relative influences of genetics and environmental factors. Psychological theories that are still evolving and being tested in the late 1990s focus on the relationship between older adults or old-old people and the broader universe. These theories will be reviewed briefly in the next sections. Because nursing addresses psychosocial, as well as physiologic, aspects of function, these theories are especially relevant to gerontological nurses. In addition to the theories discussed in this chapter, theories about stress and coping, cognitive function, and depression—also among the psychological theories of aging—are discussed in Chapters 3, 4, and 20 of this text because of their specific relevance to those chapters.

Human Needs Theory

Many psychological theories address the concept of motivation and human needs. Maslow's hierarchy of needs is one such theory that has been used by gerontologists. According to Maslow's theory (1954), five categories of basic human needs are ordered, from lowest to highest, as follows: physiologic needs, safety and security needs, love and belongingness, self-esteem, and self-actualization. Maslow believes that the attainment of lower-level needs takes priority over higher-level needs; self-actualization can occur only when lower-level needs are met to some degree. People continually move between the levels, but they always strive toward higher levels. This theory is particularly applicable to older adults because Maslow describes self-actualized people as fully mature humans who possess such desirable traits as autonomy, creativity, independence, and positive interpersonal relationships.

Life-Course and Personality Development Theories

Some psychological theories of aging, referred to as personality development theories, identify personality types as predictive forces for successful or unsuccessful aging. Other theories, referred to as life-course theories, attempt to address old age within the context of the time frame of the person's life span or life cycle. According to these theories, one's life course is divided into stages, and one moves through these stages in certain patterns. Like Maslow's human needs theory, life-course theories describe some progression through various stages and suggest that successful progression is related in some way to successful accomplishments in prior stages. There is a great deal of overlap between some of the concepts in personality development theories and those in life-course theories; indeed, these terms are often used interchangeably by different authors to refer to the same theories.

The theory of continuity, discussed in this chapter under sociologic theories of aging, also addresses the concept of personality development over the life span. Similarly, theories about personality development address the question of whether the personality changes or remains the same throughout the life course. Although most researchers agree that personality remains relatively stable over the life span, they disagree about the extent and causes of personality change or stability. Thus, personality and life-course theories of aging share many of the con-

cepts of sociologic and other psychological theories of aging.

Based on their belief that neither the activity nor the disengagement theory adequately explained personality differences, Neugarten and colleagues (1968) conducted a study of personality types. Using data from their studies, they identified four basic personality patterns in older adults: integrated, armored-defended, passive-dependent, and unintegrated. Most older adults who were subjects in their research were assigned to the mature, or integrated, personality group and had made positive adjustments to aging. They further divided this group of high-functioning older subjects into three categories based on their level of role activity: (1) reorganizers, who were engaged in a wide variety of activities, (2) focused people, who had become selective in their activities, and (3) disengaged people, who had voluntarily moved away from role commitments. People in the armored-defended group either held on to patterns of middle age as long as possible, or they closed themselves off from the world. Those with passive-dependent personalities were found to have strong dependency needs or to be apathetic "rocking-chair" people. The last type, the unintegrated personality group, formed the smallest group and were the least well adjusted. This group included those with psychological problems, those who exhibited irrational behavior, and those who failed to cope with activities of daily living (Neugarten et al., 1968).

Most theories of adult personality development are based on the theories of Carl Jung or Erik Erikson. Jung's theory (1960) considers personalities to be either extroverted and oriented toward the external world, or introverted and oriented toward subjective experiences. A balance between the two orientations, both of which are present to some degree in all people, is essential for mental health. Jung further theorized that people tend to be more extroverted in their younger years because of the nature of the demands and responsibilities associated with family and social roles. As these demands change and diminish, beginning around the age of 40 years, people become more introverted. Jung (1954) describes later adulthood as a period of taking stock, a time during which a person looks backward rather than forward and is responsible for devoting serious attention to self. Successful aging, according to Jung's theory, is dependent on accepting one's diminishing capacity and increasing number of losses.

Jung's theory set the stage for later revisions in the disengagement theory of Cumming and Henry (1961) and for Neugarten's (1968) theory of interiority. Based on studies of middle-aged and older adults, Neugarten suggested replacing the term "disengagement" with the phrase "increased interiority of the personality" (1968). Neugarten's definition of interiority was similar to Jung's definition of introversion, but she identified the middle years as beginning at 50, rather than 40 years of age. Neugarten described the middle years of life as the time when "introspection seems to increase noticeably, and contemplation and reflection and self-evaluation become characteristic forms of mental life" (Neugarten, 1968, p. 140). Like Jung, she proposed that, with increasing age, ego functions are increasingly turned toward the self and away from the outer world.

Erik Erikson's original theory (1963) about the eight stages of life has been used widely in relation to older adulthood. Erikson defines the stages of life as trust versus mistrust, autonomy versus shame and doubt, initiative versus guilt, industry versus inferiority, identity versus identify diffusion, intimacy versus self-absorption, generativity versus stagnation, and ego integrity versus despair. Each of these stages presents the person with certain conflicting tendencies that must be balanced before he or she can move successfully from that stage. As in other life-course theories, the way in which one stage is mastered lays the groundwork for successful or unsuccessful mastery of the next stage. In works published between 1950 and 1966, Erikson emphasized the life course from childhood to young adulthood; in later publications, however, he reconsidered the meaning of these stages. In 1982, when he was 80 years old, Erikson described the task of old age as balancing the search for integrity and wholeness with a sense of despair. He believed that the successful accomplishment of this task, achieved primarily through life review activities, would result in wisdom. Peck (1968) expanded Erikson's original theory and divided the eighth stage—ego integrity versus despair—into additional stages occurring during middle age and old age. The stages described by Peck as specific to old age were ego differentiation versus work-role preoccupation, body transcendence versus body preoccupation, and ego transcendence versus ego preoccupation.

Departing from those theories that begin with infancy or childhood, some of the more recently developed life-course theories concentrate on middle or later adulthood. One such theory defines the tasks of late life as (1) adjusting to decreasing physical strength and health; (2) adjusting to retirement and reduced income; (3) adjusting to the death of a spouse; (4) establishing an explicit association with one's age group; (5) adapting to social roles in a flexible way; and (6) establishing satisfactory physical living arrangements (Havighurst, 1972). Another life-course theory defines the tasks of later maturity as (1) coping with physical changes of aging; (2) redirecting energy to new roles and activities, such as retirement, widowhood, and grandparenting; (3) accepting one's own life; and (4) developing a point of view about death (Newman and Newman, 1984).

Recent and Evolving Theories

Behavioral genetic theory attempts to explain why some older people function better than others; it does not focus on average differences between groups. It attempts to answer questions such as Why do people age so differently? The focus of behavioral genetic research encompasses both genetic and environmental factors, as well as how these factors influence aging. Some theories, called developmental behavioral genetic theories, merge developmental psychology with behavioral genetics, exploring both the origins of change and the continuity in development. Studies are usually longitudinal and include twins, adoptees, and families of origin. They address issues related to longevity, personality, life events, social support, cognitive functioning, family environment, and health and disease (Bergeman and Plomin, 1996). One conclusion of these studies that is of particular relevance to gerontological nurses is that more emphasis is being placed on heterogeneity of older people and less emphasis is being placed on the inevitability of decline (Pedersen, 1996). One focus of future research is on the etiology of functional changes in older adults as their function changes and declines (Bergeman and Plomin, 1996).

Gerotranscendence is a widely recognized evolving theory that was proposed in the early 1990s by Lars Tornstam (1994). This theory proposes that human aging is a process of shifting from a rational and materialistic metaperspective to a more cosmic and transcendent vision. This shift includes the following aspects: decreased self-centeredness; decreased fear of death; increased time spent in meditation; decreased interest in material things; decreased interest in superfluous social interaction; increased feelings of cosmic union with the universe; increased feelings of affinity with past and coming generations; and a redefinition of one's perception of time, space, and objects (Ruth, 1996). One commentary on this theory states that, although it is based on limited empirical evidence, it represents a promising attempt to integrate and further develop some traditional and newer psychological theories of aging (Schroots, 1996).

The branching theory is another currently emerging psychological theory of aging. This theory is based on the principle of gerodynamics, which draws upon chaos theory and general systems theory. The basic theme of this theory is the bifurcation or branching behavior of a person at the social, biologic, or psychological level of function. Simply stated, each person passes critical points (i.e., bifurcation or branching points) and can branch off into higher- and/or lower-order processes in relation to mortality, morbidity, and quality of life. For example, traumatic life events may result in lower-order structures that result in an increased probability of dying, whereas a healthy lifestyle may result in higher-order structures that lead to a decreased probability of dying (Schroots, 1996). According to this theory, aging is defined as a series of transformations toward increasing disorder and order in form, pattern, or structure (Schroots, 1988).

Relevance for Gerontological Nursing

In caring for older adults, gerontological nurses can use psychological theories of aging as a framework for addressing certain issues, such as response to losses and continued emotional development. An excerpt from an article about the relevance of life-span development models to the nursing care of older adults underscores this point: "An understanding of the lifelong potential for development is critical to nursing interpretations of the behaviors and health needs among aging adults" (Reed, 1983, p. 18). A recent nursing article applied principles of systems theories (e.g., the branching theory) to gerontological nursing practice (Porter, 1995). Porter suggests that this kind of theory is helpful in trying to understand the behaviors of older adults as outcomes of a self-organization process (i.e., the attempt to bring order out of disorder). She further believes that gerontological nurses should (1) identify the unique ways in which older adults bring order out of disorder, (2) describe these processes in relation to each person's uniqueness, and (3) use this knowledge to develop creative nursing interventions (Porter, 1995). Theories that address the relative influence of heredity and lifestyle can be used to educate people about the importance of lifestyle and environmental measures to prevent functional declines in later adulthood.

Maslow's framework is useful for conceptualizing the nature of interventions in institutional or home settings. For instance, if older adults are unable to purchase food, it is unlikely that they will feel secure. Likewise, if older adults feel insecure about being able to meet their shelter needs, it is unlikely that they will have a sense of trust. Older adults who have already met their lower-level needs, however, can be encouraged to focus on higher-level achievements, such as self-actualization. In addition, psychological theories imply that older adults should devote some time and energy to life review and self-understanding. Nurses can facilitate this process by asking sensitive questions and by listening attentively to older adults as they share information about their past. Reminiscence is a positive experience that is essential for continued psychological development, and it can be promoted by nurses either on an individual or group basis. Last, both the sociologic and psychological theories of aging can be valuable in dispelling some of the commonly held myths about old age. An understanding of the continued potential for psychological development might help older adults and their caregivers appreciate the positive attributes, such as wisdom and creativity, that can be derived from life experiences. In addition to these implications for gerontological nurses, implications regarding specific aspects, such as coping responses and intellectual function are discussed in Chapters 3 and 4 of this text, and should be considered in the context of psychological theories of aging.

A Theory for Gerontological Nursing: The Functional Consequences Theory

Gerontological nurses derive theories from existing nursing knowledge and from relevant theories about aging, such as those discussed in this book. What is distinct about nursing theories is that they are conceptualizations of some aspect of reality, viewed from the perspective of nursing, used to describe, explain, predict, or prescribe nursing care (Meleis, 1997). Theories about aging can explain various aspects of older adulthood, but only a theory of gerontological nursing can answer the question posed by one gerontological nurse scholar: "What is there about being aged that requires a difference in nursing care?" (Wells, 1987, p. 22). A gerontological nursing theory, therefore, explains the care needs that are unique to older people and provides a basis for addressing those needs from a nursing perspective.

One approach to nursing theory development is to look for observable data and trends and generate theories to explain them. From this approach has evolved the functional consequences theory of gerontological nursing that is presented in this text. Because this theory underpins all other material presented in this text, it is the one theory of gerontological nursing that will be fully explicated. Before the functional consequences theory is discussed, however, an overview of nursing theory will be presented so as to offer a broader perspective.

Gerontological Nursing Theory in Perspective

Despite the fact that Florence Nightingale is often referred to as the first nurse-theorist, formal articulation of nursing theories did not begin until the mid-1950s. Early nursing theories were built on those borrowed from other disciplines.

Like other nurses, gerontological nurses used theories from other disciplines to underpin their beliefs and practice. By the 1980s, nurses were developing their own theories about phenomena unique to nursing, and nursing subspecialties were identifying the need for theories to explain their particular areas. During the 1990s, nurses developed mid-range theories and situation-specific theories to explain nursing phenomena that were limited in scope (Meleis, 1997).

In 1987, an issue of the *Journal of Gerontological Nursing* addressed the need for theory development in gerontological nursing (Whall, 1987). One article emphasized that this need was "based less on any perceived inadequacies in current models but rather on a call for extension of [the] current theoretical thinking that encompasses gerontological nursing" (Cowling, 1987, p. 12). Moreover, Cowling emphasized the need for theories that shed light on both the "general and unique perspectives that encompass the world of gerontological nursing practice" (p. 12). The recency of interest in gerontological nursing theory is also evident in the American Nurses Association (ANA) Standards of Gerontological Nursing Practice. In the 1976 standards, there is no reference to theory, but in the 1987 revision, there is a mandate for nurses to participate in the generation and testing of theory.

Theory Development in Nursing

Since the time of Florence Nightingale, nurses have tried to define the domain of nursing and to distinguish nursing knowledge from medical knowledge. Despite this long history, however, only recently have nurses agreed on the concepts that constitute the unique domain of nursing: nursing, health, person, and environment. In theory development, these concepts are linked, and their interrelationships are explained. These frameworks are developed along distinct research traditions, or paradigms, and each paradigm provides a different philosophical approach to theory development and research. The four research traditions or paradigms that are dominant in nursing today can be summarized as follows:

1. The *empiricist* paradigm stresses objectivity, inductive reasoning, measurable variables, and value-free assumptions (Meleis, 1997). Research follows the classic scientific method and removes, as much as possible, the variations in findings that could be caused by the uniqueness of people and their situations.
2. The *historicist* paradigm emphasizes that human phenomena necessarily exist within a sociocultural context. All truths are relative, there are always multiple truths, and the context must be taken into account when compiling findings (Meleis, 1987).
3. The *phenomenological* paradigm seeks to examine the significance of meaning in understanding human behavior, meanings for both the person and the environment that result from transactions between the two. In applying this paradigm, the nurse is considered to be part of the client's environment and the meaning of the interaction between the person and the environment is examined. Moreover, phenomenologists look for patterns of responses to variables contained in the nursing question (Meleis, 1987).
4. The *feminist,* or *gender-sensitive,* perspective is the most recently developed paradigm. The goal of this perspective is understanding, rather than simply knowing, and it can be used to develop an understanding of all nursing clients, without regard for race, gender, or culture (Meleis, 1997). Feminist methodology aims to raise the consciousness of researchers about feminist and other views of nursing phenomena, which are equal in importance to masculine and other dominant views.

Although these paradigms may seem irrelevant to nurses caring for older adults, they are reviewed here to provide a philosophical framework for understanding and evaluating the functional consequences theory of gerontological nursing. The functional consequences theory is based on the historicist perspective, and several points will be made in this regard. First, from a historicist perspective, the relevant element in evaluating a theory is its problem-solving effectiveness. Accordingly, "a theory's progress is defined by the degree to which it solves more scientific problems than its rivals" (Silva and Rothbart, 1984, p. 6). Second, data for nursing theory development include the day-to-day experiences of nurses, the common beliefs of the community of nurses, the social and psychological factors affecting the profession of nursing, and the reasoning patterns of individual nurse-theorists (Silva and Rothbart, 1984). Third, concepts pertinent to a discipline at any one time are those problems encountered by the practitioners; thus, as problems change and grow, so do the concepts that explain and inform the discipline (Ramos, 1987). These three historicist characteristics describe the context from which the functional consequences theory of gerontological nursing has evolved.

Finally, before explicating the functional consequences theory, the issue of theory testing through research must be addressed. The functional consequences theory was formulated over a period of almost 2 decades of gerontological nursing practice. As such, its approach is "from-the-ground-up" rather than "from-the-grand-down" (Wells, 1987, p. 21). It is a response to the challenge posed in the *Journal of Gerontological Nursing*: "to examine existing knowledge and, through a process of synthesis, derive models that provide directions for practice" (Wells, 1987, p. 22).

The functional consequences theory can be viewed as an example of phase one of the process model, which was proposed for constructing conceptual frameworks for clinical specialty areas (Reed, 1987). One purpose of this model is to provide enough structure to ensure congruence with nursing's metaparadigm without constricting the theoretical creativity and practical wisdom of the clinical specialty (Reed, 1987, p. 24). In phase one, concepts associated with each of the four domains are selected and then embedded in a model to form the building blocks of the framework. The selection of concepts, which may include non-nursing concepts, is guided by existing nursing theories, the needs of the particular clinical specialty, and the compatibility and logical consistency among the concepts (Reed, 1987). Phase two of the process model will involve the empirical testing of the conceptual ideas in the functional consequences theory of gerontological nursing.

The Functional Consequences Theory

The functional consequences theory postulates that older adults experience functional consequences because of age-related changes and additional risk factors. In the absence of interventions, many of the functional consequences are negative; with interventions, the functional consequences can be positive. The role of gerontological nurses is to identify the factors that cause negative functional consequences and to initiate interventions that will result in positive functional consequences. The ultimate goal of these interventions is to enable older people to function at their highest level despite the presence of age-related changes and risk factors.

This theory is diagrammed in Figure 2-1 and can be illustrated by the following example. One negative functional consequence of age-related changes affecting the eye is an increased sensitivity to glare. In practical terms, older people are less able to see clearly when they face bright lights or when lights reflect off shiny surfaces. Older adults, for instance, have increased difficulty driving into the sunlight or reading shopping mall maps that are enclosed in glass cases. In addition to this age-related change, an older adult might have a disease-related risk factor that causes similar negative functional conse-

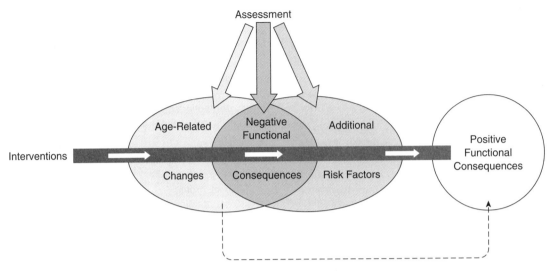

FIGURE 2-1. Functional consequences model of gerontological nursing.

quences. For instance, cataracts may cause blurred vision and increase an individual's sensitivity to glare. Environmental factors may also pose risk factors, such as when white paint, bright lights, and highly polished floors intensify the glare. These age-related changes and risk factors can interfere with the functional capacity of an older adult to the extent that the person stops performing certain activities or performs these activities in an unsafe manner.

To counteract these negative functional consequences, interventions can be initiated by the older person or suggested by a gerontological nurse. Wearing sunglasses and using other glare-reducing devices are interventions directed toward the age-related change. Cataract surgery and environmental modifications, such as the use of nonglare glass, are interventions directed toward the risk factors. The end result of these interventions is the positive functional consequence of improved and safer function of the older adult. In addition, the person's quality of life might be enhanced because of positive functional consequences. A discussion and case example illustrating the application of the func-

tional consequences theory to acutely confused, hospitalized older adults can be found in the recent nursing literature (Kozak-Campbell and Hughes, 1996).

Concepts Underlying the Functional Consequences Theory

The domain concepts of person, environment, health, and nursing are linked together in the functional consequences theory, specifically in relation to older adults. King's theory of goal attainment (1981) is the nursing theory that predominantly underpins this framework. In addition, theories from non-nursing disciplines have been incorporated to delineate the unique aspects of aging and older adults that distinguish gerontological nursing from nursing in general. The following sections will explicate the domains of nursing in the functional consequences theory. The Culture Box summarizes some cultural considerations with regard to the concepts of person, nursing, health, and environment.

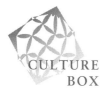

CULTURE
BOX

Cultural Considerations with Regard to the Concepts of Person, Nursing, Health, and Environment

Person
- In many cultures, a person is defined primarily in relation to his or her family and community.
- In many cultures, the concepts of interdependence and dependency hold dominance over the concepts of autonomy, independence, and individualism.

Nursing
- People in various cultural groups have different expectations of nursing care, and the role of the nurse varies accordingly.
- The nursing goal of promoting and maintaining optimal level of independence may not be universally appropriate.

Health
Most cultures hold health beliefs based on varying degrees of each of the following three major world views.
- *Magicoreligious:* Disease results from supernatural forces that cause the intrusion of a disease-producing foreign body or the entrance of a health-damaging spirit.
- *Scientific or biomedical:* Disease is viewed as a breakdown of the human machine resulting from factors such as wear and tear, external trauma, external invasion, or internal damage.
- *Holistic:* Disease results from an imbalance of various forces (Herberg, 1995).

Environment
- The concept of environment includes physical aspects, social aspects (culture), and symbolic aspects (cultural influences of art, music, history, rituals, and language) (Herberg, 1995).

Consideration of these factors is critical in providing culturally sensitive nursing care to older adults. However, before discussing those factors, the concepts of functional consequences, age-related changes, and risk factors should be examined. Display 2-1 summarizes the key concepts in the functional consequences theory of gerontological nursing.

Functional Consequences: Definition

Functional consequences are the observable effects of actions, risk factors, and age-related changes that influence the quality of life or day-to-day activities of older adults. Actions include, but are not limited to, purposeful interventions initiated by the older person or by nurses and other caregivers. Risk factors can originate in the environment, or they can arise from physiologic and psychosocial influences. Functional consequences are positive when they facilitate the highest level of performance and the least amount of dependency. Conversely, they are negative when they interfere with the person's level of function or quality of life or increase the person's dependency.

Negative functional consequences typically occur because of a combination of age-related

Functional consequences: The observable effects of actions, risk factors, and age-related changes that influence the quality of life or day-to-day activities of older adults.

Negative functional consequences: Those that interfere with the person's level of functioning or quality of life.

Positive functional consequences: Those that facilitate the highest level of performance and the least amount of dependency.

Age-related changes: Inevitable, progressive, and irreversible changes that occur during later adulthood and are independent of extrinsic or pathologic conditions.

Risk factors: Conditions that increase the vulnerability of older people to negative functional consequences. Common risk factors are diseases, environment, lifestyle, support systems, psychosocial circumstances, adverse medication effects, and attitudes based on lack of knowledge.

Older adults: People whose functional abilities are affected by the acquisition of age-related changes and risk factors. When older adults are affected by age-related changes and risk factors to the extent that they are dependent on others for daily needs, their caregivers are considered an integral focus of gerontological nursing.

Goals of gerontological nursing: To minimize the negative effects of age-related changes and risk factors and to promote positive functional consequences. Goals are achieved through the nursing process, with particular emphasis on interacting with older adults and caregivers of dependent older adults to eliminate risk factors or minimize their effects.

Health: The ability of older adults to function at their highest capacity, despite the presence of age-related changes and risk factors. This state includes quality of life and encompasses psychosocial as well as physiologic function.

Environment: External conditions, including caregivers, that influence the function of older adults. These conditions are risk factors when they interfere with function, and interventions when they enhance function.

changes and risk factors, as illustrated in the previous example of impaired visual performance. They also may be caused by interventions, in which case the interventions become risk factors. An example of a negative functional consequence caused by an intervention is the constipation that can result from use of an antidepressant medication. In this case, the medication is both an intervention for the depression and a risk factor for impaired bowel function.

Positive functional consequences are usually brought about by automatic actions or purposeful interventions. Often, older adults bring about positive functional consequences when they compensate for age-related changes without conscious intent. For example, an older person might increase the amount of light for reading or begin using sunglasses without realizing that these actions are compensating for age-related changes. At other times, interventions are initiated in response to a recognized need. In the example cited earlier, improved function would likely result from purposeful interventions, such as cataract surgery or environmental modifications. In a few instances, positive functional consequences are caused directly by age-related changes. For example, a woman may view the postmenopausal inability to become pregnant as a positive effect of aging. As a consequence, her enjoyment of sexual activities may be enhanced in later adulthood. Similarly, positive functional consequences, such as increased wisdom and maturity, can result from psychological growth in older adulthood.

Functional Consequences: Theoretical Underpinning

The concept of functional consequences draws on nursing and non-nursing theories regarding functional assessment. Non-nursing theories are derived primarily from geriatric and rehabilitative medicine (discussed in the earlier section on medical theories and in Chapter 17). In the past decade, nurses have applied a functional assessment framework to their care of chronically ill and older patients (e.g., Panicucci, 1983; Schmidt, 1985). One article describing an assessment protocol viewed functional assessment as "a cornerstone of gerontological nursing" (Brown, 1988, p. 13). In addition, nurses have identified specific "functional health patterns" (e.g., sleep, cognition, breathing, and communication) and have applied these to the assessment of older adults (e.g., Carnevali, 1993). Moreover, many gerontological nursing texts now focus on functional assessment.

The gerontological literature discusses functional assessment as a framework for research and a method for planning health services for dependent people. From a clinical perspective, health care practitioners view the multidimensional functional assessment as an important component in the care of older people. None of the literature, however, suggests an assessment of functional consequences. To date, this aspect has not been developed, and it is unique to the functional consequences theory of gerontological nursing.

The functional consequences theory draws on concepts regarding functional assessment, but it extends far beyond an assessment of function. The functional consequences theory significantly differs from functional assessment in the following ways: (1) it defines functional consequences and differentiates between positive and negative consequences; (2) it emphasizes the identification of age-related changes and risk factors that affect a person's function, rather than simply identifying a person's functional

level; (3) it attempts to distinguish between age-related changes that increase the person's vulnerability and risk factors that interfere with the person's function; and, (4) it addresses from a functional perspective not only assessment, but also interventions.

Age-Related Changes and Risk Factors

Age-related changes and risk factors are concepts crucial to the functional consequences theory because they distinguish the care of older adults from the care of other people. It is essential to differentiate between age-related changes and risk factors because the interventions for age-related changes differ from those for risk factors. It is not possible to reverse or alter the effects of age-related changes, but it is possible to compensate for their effects and to intervene so that positive functional consequences occur. By contrast, risk factors often can be modified or even eliminated, and their effects may be reversed or compensated for through interventions.

Non-nursing theories that underpin the concept of age-related changes have been addressed in earlier sections of this chapter. The biologic theories of aging, for example, are useful in understanding the concept of age-related changes. What must be emphasized here is the rapidly evolving state of knowledge regarding age-related changes. A noted geriatrician underscored this point by stating, "I find I must learn and relearn all the time, namely, to accept no symptom or loss of function in older persons as being simply 'old age.' Rather professionals should search for explanations, which will almost always be found in one or more diseases that are present, or in life style (such as incremental disuse), or in the environment" (Williams, 1986, p. 347). The functional consequences theory challenges the "what-do-you-expect-you're-old" syndrome, but it recognizes that there are not always clear distinctions between age-related and disease-related processes. Even if apparent distinctions are identified, they may be questioned at a later time as new theories evolve. With the functional consequences theory, age-related changes are not seen as the sole cause of negative functional consequences, but as factors that increase the vulnerability of older people to the negative impact of risk factors.

Nursing theories have not yet encompassed age-related changes, but at least one gerontological nurse scholar has suggested that nursing research should address this question (Wells, 1987). Nursing theories, however, have addressed risk factors in relation to health; indeed, one nursing article about risk and vulnerability is particularly applicable to the functional consequences theory (Rose and Killien, 1983). The authors analyzed the concepts of risk and vulnerability and identified their distinguishing features. The framework developed by these nurses is useful in understanding the difference between age-related changes and risk factors. Risks are conceptualized as potentially stressful environmental factors, including those in the immediate surroundings as well as those that are direct and indirect influences on the broader physical and sociocultural environment. Applying this to the functional consequences theory, examples of risk factors would be poor lighting, barriers to mobility, lack of social supports, and myths and misunderstandings about aging. Rose and Killien (1983) conceptualize vulnerability on a dynamic continuum that is affected by both constitutional and acquired factors. Constitutional factors are reflected in the person's internal environment and neurophysiology, whereas acquired factors are those resulting from experiences and life events.

Applying this to the functional consequences theory, constitutional factors would be the age-related changes that interfere with a person's ability to respond to stresses. Acquired factors would be disease-related conditions and adverse psychosocial influences, such as multiple losses in a short period. According to the functional consequences theory, however, only the constitutional factors (e.g., age-related changes) would be viewed as vulnerability characteristics, whereas the acquired factors (e.g., chronic illnesses) would be considered to be risk factors. Rose and Killien (1983) further proposed that one of the implications of this model is that interventions to improve the state of health can be directed toward either reducing the risk or changing the person's level of vulnerability. According to these authors, "It is often more feasible to modify the environment than it is to change a person's level of vulnerability, particularly if that vulnerability is primarily due to genetic or constitutional factors" (p. 68). Although their theory focuses on modification of risk factors, they also emphasize that levels of vulnerability are not static. This viewpoint is consistent with that of the functional consequences approach to gerontological nursing. The Rose-Killien model was developed from the perspective of pediatric nurses, but it provides a basis for understanding the differences, as well as the relationship, between age-related changes and risk factors in older adults.

Person

Underlying the functional consequences conceptualization of person as the focus of nursing care is the nursing theory of Imogene King (1981). According to King's theory, people are social beings who are rational and sentient and who use language to communicate thoughts, actions, customs, and beliefs. Further, they are characterized by the ability to feel, think, perceive, set goals, make decisions, choose between alternative courses of action, and select the means to achieve goals. Because they possess these characteristics, they are reacting beings. This perspective is relevant to the functional consequences theory because it emphasizes the ability of responsible people to establish and achieve goals. In the functional consequences theory, older adults are viewed as being capable of achieving positive functional consequences, despite the presence of age-related changes and risk factors. Furthermore, older adults are viewed as unique individuals who achieve positive functional consequences through interactions with their environment and with people in their environment. In particular, the interactions between nurses and older adults are of importance in achieving positive functional consequences.

The functional consequences theory of gerontological nursing is based on a holistic nursing approach that views the older adult as a complex and unique person whose functioning is influenced by the relationships between many internal and external factors. Because this theory is specific to gerontological nursing, "person" is defined in relation to the age category called "older adults." Using the non-nursing theories discussed in this text, the older adult is not defined merely by chronologic age, but also by the acquisition of physiologic and psychosocial characteristics that are associated with maturity. On the positive side, these characteristics include increased wisdom and creativity and advanced levels of personal growth based on experience. On the negative side, these characteristics include a slowing down of physiologic processes, increased vulnerability to chronic illnesses, and a diminished ability to respond to physiologic stress.

According to this conceptualization, older adults cannot be defined by strict chronologic criteria because aging is seen as a gradual process. From this perspective, a person does not discover that he or she has suddenly become an older adult at a particular chronologic age. Rather, people who live long enough are able to recognize at some point that they have developed to a mature level that is categorized as older adulthood. Although this concept has the distinct disadvantage of being difficult to mea-

sure, it has the advantage of accurately reflecting the realities of older adulthood. Because people increase in heterogeneity rather than homogeneity as they age, any definition of the older adult must, by its nature, be broad. According to the functional consequences theory, a person is considered to be an older adult when he or she manifests one or more functional consequences attributable to age-related changes alone, or to age-related changes in combination with risk factors. Stated simply, it is the accumulation of age-related functional consequences that define someone as an older adult.

The older adult is further conceptualized in the context of his or her relationships with others. A person is not an isolated entity, but a dynamic being who continually influences and is influenced by the environment and other people. This context is particularly important for older adults because the more functionally impaired a person is, the more important are the support resources. When negative functional consequences accumulate to the extent that the older adult is very dependent on others for daily needs, the caregivers may become the primary focus of gerontological nursing. Even for older people with few functional impairments, this context is important, because older people have a long history of interpersonal relationships that influence their health behaviors.

Nursing

The conceptualization of nursing in the functional consequences theory draws on many nursing theorists, beginning with Florence Nightingale, who viewed nursing as the provision of an environment conducive to healing and health promotion ([1859]1954). Modern nursing theorists agree that the focus of nursing activity is on regulating, promoting, modifying, and monitoring the interaction between the patient and the environment and communicating that interaction (Flaskerud and Halloran,

1980). In addition, the ANA statement on the scope of gerontological nursing, discussed in Chapter 1, is applicable to the definition of nursing as outlined by the functional consequences theory. Another definition that is most applicable to this theory has been proposed as follows: "The goal of gerontological nursing care is to help elderly clients function as fully as possible by realizing their highest potential" (Bahr, 1981, p. 24). Finally, King's theory of nursing is particularly relevant to the concept of nursing presented in the functional consequences theory.

King views the crux of nursing as the nurse-client transaction, which is regarded as a purposeful interaction that leads to goal attainment. Specifically, King defines nursing as "a process of action, reaction, and interaction whereby nurse and client share information about their perceptions in the nursing situation. Through purposeful communication they identify specific goals, problems, or concerns. They explore means to achieve a goal and agree to means to the goal" (King, 1981, p. 2). Outcomes of these transactions include satisfaction in performing activities of daily living, success in performing activities in one's usual roles, and achievement of immediate and long-range goals. One example of nursing activity cited by King was that of community nurses who perform health assessments of older adults and "engage in mutual goal setting to help older individuals function in their usual roles" (1981, p. 3).

King delineates the functions of nurses, emphasizing their role in teaching, guiding, and counseling individuals and groups to help them maintain health (1981). She further states: "Nurses give care to individuals who have chronic diseases and to those who need rehabilitation to help them use their potential ability to function as human beings" (1981, pp. 8–9). "Nurses use knowledge and skills to help individuals and groups cope with existential problems and learn ways of adjusting to changes in their daily activities" (1981, p. 3). Although King does not use the term "multidisciplinary

team," she clearly views the nurse as a partner in coordinating health care for individuals and groups.

According to the functional consequences theory, the goals of gerontological nursing are to minimize the effects of negative functional consequences and to promote positive functional consequences in older adults. Through the nursing process, age-related changes and risk factors are assessed, interventions are planned and implemented, and functional outcomes are evaluated. Most often, the goals are achieved through educating older adults and caregivers of dependent older adults about interventions that will eliminate risk factors or minimize their effects. The educational aspects are particularly important when myths and misunderstandings contribute to negative functional consequences. For example, when an older person believes that functional impairments are a necessary consequence of old age, the gerontological nurse can provide information about age-related changes and risk factors, assisting the older person in identifying ways of minimizing the effects of the risk factors and compensating for the effects of age-related changes.

The focus of gerontological nursing varies according to the setting. In acute care settings, the focus is on pathologic conditions that create serious risks and are expected to respond to short-term interventions. In long-term care settings, the focus is on multiple risk factors that are not immediately responsive to short-term interventions and that interfere with functional abilities to the extent that the older adult is dependent on others in several functional areas. In home and community settings, the focus is on short- and long-term interventions aimed at age-related changes and risk factors.

Health

King's nursing theory defines health as the "dynamic life experiences of a human being, which implies continuous adjustment to stressors in the internal and external environment through optimal use of one's resources to achieve maximum potential for daily living" (1981, p. 5). King emphasizes that health involves performance of the activities of daily living, but that the ultimate purpose of this performance is quality of life. Furthermore, this performance is significantly influenced by one's environment. The functional consequences theory defines health as the ability of older adults to function at their highest capacity, despite the presence of age-related changes and risk factors. It encompasses psychosocial as well as physiologic function, and it also considers the quality of life of the person. Therefore, according to this theory, health is individually determined, based on the functional capacities that are perceived as important. For example, one person might define the desired level of function as a capacity for intimate relationships, whereas another might define it as being able to perform aerobic exercise for half an hour daily.

Non-nursing theories of health can be drawn from a number of sources, but only two of these are addressed here. First, the widely used World Health Organization (WHO) definition of health is particularly relevant to the functional consequences theory of gerontological nursing. In 1959, the WHO specifically defined health in older adults: "Health in the elderly is best measured in terms of function . . . degree of fitness rather than extent of pathology may be used as a measure of the amount of services the aged will require from the community" (WHO, 1959). Second, the perspective of older people themselves has been incorporated into the functional consequences theory. There is a growing body of literature emphasizing the strong association between function and perceived well-being. It is now widely accepted that, with increased age, there is less and less association between diagnostic labels of diseases and actual functional level and well-being.

Additional evidence regarding the importance of defining health in relation to functional abilities has been derived from this author's experiences with older adults. My first formal attempt to define health from the perspective of older adults was in 1974, when I was preparing to open a clinic in an apartment complex for older adults. Because much of my emphasis would be on health promotion activities, I decided to hold a group discussion with the residents to discover how they defined health and illness. Definitions of health typically included functional aspects that were viewed as desirable, and definitions of illness typically focused on an inability to perform certain tasks. Health, for example, was variously defined as a state of being active, sociable, and productive. By contrast, typical definitions of illness involved an inability to eat, sleep, walk, or be cured. One older woman, who used a wheelchair because of severe arthritis, defined health as "being helpful to others" (Miller, 1974). In the two and a half decades since 1974, I have posed this question to older adults in hospitals, nursing facilities, community settings, and a geropsychiatric program. Repeatedly, older people have defined health in terms of function, including both physical and psychosocial aspects.

Environment

King's theory helps to explain the concept of environment as it is defined in the functional consequences theory, of gerontological nursing. The *internal environment* transforms energy to enable human beings to adjust to continual external environmental changes. The *external environment* is defined as "an organized boundary system of social roles, behaviors, and practices developed to maintain values and the mechanisms to regulate the practices and rules" (King, 1981, p. 115). King views the nurse as part of the environment as well.

In the functional consequences theory, the concept of environment takes on several meanings, and some might even seem contradictory. For example, environment can be both a risk factor for negative functional consequences and a source of interventions for positive functional consequences. The environment also includes the setting where the care is provided. For dependent older adults, the environment includes their caregivers. These conceptualizations are consistent with King's theory, in which a transaction is defined as observable behavior of human beings interacting with their environment. According to King, the purpose of transactions is to attain goals, which focus on improved function in activities of daily living. In turn, the hoped-for outcome is a "relatively useful, satisfying, productive, and happy life" (King, 1981, p. 4).

A non-nursing theory that sheds light on the concept of environment in the functional consequences theory is Lawton's adaptation theory (discussed in the Sociologic Theories section of this chapter). Gerontologists have used this theory, along with the person-environment congruence model of Kahana (1975), to examine the specific attributes of the environment that are important in the interactions between older people and their environments (Windley and Scheidt, 1980). Among the considerations that have been identified by these gerontologists and that are applicable to the functional consequences theory are the following:

1. Is the environment comfortable?
2. How does the spatial organization influence orientation and direction finding?
3. Can the type and amount of visual and auditory stimuli be controlled?
4. How does the environment compensate for sensory deficits?
5. Does the environment allow for choices in the degree of privacy and personal use of space?
6. How does the environment affect activities of daily living?

These attributes are central components of the environment, as viewed in light of the functional consequences theory, because they represent specific environmental factors that directly influence the functional status of older people. In summary, environmental characteristics can cause negative functional consequences, but with interventions, they can also be the best sources of positive functional consequences.

Chapter Summary

The functional consequences theory of gerontological nursing is consistently used in this text to explain nursing care of older adults. It is applicable to physiologic function as well as psychosocial function; that is, it can explain why older adults might be incontinent, as well as why they might be depressed. Most important, it provides a specific, practical, and theory-based approach to nursing care of older adults. It answers two crucial questions: What is unique about the care needs of older adults? and How can gerontological nurses effectively care for older adults?

As a mid-range theory for gerontological nursing, the functional consequences theory is intended to be used in conjunction with other theories that explain nursing from a broader perspective. It is not intended to explain all aspects of nursing care of older adults, but only those aspects that distinguish care of older adults from the care of other populations. In this book, therefore, there is very little discussion of pathologic conditions, such as cancer, that commonly occur in older adults. The rationale for this exclusion is that disease processes are not different in older adults, but the impact of diseases is different because of age-related changes and additional risk factors. Information in this book does not duplicate information about medical-surgical nursing care or about diseases of adults. Rather, it addresses the unique aspects of the nursing care of older adults, no matter what their level of health or illness. It is applicable to the nursing care of all older people, whether they are in intensive care units or community settings. What differs according to the level of health or illness is the additional theory base that the nurse applies in conjunction with the functional consequences theory. A nurse practicing in an intensive care unit, for example, would use critical care theories along with the functional consequences theory, whereas a nurse working in a community setting would use theories relating to community health nursing in conjunction with the functional consequences theory. In sum, the functional consequences theory explains what is unique about the responses of older adults to actual or potential health problems; as such, it is a theory for the practice of gerontological nursing.

Critical Thinking Exercises

You are doing an admission assessment on an 87-year-old woman who is being admitted to the hospital with congestive heart failure for the 3rd time in the past 2 years. She does not have any cognitive impairment and she lives alone in her own home. When you ask her why she came to the hospital, she states, "I'm 87 years old, you know, isn't that a good enough reason to be sick? Don't you think you'll be in the hospital when you're my age?"

1. How do you respond to her?
2. What additional assessment information would you want?
3. What health teaching would you think about incorporating into your care plan?

Educational Resources

Alliance for Aging Research
2021 K Street, NW, Suite 305, Washington, DC 20000
(202) 293–2856

National Institute on Aging
US Department of Health and Human Services, Public Health Services, Building 31, Room 5C27, Bethesda, MD 20892
(301) 496–1752
www.nih.gov/nia

References

Achenbaum, W. A., & Bengston, V. L. (1994). Re-engaging the disengagement theory of aging: On the history and assessment of theory development in gerontology. *The Gerontologist, 34,* 756–763.

Bahr, S. R. T. (1981). Overview of gerontological nursing. In M. O. Hogstel (Ed.), *Nursing care of the older adult* (pp. 3–29). New York: John Wiley & Sons.

Baker, G. T., & Martin, G. R. (1997). Molecular and biologic factors in aging: The origins, causes, and prevention of senescence. In C. K. Cassel, H. J. Cohen, E. B. Larson, D. E. Meier, N. M. Resnick, L. Z. Rubenstein, & L. B. Sorenson (Eds.), *Geriatric medicine* (3rd ed., pp. 3–28). New York: Springer.

Becker, P. M., & Cohen, H. J. (1984). The functional approach to the care of the elderly: A conceptual framework. *Journal of the American Geriatrics Society, 32,* 923–929.

Bergeman, C. S., & Plomin, R. (1996). Behavioral genetics. In J. E. Birren (Ed.), *Encyclopedia of Gerontology: Age, aging, and the aged* (Vol. 1, pp. 163–172). San Diego: Academic Press.

Brody, H. (1987). Lipofuscin. In G. L. Maddox (Ed.), *The encyclopedia of aging* (p. 404). New York: Springer.

Brown, M. D. (1988). Functional assessment of the elderly. *Journal of Gerontological Nursing, 14*(5), 13–17.

Burns, R., Pahor, M., & Shorr, R. I. (1997). Evidence-based medicine holds the key to the future for geriatric medicine. *Journal of the American Geriatrics Society, 45,* 1268–1272.

Carnevali, D. (1993). Health care for the elderly: Nursing's area of accountability. In D. L. Carnevali & M. Patrick (Eds.), *Nursing management for the elderly* (pp. 3–13). Philadelphia: J. B. Lippincott.

Cowling, R. W. (1987). Metatheoretical issues: Development of new theory. *Journal of Gerontological Nursing, 13*(9), 10–13.

Crimmins, E. M., & Saito, Y. (1993). Getting better and getting worse. *Journal of Aging and Health, 5*(1), 3–36.

Cristofalo, V. J. (1996). Ten years later: What have we learned about human aging from studies of cell cultures? *The Gerontologist, 36,* 737–741.

Cumming, E., & Henry, W. (1961). *Growing old: The process of disengagement.* New York: Basic Books.

Erikson, E. H. (1963). *Childhood and society* (2nd ed.). New York: W.W. Norton.

Evans, J. G. (1993). The aging-disease dichotomy is alive, but is it well? *Journal of the American Geriatrics Society, 41*, 1272–1273.

Field, D. (1991). Continuity and change in personality in old age—Evidence from five longitudinal studies: Introduction to a special issue. *Journal of Gerontology: Psychological Sciences, 46*(6), P271–P274.

Field, D., & Millsap, R. E. (1991). Personality in advanced old age: Continuity or change? *Journal of Gerontology: Psychological Sciences, 46*(6), P299–P308.

Flaskerud, J. H., & Halloran, E. J. (1980). Areas of agreement in nursing theory development. *Advances in Nursing Science, 3*(1), 1–7.

Fozard, J. L., Metter, E. J., & Brant, L. J. (1990). Next steps in describing aging and disease in longitudinal studies. *Journal of Gerontology: Psychological Sciences, 45*(4), P116–P127.

Gordon, P. (1974). Free radicals and the aging process. In M. Rockstein (Ed.), *Theoretical aspects of aging* (pp. 61–81). New York: Academic Press.

Hagberg, B., Samuelsson, G., Lindberg, B., & Dehlin, O. (1991). Stability and change of personality in old age and its relation to survival. *Journal of Gerontology: Psychological Sciences, 46*(6), P285–P291.

Hardy, M. E. (1978). Perspectives on nursing theory. *Advances in Nursing Science, 1*(1), 37–48.

Harman, D. (1956). Aging: A theory based on free radical and radiation chemistry. *Journal of Gerontology, 11*, 298–300.

Havighurst, R. J. (1972). *Developmental tasks and education* (3rd ed.). New York: David McKay.

Havighurst, R. J., & Albrecht, R. (1953). *Older people.* New York: Longmans, Green.

Havighurst, R. J., Neugarten, B. L., & Tobin, S. S. (1963). Disengagement, personality and life satisfaction in the later years. In P. Hansen (Ed.), *Age with a future* (pp. 419–425). Copenhagen: Munksgoard.

Hayflick, L. (1965). The limited in vitro lifetime of human diploid cell strains. *Experimental Cell Research, 37*, 614–636.

Hayflick, L. (1974). The longevity of cultured human cells. *Journal of the American Geriatrics Society, 22, 1–12.*

Hayflick, L. (1988a). Aging in cultured human cells. In B. Kent & R. N. Butler (Eds.), *Human aging research: Concepts and techniques.* New York: Raven Press.

Hayflick, L. (1988b). Why do we live so long? *Geriatrics, 43*(10), 77–87.

Heidrick, M. L. (1987). Autoimmunity. In G. L. Maddox (Ed.), *The encyclopedia of aging* (pp. 50–51). New York: Springer.

Herberg, P. (1995). Theoretical foundations of transcultural nursing. In M. M. Andrews & J. S. Boyle (Eds.), *Transcultural concepts in nursing care.* Philadelphia: J. B. Lippincott.

Jung, C. G. (1954). Marriage as a psychological relationship. In W. McGuire, H. Reed, M. Fordham, & G. Adler (Eds.) (R. F. C. Hull, trans.), *Collected works: Vol. 17. The development of personality* (pp. 187–201). New York: Pantheon Books.

Jung, C. G. (1960). The stages of life. In W. McGuire, H. Reed, M. Fordham, & G. Adler (Eds.) (R. F. C. Hull, trans.), *Collected works: Vol 8. The structure and dynamics of the psyche* (pp. 387–403). New York: Pantheon Books.

Kahana, E. (1975). A congruence model of person-environment interaction. In P. G. Windley, T. Byerts, & E. G. Ernst (Eds.), *Theoretical developments in environments for aging* (pp. 181–214). Washington, DC: Gerontological Society of America.

Katz, S., Branch, L. G., Branson, M. H., Papsidero, J. A., Beck, J. C., & Greer, D. S. (1983). Active life expectancy. *The New England Journal of Medicine, 309*, 1218–1224.

Kennie, D. C. (1983). Good health care for the aged. *Journal of the American Medical Association, 249*, 770–773.

Kenyon, G. M. (1996). Philosophy. In J. E. Birren (Ed.), *Encyclopedia of gerontology: Age, aging, and the aged* (Vol. 2, pp. 307–316). San Diego: Academic Press.

King, I. M. (1981). *A theory for nursing.* New York: John Wiley & Sons.

Kohn, R. R. (1982). Cause of death in very old people. *Journal of the American Medical Association, 247*, 2793–2797.

Kozak-Campbell, C., & Hughes, A. M. (1996). The use of the functional consequences theory in acutely confused hospitalized elderly. *Journal of Gerontological Nursing, 22*(1), 27–36.

Lawton, M. P. (1982). Competence, environmental press, and the adaptation of older people. In M. P. Lawton, P. G. Windley, & T. O. Byerts (Eds.), *Aging and the environment: Theoretical approaches* (pp. 33–59). New York: Springer.

Lawton, M. P., Weisman, G. D., Sloane, P., & Calkins, M. (1997). Assessing environments for older people with chronic illness. *Journal of Mental Health and Aging, 3*(1), 83–100.

Leaf, A. (1973a). Every day is a gift when you are over 100. *National Geographic, 93*, 110–143.

Leaf, A. (1973b). Getting old. *Scientific American, 229*, 45–52.

Leaf, A. (1973c). Unusual longevity: The common denominators. *Hospital Practice, 8*(10), 74–86.

Lemon, B. W., Bengston, V. L., & Peterson, J. A. (1972). An exploration of the activity theory of aging: Activity types and life satisfaction among in-movers to a retirement community. *Journal of Gerontology 27*, 511–523.

Lints, F. A. (1978). *Genetics and ageing.* Basel, Switzerland: S. Karger.

Longino, C. F., & Kart, C. S. (1982). Explicating activity theory: A formal replication. *Journal of Gerontology, 37*, 713–722.

Lynott, R. J., & Lynott, P. P. (1996). Tracing the course of theoretical development in the sociology of aging. *The Gerontologist, 36*, 749–760.

Marshall, V. W. (1996). Theories of aging: Social. In J. E. Birren (Ed.), *Encyclopedia of gerontology: Age, aging, and the aged* (Vol. 2, pp. 569–572). San Diego: Academic Press.

Maslow, A. H. (1954). *Motivation and personality*. New York: Harper & Row.

Meleis, A. I. (1987). Theoretical nursing: Today's challenges, tomorrow's bridges. *Nursing Papers/Perspectives on Nursing, 19*(1), 45–57.

Meleis, A. I. (1997). Theoretical nursing: Development and progress (3rd ed.). Philadelphia: J. B. Lippincott.

Miller, C. A. (1974, August 28). Healthy aging. Unpublished notes from a group discussion with residents of Lakeview Towers, Cleveland, OH.

Miller, R. A. (1997). When will the biology of aging become useful? Future landmarks in biomedical gerontology. *Journal of the American Geriatrics Society, 45*, 1258–1267.

Neugarten, B. L. (1968). Adult personality: Toward a psychology of the life cycle. In B. L. Neugarten (Ed.), *Middle age and aging* (pp. 137–147). Chicago: University of Chicago Press.

Neugarten, B. L., Havighurst, R. J., & Tobin, S. S. (1968). Personality and patterns of aging. In B. L. Neugarten (Ed.), *Middle age and aging* (pp. 173–177). Chicago: University of Chicago Press.

Newman, B. M., & Newman, P. R. (1984). *Development through life: A psychosocial approach* (3rd ed.). Homewood, IL: Dorsey Press.

Newquist, D. D. (1987). Voodoo death in the American aged. In J. E. Birren & J. Livingston (Eds.), *Cognition, stress, and aging* (pp. 111–133). Englewood Cliffs, NJ: Prentice-Hall.

Nightingale, F. (1954). Notes on nursing: What it is and what it is not. In L. R. Seymer (Ed.), *Selected writings of Florence Nightingale* (pp. 123–220). New York: Macmillan. (Original work published 1859).

Onega, L. L., & Tripp-Reimer, T. (1997). Expanding the scope of continuity theory: Application to gerontological nursing. *Journal of Gerontological Nursing, 23*(6), 29–35.

Palmore, E. B. (1987). Centenarians. In G. L. Maddox (Ed.), *The encyclopedia of aging* (pp. 107–108). New York: Springer.

Panicucci, C. L. (1983). Functional assessment of the older adult in the acute care setting. *Nursing Clinics of North America, 18*, 355–363.

Peck, R. C. (1968). Psychological developments in the second half of life. In B. L. Neugarten (Ed.), *Middle age and aging* (pp. 88–92). Chicago: University of Chicago Press.

Pedersen, N. L. (1996). Gerontological behavior genetics. In J. E. Birren & K. W. Schaie (Eds.), *Handbook of the psychology of aging* (4th ed.). San Diego: Academic Press.

Pelletier, K. R. (1986). Longevity: What can centenarians teach us? In K. Dytchwald (Ed.), *Wellness and health promotion for the elderly* (pp. 201–217). Rockville, MD: Aspen.

Porter, E. J. (1995). Non-equilibrium systems theory: Some applications for gerontological nursing practice. *Journal of Gerontological Nursing, 21*(6), 24–31.

Ramos, M. C. (1987). Adopting an evolutionary lens: An optimistic approach to discovering strength in nursing. *Advances in Nursing Science, 10*(1), 19–26.

Reed, P. G. (1983). Implications of the life-span developmental framework for well-being in adulthood and aging. *Advances in Nursing Science, 6*, 18–25.

Reed, P. G. (1987). Constructing a conceptual framework for psychosocial nursing. *Journal of Psychosocial Nursing and Mental Health Services, 25*(2), 24–28.

Riley, M. W. (1996). Age stratification. In J. E. Birren (Ed.), *Encyclopedia of gerontology: Age, aging, and the aged* (Vol. 1, pp. 81–92). San Diego: Academic Press.

Riley, M. W., Johnson, M., & Foner, A. (1972). *Aging and society. Vol. 3: A sociology of age stratification*. New York: Russell Sage Foundation.

Rockstein, M., & Sussman, M. L. (1979). *Biology of aging* (pp. 3–45). Belmont, CA: Wadsworth.

Rose, A. M. (1965). The subculture of the aging: A framework for research in social gerontology. In A. M. Rose & W. Peterson (Eds.), *Older people and their social worlds*. Philadelphia: F. A. Davis.

Rose, M. H., & Killien, M. (1983). Risk and vulnerability: A case for differentiation. *Advances in Nursing Science, 5*, 60–73.

Ruth, J. E. (1996). Personality. In J. E. Birren (Ed.), *Encyclopedia of gerontology: Age, aging, and the aged* (Vol. 2, pp. 281–294). San Diego: Academic Press.

Schaie, K. W., & Willis, S. L. (1991). Adult personality and psychomotor performance: Cross-sectional and longitudinal analysis. *Journal of Gerontology: Psychological Sciences, 46*(6), P275–P284.

Schmidt, M. D. (1985). Meet the health care needs of older adults by using a chronic care model. *Journal of Gerontological Nursing, 11*(8), 30–34.

Schroots, J. J. F. (1988). On growing, formative change, and aging. In J. E. Birren & V. L. Bengston (Eds.), *Emergent theories of aging* (pp. 299–332). New York: Springer.

Schroots, J. J. F. (1996). Theoretical developments in the psychology of aging. *The Gerontologist, 36*, 742–748.

Silva, M. C., & Rothbart, D. (1984). An analysis of changing trends in philosophies of science on nursing theory development and testing. *Advances in Nursing Science, 6*(2), 1–13.

Siu, A. L., Beers, M. H., & Morgenstern, H. (1993). The geriatric "medical and public health" imperative revisited. *Journal of the American Geriatrics Society, 41*, 78–84.

Smith, D. W. E. (1997). Centenarians: Human longevity outliers. *The Gerontologist, 37*, 200–207.

Tornstam, L. (1994). Gerotranscendence—A theoretical and empirical exploration. In L. E. Thomas & S. A. Eisenhandler (Eds.), *Aging and the religious dimension*. Westport, CT: Greenwood.

Vercruyssen, M., Graafmans, J. A. M., Fozard, J. L., Bouma, H., & Rietsema, J. (1996). Gerotechnology. In J. E. Birren (Ed.), *Encyclopedia of gerontology: Age, aging, and the aged* (Vol. 1, pp. 593–603). San Diego: Academic Press.

Wells, T. J. (1987). Nursing model and research compatibility: Concerns and possibilities. *Journal of Gerontological Nursing, 13*(9), 20–23.

Whall, A. (1987). Nursing model development: Conceptual model directions. *Journal of Gerontological Nursing, 13*(9), 6–7.

Williams, T. F. (1986). Geriatrics: The fruition of the clinician reconsidered. *The Gerontologist, 26,* 345–349.

Williams, T. F. (1987). Aging or disease? *Clinical Pharmacology and Therapeutics, 42,* 663–665.

Windley, P. G., & Scheidt, R. J. (1980). Person-environment dialectics: Implications for competent functioning in old age. In L. W. Poon (Ed.), *Aging in the 1980s* (pp. 407–423). Washington, DC: American Psychological Association.

World Health Organization (WHO). (1959). *The public health aspects of the aging of the population.* Copenhagen: WHO.

Yates, F. E. (1996). Theories of aging: Biological. In J. E. Birren (Ed.), *Encyclopedia of gerontology: Age, aging, and the aged* (Vol. 2, pp. 545–555). San Diego: Academic Press.

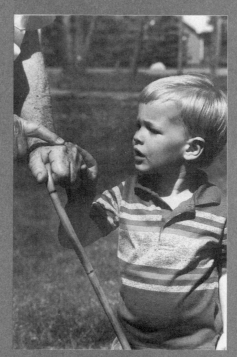

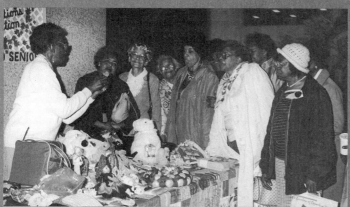

*Changes, Consequences,
and Care Related to
Psychosocial Function*

Psychosocial Function

Chapter

3

Learning Objectives

1. *Delineate age-related changes that affect psychosocial function.*
2. *Discuss theories regarding stress and coping as they apply to older adults.*
3. *Examine risk factors that influence psychosocial function in older adults.*
4. *Discuss the functional consequences of age-related changes and risk factors that affect psychosocial function.*
5. *Identify interventions directed toward assisting older adults develop coping resources, use effective coping mechanisms, and minimize the functional consequences of stress.*

Although the physiologic changes and chronic illnesses associated with older adulthood may affect a person's functional abilities, the psychosocial changes are often the most challenging and demanding in terms of coping energy. Of course, some of the psychosocial challenges arise from physical changes, but many are attributable to changes in roles, relationships, and living environments. Like many of the age-related physiologic changes, many of the psychosocial changes are inevitable and somewhat predictable. Therefore, older adults can prepare for and respond to psychosocial changes by developing and using effective coping strategies. Using the functional approach, nurses can identify both the age-related psychosocial changes and the risk factors that cause negative functional consequences for the older adult. Interventions can then be directed toward supporting effective coping mechanisms and assisting in the development of new coping strategies.

Age-Related Psychosocial Changes

Certain life events demand an emotional adjustment on the part of the person experiencing the event, and different challenges are likely to occur during different periods in one's life. For example, younger adults are likely to experience the following life events: establishing a career, moving away from the nuclear family, committing to a partner, buying a house, and beginning a family. The major life events of younger adulthood are familiar to us either through personal experiences or the shared experiences of friends. These events generally are viewed positively, and they are likely to be chosen purposefully. By contrast, the life events of older adulthood might be unknown, unexpected, and, in fact, unwanted or even feared. Also, in contrast to the life events of younger adulthood, many life events associated with old age involve losses, rather than gains. In addition, the losses of older adulthood are likely to be losses of significant others and objects that have been part of life for many decades.

Life Events of Older Adulthood

The life events most likely to occur in older adulthood have several characteristics that distinguish them from the life events and adjustments associated with younger adulthood. These distinguishing features include the following:

1. They are viewed as losses, rather than gains.
2. They are most likely to occur close together, with less time available to adjust to each event.
3. They are longer lasting and often become chronic problems.
4. They are inevitable, evoking a feeling of powerlessness.

Some examples of common events requiring psychosocial adjustments in older adulthood are widowhood, retirement, confronting ageist attitudes, chronic illness and functional impairments, decisions about driving a car, death of friends and family, and relocation from the family homestead. The longer a person lives, the more likely it is that all of these events will happen.

Widowhood

The example of widowhood as a life event of older adulthood illustrates all of the characteristics just listed. For most older couples, widowhood is inevitable for one of the two partners, and the chances are greater that the woman will be widowed rather than the man. When widowhood occurs, additional consequences may follow. Common additional consequences include loss of one's sexual partner; loss of companionship and intimacy; feelings of grief, loneliness, and emptiness; increased responsibilities and increased dependency on others; loss of income and less efficient financial management; and changes in relationships with children, married friends, and other family members. When a marriage has lasted for many decades, as is common in people who are in their seventies and eighties, the impact of the loss can be tremendous, and the feelings of grief, loneliness, and emptiness may be overwhelming.

Another characteristic of widowhood in older adulthood is that the chance of remarriage diminishes with advancing age, especially for women. Thus, there is little potential for resuming the married lifestyle. Last, if the married couple had clearly divided roles, as is common

in the cohort of people who are old today, loss of the partner means an adjustment in important day-to-day tasks. For example, older couples often divide tasks so that only one of the two manages money, drives the car, cleans the house, shops for groceries, and does household repairs and maintenance. When the person responsible for a task can no longer function in this role, the other person may be unable, unwilling, or unprepared to assume this role.

Confronting Ageist Attitudes

A life adjustment that, by its nature, is unique to older adulthood is the acceptance of being considered old. Because of the ageist attitudes common in modern industrialized societies, many older adults deny that they are old. Even if a person has a good self-acceptance of being old, it may be socially unacceptable to admit that it is okay to be old. Thus, old age in our society is often accompanied by feelings of devaluation and degradation.

Because of these attitudes, older adults may be confronted with age-determined expectations that dictate appropriate social behaviors. For example, public displays of affection are viewed as socially appropriate for teenagers and younger adults. But when older adults hold hands or kiss in public, observers are likely to make comments like, "Isn't that cute, look at that old couple holding hands." Having sexual relationships outside of a marriage is another action that is generally overlooked when done by young adults, but that is increasingly likely to be criticized when done by older adults.

As an example of age-determined expectations, consider the following scene:

A gray-haired man, who was clearly an older adult, was wearing headphones and listening to music on a portable radio. He was briskly moving along in a combination dance-walk tempo on a public sidewalk in an urban area. Observers remarked that the old man looked like he needed psychiatric care, whereas they ignored several teens nearby who were exhibiting the same type of behavior.

The only apparent difference between the older adult and the teens was that the younger people were listening to louder music and demonstrated less control in their movements. The primary difference, however, was in the age-determined expectations in the eyes of the beholders!

Retirement

Societal attitudes can influence one's adjustment to retirement, which is usually an age-related life event. In societies like that of the United States, where a strong work ethic is held, people are valued based on their contribution to the work force. Working people have a higher social status than unemployed people. Moreover, among working people, status is based on the kind of job one holds and the salary one earns. Therefore, when people retire, they inevitably cope with a change in social status. This challenge may be the greatest for people whose self-concept is based on high job status. For married couples, the spouse, as well as the worker, must adjust to the changes related to retirement; indeed, the adjustment might be even more difficult for the spouse than for the retiree. Studies suggest that retirement may be particularly stressful for people who experience health or financial problems at the time of retirement, in contrast to people who plan their retirement and do not experience financial burdens (Bosse et al., 1991).

Chronic Illness and Functional Impairments

Another major life adjustment for many older adults is coping with chronic illnesses and functional limitations, particularly limitations that curtail their independence. Although chronic illnesses are not an inevitable part of aging, 85% of people older than 65 years of age have one chronic illness, and 50% have two or more. Most older adults are able to function with little or no assistance in daily activities; however, the longer a person lives, the more likely it is that he or she will experience functional limitations.

Most functional limitations necessitate only minor adjustments in daily living, but some functional consequences, such as immobility or sensory impairments, significantly increase a person's dependency on others. Other consequences of chronic illnesses include altered self-concept; changes in lifestyle; trips to primary care providers and hospitals; unpredictability about one's ability to do what one wants; expenditures for assistance, medications, and medical care; and adverse medication effects, which sometimes cause further functional impairments. People who have functional impairments also are more vulnerable to personal crimes and may feel more fearful of crime.

Decisions About Driving a Car

Age-related and disease-related changes in visual abilities, cognitive abilities, musculoskeletal function, and central nervous system function can affect the older adult's ability to drive safely. One study found that the following medical conditions were significant factors in the decision to give up driving: stroke, macular degeneration, Parkinson's disease, retinal hemorrhaging, and any activity limitation (Campbell et al., 1993). Another study found that the following factors increased the risk of driving cessation for community-living older adults: cataracts, increasing age, decreased income, unemployment, neurologic disease, lowered physical activity level, and functional disability (Marottoli et al., 1993).

Most commonly, older drivers gradually change their driving behavior to compensate for physical changes. For example, they may stop driving at night or in heavy or fast traffic (Persson, 1993). Older adults are more likely to reduce their driving than to stop driving altogether, and people aged 70 years and older drive about one third the distance that people aged 35 to 39 years do (Evans, 1988). For the older adult, however, even this reduction in the amount of driving has consequences, such as social isolation and dependence on others.

Decisions about driving a car represent one of the most emotionally charged issues relating to functional impairment that older adults and their families face. In the United States, access to an automobile and the possession of a valid driver's license not only provide transportation but also serve as significant indicators of autonomy. In fact, the ability to drive is synonymous with independence. Indeed, one article about older drivers stated that "possession of a driver's license, even one that goes unused, protects the older adult from public or personal disruption of identity because it is tangible proof that one is integrated into the heterogeneous world of others" (Eisenhandler, 1990, p. 4). One conclusion of Eisenhandler's interviews with older adults was that retaining a driver's license and the ability to drive, even if the driving is restricted, is a powerful means of warding off an old age identity.

The loss of an independent means of transportation affects every aspect of an older person's life, from the acquisition of food and medicine to opportunities for social interaction. Because of this global impact, families and older persons may avoid dealing with driving-related issues. Family members may be reluctant to suggest that an older relative give up driving for a number of reasons. For example, family members may not want to assume an authority role, or they may lack acceptable alternatives for transportation. It is not surprising, then, that older adults and their families may avoid or resist the decision to stop driving. Neither is it surprising that when older adults give up or significantly curtail their driving, they face a difficult psychosocial challenge.

Relocation

Another area of psychosocial adjustment for older adults is the decision to move from the family home. As people grow older and their family situations change, a relocation from the family home is likely to be a major decision. Older people in urban areas often find they are living in unsafe or isolated conditions because the neighborhood around them has changed gradually. For example, many older people live in urban areas that were originally settled by

people of the same ethnic background. Neighbors who were of the same cultural background may have moved away, leaving one or two socially isolated older people. For people in rural areas, the geographic distance and lack of supportive services may lead to serious consequences for older adults who are functionally impaired, especially if they have few social supports.

Additional problems arise when a home needs extensive repairs and the older homeowner is less able physically and financially to maintain the house and pay for utilities. Although the purchase of a house in younger adulthood usually signifies a step upward in social status, the move from the family household in older adulthood often means a step toward more dependent living arrangements.

Relocation to a nursing home is a common and significant life event for older adults. Although only 5% of people aged 65 years or older in the United States are in a nursing facility at any one time, the chance of being admitted to a nursing facility at some time is about 50% for a person aged 65 years. Because most of these admissions are for short-term stays, nurses caring for older adults in hospitals and nursing homes frequently deal with the relocation adjustments of older adults and their families.

In 1963, the first study on the effects of relocation from one nursing home to another stirred much attention with its findings that a high mortality rate was associated with relocation (Aldrich and Mendkoff, 1963). This study, which was widely quoted, led to the use of phrases such as "transfer trauma" and "transplantation shock." In recent years, the interpretation of this study has been questioned as too simplistic, and researchers have instead focused on the variables that influence adjustment to relocation. Today, gerontologists do not consider an increased risk of mortality to be an inevitable consequence of relocation per se, and the older adult's degree of willingness to move and level of involvement in decision making are seen as important variables.

In the American health care system, the decision regarding nursing home care is too often viewed as strictly a medical decision, rather than a medical-psychosocial decision with serious psychosocial consequences. Medical professionals do not always address the serious financial and emotional significance of decisions regarding long-term care, and it is often the gerontological nurse who deals with these decisions from a holistic perspective. In fact, nurses are the health care professionals who are likely to have the most important role in assisting older adults with this major life event.

Death of Friends and Family

Like other life events of older adulthood, the loss of friends and family becomes more inevitable with each advancing year. Many people who are in their eighties or nineties have outlived most, if not all, of their friends and many of their relatives. Indeed, people who are in their nineties may not even know anyone who is older than they are. Loneliness and social isolation are two consequences of these losses. Moreover, as people are confronted with the death of others who are younger than or similar to them in age, they become increasingly aware of their own mortality. Older people may read obituaries and death notices in the newspaper as a daily activity. Although families may view this activity as a morbid preoccupation, it may, in fact, be an effective way for older people to learn what is happening to their friends.

Figure 3-1 illustrates some of the major life events that are likely to occur in older adulthood, as well as the related consequences. The illustration attempts to show the interrelatedness between the life events of older adulthood.

Impact of Age-Related Changes on Stress and Coping

Psychological theories of aging address a variety of questions. What influences the way older adults respond to life events? Are certain life events more stressful for older adults? How do coping patterns change in older adulthood? Although numerous psychological theories have attempted to explain stress and coping, there is very little agreement about the relationship between age and these concepts. In the following sections, a few of the more widely accepted theories about stress and coping are discussed. In keeping with the perspective of this text, these theories are used to explain the age-related changes that can cause positive or negative functional consequences with regard to psychosocial function. The term *stress* refers to the difference between the demands placed on someone and his or her potential capacity to meet those demands. The term *coping* refers to the process an individual uses to manage stressful events. In addition, some of the recent conclusions, as well as the unanswered questions, about the response of older adults to stressful events are discussed. The reader must keep in mind that, although this area of research is evolving rapidly, it is still in its infancy, and the answers to many questions about the interrelationships between stress, coping, and aging are still being explored.

Theories Regarding Stress

Hans Selye's stress theory, first proposed in 1956, laid the groundwork for contemporary theories of stress. Selye defined stress as the sum of all the nonspecific effects of factors that act on the body (Selyer, 1956). These factors, including normal activities as well as disease states, are called stressors, and they are considered to be equally important regardless of whether they are pleasant or unpleasant. According to Selye's theory, people respond to stressors in three stages: alarm, resistance, and exhaustion. A major criticism of Selye's theory is his application of the term *stress* to the external stimuli, the internal consequences, and the actions taken to prevent or neutralize the event. Additional limitations of Selye's theory center on his lack of distinction between pleasant and unpleasant

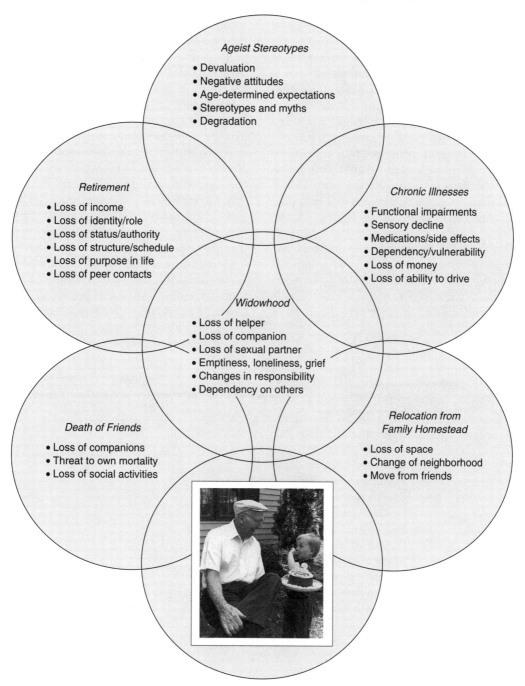

FIGURE 3-1. Psychosocial challenges of older adulthood.

stressors and his failure to address the meaning of events for the person.

In addition to the work of Selye, the work of Holmes and Rahe (1967) is often used as a theoretical basis for investigating stress. According to this framework, stress is viewed as a mediator between a life event and adaptation to that event. Life events are defined as discrete and identifiable changes in life patterns that create stress and that can lead to negative health outcomes. According to this theory, stress causes physical and psychological harm that is in proportion to the intensity of the impact on and duration of a disruption in one's usual life pattern. Holmes and Rahe developed the Social Readjustment Rating Scale (SRRS) as a tool for measuring the duration and intensity of specific life events. The SRRS is a checklist of 43 life events, with relative weights assigned to each

according to the usual amount of adaptive effort required by each event.

Because one of the criticisms of the SRRS is its assumption that life events always have a negative impact, researchers have been prompted to consider the meaning of life events for individuals. There is much agreement now that the response of different individuals to the same stressful event will show tremendous variability. Variations of the SRRS have taken into account the meaning of life events for the person. Lazarus (1966), for instance, proposed a scale based on his cognitive appraisal approach. According to Lazarus, people initially appraise the significance of an event according to the way it actually or potentially affects their well-being. Secondarily, they appraise the event according to the personal and social resources that are available for coping, as well as the cost of these

TABLE 3-1
Strokes/Gordon Stress Scale: Selected Items

Rank	Event or Situation	Weight
1	Death of a son or daughter (unexpected)	100
2	Decreasing eyesight	99
2	Death of a grandchild	99
3	Death of spouse (unexpected)	97
4	Loss of ability to get around	96
4	Death of son or daughter (expected, anticipated)	96
5	Fear of your home being invaded or robbed	93
5	Constant or recurring pain or discomfort	93
6	Illness or injury of close relative	92
7	Death of spouse (expected, anticipated)	90
7	Moving in with children or other family	90
7	Moving to an institution	90
8	Minor or major car accident	89
8	Needing to rely on cane, wheelchair, walker, hearing aid	89
8	Change in ability to do personal care	89
10	Loneliness or aloneness	87
11	Having an unexpected debt	86
11	Your own hospitalization (unplanned)	86
12	Decreasing hearing	85

TABLE 3-1
Strokes/Gordon Stress Scale: Selected Items (Continued)

Rank	Event or Situation	Weight
13	Fear of abuse from others	84
13	Being judged legally incompetent	84
13	Not feeling needed or having a purpose in life	84
14	Decreasing mental abilities	84
15	Giving up long-cherished possessions	82
15	Wishing parts of your life had been different	82
16	Using your savings for living expenses	80
17	Change in behavior of family member	79
18	Taking a relative or friend into your home to live	78
19	Concern about elimination	77
19	Illness in public places	77
20	Feeling of remaining time being short	76
20	Giving up or losing driver's license	76
20	Change in your sleeping habits	76
21	Difficulty using public transportation system	75
23	Uncertainty about the future	73
25	Fear of your own or your spouse's driving	71
27	Concern for completing required forms	69
27	Death of a loved pet	69
29	Reaching a milestone year	67
32	Outstanding personal achievement	64
33	Retirement	63
35	Change in your sexual activity	59

Adapted, with permission, from Shirlee A. Stokes and Susan E. Gordon, (1988), *User's manual, SGSS,* Pace University.

resources in relation to positive and negative outcomes. Using these concepts, Folkman and Lazarus (1980) proposed the Ways of Coping Checklist to measure individual thoughts, feelings, and actions in response to specific stressful situations.

In addition to questioning the impact of major life events, researchers also are questioning the impact of daily stresses. Older adults may experience more stress from the ordinary stressors of daily living, called hassles or chronic stress, than from stressful events (Blazer, 1998). Older adults are likely to experience stressful hassles related to their health, home maintenance, and social and environmental issues. Re-searchers now are looking at daily hassles as well as life events as sources of acute and chronic stress for older adults.

As life event scales have become more popular, the need for a scale specific to older adults has been identified. Most scales address issues that are pertinent to younger and middle-aged adults, excluding important life events that are relevant to older adults. In 1988, two nurses proposed the Stokes/Gordon Stress Scale (SGSS) for research of and clinical use with older adults (Stokes and Gordon, 1988). The SGSS is a 104-item checklist that can be self-administered and then scored according to a scoring sheet. The end result is a stress score, which can be used as a measure of the level of stress an older person is experiencing at a given time. The items in this checklist were identified through interviews with older adults, a literature review, and consultations with gerontological nurses. Some of the significant stresses, such as decreasing eyesight and hearing, can be addressed through nursing interventions aimed at improving functional abilities. Other significant stresses, such as losses of or changes in relationships, can be addressed through the psychosocial interventions discussed in this chapter. Table 3-1 identifies some of the SGSS items and their corresponding relative weights. The SGSS and a user's guide can be obtained from the Stokes/Gordon Stress Study (the address for which is listed in the Educational Resources section of this chapter).

Theories Regarding Coping

Before the 1980s, it was assumed that the impact of major life events associated with older adulthood was negative. Based on this assumption, researchers tried, but failed, to identify specific changes that adversely affect older adults. There is now much agreement that no one life event has a greater or consistently negative impact on older adults. Rather, it is the occurrence of several events close together, along with the chronic hassles of daily life, that influence the person's ability to cope. Wan (1982) studied the impact of major role losses and found that the concurrence of retirement and widowhood in a single time period was likely to cause an adjustment problem, whereas retirement alone would not have a negative effect on health. A more recent study suggests that life events that are associated with more important roles in life have a more negative impact on well-being (Krause, 1994). Thus, even a seemingly insignificant event might represent a breaking point for an older adult who has experienced several prior events that demand coping energy.

In addition to the influence of the timing of particular events, the degree of anticipation of

a certain event can influence its impact. People who are able to rehearse or work through anticipated stressful events are likely to cope more effectively than those who avoid thinking about the pending occurrence. A study of bereaving and nonbereaving older adults found that the anticipated death of a loved one might not be as stressful as unexpected disruptions in daily routines (Willis et al., 1987). Willis and his colleagues concluded that "expectancy and perceived control over life circumstances may be powerful predictors of outcome for elderly persons following a stressful life event" (1987, p. 629). Research continues to confirm the fact that perceived control over events is essential to psychological and physical well-being (Menec and Chipperfield, 1997a).

There is increasing evidence that a person's response to stressful events depends on the personal resources available at the time the event occurs. A recent study found that wisdom—defined as the person's degree of psychological development—has a stronger effect on life satisfaction than objective circumstances (Ardelt, 1997). The following personal resources have been found to facilitate effective coping in younger adults: high income, high self-efficacy, high occupational status, a marriage partner, the availability of a confidant(e) and a large social network, and a commitment to religious beliefs and involvement in religious activities (Simons and West, 1984–85). These researchers found that, of these seven variables, only income served as a coping resource for older adults. They also found that high occupational status and feelings of high self-efficacy impeded, rather than facilitated, effective coping of this age group during times of stress. Under usual circumstances, high self-efficacy and occupational status were assets for the older adult, but during times of significant life changes, these influences were liabilities. Simons and West speculate that people with high status suffer a greater blow to their ego than do those of lower status when faced with the kinds of inevitable life events that are typical of older adulthood, which are "powerful status levelers" (p. 183). A more recent study found that perceived control had a positive buffering effect for old-old adults (80+ years of age), but not for young-old adults (65–79 years of age) (Menec and Chipperfield, 1997b). In this study, high perceived control was of benefit in reducing hospitalization and mortality in old-old adults who had little functional impairment. These researchers have further speculated that old-old adults who have significant functional impairments may be too impaired for perceptions of control to have any impact.

The influence of social supports as a coping resource has been a topic of research and debate since the 1970s. Initially, it was thought that large and diverse social networks provided the greatest level of support in times of crisis. This conclusion has been questioned, however, and data from several studies have been inconsistent. For older adults, the stress-buffering influence of social supports may be associated with the positive effect of such supports on self-esteem or on feelings of increased personal control. In one study, it was determined that social resources directly and significantly reduced stress and mediated the detrimental effects of social stressors on distress (Ensel and Lin, 1991).

In addition to studying age-related differences in coping resources, researchers have studied the internal mechanisms used in dealing with stressful situations. These mechanisms include seeking information; maintaining a hopeful outlook; using stress-reduction techniques; denying or minimizing the threat; channeling energy into physical activity; creating fantasies about various outcomes; finding reassurance and emotional support; identifying limited and realistic goals; identifying a positive purpose for the event; getting involved in other activities, such as work and family; and expressing oneself creatively, such as through music, art, or writing.

In the late 1970s, two opposing theories were proposed to explain age-related differences in coping mechanisms. Pfeiffer (1977) theorized that older adults used more primitive defense mechanisms, such as denial, anxiety, and depression-withdrawal. By contrast, both Haan (1977) and Vaillant (1977) assert that the use of different coping mechanisms depends on the person's degree of maturity. They maintained that less mature people use mechanisms such as denial and projection, whereas more mature people use mechanisms such as humor and sublimation. In an attempt to address these divergent views, McCrae (1982) studied the response of older and younger adults to stressful life events. McCrae concluded that the difference in the use of coping mechanisms in these populations was not related to the age of the person, but to the type of stress with which the person was coping. A more recent study, designed to address the complexities of this issue, concluded that the type of coping and defense strategies used depends both on the level of ego maturity of the person and the source of stress (Labouvie-Vief et al., 1987).

One approach to categorizing coping styles is to distinguish between problem-focused and emotion-focused behaviors. Problem-focused coping is directed toward altering the stress-provoking event, whereas emotion-focused coping is directed toward regulating one's emotional response to the event. Within these two categories, specific coping methods include confrontive and cognitive types of problem-focused coping; distancing, self-control, escape-avoidance, accepting responsibility, and positive reappraisal methods of emotion-focused coping; and, for both categories, the seeking of social support (Folkman et al., 1987). The choice of a coping style and method depends, in part, on the way people appraise the situation in terms of its personal significance and their ability to alter the outcomes. Studies that have applied this framework have revealed that, when people appraise a situation as high in potential for change (in contrast to having little or no such potential), they tend to use confrontation, positive reappraisal, and planned problem solving and are less likely to use escape-avoidance (Folkman et al., 1986). A study of coping strategies used by men and women older than 84 years of age found that older men were most likely to use problem solving, whereas older women were most likely to use positive reappraisal (Dunkle et al., 1992).

One study of coping styles found "striking and consistent" differences between younger subjects, who were found to use predominantly active and problem-focused forms of coping, and older subjects, who were found to use predominantly passive and emotion-focused coping strategies (Folkman et al., 1987). Coping mechanisms of older subjects included distancing, positive appraisal, and acceptance of responsibility.

The authors suggested that these differences had more to do with the types of stress than with the age differences in the two groups. That is, the coping patterns of older people were consistent with and appropriate for the less changeable types of problems with which they were coping.

A study of coping mechanisms of people aged 85 years and older identified two adaptive techniques that helped sustain a sense of well-being despite experiences of physical and social losses. First, older adults in the study directed their coping strategies toward specific losses (e.g., daily activities were incorporated into a routine to make them more manageable). Second, these older adults developed a sense of control over their lives by redefining their optimal health and functional level and their desired level of social

---

DISPLAY 3-1
Factors That Influence Coping in Older Adulthood

The Impact of Life Events on Coping

- The unique meaning of a life event must be considered for each person.
- The timing of events can significantly influence a person's ability to cope, with several events in a short period of time having an extremely detrimental effect.
- No one life event has been found to have a consistently negative impact on the older adult.
- The amount of anticipation about an event can influence the ability to cope, with more stress being associated with events that are least anticipated.
- Daily hassles may demand greater coping energy than major life events.

Coping Resources

- Financial assets are an important buffer against stressful life events for older adults.
- Although high social status and high feelings of self-efficacy are assets for older adults under normal circumstances, they may be deleterious factors at the time of stressful life events.

- Social supports may be a buffer against stress, particularly through their positive effects on self-esteem and feelings of personal control.

Coping Styles

- The choice of coping mechanisms is influenced more by the individual's level of maturity than by chronologic age.
- Passive, emotion-focused coping styles are effective in dealing with situations that have a low potential for change.
- Active, problem-focused coping styles are effective in dealing with situations that can be changed.
- Older adults report that religious beliefs and activities are two of their most effective coping behaviors.
- Activities that distract attention from the stressful problem are helpful to older adults.

integration (Johnson and Barer, 1993). Another study has suggested that coping with health problems can be a source of efficacy for older adults if they perceive health problems as manageable rather than uncontrollable (Aldwin, 1991).

Conclusions Regarding Stress and Coping in Older Adulthood

Conclusions about stress and coping in older adulthood must be considered in relation to the rapidly evolving knowledge about these phenomena. One recent study that addressed some of the controversies concerning the interrelationships between age, stress, and coping found that old-old subjects (ages 75 to 91 years) were least likely to view their lives as having problems, and they expended less effort in coping. The authors suggested that this finding could be attributed to either or both of the following explanations. One explanation is that the perspective and life experiences of older adults may render most problems trivial, resulting in a less stressed attitude toward problems and their resolutions. The other explanation is that older adults develop routine stress management skills that are appropriate for responding to the stresses that have become chronic rather than episodic (Aldwin et al., 1996). Additional conclusions that can be drawn from studies on stress and coping in older adults are summarized in Display 3-1. The Culture Box summarizes information about cultural influences on stress and coping.

Religion, Spirituality, and Aging

Although it is difficult to identify specific age-related changes in religious and spiritual needs,

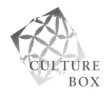

CULTURE BOX

Cultural Influences on Stress and Coping

Cultural factors may influence perceptions of stress in caregiving situations.

- In Latino families the stress of caregiving may be appraised in relation to the degree of disruption to the family rather than the degree of interference with a person's perceived control over life circumstances (Aranda and Knight, 1997).
- In Chinese families the stress of caregiving may be increased or decreased by cultural ideals promoting filial piety, family interdependence, veneration of elderly family members, and acceptance of family caregiving roles (Shaw et al., 1997; Dai and Diamond, 1998).

Cultural factors may influence the coping strategies that are used in caregiving situations.

- Prayer and religious beliefs may be more predominant among African Americans and other groups.
- Passive coping styles may be more predominant among American Indians and other groups.

Cultural factors often create barriers to the use of formal support services by ethnic elders (Tennstedt and Chang, 1998).

Cultural barriers to the use of formal support services may increase the feelings of burden experienced by caregivers who feel they cannot use these services.

this topic is addressed here because of its importance as a component of psychosocial function. Also, for many older adults, religion and spirituality acquire increased importance as resources, and should be identified as part of a comprehensive psychosocial assessment.

Florence Nightingale viewed spirituality as intrinsic to human nature and emphasized that it was an individual's deepest and most potent resource for healing. A recent discussion of her views concluded that nurses can foster spirituality by helping patients clarify the most valuable qualities they can bring forth from within, the circumstances that are most helpful for the unfolding of these qualities, and the interventions that bring about these best conditions into their lifestyles (Macrae, 1995). Certainly, this perspective is most appropriate to nurses who are addressing psychosocial needs of older adults.

Religion and spirituality are closely related but distinct concepts. Religion and religiosity refer to the beliefs, feelings, and behaviors that are associated with a faith community. Religion has a strong social component. Gerontologists have looked at various aspects of the role of religion as an aspect of psychosocial function in older adulthood. Some of the current research findings are as follows: (1) more than 75% of older adults say that religion is very important to them; (2) more than 50% of all older people watch religious television programs at least occasionally; (3) about 50% of older adults attend religious services at least once weekly; (4) older adults are likely to identify religion as their primary way of coping with difficult life events; (5) Hispanics, African Americans, and Native Americans are among the ethnic groups that report high levels of involvement of older adults in both organizational and nonorganizational religious activities; and (6) for older adults, religion contributes to significantly higher levels of adjustment as measured by anxiety, depression, alcohol abuse, and suicide rates (McFadden, 1996). Based on these findings, it is important for gerontological nurses to assess religious af-

filiation as a social resource and a component of mental health for older adults, as discussed in Chapter 5.

Spirituality generally is viewed as a broader concept than religion. For many people, religion is a part of their spirituality; for others, it is not. Definitions of spirituality generally include the following concepts: healing; wholeness; social justice; personal growth; interpersonal relationships; a sense of meaning and purpose to life; a transcendent relationship with a higher being; an association with reverence, mystery, and inspiration; connectedness with nature, other people, and the universe; and feelings of and behaviors arising from love, faith, hope, trust, and forgiveness. The current nursing literature reflects a growing awareness of the importance of routine assessment of spiritual needs as a basis for planning interventions to address these needs (e.g., Barry and Joyce, 1996; Hungelmann et al., 1996). The nursing literature also focuses on the importance of providing spiritual care for older adults who are on a journey and are capable of spiritual growth (Berggren-Thomas and Griggs, 1995). Additionally, spirituality is viewed by holistic nurses as an essential component of their role as healers (e.g., Burkhardt and Nagai-Jacobson, 1997). Based on this perspective of spirituality, religious practices are one way of expressing spirituality, and an affiliation with a religious denomination provides a vehicle for formalized religious practices. Other expressions of spirituality discussed in the nursing literature include prayer, meditation, centering, forgiveness, love and caring, creative activities, storytelling and reminiscence, work as a service to others, and rituals and other activities that nourish the spirit.

Older adults are likely to express spiritual needs when they are coping with the loss of a significant relationship or dealing with news about a serious or terminal illness. Older adults who are caregivers for others, especially a spouse, are likely to express spiritual needs in relation to decisions about the care of the other person. Feelings of guilt about not being able to meet the needs of a dependent loved one, or feelings of "playing God" in regard to decisions about mentally incompetent loved ones may reflect spiritual distress. In these circumstances, support and reassurance from a nurse who has dealt with these decisions in professional experiences may be more effective than the counseling of a clergy person. At times, such spiritual distress may be alleviated through information from the primary care provider, especially when family members want the primary care provider's permission or guidance about long-term care decisions. In these cases, the nurse may be able to facilitate communication between the primary care provider and the family to alleviate the spiritual distress. Often, the spiritual needs of older adults and their caregivers can be met by intentionally conveying caring and compassion through attentive listening and other communication techniques.

Risk Factors

From the functional consequences perspective, any factor that interferes with coping abilities can be considered to be a risk factor for impaired psychosocial function. Conclusions about these factors can be drawn from the theories of stress and coping and from knowledge about causes of impaired mental health in older adulthood. Therefore, risk factors that influence psychosocial function are categorized into two subgroups: those that contribute to high levels of stress and poor coping, and those that may impair mental health in older adulthood.

Risk Factors for High Levels of Stress and Poor Coping

The following factors have been identified as risks for high levels of stress and poor coping in older adults: diminished economic resources, an immature developmental level, the occur-

rence of unanticipated events, the occurrence of several daily hassles at the same time, the occurrence of several major life events in a short period of time, and high social status and high feelings of self-efficacy in situations that cannot be changed. People who have a rigid set or narrow range of coping skills are more at risk for impaired coping because different types of coping strategies are effective in different situations. People who cannot realistically appraise a situation also may be at increased risk for poor coping because the choice of effective coping behaviors depends partially on the ability to determine the potential for change.

An accurate appraisal is particularly important with regard to health problems, and it depends on the person's knowledge about health changes and potential interventions. For example, older adults who experience urinary incontinence or difficulties with sexual function may consider these changes to be inevitable consequences of age. Based on this appraisal, older adults may use passive, emotion-focused coping mechanisms, trying simply to accept the situation. The outcome will be an unnecessary and unfortunate functional impairment and a diminished quality of life for the older adult. By contrast, if the situation is appraised more accurately as a potentially treatable condition, more active, problem-focused coping mechanisms are likely to be used. Even if the health problem is accurately appraised as changeable, however, older adults must identify health professionals who understand the problem and who will attempt to find solutions. It is only when both the older adult and the health care professional accurately appraise the situation as changeable that interventions can be initiated to effect positive functional consequences.

Risk Factors for Impaired Mental Health

The following factors have been found to be detrimental to the mental health of older adults:

poor physical health, impaired functional abilities, lack of social and financial resources, lack of good housing and transportation, and widowed or divorced marital status. For community-living older adults, there is a strong correlation between impaired mental health and impaired physical health or the inability to perform activities of daily living. The inability to perform activities of daily living also increases the potential for being hospitalized for psychiatric care. One of the earliest studies of the reasons older adults were being hospitalized for psychiatric illness revealed that the degree of psychiatric disturbance or manifestation of eccentric behavior did not account for the hospitalization. Instead, people were likely to be hospitalized when the disturbance interfered with their ability to meet their personal needs (Lowenthal et al., 1967). A recent commentary on these findings suggests that, for older adults, "taking care of one's self may be the functional and social equivalent of work performance among younger people" (Fiske, 1980, p. 348). Thus, for older adults, impaired functional abilities may be the most important risk factor for impaired mental health.

Functional Consequences

High levels of stress and poor coping can cause mental and physical health impairments. The interrelationships between stress and coping, and between mental and physical health, however, are difficult to define because impaired physical health is both a risk factor for and a negative consequence of impaired mental health. In addition, stress is viewed as both a risk factor for and a negative consequence of physical and mental health impairments. Because of the cyclic nature of these interrelationships, and the fact that many aspects of the interrelationships were discussed in previous sections, this discussion of functional consequences is limited to some of the findings regarding the effects of stressful events on older adults.

Since the life events scale of Holmes and Rahe was first proposed in 1967, many studies have been conducted to measure the negative impact of stressful events on physical health. Some studies have found an association between a high SRRS rating and the occurrence of certain diseases, such as heart attacks. Other researchers, however, point out that the association between illness and life events is not strong. One review of the literature summarized the association as "quite modest. That is, many individuals who experience substantial life change do not become ill, and many persons who become ill have experienced only a moderate amount of life change" (West and Simons, 1983, p. 236). One of the few studies of the relationship between stress and health in older adults concluded that physical health/function before the occurrence of a life event was the most significant factor in influencing the health status of the person after the stressful event (Wan, 1984).

Depression is another negative functional consequence of stress. The relationship between stress and depression has been articulated by one group of researchers as follows: "Depression has been demonstrated as being related to such negative life events as physical impairment, social dissatisfaction, reduced function, low income, and loss of social support, all of which are particularly frequent among elderly people" (Rozzini et al., 1988, p. 229). This study further concluded that "depression in elderly people is strongly related to the appearance of somatic symptoms, which, in turn, are linked with factors such as physical impairment, social satisfaction, Instrumental Activity of Daily Living, income, and family structure" (p. 232). Although this study did not confirm a causal relationship, it points to the cyclical relationship between stressful events, mental health, and physical illness.

Finally, stress may have negative functional

consequences in terms of intellectual abilities. A study of healthy older women found that high levels of stress contributed to a decline in intellectual function (Sands, 1981–82). This study also identified a relationship between intellectual function and several specific stressful events. That is, changes in personal health or the health of a family member were positively related to declines in intellectual function, whereas vacations were negatively related to a decline in this area of function.

Conclusions About Functional Consequences

Little is known about the causal relationship, if any, between stressful events, coping, and consequences, and less is known about these interrelationships in older adulthood. Perhaps the most accurate conclusions thus far are that (1) the experience of a stressful event is commonly associated with the occurrence of physical illness, and (2) the occurrence of more than one stressful event in a short period of time is likely to have a negative effect on psychosocial health and function. Until more research is done in this area, these conclusions must be accepted, and the psychosocial adjustments of older adulthood must be addressed in much the same way as are issues for adults in general. That is, nurses can help a person cope with the uncomfortable and emotionally painful feelings associated with stressful events. They also can assess the psychosocial adjustments of older adults with sensitivity to the unique meaning of a particular event for the older person, and with awareness of the tremendous impact of more than one life event during a short period of time.

Nursing Assessment

Psychosocial adjustments of older adulthood cannot be separated from other aspects of psychosocial function. Therefore, the assessment of psychosocial function has been addressed comprehensively in a separate chapter. Readers are directed to Chapter 5 for a thorough review of the assessment of psychosocial adjustments, which are discussed in conjunction with other aspects of psychosocial function.

Nursing Diagnosis

Self-Concept Disturbance is a nursing diagnosis that might be used to address the psychosocial adjustment issues of older adults relating to disturbances of body image, personal identity, or self-esteem. This nursing diagnosis is defined as "the state in which the individual experiences or is at risk of experiencing a negative state of change about the way he feels, thinks, or views himself. It may include a change in body image, self-ideal, self-esteem, role performance, or personal identity" (Carpenito, 1997, p. 756). Related factors might be the internalization of ageist attitudes, the loss of roles or financial security, the need for a change to a more dependent living arrangement, and chronic illnesses that affect one's abilities and role identities.

If the nursing assessment identifies threats to the older person's sense of control, an appropriate nursing diagnosis is Powerlessness. This is defined as "the state in which an individual or group perceives a lack of personal control over certain events or situations that affects outlook, goals, and lifestyle" (Carpenito, 1997, p. 658). Common related factors for older adults are forced retirement, loss of the ability to drive a car, lack of involvement in decision making, untreatable illnesses that interfere with one's functional status (e.g., dementia), and institutional constraints, such as lack of privacy and the need to follow schedules that do not meet the needs of the individual.

Impaired Adjustment is another nursing diagnosis that addresses the psychosocial needs of older adults. This is defined as "the state in which the individual is unwilling to modify his or her life-style/behavior in a manner consistent with a change in health status" (Carpenito, 1997, p. 124). For example, this nursing diagnosis would be applicable to an older adult who is driving unsafely because of cognitive or other functional deficits, but who refuses to give up driving. Another nursing diagnosis that might be applied to the psychosocial needs of older adults is Ineffective Individual Coping. Carpenito defines this as "a state in which the individual experiences, or is at risk to experience, an inability to manage internal or environmental stressors adequately due to inadequate resources (physical, psychological, behavioral, and/or cognitive)" (1997, p. 258). She suggests that the diagnosis of Impaired Adjustment might be appropriate during the initial period after a stressful event, whereas the diagnosis of Ineffective Individual Coping would be more applicable to longer-term coping problems.

Nurses who are addressing the spiritual needs of older adults might find the diagnosis of Spiritual Distress useful and appropriate if the older person is experiencing conflicts with his or her belief system. Spiritual Distress is defined as "the state in which the individual or group experiences or is at risk of experiencing a disturbance in the belief or value system that provides strength, hope, and meaning to life" (Carpenito, 1997, p. 852). If nursing care is directed toward promoting spiritual growth for an older adult, the appropriate nursing diagnosis would be Potential for Enhanced Spiritual Well-Being.

Nursing Goals

One nursing goal for older adults with Self-Concept Disturbance is to enhance their self-esteem. This is accomplished through nursing interventions that challenge ageist attitudes and by any interventions that improve the functional abilities of older adults. Other ways of enhancing self-esteem include identifying meaningful roles

and acknowledging past and present achievements. A nursing goal for older adults who experience Powerlessness would be to promote a sense of control. This is achieved by including older adults in decisions about their care and by using interventions that increase the older adult's perception of control over the environment. Current gerontological nursing literature increasingly reflects the need to individualize the care of residents of long-term care facilities and to develop interventions that address their sense of powerless. Recent articles by Evans (1996) and Tolley (1997) provide excellent examples of assessments and interventions that address the goal of improving self-esteem in nursing home residents. Additional nursing interventions that can be used to enhance the self-esteem of nursing home residents are discussed in articles by Nores (1997) and Smith and Sullivan (1997).

A lack of social supports and other important coping resources is a common related factor for older adults with a nursing diagnosis of Ineffective Individual Coping. Thus, a goal for older adults with this diagnosis might be to foster social supports. Although many of the important coping resources, such as financial assets, usually are not addressed through nursing interventions, nurses have many opportunities to foster the development of social networks for older adults. In some situations, particularly in home and nursing home settings, nurses often become an integral part of the older person's social network. Specific ways of fostering social supports and implementing other interventions to address the psychosocial needs of older adults are discussed in the Nursing Interventions section of this chapter, and are summarized in Display 3-2.

The nursing goals for older adults with a diagnosis of Impaired Adjustment would include assisting the older adult to use effective coping mechanisms and to minimize the negative functional consequences of the stressor. Healthy aging classes, described in detail in the interventions section, is one nursing model of a group

Using Communication to Enhance Self-Esteem

- Consciously communicate positive regard through your actions (e.g., recognize the presence of someone as you walk past).
- Acknowledge a person by using his or her preferred name and title.
- Be cautious about communicating ageist attitudes, even inadvertently.
- Do not use names or phrases that reflect ageist attitudes (e.g., "little old lady" or "dirty old man").
- Use the same tone of voice as you use for your colleagues.
- Do not raise your voice except when necessary to facilitate communication with someone who has impaired hearing.
- When labeling clothing, put the person's name in an inconspicuous place.
- Do not use terms that are associated with babies (e.g., *diapers, baby food*).
- Do not use *we* or *us* unless the term is accurate. (For example, do not say "Let's take our medicine now.")
- Do not label people as "senile."
- Provide positive feedback for individual accomplishments, even in daily self-care tasks.
- Focus the conversation on the person's strengths and positive attributes, rather than on their limitations.
- Acknowledge positive relationships by asking about family pictures and items, such as greeting cards, that reflect caring relationships.
- When negative functional consequences are attributed to old age, offer an alternative explanation and identify a contributing factor that is amenable to change.
- Identify new roles for people and acknowledge those past and present roles that are viewed positively.
- For people who have physical impairments, focus on nonphysical attributes, such as personality characteristics or interpersonal relationships.
- Apply all the communication techniques discussed in the chapter on psychosocial assessment (Chapter 5).

Facilitating Maximum Independence

- Make sure that the person has access to all necessary assistive devices and personal accessories (e.g., wigs, canes, dentures, walkers, and hearing aids).
- Allow enough time for the person to perform tasks at her or his own pace, and avoid unnecessary dependence that results from an overemphasis on time efficiency.
- Make sure that the environment has been adapted as much as possible to compensate for sensory losses and other functional impairments.

Promoting a Sense of Control

- Ask about likes and dislikes and try to address personal preferences.
- Whenever possible, allow the person to choose between two alternatives, even if the options are in a very narrow range (e.g., "Would you prefer to wear the yellow sweater or the pink one today?").
- Ensure as much privacy, or perceived privacy, as possible.
- Knock on the door and ask permission before entering a bedroom, even in institutional settings.
- Allow as much expression of individuality as possible in the personal environment (e.g., use personal furniture when possible and display family pictures in full view).
- Make sure that the call light is accessible for people who are confined.
- Do not talk about someone in his or her presence as if he or she does not exist.
- Involve older adults as much as possible in decisions, especially those that affect their care most directly.
- Avoid referring to nursing home *placement*. Refer instead to an *admission*, and include the person in the decision-making process.

Fostering Social Supports

- Use interventions to deal with hearing impairments and other communication barriers (see Chapter 6).
- Encourage participation in group activities.
- For people in wheelchairs, especially those who cannot move independently, position the chair in a way that promotes social interaction.
- For nursing home residents, plan table and room arrangements in such a way that social relationships are fostered.

TABLE 3-2
Coping Strategies for the Challenges of Older Adulthood

Psychosocial Adjustment	Coping Strategy
Ageist stereotypes	Develop a firm self-identity, challenge the myths, question any behaviors that are based on age-determined expectations.
Retirement	Develop new skills, use time for hobbies and personal pursuits, become involved with meaningful volunteer activities.
Reduced income	Take advantage of discounts for seniors.
Declining physical health	Maintain good health practices (nutrition, exercise, rest).
Functional limitations	Adapt the environment to ensure safety and optimal functional status, take advantage of assistive devices and equipment, accept help when necessary.
Changes in cognitive skills	Take advantage of educational opportunities, enroll in classes, keep mentally stimulated, join a discussion group, use the library, avoid dwelling on the things you cannot do and focus on your abilities, take advantage of increased potential for wisdom and creativity.
Death of spouse, friends, and family members	Allow yourself to grieve appropriately, take advantage of opportunities for group or individual counseling and support, establish new relationships, renew old friendships, cherish the happy memories of the past, realize new freedoms.
Relocation from family home	Look into the broad range of options for housing, appreciate the relief from the responsibilities of home ownership, take advantage of new services and opportunities for socialization.
Other challenges to mental health	Maintain a sense of humor, use stress-reduction techniques, learn assertiveness skills, participate in support groups.

intervention for assisting older adults to adjust to the challenges typical of older adulthood. Specific coping strategies are summarized in Table 3-2.

Nursing Interventions

Nurses have many opportunities to help older adults develop effective coping strategies, the end result of which is twofold: a reduced level of stress and anxiety and an improved quality of life. A recent nursing article presents a model for promoting anticipatory coping for older adults (Moneyham and Scott, 1995). This model emphasizes the importance of health care providers communicating their own positive views of aging, as well as their confidence in the older adult's ability to cope, during the course of their work with older clients. The following nursing interventions include strategies that enhance self-esteem, promote a sense of control, foster social supports, and strengthen coping mechanisms.

Enhancing Self-Esteem

Self-esteem has been addressed in the nursing literature perhaps more than any other aspect of psychosocial function, and it is considered to be an essential component of nursing care. In a commentary on the importance of self-esteem as a consideration in nursing care, Meisenhelder (1985, p. 127) stated, "Since self-esteem is such a universal human health need, creating and maintaining a [sic] positive self-esteem becomes an automatic goal for each client and [a legitimate] concern of each nurse." In reference to the care of older adults, Whall (1987, p. 41) commented, "If we, as nurses, can enhance only one aspect of our clients' mental health, we should strive to enhance their self-esteem."

As emphasized in Chapter 5, older adults do not necessarily experience diminished self-esteem, despite ageist attitudes and other influences that are likely to have a negative impact on their self-esteem. When loss of self-esteem occurs, it may be the result of increased rigidity and/or an inability to find new coping strategies (Coleman et al., 1993). Thus, an important nursing intervention is to assist older adults in identifying effective coping skills, as presented in the discussion of Healthy Aging Classes that appears later in this chapter.

The following potential threats to self-esteem are likely to occur in older adulthood and can be addressed through nursing interventions: dependence, infantalization, devaluation, depersonalization, functional impairments, and lack of control over one's environment. Many of these actual and potential threats arise from the staff and environments of the institutions where older adults receive their care. Other threats arise from the negative functional consequences that are discussed throughout this text. Thus, to enhance self-esteem in older adults, nursing interventions must address the many threats to self-esteem that are within the scope of nursing care.

Self-esteem depends partially on the perceived appraisal of significant others, which is communicated through verbal as well as nonverbal messages. Nurses must be aware of their ageist attitudes and avoid reflecting these attitudes in verbal statements. For example, even a remark such as "You certainly look good for 85 years old," although said with good intentions, can reinforce ageist attitudes. Hidden messages in this statement may be that it is better to look younger, and that when you are old, you generally do not look good. If ageism is going to be curbed, even subtle messages communicating negative attitudes about old age must be avoided. For instance, a statement such as the following might enhance an older person's self-esteem and challenge ageist attitudes: "At 85 years old, you must have a lot of wisdom. What advice can you give about successful aging?" Additional messages designed to promote self-esteem are identified in Display 3-2 and are discussed in the section on Communication in Chapter 5.

Because self-esteem is based primarily on the perceived appraisal of significant others, nonverbal communication may influence self-esteem even more than verbal communication. For example, if a nurse walks past an older person sitting in a hallway without acknowledging his or her presence, the action may be perceived as an indication that the older person is not valued by the nurse. Even though the nurse may have been attending to responsibilities and had no intention of communicating this negative message, this action may negatively affect that older person's self-esteem. In influencing the self-esteem of others, nurses must keep in mind that the perception of their actions is often more important than their actual intent. Therefore, if nurses are aiming to enhance the self-esteem of older adults, they must be aware of any messages that might influence the older person's perceptions. In addition, they must use both verbal and nonverbal messages to communicate feelings of positive regard whenever possible.

Another intervention aimed at challenging ageist attitudes is the redirecting of the negative attributions associated with aging to external factors, such as the environment. Many studies have confirmed the importance of modifying the way people perceive and explain events, shifting attention to factors that can be changed or controlled. In the classic study by Rodin and Langer (1980), whenever a nursing home resident attributed a problem to being old, the staff provided another explanation and identified a causative factor that was amenable to change. For example, when residents attributed feelings of fatigue to being old, they were reminded that they were awakened at 5:30 A.M. (Rodin and Langer, 1980). In a commentary on the relevance of this study for nurses, Taft states, "Nurses can improve self-esteem in the elderly by changing negative, defeatist attitudes into hopeful, problem-solving approaches" (1985, p. 83). Recent studies have confirmed the importance of providing opportunities for choice and promoting perceived self-efficacy for nursing home residents (Kane et al., 1997; Johnson et al., 1998). This approach also can assist older adults in developing problem-focused coping mechanisms as a preferred alternative to passive acceptance of the negative functional consequences of older adulthood. A recent study of community-living older adults found that an increase in one's perceived level of control was positively related to participation in physical exercise and leisure activities, which, in turn, were predictive of improved perceived health and increased life satisfaction (Menec and Chipperfield, 1997a).

Self-esteem is closely associated with physical health and functional abilities; it is diminished at times of illness. Therefore, any intervention directed toward improving functional abilities also can be effective in enhancing self-esteem. Throughout this text, in all the discussions of physiologic function, numerous interventions are discussed for improving functional abilities. An additional intervention that has been found to be effective in improving the physiologic function of older adults, as well as their self-esteem, is participation in an aerobic exercise program. In one study, older adults who participated in a 14-week aerobic exercise program showed significant improvements in self-concept and perceived internal locus of control, compared with subjects in a nonparticipating control group (Perri and Templer, 1984–85). The participants also experienced improved feelings of well-being, improved physical health and appear-

ance, and a sense of accomplishment and success.

Another mechanism for increasing self-esteem is the identification of roles for the older adult. Studies have found that people with a great number of role identities have improved perceptions of their own worth and efficacy, which are two components of self-esteem (Dietz, 1996). The nurse can ask older persons about their responsibilities as parents, grandparents, or roommates as a strategy for improving their self-perception. In long-term care settings, the nurse can create meaningful roles, such as helper or assistant, for older adults by involving them in tasks that are viewed as productive. When older adults volunteer to assist others, nurses can enhance their self-esteem by acknowledging this contribution with a remark such as, "You certainly help us a lot when you help take Mrs. Smith to the dining room in her wheelchair."

An often overlooked but essential aspect of self-esteem in older adulthood is the acknowledgment of present achievements. When people are dependent on others, they often have difficulty feeling a sense of accomplishment, or even a sense of basic usefulness. Therefore, an intervention to increase the self-esteem of people who are physically impaired is to focus attention on nonphysical assets, such as family relationships or a good sense of humor. One way of focusing attention on positive relationships is to acknowledge the receipt of flowers, greeting cards, and other visible signs of concern expressed by others. Asking about a get-well card that someone has received will provide an opportunity for a discussion of positive relationships, and it may also remind that person that others care.

In addition to focusing on present roles and positive relationships, another intervention designed to enhance self-esteem is to focus on past achievements. This may be done within the context of a group exchange or on an individual basis. This intervention may be especially effective for people who have difficulty identifying current accomplishments. On an individual basis, nurses can ask older adults about their past accomplishments in areas such as work and family. Asking questions about family pictures is one way of opening a discussion of successful and positive relationships. Encouraging older people to talk about grandchildren and great-grandchildren is another intervention that may enhance their feelings of accomplishment. Nurses can further enhance self-esteem with comments such as, "You must be proud of your grandchildren" or "You certainly have accomplished a lot."

In terms of group interventions, the reminiscence group is one of the most widely used therapy models for older adults, and it is used often by nurses. The theory underlying the use of reminiscence groups was first explicated by Robert Butler in 1961. According to Butler (1961), reminiscence is part of a normal life review process for older adults, and it is based on the realization that the end of life is approaching. Life review is characterized by a progressive return to consciousness of unresolved conflicts that can then be reexamined and reintegrated. Among the positive outcomes of a life review are a sense of pride in one's accomplishments and a feeling of having done one's best (Butler and Lewis, 1991, pp. 111–113).

Although the two processes are distinct, reminiscence and life review are often mistakenly viewed as being synonymous. In contrast to life review, reminiscence is a less formal and less intense intervention that, nonetheless, is based on the same theoretical framework. An additional difference is that life review addresses both pleasant and unpleasant issues of the past, whereas reminiscence focuses primarily on pleasant and positive experiences. Although life review interventions require the involvement of a person with advanced mental health skills, reminiscence interventions can be done by an astute and caring person who has some understanding of older adulthood. Nursing models

of reminiscence groups interventions have been presented frequently in the literature (e.g., Haight and Burnside, 1992; Lashley, 1993; Burnside, 1994; Burnside and Schmidt, 1994; Puentes, 1998).

Reminiscence groups provide a structured intervention for enhancing the self-esteem of older adults by focusing attention on past events. One study reported the effects of two types of group interventions—reminiscence groups and current-event discussion groups—on older adults living in long-term care institutions (Lappe, 1987). The major variable between the two groups was the time frame upon which each focused: present events or remote past events. The nurse-researcher concluded that "group sessions utilizing reminiscing [increased] the self-esteem scores of elderly institutionalized clients to a greater degree than [did] group sessions utilizing discussion of current events. . . . The results imply that the intervention of reminiscing, rather than the group process alone, produced the increase in self-esteem scores" (p. 15). Lappe emphasizes that nurses do not require specialized skills, or a skill level exceeding that acquired during undergraduate nursing education, to lead reminiscence groups. According to Lappe, "Nurses who take an interest in their clients, [who] are good listeners, and [who] are able to use a structured supportive approach have the potential to conduct an effective reminiscence group" (p. 16). For a comprehensive discussion of reminiscence and other group therapies for older adults, with particular emphasis on the role of the nurse, the reader should consult *Working with Older Adults: Group Process and Techniques* (Burnside and Schmidt, 1994).

Promoting a Sense of Control

Loss of control over one's environment has been associated with a variety of negative consequences, such as increased mortality rates, impaired physical and mental health, and decreased personal and social well-being (Slivinske and Fitch, 1987). Similarly, a recent study of community-living older adults found that lower self-efficacy was related to a decline in functional status over an 18-month period (Mendes de Leon, 1996). The researchers found that high self-efficacy is a major factor in enabling older adults to carry out self-care activities, even when their ability to do so was compromised by functional impairments.

Perceived control of events and independence when performing personal activities also has been found to buffer the effects of stress on well-being (Roberts et al., 1994). In addition, one's feelings of self-efficacy, or possession of an internal locus of control, are thought to influence one's response to stressful situations. Simply stated, people who feel more control over their environment and the decisions affecting them can accept their situation more readily. Therefore, in addition to using interventions to enhance self-esteem, nurses use interventions to involve older adults in decisions and to improve their perceived control over the environment. In institutional settings, it is particularly important to create opportunities for decision making because residents generally desire more choice than they are given (Jirovec and Maxwell, 1993).

Older persons frequently are left out of the decision-making process, even for those decisions that most profoundly affect their lives, such as moving to a nursing home. One study found that 59% of skilled nursing facility residents did not perceive themselves as having made the decision to be admitted, either by themselves or with the help of others (Reinardy, 1992). This lack of involvement occurs for a variety of reasons, related both to the older adult and to the decision makers. Some of the barriers within the older adult are dementia, depression, long-term passivity regarding decisions, and hearing impairments or other communication barriers. Some of the barriers within the decision makers that may thwart the decision-making process include stereotypes of older people as incompetent, perceptions that the older adult is

not interested in or capable of making decisions, and an unwillingness to deal with the older person's anticipated resistance to the desired outcome.

Many of the reasons for excluding older adults from the decision-making process are related to the attitudes of the family and of professional caregivers, so one nursing intervention is to challenge these attitudes. For example, in acute care settings, nurses can facilitate communication between older patients and their primary care provider to ensure that the older person is included in decisions about medical treatment and discharge plans. In long-term care settings, nurses have numerous opportunities to involve older adults in decisions about their daily care, medical interventions, and discharge plans. In home settings, nurses might work with family members as well as older adults to ensure that the latter are involved in decisions about their care and that their rights are respected. In any setting, nurses may have to remind health professionals, as well as family members and other caregivers, that although people may gain rights by virtue of being a certain age, they do not lose their rights just because they reach a certain age. For a comprehensive discussion of the nurse's role in decisions regarding long-term care for people with dementia, refer to Chapter 19.

Other aspects of decision making that can be addressed in nursing interventions are one's verbal interactions and choice of terminology. With regard to verbal communication, health professionals often talk *about* older adults when in their presence rather than addressing questions *to* them and focusing the conversation *on* them. With regard to terminology, the word *"placement"* often is used in reference to an older adult's admission to a nursing home. This term denotes a passivity on the part of the older adult; it is closer to the terminology used when objects are placed on a shelf than to words normally used in reference to human beings. Nurses would communicate more positive feelings and a greater sense of control if they referred to an *admission* to a nursing home. The term admission suggests that certain criteria have been met and that an active decision has been made to determine whether the person meets these criteria. Even more important than using the correct terms, nurses must ensure that older adults are, in fact, actively involved in the decision-making process, rather than passively being "placed." Other interventions aimed at diminishing the anxiety about a move to a nursing home include initiating discussion of the topic, correcting misconceptions about nursing homes, and providing accurate and current information through the use of videotapes (Kaisik and Ceslowitz, 1996).

Another area affecting one's perceived control over the environment involves the lack of privacy and loss of individuality that often occur in institutional settings. Nurses can show respect for privacy by knocking on bedroom doors and asking permission before entering, by closing doors when privacy is desired, by asking permission before pulling bed curtains open, and by being careful about moving personal belongings without permission from the older person. Concern for individuality is shown by allowing the person to have personal belongings and to arrange these belongings in whatever fashion is desired.

The effects of control-enhancing interventions were studied in a group of older people in a retirement community and compared to those in a control group (Slivinske and Fitch, 1987). The primary intervention was involvement in a physical fitness program and a class designed to help participants increase their mastery of the environment. In addition to exhibiting an increase in perceived control, the subjects who participated in these interventions perceived a significant improvement in their physical health, economic resources, level of spirituality, and quality of social resources. These researchers concluded that "declines in perceived control and well-being usually attributed to advancing age may actually be produced by environmental forces, the reaction of people to them, or both." This conclusion underscores the importance of nursing interventions directed toward negative consequences in all areas of function. These interventions have been discussed throughout this text and can be viewed as interventions for improving the older person's perceived sense of control over the environment.

Fostering Social Supports

Social isolation is likely to occur because of any of the following factors that commonly occur in older adulthood: hearing impairments and other communication barriers; chronic illnesses that limit activity or energy; lack of opportunities because of caregiving responsibilities; mobility limitations, including an inability to drive a car; mental or psychosocial impairments that interfere with relationships; and loss of spouse, friends, or family through death, illness, or physical distance. Therefore, any intervention directed toward these risk factors also can be an intervention to improve social supports. Because these interventions have been discussed throughout this text, they will not be addressed in this section. However, nurses should appreciate the potential positive effects on social supports that are associated with interventions that improve the functional status of an older person.

In long-term care settings, nurses can create opportunities for social interaction through the use of group therapy and the encouragement of conversations at mealtimes. Sometimes, a very simple intervention, such as positioning wheelchairs so people can interact with each other, can significantly influence social contacts, either positively or negatively. Whenever possible, nurses should arrange room assignments to encourage opportunities for support and social interactions. Reminiscence groups, discussed as an intervention to enhance self-esteem, can also be effective as an intervention for fostering social supports. One study of the effects of reminiscence groups on community-living older adults revealed that these groups can lead to the formation of new friendships, as well as the development of ongoing peer support groups (Sherman, 1987).

In home settings, nurses can identify community resources, such as volunteer friendly visitor and meal programs, to decrease social isolation. Support and education groups that primarily focus on coping with a chronic illness (e.g., stroke clubs, or better breathing groups) also provide excellent opportunities for social contact and the development of friendships with people who are in similar situations. For people who are socially isolated because of caregiving responsibility, caregiver support groups can enhance coping abilities and provide social support.

Display 3-2 summarizes the interventions for fostering social supports, enhancing self-esteem, and promoting a sense of control over the environment.

Healthy Aging Classes

When older adults need assistance in coping with specific functional consequences, or when they need education to clarify myths and misunderstandings about age-related changes, individual counseling may be the best intervention. When older adults need counseling about psychosocial adjustments, however, this may be done most effectively through educational groups. Indeed, one model developed to teach resourcefulness skills to older adults found that the group members improved, as measured by adaptive function and life satisfaction, as a result of their participation in the group. This nurse-led group focused on helping the members develop strategies to enhance self-control, problem-solving skills, and self-efficacy behaviors that would be useful in coping with distress and managing daily activities (Zauszniewski, 1997).

Another example of a nurse-led group intervention that allows for sharing of experiences among peers is the healthy aging class, developed by this author and used successfully during the past 2 decades in a variety of settings with older adults at various functional levels. This model is based on the belief that older adults who are beginning to recognize age-related physical and psychosocial changes or who are already dealing with such changes can benefit from sharing their experiences with their peers. This model will be described in detail, as the healthy aging class is an intervention designed to enhance the coping skills of older adults who are adjusting to any of the challenges of older adulthood.

Goals

The goals for older adults who participate in healthy aging classes are as follows: (1) to recognize the impact of common age-related physical and psychosocial changes; (2) to support and encourage any effective coping mechanisms already being used; (3) to develop coping mechanisms that are not being used, but which may prove effective for a particular situation; (4) to obtain information that will facilitate problem-focused coping mechanisms for stressful situations that are amenable to change; and (5) to provide an opportunity for the sharing of similar experiences with peers.

Setting

Healthy aging classes can be initiated by nurses in any setting, but long-term care institutions are perhaps the most conducive setting for several reasons. First, nurses have many opportunities to establish and lead groups. Second, the residents of long-term care facilities provide a captive audience from which to select group members. Third, residents of long-term care institutions usually are not acutely ill, and they are dealing with psychosocial adjustments that are readily identified. Finally, residents of long-term care settings have in common at least one major life event, which is a temporary or permanent move to a more dependent setting.

Community settings also are quite conducive to successful healthy aging classes, but nurses may have to be more creative in gathering the group members. Nurses who provide nursing services or health education programs for senior centers or assisted living facilities might be able to establish ongoing healthy aging classes as part of their nursing responsibilities. In these settings, a healthy aging class may be an efficient, as well as effective, way of providing health education using a format that has the additional advantage of enhancing coping mechanisms.

In acute care settings, nurses usually do not plan and implement group therapies, but in rehabilitative settings, nurses may have the opportunity to initiate healthy aging classes. In psychiatric units, often there are enough older adults among the patients to warrant the implementation of healthy aging classes as a form of group therapy.

Membership Criteria

The primary criteria for group membership are that the person be willing to acknowledge age-related changes and be capable of acquiring insight into his or her adjustment to these changes. This author has led groups ranging from highly functional older adults in community settings to seriously impaired older adults in a hospital-based medical geropsychiatric unit. Group members may be coping with similar psychosocial stresses, but this is not necessarily a criterion for participation. For example, a healthy aging class may be composed of older adults who all have some degree of depression or who are coping with a particular stressful event, such as widowhood. An ideal group includes members who are coping with various life events commonly associated with older adulthood and who are motivated to learn effective coping styles.

The group usually works best if the membership is stable and closed, but this is not always possible. A major disadvantage of an open group is that it is very difficult to develop cohesiveness. If the membership is open and chang-

ing, the leader must be more directive, and the group as a whole will not be able to establish ongoing priorities for discussion topics. In addition, with changing membership, the leader has to focus more attention on the exchange of information about group members at the beginning of each session.

Size of Group and Length, Duration, and Frequency of Sessions

Group size can range from 5 to 12 members, with the ideal class numbering about 8 members. Groups can either be ongoing or time-limited. When the membership is changing, such as in psychiatric or rehabilitative settings, the group session can be offered as an ongoing mode of therapy. In long-term care or community settings, it is best to schedule group meetings for a predetermined length of time, such as 8 to 10 weeks, and allow for changes in membership at the end of each period. It is recommended that sessions be held at weekly intervals, and that the time and place for each meeting be consistent. The length of each session should be approximately 1 hour. In community settings, the groups might be scheduled to meet in conjunction with a meal program, because social relationships usually are formed among participants in these programs. As in institutional settings, a community center offers an audience from which to select the group members, and transportation usually is not a problem. Other potential community-based sites include assisted living facilities and group settings, such as adult care homes (also called board-and-care homes).

Criteria for and Responsibilities of Group Leaders

Group sessions can be led by one nurse, but it is often helpful to have a co-leader who has had social service training. An older adult who has made a positive psychosocial adjustment and who can serve as a role model also can be a good co-leader. The nurse must be able to clarify myths and misunderstandings about age-related changes and be skilled in group dynamics. As with the reminiscence group, the healthy aging class is not an intense psychotherapy session; therefore, the group leader is not required to be specially trained in mental health. To lead a healthy aging class, however, a good understanding of both the physiologic and psychosocial aspects of aging is essential.

The primary responsibilities of the group leaders are to facilitate the discussion of psychosocial adjustments of older adulthood and to provide feedback and clarification to the members. As with other groups, the leader must ensure that all members have an opportunity to participate and that the members attend to the identified topic. The leaders also must ensure that some conclusions are reached before the end of each session so that members leave with a feeling of accomplishment relating to at least one psychosocial challenge of older adulthood.

Format

As in all educational groups, the leader begins with an explanation of the purpose of the group and an introduction of the leaders and members. The leader might also review the details of the sessions, such as their length, the duration of the group, the role of the leader, and the expectations of the members. After the introductory material has been discussed and any questions have been answered, the leader introduces the concepts of life events and adjustments to the challenges of older adulthood. A statement similar to the following can be used: "Throughout life, certain events are likely to occur that affect us emotionally. These events may involve our health, our personal relationships, the place where we live, job or career responsibilities and opportunities, or other events that require an adjustment on our part. These are sometimes referred to as major life events, and they often occur at certain points of life. To begin our discussion today, let's look at some of the major life events that are likely to occur in younger adulthood, around the age of 20 to 30 years." The group then identifies various life events,

such as finding a job, moving from the family home, finding a partner, and starting a family. The members then are asked to identify life adjustments that are likely to occur between 30 and 50 years of age.

After the members have identified these life events, the leader emphasizes that one purpose of the healthy aging class is to identify the life events of older adulthood so as to adjust successfully to the challenges they present. The term *challenges* should be used so as to communicate an active mode of addressing issues. The leader may want to discuss the phrase "challenges of older adulthood" and allow the group members to comment on what they see as challenges in their lives. As the members identify the life events of older adulthood, the leader writes the events on a board or paper so all the members can see the list. The leader can then ask about events that the members have experienced, as well as those events that the members think they are likely to experience in the next few years. As events are identified, the members also are asked to identify the consequences of the events that require an adjustment. Examples of these life events and consequences have been discussed earlier in this chapter, and they are summarized in Figure 3-1. If not all the major life events are identified by group members, the leader may ask about a certain event, such as coping with one's own or a spouse's retirement. This discussion should continue until all the events and consequences in Figure 3-1 have been identified.

If the group is a closed one with a stable membership, the leader may devote the majority of the first meeting to this discussion. The leader should emphasize that the rest of the meetings will be devoted to discussions of the identified issues, and that the first meeting will set the stage for future sessions. If the group is open and has a changing membership, the leader may need to be more directive during this first phase in order to limit the time spent on this topic. With changing membership, this initial identification of issues would be limited to the first

20 to 30 minutes. The discussion of problem-focused coping mechanisms for one specific issue can then be slated for the latter half of the meeting.

After the issues have been identified, the leader should summarize the discussion, referring to the list of challenges written for the members to see. The members are then asked to share ideas about coping strategies that they have found to be helpful in adjusting to these changes. The leader may begin this part with a statement such as: "Now that we've identified the challenges of older adulthood, let's look at what things are helpful in responding to these challenges. I'd like each of you to share with the group one thing you do, in general, to help you face difficult challenges." After members have identified general coping mechanisms, the leader can suggest that the group choose one specific life event of older adulthood and discuss specific coping mechanisms that might be used to address this challenge. Examples of coping strategies that might be discussed in relation to specific life events are summarized in Table 3-2. As these coping strategies are identified, they should be written on a board, and members should be encouraged to relate their own personal experiences.

As the cohesiveness and trust level among members increases, particularly in closed groups, the sharing of experiences may become very open and revealing. The task of the leader, then, is to keep the discussion focused on appropriate coping mechanisms. In cohesive groups with highly functional members, the leader might have an opportunity to discuss the difference between emotion-focused and problem-focused mechanisms. The depth of discussion will depend on the degree of group cohesiveness and trust, the functional level of the members, and the comfort level and willingness of the leader to deal with the identified issues.

During the last 10 minutes of each session, the leader should attempt to bring the discussion to some closure on at least one issue. This may be accomplished by summarizing the issues and coping mechanisms that were identified. In open groups, the leader would end by encouraging those members who do not return to the group to look at coping mechanisms for their own specific issues, either by themselves or with a friend or confidant(e). For ongoing groups, the leader would end the session by coming to some agreement on the issues that will be discussed during the next session. The leader also can encourage group members to think about the identified issues in the interim.

Evaluating Nursing Care

Nursing care of older adults with Self-Concept Disturbance is evaluated by determining the extent to which older adults express positive views of themselves. Another measure of effective nursing care of older adults with such a diagnosis is that they no longer verbalize ageist attitudes. Nursing care of older adults who express a sense of Powerlessness is evaluated by the extent to which these individuals become involved in decisions that affect them. Another such measure would be the degree to which such older adults express feelings of control over their lives and their futures. Nursing care for older adults with Ineffective Individual Coping would be evaluated by observing behaviors that reflect the use of a variety of coping strategies. For example, an older adult might learn to use problem-focused coping strategies for a situation that they previously viewed as hopeless and unchangeable.

Chapter Summary

Older adults face many psychosocial challenges that are associated with the life events of later adulthood (e.g., functional limitations and loss of significant relationships). Factors that influence the response of older adults to stressful events include the meaning of the event, the timing of the event, and the degree of anticipation of the event. Social resources and long-term coping styles also influence the response of an older individual to stress. Factors that increase the risk of poor coping responses include lack of economic resources and the occurrence of several major life events within a short period of time. Functional consequences of high levels of stress and poor coping include depression and mental changes.

Nursing diagnoses that might be applicable to psychosocial adjustment issues include Self-Concept Disturbance, Powerlessness, Impaired Adjustment, and Ineffective Individual Coping. Nursing goals are directed toward enhancing self-esteem, promoting a sense of control, fostering social supports, and assisting the older adult with the use of effective coping mechanisms. Nursing interventions to achieve these goals include individual and group therapy and education. Communication techniques are other interventions that are directed toward enhancing self-esteem and challenging ageist attitudes. Evaluation criteria include observations that the older adult expresses positive self-esteem, some degree of control over his or her life, and effective coping mechanisms.

Critical Thinking Exercises

1. Take a sheet of paper and draw two vertical lines to make three equal columns. Think of someone you know in your personal life or professional practice who is 80 years old or older. In the left column, list three or more life events that this person has experienced in later adulthood. In the center column, describe the impact of the life event on the person's daily life. In the right column, list the coping mechanisms the person has used to deal with the life event. You can guess at the information, as needed, to complete the information in the center and right columns.

2. Think of a recent life event in your own life and answer the following questions: How close in time was the life event to other stressful events in your life? What impact did the life event have, and what were the manifestations of stress in your life (e.g., in your work, your health, your personal life, your relationships with other people)? What coping mechanisms did you use? Were the coping mechanisms effective? What coping mechanisms would you like to develop to prepare yourself for older adulthood?

3. You are asked to lead a 1-hour discussion entitled "Mental Health and Aging" for a group of 10 people at a senior citizen center. Describe your approach to this topic. What would your goals for the class be? How would you involve the participants? What visual aids would you use?

Case Example and Nursing Care Plan

Pertinent Case Information

Mr. P. is 86 years old and has recently been admitted to a nursing facility for long-term care. His medical diagnoses are diabetes, glaucoma, retinopathy, and dementia of the Alzheimer's type. Mr. P. lived with his wife until 6 months ago when she died after a brief illness. After her death, he needed help with all his activities of daily living, and his daughter arranged home care assistance for 6 hours daily. About 1 month ago he started getting up and wandering outside at night. Once, he wandered off at 3:00 A.M., and the police had to take him home. After this episode, he was afraid to be alone, and he agreed to go to a nursing facility because he could not afford to pay for 24-hour assistance at home.

During the first week in the nursing facility, Mr. P. was cooperative with the staff and sociable with the other residents. He was resistant to the morning schedule of getting up at 6:00 A.M. and eating breakfast in the dining room at 7:30 A.M., but he passively complied when the staff firmly directed him. His daughter visited him daily and accompanied him to social and recreational activities with other residents. Mr. P. has been in the nursing facility for 10 days, and he is becoming very resistant to staff efforts to get him dressed for breakfast. When he attends group activities, he is very disruptive and stands up and yells about being a hostage in a monastery. Mr. P. tells other residents that he was tricked into coming to this place, and that the only reason he has to stay is because his daughter has taken over his house and is living there with her family. He frequently paces up and down the corridors and says he has to find his daughter to take him home because his wife is sick and she needs him to take care of her. When you walk up and down the hallway with him he says, "I don't know why they keep me locked up here, I can't do anything like I used to do at home. It's like a monastery where you have to get up in the middle of the night and they make you get cleaned up and eat breakfast when it's still dark out."

Nursing Assessment

Your nursing assessment reveals that Mr. P. needs supervision in all activities of daily living because of poor vision and memory impairment. He needs some assistance with personal care, but he can dress himself if his clothes are set out for him. When Mr. P. was admitted to the nursing facility, he was assigned to the "night shift wakers" group, which means that the night shift is responsible for waking him and getting him ready for breakfast by 7:30 A.M.. The night shift nursing assistants help him with showering, shaving, and dressing.

During the admission interview, Mr. P.'s daughter, Jane, said that his typical morning routine at home was to get up around 8:30 A.M. and get dressed independently, using the clothes that were set out for him by the home health aide. He ate breakfast around 9:30 A.M. and then spent the day "working on his papers." Jane, who lives out-of-town, would call her father 4 times a week. When Jane talked with him on the phone, he always told her how busy he was working on his papers. Although Jane was paying all his bills from a joint bank account, Mr. P. would spend hours and hours with bill stubs, old bank statements, and an inactive checking account, thinking he was paying his bills.

Jane had been staying at her father's house for the 2 weeks prior to admission and the 1 week after his admission to the nursing facility. She plans to return to town for a couple of days every other month and will visit her father at those times. The only nearby relative is a sister-in-law who comes to visit Mr. P. every 2 weeks.

Nursing Diagnosis

You use the nursing diagnosis of Powerlessness related to relocation to a nursing facility and lack of control over activities of daily living. You select this diagnosis, rather than Impaired Adjustment or Ineffective Individual Coping, because Mr. P. focuses on a theme of loss of control. Your assessment identifies several factors that contribute to his powerlessness, and you address these factors in your nursing care plan.

Goals	Nursing Interventions	Evaluation Criteria
Mr. P. will feel he has greater control over his morning schedule.	Take Mr. P. off the "night shift wakers" list and allow him to sleep until 8 A.M. Allow Mr. P. to wear his pajamas and robe to breakfast and to shower, bathe, and dress after breakfast.	Mr. P. will no longer verbalize feelings of being locked up in a monastery or a prison.
Mr. P. will be as independent as possible in his activities of daily living.	The staff will set out Mr. P.'s clothing for the day and allow him to dress himself. The staff will give Mr. P. positive feedback for dressing himself.	Mr. P. will dress himself with minimal supervision. Mr. P. will carry out his personal care activities at a pace that is comfortable for him.
Mr. P. will engage in a familiar activity that gives him a meaningful role.	Ask Jane to send a set of bill stubs, old bank statements, and the inactive checkbook so that Mr. P. can do his "work." Encourage Mr. P. to "work with his papers" in the activity room, where he can interact with other residents. Give Mr. P. positive feedback when he interacts with other residents. Talk to Mr. P. about his paperwork.	Mr. P. will resume his former routine of "working with his papers" and will interact with other residents.

Educational Resources

National Senior Service Corps
1100 Vermont Avenue, NW, Washington, DC 20525
(800) 424–8867
www.seniorcorps.org

Stokes/Gordon Stress Scale
Pace University, Lienhard School of Nursing
861 Bedford Road, Pleasantville, NY 10570
(914) 773–3200

References

Aldrich, C., & Mendkoff, E. (1963). Relocation of the aged and disabled: A mortality study. *Journal of the Geriatric Society, 11*(3), 185–194.

Aldwin, C. M. (1991). Does age affect the stress and coping process? Implications of age differences in perceived control. *Journal of Gerontology: Psychological Sciences, 46*(4), P174–P180.

Aldwin, C. M., Sutton, K. J., Chiara, G., & Spiro A. III. (1996). Age differences in stress, coping, and appraisal: Findings from the normative aging study. *Journal of Gerontology: Psychological Sciences, 51B*(4), P179–P188.

Aranda, M. P., & Knight, B. G. (1997). The influence of ethnicity and culture on the caregiver stress and coping process: A sociocultural review and analysis. *The Gerontologist, 37,* 342–354.

Ardelt, M. (1997). Wisdom and life satisfaction in old age. *Journal of Gerontology: Psychological Sciences, 52B*(1), P15–P27.

Barry, R., & Joyce, D. J. (1996). Gerontology, spirituality, and nursing. In V. Burggraf & R. Barry (Eds.), *Gerontological nursing: Current practice and research* (pp. 47–53). Thorofare, NJ: SLACK.

Berggren-Thomas, P., & Griggs, M. J. (1995). Spirituality

in aging: Spiritual need or spiritual journey? *Journal of Gerontological Nursing, 21*(3), 5–10.

Blazer, D. (1998). *Emotional problems in later life* (2nd ed.). New York: Springer.

Bosse, R., Aldwin, C. M., Levenson, M. R., & Workman-Daniels, K. (1991). How stressful is retirement? Findings from the normative aging study. *Journal of Gerontology: Psychological Sciences, 46*(1), P9–P14.

Burkhardt, M. A., & Nagai-Jacobson, M. G. (1997). Spirituality and healing. In B. M. Dossey (Ed.), *Core curriculum for holistic nursing* (pp. 42–51). Gaithersburg, MD: Aspen.

Burnside, I. (1994). Group work with older persons. *Journal of Gerontological Nursing, 20*(1), 43–45.

Burnside, I., & Schmidt, M. G. (1994). *Working with older adults: Group process and techniques* (3rd ed.). Boston: Jones and Bartlett.

Butler, R. N. (1961). Reawakening interest. *Nursing Homes, 10,* 8–19.

Butler, R. N., & Lewis, M. I. (1991). *Aging and mental health* (4th ed.). New York: Merrill.

Campbell, M. K., Bush, T. L., & Hale, W. E. (1993). Medical conditions associated with driving cessation in community-dwelling, ambulatory elders. *Journal of Gerontology: Social Sciences, 48*(4), S230–S234.

Carpenito, L. J. (1997). *Nursing diagnosis: Application to clinical practice* (7th ed.). Philadelphia: J.B. Lippincott.

Coleman, P. G., Ivani-Chalian, C., & Robinson, M. (1993). Self-esteem and its sources: Stability and change in later life. *Ageing and Society, 13,* 171–192.

Dai, Y-T., & Dimond, M. F. (1998). Filial piety: A cross-cultural comparison and its implications for the well-being of older parents. *Journal of Gerontological Nursing, 24*(3), 13–18.

Dietz, B. E. (1996). The relationship of aging to self-esteem: The relative effects of maturation and role accumulation. *International Journal of Aging and Human Development, 43*(3), 249–266.

Dunkle, R. E., Roberts, B., Haug, M., & Raphelson, M. (1992). An examination of coping resources of very old men and women: Their association to the relationship between stress, hassles, and function. *Journal of Women & Aging, 43*(3), 79–104.

Eisenhandler, S. A. (1990). The asphalt identikit: Old age and the driver's license. *International Journal of Aging and Human Development, 301*(1), 1–14.

Ensel, W. M., & Lin, N. (1991). The life stress paradigm and psychological distress. *Journal of Health and Social Behavior, 32,* 321–341.

Evans, L. K. (1996). Knowing the patient: The route to individualized care. *Journal of Gerontological Nursing, 22*(3), 15–19.

Evans, R. (1988). Older driver involvement in fatal and severe traffic crashes. *Journal of Gerontology: Social Sciences, 43*(6), S186–S193.

Fiske, M. (1980). Tasks and crises of the second half of life: The interrelationship of commitment, coping, and adaptation. In J. E. Birren & R. B. Sloan (Eds.), *Handbook of mental health and aging* (pp. 337–373). Englewood Cliffs, NJ: Prentice-Hall.

Folkman, S., & Lazarus, R. S. (1980). An analysis of coping in a middle-aged community sample. *Journal of Health and Social Behavior, 21,* 219–239.

Folkman, S., Lazarus, R. S., Dunkel-Schetter, C., DeLongis, A., & Gruen, R. (1986). The dynamics of a stressful encounter: Cognitive appraisal, coping, and encounter outcomes. *Journal of Personality and Social Psychology, 50,* 992–1003.

Folkman, S., Lazarus, R. S., Pimley, S., & Novacek, J. (1987). Age differences in stress and coping processes. *Psychology and Aging, 2,* 171–184.

Haan, N. (1977). *Coping and defending: Processes of self-environment organization.* New York: Academic Press.

Haight, B. K., & Burnside, I. (1992). Reminiscence and life review: Conducting the processes. *Journal of Gerontological Nursing, 18*(2), 39–42.

Holmes, T. H., & Rahe, R. H. (1967). The social readjustment rating scale. *Journal of Psychosomatic Research, 11,* 213–218.

Hungelmann, J., Kenkel-Rossi, E., Klassen, L., & Stollenwerk, R. (1996). Focus on spiritual well-being: Harmonious interconnectedness of mind-body-spirit—Use of the JAREL Spiritual Well-Being Scale. *Geriatric Nursing, 17,* 262–266.

Jirovec, M. M., & Maxwell, B. A. (1993). Nursing home residents' functional ability and perceptions of choice. *Journal of Gerontological Nursing, 19*(9), 10–14.

Johnson, B. D., Stone, G. L., Altmaier, E. M., & Berdahl, L. D. (1998). The relationship of demographic factors, locus of control and self-efficacy to successful nursing home adjustment. *The Gerontologist, 38,* 209–216.

Johnson, C. L., & Barer, B. M. (1993). Coping and a sense of control among the oldest old: An exploratory analysis. *Journal of Aging Studies, 7*(1), 67–80.

Kaisik, B. H., & Ceslowitz, S. B. (1996). Easing the fear of nursing home placements: The value of stress inoculation. *Geriatric Nursing, 17,* 182–186.

Kane, R. A., Caplan, A. L., Urv-Wong, E. K., et al. (1997). Everyday matters in the lives of nursing home residents: Wish for and perception of choice and control. *Journal of the American Geriatrics Society, 45,* 1086–1093.

Krause, N. (1994). Stressors in salient social roles and well-being in later life. *Journal of Gerontology: Psychological Sciences, 49*(3), P137–P148.

Labouvie-Vief, G., Hakim-Larson, J., & Hobart, C. J. (1987). Age, ego level, and the life-span development of coping and defense processes. *Psychology and Aging, 2,* 286–293.

Lappe, J. M. (1987). Reminiscing: The life review therapy. *Journal of Gerontological Nursing, 13*(4), 12–16.

Lashley, M. E. (1993). The painful side of reminiscence. *Geriatric Nursing, 14*(3), 138–141.

Lazarus, R. S. (1966). *Psychological stress and the coping process.* New York: McGraw Hill.

Lowenthal, M. F., Berkman, P. L., Pierce, R. C., Buehler, J. A., Brissette, G. G., Robinson, B. D., & Trier, M. T. (1967). *Aging and mental disorder in San Francisco.* San Francisco: Jossey-Bass.

Macrae, J. (1995). Nightingale's spiritual philosophy and its significance for modern nursing. *Image: Journal of Nursing Scholarship, 27*(1), 8–10.

Marottoli, R. A., Ostfeld, A. M., Merrill, S. S., Perlman,

G. D., Foley, D. J., & Cooney, L. M. (1993). Driving cessation and changes in mileage driven among elderly individuals. *Journal of Gerontology: Social Sciences.* 48(5), S255–S260.

McCrae, R. M. (1982). Age differences in the use of coping mechanisms. *Journal of Gerontology, 37,* 454–460.

McFadden, S. H. (1996). Religion and spirituality. In J. E. Birren (Ed.), *Encyclopedia of gerontology: Age, aging, and the aged* (Vol. 2, pp. 387–397). San Diego: Academic Press.

Meisenhelder, J. B. (1985). Self-esteem: A closer look at clinical interventions. *International Journal of Nursing Studies, 22,* 127–135.

Mendes de Leon, C. F., Seeman, T. E., Baker, D. I., Richardson, E. D., & Tinetti, M. E. (1996). Self-efficacy, physical decline, and change in functioning in community-living elders: A prospective study. *Journal of Gerontology: Social Sciences, 51B*(4), S183–S190.

Menec, V. H., & Chipperfield, J. G. (1997a). Remaining active in later life: The role of locus of control in seniors' leisure activity participation, health, and life satisfaction. *Journal of Aging and Health, 9*(1), 105–125.

Menec, V. H., & Chipperfield, J. G. (1997b). The interactive effect of perceived control and functional status on health and mortality among young-old and old-old adults. *Journal of Gerontology: Psychological Sciences, 52B*(3), P118–P126.

Moneyham, L., & Scott, C. B. (1995). Anticipatory coping in the elderly. *Journal of Gerontological Nursing, 21*(7), 23–28.

Nores, T. H. (1997). What is most important for elders in institutional care in Finland? *Geriatric Nursing, 18,* 67–69.

Perri, S., & Templer, D. I. (1984–1985). The effects of an aerobic exercise program on psychological variables in older adults. *International Journal of Aging and Human Development, 20*(3), 167–172.

Persson, D. (1993). The elderly driver: Deciding when to stop. *Gerontologist, 33*(1), 88–91.

Pfeiffer, E. (1977). Psychopathology and social pathology. In J. E. Birren & K. W. Schaie (Eds.), *Handbook of the psychology of aging* (pp. 650–671). New York: Van Nostrand Reinhold.

Puentes, W. J. (1998). Incorporating simple reminiscence techniques into acute care nursing practice. *Journal of Gerontological Nursing, 24*(2), 14–20.

Reinardy, J. R. (1992). Decisional control in moving to a nursing home: Postadmission adjustment and well-being. *Gerontologist, 32*(1), 96–103.

Roberts, B. L., Dunkle, R., & Haug, M. (1994). Physical, psychological, and social resources as moderators of the relationship of stress to mental health of the very old. *Journal of Gerontology: Social Sciences, 49*(1), S35–S43.

Rodin, J., & Langer, E. (1980). Aging labels: The decline of control and the fall of self-esteem. *Journal of Social Issues, 36*(2), 12–29.

Rozzini, R., Bianchetti, A., Carabellese, C., Inzoli, M., & Trabucci, M. (1988). Depression, life events and somatic symptoms. *The Gerontologist, 28,* 229–232.

Sands, J. D. (1981–1982). The relationship of stressful life events to intellectual functioning in women over 65. *International Journal of Aging and Human Development, 14,* 11–22.

Selye, H. (1956). *The stress of life.* New York: McGraw-Hill.

Shaw, W. S., Patterson, T. L., Semple, S. J., et al. (1997). A cross-cultural validation of coping strategies and their associations with caregiving distress. *The Gerontologist, 37,* 490–504.

Sherman, E. (1987). Reminiscence groups for community elderly. *The Gerontologist, 27,* 569–572.

Simons, R. L., & West, G. E. (1984–1985). Life changes, coping resources, and health among the elderly. *International Journal of Aging and Human Development, 20,* 173–189

Slivinske, L. R., & Fitch, V. L. (1987). The effect of control enhancing interventions on the well-being of elderly individuals living in retirement communities. *The Gerontologist, 27,* 176–181.

Smith, M. K., & Sullivan, J. M. (1997). Nurses' and patients' perceptions of most important caring behaviors in a long-term care setting. *Geriatric Nursing, 18,* 70–73.

Stokes, S. A., & Gordon, S. E. (1988). Development of an instrument to measure stress in the older adult. *Nursing Research, 37,* 16–19.

Taft, L. B. (1985). Self-esteem in later life: A nursing perspective. *Advances in Nursing Science, 8*(1), 77–84.

Tennstedt, S., & Chang, B-H. (1998). The relative contribution of ethnicity versus socioeconomic status in explaining differences in disability and receipt of informal care. *Journal of Gerontology: Social Sciences, 53B,* S61–S70

Tolley, M. (1997). Power to the patient. *Journal of Gerontological Nursing, 23*(10), 7–12.

Vaillant, G. E. (1977). *Adaptation to life.* Boston: Little, Brown.

Wan, T. H. (1982). *Stressful life events, social-support networks and gerontological health.* Lexington, MA: D. C. Heath.

Wan, T. H. (1984). Health consequences of major role losses in later life. *Research on Aging, 6,* 469–489.

West, G. E., & Simons, R. L. (1983). Sex differences in stress, coping resources, and illness among the elderly. *Research on Aging, 5,* 235–267.

Whall, A. L. (1987). Self-esteem and the mental health of older adults. *Journal of Gerontological Nursing, 13*(4), 41–42.

Willis, L., Thomas, P., Garry, P. J., & Goodwin, J. S. (1987). A prospective study of response to stressful life events in initially healthy elders. *Journal of Gerontology, 42,* 627–630.

Zauszniewski, J. A. (1997). Teaching resourcefulness skills to older adults. *Journal of Gerontological Nursing, 23*(2), 14–20.

Cognitive Function

Chapter

4

Learning Objectives	1. *Describe theories about adult intellectual development and age-related cognitive changes, including memory changes.*
	2. *Examine risk factors that influence cognitive function in older adults.*
	3. *Discuss the functional consequences that affect cognition in older adults.*
	4. *Identify interventions directed toward reversing any cognitive declines that are remediable and compensating for those that are irreversible.*
	5. *Describe guidelines for educational interventions for older adults.*

*T*he question whether cognitive function declines in old age is one of the most controversial areas of psychology, and the debate is becoming more heated as newer theories of cognitive aging are developed. In the late 1970s, psychologists thought that a decline in cognitive abilities was a normal part of the aging process. By the mid-1980s, this conclusion was being challenged, particularly because it was based on cross-sectional rather than longitudinal studies of intelligence. Currently, researchers in the field of cognitive aging are looking not only at measures of cognitive ability, but also at measures of an older adult's capacity to maintain intellectual skills despite the age-related changes and risk factors that are likely to interfere with cognitive function. Some of the questions that researchers are attempting to answer are, Why do some people show intellectual decrement in early adulthood, whereas others maintain or increase their intellectual skills well into old age? and Can interventions prevent, retard, or reverse intellectual decline? Additionally, an emerging question is, How can we enhance cognitive abilities, even in those people who are intellectually intact? (Whitehouse et al., 1997).

Theories About Adult Intelligence

Many of the questions and much of the controversy about cognitive aging stem from the various ways of defining and measuring intelligence. A few of the distinct aspects of cognition that have been identified include visualization, auditory thinking, quantitative thinking, fluid intelligence, crystallized intelligence, speed of thinking, short-term apprehension and retrieval, and storage and retrieval from long-term memory. Intellectual abilities are formally measured with psychometric tests, but many questions have been raised about conclusions based on these measures. In the following sections, several theories about cognitive aging and some of the controversial issues about measurement of adult intelligence are reviewed.

Measures of Adult Intelligence

A literature review of aging and cognition identified four distinct phases in the use of psychometric tests to measure adult intelligence (Woodruff, 1983). During phase I, adult intelligence was measured with tests designed to predict school performance in children. In cross-sectional studies using these tests, younger adults consistently scored higher than older adults. Based on these results, it was concluded that intelligence begins to decline in early adulthood. Phase II studies began in the mid-1950s, when questions were raised about the validity of cross-sectional studies. Phase II longitudinal studies, developed to identify patterns of adult intellectual development, consistently revealed that intellectual function remained the same or improved up to the age of 50 or 60 years, after which it gradually declined. A landmark 21-year study that included both longitudinal and cross-sectional data confirmed the findings of the previous studies. That is, the cross-sectional studies showed that adult intelligence peaks around the age of 35 years and then sharply declines, whereas the longitudinal studies indicate that adult intelligence peaks around the age of 60 years and then declines slightly until the ages of 74 to 81 years (Schaie and Willis, 1986, p. 299).

Phase III studies, begun in the 1970s, were designed to address the question whether life experiences account for some of the age differences reflected in intelligence scores. Studies were developed that modified adult cognition to test the effects of experience and environment. This approach had the practical benefit of identifying ways to improve cognitive abilities (Woodruff, 1983). According to Botwinick (1984), this approach used modification studies to explore individual plasticity, or the person's possible range of tested behavior. Typically, this testing method involved administration of an initial test, followed by a period of training, and then by a retest using a different type of test. Although this kind of study is still being evaluated and refined, Botwinick (1984, p. 271) concludes that "these studies have shown that the old, like the young, have more potential than is typically measured by the tests."

Phase IV studies, first developed in the 1980s, are based on the discovery that performance on intelligence tests could be improved through interventions. In this phase, researchers have tried to identify cognitive skills that develop over the adult life span, such as those based on wisdom and experience (Woodruff, 1983). Phase IV studies also address new questions about the complex relationship between cognition and other factors, such as speed of response. For example, the results of these studies suggest that older people respond more quickly with practice, and, in fact, improve more than do younger people (Botwinick, 1984, p. 246). Researchers are now trying to identify those people who are at risk for developing cognitive impairment and to identify intervention strategies that can help maintain high levels of intellectual function in later adulthood. For example, a recent study found that physical fitness may be a buffer for age-related declines in some measures of fluid intelligence (Etnier and Landers, 1997). One conclusion derived from recent studies about cognitive function is that successful aging is more concerned with adaptation to change across the life span than to the elimination of such changes (Smith, 1996).

Another question that has been posed by researchers concerns the possible influence of preclinical dementia on estimates of age-related changes in cognitive function. One recent study revealed that at least one fifth of subjects between the ages of 75 and 85 years developed clinically diagnosed dementia an average of 4 years after baseline, and that this was undetectable at the time of screening (Sliwinski et al., 1996). The authors emphasize that inclusion of older adults with preclinical dementia may result in overestimation of the effect of age on cognitive function.

Theory of Fluid and Crystallized Intelligence

Cattell and Horn's theory of fluid and crystallized intelligence has been used to explain age-related declines in some cognitive abilities

(Horn, 1982). Crystallized intelligence refers to those cognitive skills that are acquired through culture, education, informal learning, and other life experiences. Crystallized intelligence is strongly associated with wisdom, judgment, and life experiences. By contrast, fluid intelligence depends primarily on a person's inherent abilities, such as memory, pattern recognition, and the central nervous system. Fluid intelligence is associated with an ability to identify complex relationships and to draw conclusions from these relationships.

Horn (1970) hypothesized that fluid and crystallized intelligence develop concurrently during infancy and childhood and, in fact, are indistinguishable as the central nervous system is maturing. During early adulthood, fluid intelligence begins to decline because of the progressive age-related deterioration of neural structures. Horn subsequently concluded that this decline in fluid intelligence reflected a diminished ability to maintain spontaneous alertness, focused intensive concentration, and an awareness of possible organization for otherwise unorganized information (Horn 1982). By contrast, crystallized intelligence continues to develop throughout adulthood because of accumulated experiences and learning. Crystallized intelligence, except for those processes that depend on speed of response, does not change with age, and it may even increase because of adult educational experiences.

In applying this theory to cognitive aging, specific aspects of fluid and crystallized intelligence can be compared to aspects of traditional tests of intellectual function. For example, components of fluid intelligence, such as reasoning and abstraction, coincide roughly with the Wechsler Adult Intelligence Scale (WAIS) Performance Scale measures, and are thought to decline in older adulthood. Similarly, the components of crystallized intelligence, such as information and comprehension, correspond roughly with the WAIS Verbal Scale measures, which do not exhibit a decline with advancing years. Based on this theory, cognitive aging is

caused by a disintegration of higher-order functions that normally facilitate the transfer and integration of information. A recent study of the relationship between sensory and cognitive functions found that sensory function was highly connected to intellectual function, particularly to fluid intellectual abilities, in older adults (Baltes and Lindenberger, 1997).

Stage Theory of Adult Cognitive Development

Schaie (1977–1978), expanding on Piaget's theory of intellectual development in childhood and adolescence, proposed a theory of stages relating to adult cognitive development. Schaie reasoned that, if the focus of childhood and adolescence is the acquisition of knowledge, then the focus of adulthood is the application of knowledge. The achieving stage of adult cognitive development, which marks the onset of adult cognitive maturity, is characterized by a striving to apply one's newly acquired knowledge to demands and commitments, such as career and family. In this stage, young adults use their intellectual abilities to establish their independence and develop goal-oriented behaviors. The second stage of adult cognitive development, called the responsible stage, extends in age from the late thirties to the early sixties. During this stage, people focus on integrating their long-range goals and attending to the needs of their family and society. Some people in this stage have high levels of social responsibilities; these individuals are categorized as being in the executive stage. The tasks of the last stage, called the reintegrative stage, are to simplify life and to select only those responsibilities that have meaning and purpose. During this stage, rather than asking, What should I know? the older adult asks, Why should I know?

Theory of Cognitive Growth in Adulthood

The theory of cognitive aging and psychological growth postulates that the thinking of older adults becomes increasingly complex and shows progressive reorganization of intellectual skills (Labouvie-Vief and Blanchard-Fields, 1982). Because these skills differ from those of younger adults, they cannot be measured with traditional intelligence tests. Labouvie-Vief and Blanchard-Fields cite numerous examples of studies in which conclusions about cognitive decline are based on standards of youth-oriented cognitive patterns. They suggest that if these studies were interpreted in relation to the advanced psychological development that occurs with mature aging, the conclusions would be different.

As we enter the third millennium, more and more studies are focusing on the potential for intellectual growth in older adulthood. There is a growing recognition that later life holds the potential for continuing self-actualization that can be enhanced by the cumulative effects of wisdom and life experiences. Along with this awareness comes the recognition that educational programs should be available for older adults and adapted to their needs (Manheimer, 1996).

Theories About Memory

Memory function raises more questions and stirs more emotions than any other aspect of cognition. Older adults often believe their memory is not as good as it used to be, and this belief is reinforced by trite statements, such as "You can't teach an old dog new tricks." Even among gerontological practitioners, it is not unusual to hear statements such as "Of course your memory isn't as sharp as it used to be; you're 82 years old." Despite the prevalence of such beliefs, very little is known about age-related changes in the processes involved in learning and memory. For several decades, memory has been viewed as a process involving three phases: encoding, storage, and retrieval. In recent years, however, questions have been raised about conclusions based on this theory, and additional theories are being developed in an attempt to explain memory processes. Several of these theories are summarized in the following sections.

Multiphase, Multistore Theory

According to the multiphase, multistore theory, memory is a computer-like information-processing system. Information is first perceived, then stored, and lastly, it is retrieved when needed or wanted. Researchers have attempted to identify changes in one or more of these phases to explain age-related differences in memory and learning. The following are age-related encoding deficits that have been identified: (1) verbal elaboration, or the degree to which different items are distinctly encoded; (2) visual elaboration, or the use of visualization for encoding; and (3) organization, or the degree to which the items are related to each other for encoding (Poon, 1985, p. 443). Primary memory has a short duration and a very small capacity. It has been described as more of a holding tank for events of the immediate past few seconds, rather than as a true memory storage system (Botwinick, 1984, p. 332). Information in the primary memory can either be recalled for a brief time or be transmitted to long-term storage. Studies on primary memory and aging are controversial. Some studies have not identified significant age-related changes in this aspect of memory function. When age differences have been identified, they have been attributed to the influence of a large number of items, or to the speed of recall for the most recently presented items in a list (Botwinick, 1984, pp. 325–326; Poon, 1985, p. 341). In contrast to these findings, a recent review of the literature on memory aging revealed significant age differences in studies on recall from short-term memory. The authors of this literature review concluded that research results of adult age differences in memory function are quite diverse and still controversial (Verhaeghen et al., 1993). A recent study suggests: (1) that older adults are less effective in encoding new material, (2) that their associations are more affected by interference from other associations, or (3) that both factors are possible (Fisk and Warr, 1998).

In contrast to primary memory, secondary memory is longer-term and therefore is more important in terms of the retrieval, as well as storage, of information. Secondary memory has been the focus of many studies of age differences in memory function and is the aspect that shows the most age-related decline (Poon, 1985, p. 437).

The third process in the multiphase model involves the ability to access information from storage. This memory is variously called the remote, tertiary, or very long-term memory, and the skills involved are classified as recall memory and recognition memory. A discussion of studies on recall and recognition suggests that both types of memory may decline equally in older adulthood (Botwinick, 1984, p. 332). In addition to looking at differences in recall and recognition, studies have compared remote and recent memory. A popular belief is that older people remember events of long ago better than events of the immediate past. This belief, however, has not consistently been supported in studies. Botwinick summarizes the current understanding of age-related changes as follows: "TM [tertiary memory] may or may not hold with age, but even if not, the old have a large store of information, as large as that of younger people. This store is largely of occurrences of long ago" (1984, p. 333).

Levels of Processing Theory

Another theoretical approach is to disregard the storage and retrieval aspects of memory and emphasize the encoding and analyzing aspects. Memory is viewed as a continuum of processing, ranging from shallow to deep levels, and the duration of a particular memory depends on the depth of the processing. According to this theory, the deeper the level at which information is stored, the longer the memory will last. Duration of storage can be influenced by any of the following: (1) the processing techniques, ranging

from the shallowest levels used for sensory information to the deepest levels used for highly abstract information; (2) the elaboration, or quality, of processing carried out at any depth level; (3) the distinctiveness of the information, which depends partially on how well it is learned; and (4) the depth and elaboration of retrieval processes (Botwinick, 1984, pp. 336–338). Several studies based on this framework have concluded that the memory function of older adults is decreased because of faulty processing mechanisms (Botwinick, 1984, p. 355).

Automatic and Effortful Processing Theory

The automatic and effortful processing theory views memory as a continuum (Hasher and Zacks, 1979). At the one end is automatic processing, or those tasks that do not require attention or awareness and do not improve with practice. At the other end is effortful processing, or those tasks that demand high levels of attention and cognitive energy. With practice, effortful tasks require less attention and become more automatic. According to this theory, automatic memory would not be affected by age because these tasks require little or no cognitive energy. Effortful memory, however, would decline with age because only a limited amount of cognitive resources are available for memory functions, and these resources gradually decline, beginning in early adulthood. Studies of automatic processing activities in older adults support the theory of little or no decline in automatic processing and some deficits in effortful encoding tasks (Botwinick, 1984, pp. 342–346; Rohling and Scogin, 1993). Older adults may have memory deficits because they do not comprehend information as well, but when given clues, they can remember as well as younger adults (Botwinick, 1984, p. 350).

Contextual Theories

In recent years, the information-processing model has been viewed as too simplistic because it ignores the milieu in which the memory operates. Newer theories, called contextual theories, have expanded the information-processing model, addressing some of the variables that may affect memory. Some of the factors that may influence memory function, regardless of age, are motivation, expectations, experiences, education, personality, task demands, learning habits, intellectual skills, sociocultural background, physical and mental health, and style of processing information. Studies of specific factors have found that the following variables interact with chronologic age to influence memory function in older adults: verbal abilities, monetary incentives, item familiarity, and motivation and motivation-related variables (Poon, 1985, p. 444). A recent study that addressed a variety of contextual factors in adults older than 70 years of age found that general processing speed was the major mediator of age-related variance in several memory tasks (Luszcz et al., 1997).

Metamemory

Metamemory is an evolving concept that refers to self-knowledge about memory or cognitive functions. It includes all of one's knowledge and perceptions about the function and development of memory. Interest in metamemory is based on the belief that metacognitive processes enable a person to influence and regulate the memory processes consciously. Metamemory is important in everyday activities because if people know what they can remember and how much effort they will need to remember certain things, they can plan efficient and effective strategies for remembering. Moreover, negative beliefs about memory capacity have far-reaching consequences, including anxiety, depression, decreased effort and motivation, and increased dependency on others (Lachman et al., 1992). Studies have revealed that older adults tend to perceive themselves as less competent in some cognitive skills than they actually are, and as less competent than younger

adults in many cognitive tasks (Hultsch and Dixon, 1990; Schaie et al., 1994). Recently, psychologists have begun to look at metamemory, or memory self-evaluation, as one indicator of future cognitive decline. The results of a longitudinal study of adults older than 84 years of age indicate that self-reported memory function has some predictive value for decline on several memory tests, as well as for subsequent diagnosis of dementia (Johansson et al., 1997).

Risk Factors

Central Nervous System Changes

Questions about brain aging are particularly difficult to answer because much of the research necessarily utilizes brain tissue derived from autopsies, rather than from living subjects. When changes have been identified in older brains, questions have been raised about whether these changes are age-related or disease-related. Some changes that were once thought to be age-related are now thought to be disease-related; other changes are present to a small degree in nondiseased brains but to a greater degree and with different patterns of distribution in diseased brains. Some of the changes that have been identified in older brains are loss of neurons, diminished blood flow, accumulation of lipofuscin, reduction of brain weight, decline in synaptic function, changes in neurotransmitter activity, decreased use of glucose and oxygen, and the presence of senile plaques and neurofibrillary tangles. Other central nervous system changes that can influence cognition in older adults include diminished sensory abilities and slower speed of response. Recent studies support the conclusion that an age-related slowing of processing speed is associated with deficits in memory and other cognitive abilities (Salthouse and Coon, 1993). Increasing task difficulty or complexity may exaggerate this slowing (Fozard et al., 1994).

Personal Characteristics and Mental Health

Cognitive abilities in people of any age are significantly influenced by numerous personal and environmental factors. Level of education has consistently been found to be one of the most significant factors affecting cognitive performance. Self-perceptions and expectations also significantly affect cognitive skills and performance on intelligence tests. This concept is evident in much of the popular self-help literature, which suggests that "if you expect to succeed, you will; if you expect to fail, you will." Studies indicate that learned helplessness and perceived locus of control may contribute to the decline in memory function in older adults (Perlmutter et al., 1987). Studies also have identified as a negative influence on memory the ageist labels and diminished expectations of older adults in modern societies (Ryan and See, 1993). Other research has focused on the finding that older adults score lower on tests of intellectual function than younger subjects, and questions have been raised regarding differences in the relevance of the material for older and younger subjects and in their motivation.

Mental health can significantly influence cognitive abilities, and anxiety and depression are the two mental health factors most consistently identified as risks for poor cognitive function. Indeed, one literature review concluded that "the poorer performance of older adults on memory tasks may be the consequence of the anxiety and/or depression prevalent in this age group" (Perlmutter et al., 1987, pp. 67–68). This literature review cited the following specific findings: (1) anxiety inhibits performance through excessive self-focusing and worrying; (2) depression can influence behavior because of decreased concentration, attention deficits, and negative expectations; and (3) memory deficits improve after interventions to reduce anxiety and alleviate depression in older adults. A recent study found that memory complaints of older adults were associated with increased feelings of anxiety about their physical health

and increasingly negative feelings about their own capabilities (Hänninen et al., 1994). Similarly, a recent study found that a combination of depression and increased age negatively affected cognitive performance (Lyness et al., 1994).

Sensory Function and Physical Health

Because the acquisition of information is highly dependent on sensory input, particularly vision and hearing, cognitive processes are affected by sensory function. Age-related changes in hearing and vision are fully discussed in Chapters 6 and 7. The impact of these changes on cognition is attributable to the reduced quantity and quality of information from the environment. A study of various functional impairments on self-reported memory problems indicated that hearing deficits had the strongest net effect (Cutler and Grams, 1988). Although much is known about age-related changes in vision and hearing, little is known about how older adults compensate for these deficits. Botwinick (1984, p. 224) suggests that the increase in cautiousness that characterizes older adults may be a compensatory mechanism for declining sensory skills.

Studies indicate that good health and self-reported health are positively correlated with higher scores on intelligence tests. In fact, self-reported health has been found to account for a great portion of individual differences in older versus younger adults' performances on intelligence tests (Perlmutter and Nyquist, 1990). One study revealed that health and functional impairments best predicted everyday memory problems (Cutler and Grams, 1988). In addition, one literature review concluded that "memory deficits may be at least partially due to poor physical fitness, a transient state that is potentially reversible through exercise therapy" (Perlmutter et al., 1987, p. 70). Some studies have identified an association between specific health problems (e.g., diabetes) and lower scores on intelligence tests (Boxtel, 1998). There is increasing evidence that aerobic exercise and good physical conditioning may improve cognitive abilities, possibly owing to the effect of exercise on reaction time.

Nutritional status has been singled out as a physical health variable that influences cognitive function, particularly memory performance, regardless of a person's age. Although few studies have addressed the relationship between nutrition and cognition in older adults, one study has reported a significant association between low serum levels of vitamins C and B_{12} and lower scores on the Wechsler Memory Scale for healthy older adults (Goodwin et al., 1983). A more recent longitudinal study revealed that higher levels of ascorbic acid and beta-carotene were associated with better memory performance in older adults (Perrig et al., 1997). Other studies have shown an association between reversible memory disorders and deficiencies of folate, niacin, thiamine, vitamin B_{12}, vitamin C, and multiple vitamins (Perlmutter et al., 1987, p. 71). Interest in the role of choline and lecithin stems from the theory that cognitive and memory deficits may be caused by a disruption of normal acetylcholine transmission in the brain. Although the consumption of foods rich in choline or lecithin can increase plasma choline levels, the effectiveness of these interventions has not been determined.

Chemical Effects: Alcohol and Medications

Much of the research on the relationship between alcohol consumption and cognitive function is not age-specific, but conclusions can be applied to older adults as well as younger adults. For example, moderate consumption of alcohol may interfere with short-term memory, but not with immediate or long-term memory. Long-term consumption of alcohol in excessive amounts may interfere with memory performance, even during periods of abstention from alcohol.

Prescription and over-the-counter medications can interfere with memory and other cognitive functions in a variety of ways. Anticholinergic ingredients, contained in numerous prescription and over-the-counter medications, affect memory and other cognitive functions. A recent study supports many other studies concluding that "cognitive toxicity" may be an adverse effect of over-the-counter and prescription medications containing anticholinergic ingredients (Katz et al., 1998). Mechanisms of medication action that can interfere with cognitive function are described in detail in Chapter 18.

Functional Consequences

Very few changes in cognition are attributable to age-related factors alone, but like many other aspects of function, cognitive deficits are linked to risk factors. In healthy, mentally stimulated, older adults, deficits are generally minimal and do not interfere with activities of daily living. The terms "benign senescent forgetfulness" or "age-associated memory impairment" refer to memory deficits that are thought to occur in older adults, even in the absence of any risk factors. These deficits are minor and nonprogressive, and they are most noticeable in association with stressful conditions. In actuality, they are not much different from the kind of forgetfulness that all people experience at times. The major difference is that, when they occur in older people, they may be taken more seriously or viewed as evidence of so-called senility.

Some of the conclusions drawn from studies of cognitive aging that have generated the greatest accord are summarized in Display 4-1. Information about factors that influence learning in older adults also is included in Display 4-1, as these factors are important considerations in determining appropriate educational interventions in nursing care plans. It is important to keep in mind that conclusions about cognitive aging do not address cultural factors, and therefore are limited by the factors cited in the Culture Box. Figure 4-1 summarizes the age-related changes,

---

DISPLAY 4-1
Functional Consequences Affecting Cognition

Intellectual Abilities
- Healthy older adults show no decline, and perhaps improve, in some cognitive skills, such as wisdom, judgment, creativity, common sense, coordination of facts and ideas, and breadth of knowledge and experience.
- Most older adults show a slight and gradual decline in some cognitive skills, such as abstraction, calculation, word fluency, verbal comprehension, spatial orientation, and inductive reasoning.
- Age-related cognitive declines are thought to begin around the age of 60 years.

Memory
- Short-term memory shows a modest decline in older adulthood.
- Remote memory may or may not be better than recent memory in older adults, but regardless of whether it changes, older adults have a larger store of information about the past than do younger adults.

- The following factors influence cognitive function: motivation, expectations, personality, task demands, learning habits, intellectual skills, educational level, sociocultural background, style of processing information, and actual and self-reported health status.

Learning Abilities of Older Adults
- Older adults are as capable of learning new things as younger people, but the speed with which they process information is slower.
- Older adults are more cautious in their responses and make more errors of omission.
- Potential barriers to learning in older adults include sensory deficits, lack of relevance, teacher-learner age differences, and values that are incongruent with new knowledge.

---

risk factors, and functional consequences that may affect cognitive function.

Nursing Assessment

Formal assessment of intellectual performance is accomplished by administering psychometric tests, but nurses can informally assess memory and cognitive skills using the functional approach. In addition to assessing the intellectual performance of older adults, nurses can assess individuals for risk factors that might contribute to cognitive deficits. A recent nursing study of the relationships between loneliness, social support, and decline in cognitive function in hospi-

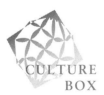
CULTURE BOX

Cultural Factors and Cognitive Function

- It is important to recognize that the standards of intellectual performance used in the United States have been developed for English-speaking White Americans.
- It is important to recognize that cognitive abilities are highly influenced by health, education, and socioeconomic status and that these factors and cultural factors are interrelated.
- Cultural and language factors may influence an older adult's perception and description of memory problems.

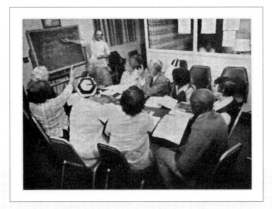

AGE-RELATED CHANGES

- Older adults may show declines in some intellectual skills, but they are capable of cognitive growth and intellectual development throughout adulthood

NEGATIVE FUNCTIONAL CONSEQUENCES

- Slight decline in short-term memory
- No decline in crystallized intelligence (e.g., wisdom, creativity, common sense, breadth of knowledge)
- Slight, gradual decline in fluid intelligence (e.g., abstraction, calculation, spatial orientation, inductive reasoning)
- Slower processing of information

RISK FACTORS

- Impaired sensory function
- Alcohol consumption
- Medications (e.g., anticholinergics)
- Physiologic disorders (e.g., malnutrition)
- Psychosocial influences (e.g., anxiety, depression)
- Environmental distractions
- Lack of motivation
- Lack of stimulation

FIGURE 4-1. Cognitive function in older adults.

talized elderly emphasized the need to thoroughly assess cognitive status as well as social support to identify risk factors for negative consequences of hospitalization (Ryan, 1998). Nursing assessment of cognition is an integral part of the psychosocial assessment, and is discussed in Chapter 5.

Nursing Diagnosis

Because age-related changes in cognitive function do not significantly affect activities of daily living, the only nursing diagnosis that might be applicable is Health-Seeking Behaviors. This diagnosis is defined as "the state in which an individual in stable health actively seeks ways to alter personal health habits and/ or the environment in order to move toward a higher level of wellness" (Carpenito, 1997, p. 450). This diagnosis could be applied to older adults who are aware of some decline in their intellectual abilities and who wish to preserve specific cognitive abilities, such as memory. Nurses working in community settings may have opportunities to address this health-related concern of older adults, perhaps through group health education. The case example and nursing care plan at the end of this chapter illustrate interventions related to cognitive function in older adulthood that might be used for individual or group health education.

Nursing Goals

Interventions for older adults with age-related cognitive changes are directed toward reversing those declines that are remediable and compensating for those that are irreversible (Willis, 1987, pp. 180–182). Willis describes two types of remediation interventions: remediation-in-kind, which directly improves a cognitive skill (e.g., practicing to improve perceptual speed skills); and remediation-with-compensa-

tion, which involves the improvement of one skill to compensate for a decline in another (e.g., increasing one's level of caution to compensate for a slower speed of performance). Compensation interventions for irreversible declines often include the use of external devices. In addition to remediation and compensation interventions, other interventions are directed toward maintaining skills or even improving skills. In most settings where nurses care for older adults, the goal is to help older adults develop compensatory mechanisms for impaired cognitive function.

Nursing Interventions

In the 1980s, the Penn State Adult Development and Enrichment Project (ADEPT) was devised to answer the question, To what degree and under what conditions do older adults maintain a capacity to raise their level of function in fluid intelligence? (Baltes et al., 1986, p. 176). The findings of the initial ADEPT studies emphasized that performance is only one level of achievement, and that, at any age, there is room for performance enhancement (Baltes and Willis, 1982). Later studies supported this finding and concluded that the "reserve capacity of many older individuals in fluid intelligence is even more extensive than indicated in previous research" (Baltes et al., 1986, p. 176). These researchers further concluded that the benefits accrued from training are not solely confined to improved response time, but also include the improvement of cognitive skills. These studies prompted the development of cognitive training methods with an emphasis on practical intelligence rather than on academically measured intelligence. The nursing interventions discussed in this section review some of the approaches that nurses can use to assist older adults in maintaining and developing cognitive skills that focus on practical intelligence.

In addition to using the interventions discussed here, nurses can encourage older adults to take advantage of the many educational programs that are geared specifically for them. For example, some universities and colleges (particularly community colleges) offer reduced-rate or no-fee courses for students aged 60 years and older. Some programs also offer associate degrees, certification programs, or a General Equivalency Diploma (GED). Elderhostel is a national organization that provides numerous opportunities for individuals aged 55 years and older to become involved in educational and social action groups in the United States and worldwide. These educational activities involve short-term residential programs that usually last 4 to 5 days in the United States and 2 to 4 weeks in other countries. Institutes for Learning in Retirement (ILR) is a community-based organization for retirement-age learners that develops and implements educational programs in affiliation with a college or university. These sessions typically involve homework and usually are held for a couple hours weekly for several months. (See the Educational Resources section for information about Elderhostel and ILR). Less formal education programs often are available through local senior centers and adult education programs affiliated with local school districts.

Education About Memory and Cognition

The concept of metacognition suggests that an understanding of one's own cognitive processes is an important type of knowledge that influences performance. The following interventions, therefore, are essential for optimal cognitive function: (1) correction of misinformation and negative expectations; (2) provision of accurate information about age-related changes; and (3) provision of information about techniques to enhance cognitive abilities. These principles have been described specifically in relation to memory function in older adults (Perlmutter et al., 1987, pp. 62–63). One example cited is that if someone wants to remember a list of names, both the intent to remember and a knowledge about techniques for remembering would be necessary. In addition, the person's performance would be improved even more if he or she knew which techniques were most effective. Thus, just as nurses educate older adults about techniques for improving physical health, they can also educate them about techniques for improving cognitive health. Recent studies conclude that "older adults benefit from cognitive exercise more than the negative aging stereotypes or decline theories would suggest" (Baltes, 1993, p. 583).

In community and long-term care settings, group sessions can be effective and efficient ways of addressing many psychosocial aspects of aging, including cognitive function. For example, the healthy aging class, which was described in Chapter 3, can be used as a model for health education about age-related cognitive changes. Other models for nurse-led groups relating to memory training may be found in the gerontological nursing literature (e.g., Clites, 1984). The model developed by Turner Geriatric Services at the University of Michigan can be used for either a single- or multiple-session program for older adults. A training manual provides information about developing memory training programs, and it includes lesson plans and handouts for group leaders (Fogler and Stern, 1994). Display 4-2 outlines a sample presentation for older adults based on the material from the Turner Geriatric Clinic. This display can be used readily by nurses to educate older adults about techniques for memory enhancement.

Concentration and Attention Enhancement Techniques

When one's ability to attend to the environment and concentrate on visual and auditory cues is limited, the ability to learn and remember is also impaired. Thus, techniques, such as relaxation and imagery, that enhance attention and concen-

DISPLAY 4-2
Memory Training for Older Adults

Introduction

- Forgetting is a normal part of life for all people, but memory skills can be learned. The purposes of this program are to look at some reasons people forget things and to discuss ways of improving memory skills.
- When older adults are forgetful, they may blame it on old age, rather than seeing it as something that happens to everyone, regardless of age.
- Memory problems can be viewed as a challenge. Anyone can improve their memory, but as with any other skill, an effort must be made.

Stages of Memory

- *Sensory memory* lasts only a few seconds. It involves the awareness of information obtained through vision, hearing, smell, taste, and touch.
- *Short-term memory* is your working memory, or what's in your conscious thoughts. This, too, is very brief and contains small amounts of information. For example, this type of memory allows you to recall a telephone number as you dial it.
- *Long-term memory* is the memory bank, or what you depend on whenever you need to retrieve information. This memory bank is almost limitless and contains information you just learned, as well as information from long ago.

Memory Changes and Aging

- Aging is blamed for a lot of memory problems, but very few changes occur solely because of aging.
- In older adulthood, the processes of learning new information and recalling old information slow down a little. The overall ability to learn and remember, however, is not significantly affected in healthy older people.

Factors That Interfere with Memory

As people grow older, an increasing number of factors may interfere with their ability to remember, including the following:

- Not being attentive to the situation. This might be attributable, for example, to the fact that the situation is not relevant to you.
- Being distracted by a lot of things that interfere with your ability to concentrate. For example, this might be the result of worry or anxiety.
- Feeling stressed
- Having a physical illness or being tired
- Having vision, hearing, or other functional impairments that interfere with the ability to obtain information
- Feeling sad or depressed, or coping with loss or grief
- Not being intellectually stimulated (principle of "use it or lose it!")
- Not having cues to help you remember
- Not organizing information for easy retention; not being organized in daily life
- Taking medications or alcohol that interfere with mental abilities
- Not being physically fit (e.g., as a result of poor nutrition or lack of exercise)

Ways of Improving Memory Skills

- Write things down (e.g., use lists, calendars, and notebooks).
- Use auditory cues (e.g., timers, alarm clocks) in conjunction with written cues.
- Use environmental cues. (For instance, you might remove something from its usual place, then return it to its normal location after it has served its purpose as a reminder.)
- Assign specific places for specific items and keep the items in their proper place (e.g., keep keys on a hook near the door).

(continued)

DISPLAY 4-2
Memory Training for Older Adults (Continued)

- Put reminders in appropriate places (e.g., place shoes that need to be repaired near the door).
- Use visual images. ("A picture is worth a thousand words.") Create a picture in your mind when you want to remember something; the more bizarre the picture, the more likely it is that you will remember.
- Use active observation: pay attention to details of what's going on around you and be alert to the environment.
- Make associations, or mental connections. (For example, the phrase "spring ahead, fall back" can be recalled to ensure accuracy in changing clocks for seasonal time changes [from daylight savings time to standard time and vice versa].)
- Make associations between names and mental images (e.g., Carol and Christmas carol).
- Rehearse items you want to remember by repeating them aloud or writing the information on paper.
- Use self-instruction; say things aloud (e.g., "I'm putting my keys on the counter so I remember to turn off the stove before I leave.").
- Divide information into small parts that can be remembered easily. (For instance, to remember an address or a zip code, divide it into groups [seven hundred sixty, fifty five]).
- Organize information into logical categories (e.g., shampoo and hair spray, toothpaste and mouthwash, soap and deodorant).
- Use rhyming cues (e.g., "In 1492, Columbus sailed the ocean blue.").
- Use first-letter cues and make associations. (For example, to remember to buy carrots, apples, radishes, pickles, eggs, and tea bags, remember the word CARPET).

- Make word associations. (For instance, to remember the letters of your license plate, make a word, such as camel, out of the letters CML.)
- Search the alphabet while focusing on what you're trying to remember. (For example, to remember that someone's name is Martin, start with names that begin with A and continue naming names through the alphabet until your memory is jogged for the correct one.)
- Make up a story to connect things you want to remember. (For instance, if you have to go to the cleaners and the post office, create a story about mailing a pair of pants.)

Conclusion

- Don't try to remember all of these techniques—you'll need another method just to remember them all!
- Select a few techniques that you like, and use these whenever appropriate or needed.
- Minimize any distractions; pay attention to one thing at a time.
- Give yourself time to remember; forgetfulness is most likely to occur when you are in a hurry. Try to prepare in advance, when you have time to concentrate.
- Maintain some sense of organization in your daily life, and devise systems to organize routine tasks, like taking medications.
- Carry a note pad or calendar, and use written records so you don't have to rely entirely on mental cues.
- Relax and maintain a sense of humor. If you become anxious about your memory and are convinced you can't remember, then you will create a self-fulfilling prophecy.

Adapted, with permission, from J. Fogler and L. Stern, (1994), *Improving Your Memory: How to Remember What You're Starting to Forget* (Baltimore, MD: Johns Hopkins University Press).

tration may also improve memory and learning. Likewise, any method that reduces environmental distractions may also improve one's cognitive abilities. Many of the popular self-help books describe methods of relaxation as a way of opening the mind to new learning. The relaxation technique outlined in Chapter 14 can be taught to older adults for a variety of uses, including the enhancement of mental skills. Nurses can encourage older adults to use these techniques as mental health practices that can improve cognitive abilities.

Adapting Health Education to Older Adults

Much of the research on cognitive aging has centered on factors that affect learning in older adulthood. Because many nursing interventions include patient teaching or health education, principles regarding cognitive aging can be used to adapt educational methods and materials to older adults. The suggestions presented in this text for communicating with older adults and

compensating for hearing and vision deficits can be applied to health education. Display 4-3 summarizes guidelines that can be applied to educational interventions for older adults. Examples of models of educational materials that have been adapted to meet the unique learning styles of older adults can be found in the nursing and gerontology literature (e.g., Ressler, 1991; Weinrich and Boyd, 1992).

Evaluating Nursing Care

Nursing care of older adults who want to maintain a high level of cognitive function is evaluated by the degree to which these adults express satisfaction with their cognitive abilities, such as memory skills. Objectively, it is evaluated by the degree to which they use their cognitive abilities to meet their daily needs. For example, an older adult who forgets to keep appointments might learn to use a calendar or other organizational aids to remember the appointments. In this situation, the effectiveness of interventions

---

DISPLAY 4-3
Educational Interventions for Older Adults

Conditions That Are Most Conducive to Learning

- Contexts that are supportive and rewarding (e.g., praise), in contrast to those that are neutral, challenging, or critical
- An environment that is pleasant, familiar, and has the least number of distractions possible
- Information that relates to prior experiences and is personally relevant, rather than meaningless
- Information that is concrete rather than abstract

Presentation Methods Most Conducive to Learning

- A self-paced, rather than externally paced, rate

- Emphasis on the integration and application of knowledge and experience, rather than on the acquisition of large amounts of new information
- Use of visual methods for material that is meaningful and lends itself to thoughtful analysis
- Use of auditory methods, alone or in combination with visual ones, for information that is factual and straightforward
- Provision of advance organizers, such as outlines, written cues, and introductory overviews
- Reinforcement of the value of organizing aids

would be measured by how well the person remembers to keep appointments.

Chapter Summary

Age-related changes affecting some intellectual skills are noticed around the age of 60 years, even in healthy adults. These changes are minor and do not interfere significantly with daily function, especially if compensatory interventions are used. Factors that influence cognitive abilities in older adulthood include chemical effects (e.g., medications), personal characteristics (e.g., educational level), and physical and mental health status (e.g., sensory function). Any major decline in cognitive function is caused by disease conditions, such as dementia or other risk factors, as discussed in Chapter 19. Functional consequences affecting cognition include a slight and gradual decline in some intellectual abilities, such as short-term memory (refer to Display 4-1).

Nursing assessment of cognition is reviewed in Chapter 5 as part of the comprehensive psychosocial assessment. Health-Seeking Behaviors is a nursing diagnosis that might be used for older adults with age-related changes in cognitive function. A nursing goal is to reverse or compensate for declines in cognitive function. This is accomplished through educational interventions, such as memory training (refer to Display 4-2). Nursing care is evaluated by the degree to which the older adult successfully uses memory training skills to improve his or her functional level.

Critical Thinking Exercises

1. Identify the factors in your own life that interfere with cognitive function.
2. What memory aids do you use in your life? Are they effective? Would you like to develop additional memory aids?
3. You are working in a senior center and have suggested that the center sponsor a series of classes on the memory problems of older adults. This suggestion is based on your observation that many of the older adults have asked you questions about memory problems, Alzheimer's disease, and the recent news articles about Ginkgo biloba. Address each of the following issues:
   a. The center director is a firm believer in the adage, "You can't teach an old dog new tricks." How would you convince the director that the classes you wish to offer are worthwhile?
   b. How would you structure the sessions (number and length of sessions, number of participants, and so forth)?
   c. Describe the content you would cover and the approach you would use for each topic. Include information about normal cognitive aging, risk factors for impaired cognitive function, and techniques for improving memory and other aspects of cognition.
   d. What audiovisual aids, including written materials, would you use?
   e. How would you adapt your teaching method and materials for the group?
   f. How would you evaluate the sessions?

Case Example and Nursing Care Plan

Pertinent Case Information

Mrs. C. is 71 years old and lives alone in her own home. She attends a local "Senior Wellness" clinic for blood pressure checks, health screenings (e.g., cholesterol levels), and her annual flu shot. During her monthly visit for a blood pressure check, she confides that she is embarrassed about missing a doctor's appointment last week. She says she has been noticing increased difficulties with memory, and one of her friends has told her that she might have Alzheimer's disease. She asks if there's a place where she can get a test for Alzheimer's.

Nursing Assessment

Your focused nursing assessment indicates that Mrs. C. has missed a couple of health care appointments during the past year. She has stated that she missed a dental appointment 6 months ago when she was very worried about her daughter, who was undergoing diagnostic tests for a lump in her breast. Last week, when she missed her doctor's appointment, she had been very busy shopping for presents for her grandson's wedding. When you ask about additional problems with memory, Mrs. C. admits that she has more difficulty remembering people's names than she used to have. You do not identify any risk factors that might affect Mrs. C.'s cognitive abilities (e.g., depression, medication effects, poor nutrition). Mrs. C. has never used calendars, and she says she remembers her doctor's appointments by keeping the appointment cards in her desk drawer along with her bills and her checkbook. She says that she checks her appointment cards every month, but she hadn't noticed the cards for the two appointments she missed.

Nursing Diagnosis

You use the nursing diagnosis of Health-Seeking Behaviors because Mrs. C. is interested in learning about memory training skills to assist her in remembering appointments. Mrs. C. has a poor understanding of age-related cognitive changes, and she indicates that she is interested in learning about ways to improve her memory.

Goals	Nursing Interventions	Evaluation Criteria
Mrs. C. will express an interest in improving her memory skills.	Use information in Display 4-1 to teach Mrs. C. about age-related changes that affect cognitive abilities.	Mrs. C. will agree to participate in a discussion of memory training skills.
	Discuss the difference between dementia and age-associated memory impairment.	

Emphasize that memory skills can be developed through memory training techniques.

Mrs. C. will use memory training techniques to improve her functional level.	Give Mrs. C. a copy of Display 4-2 and review the information. Assist Mrs. C. in identifying one or two strategies for remembering appointments (e.g., begin using a calendar). Assist Mrs. C. in identifying one or two strategies for remembering the names of people she meets (e.g., using visual images).	Mrs. C. will report success in using a method for remembering appointments. Mrs. C. will report success in using a method for remembering names of people.

Educational Resources

Elderhostel, Institute for Learning in Retirement
75 Federal Street, Boston, MA 02110–1941
Elderhostel: (617) 426–8056; Institute: (617) 422–0784
www.elderhostel.org
• Provides a wide-range of short-term learning opportunities for people who are age 55 years and older

Turner Geriatric Clinic, University of Michigan Health Systems
1500 East Medical Center Drive, Ann Arbor, MI 48109
(734) 764–2556
• *Improving Your Memory: How to Remember What You're Starting to Forget* (self-help manual or a text for a memory-improvement course)
• *Teaching Memory Improvement to Adults* (training manual for professionals who want to offer memory improvement programs for older adults)

References

Baltes, P. B. (1993). The aging mind: Potential and limits. *Gerontologist, 33*(5), 580–594.

Baltes, P. B., Dittmann-Kohli, F., & Kliegl, R. (1986). Reserve capacity of the elderly in aging-sensitive tests of fluid intelligence: Replication and extension. *Psychology and Aging, 1,* 172–177.

Baltes, P. B., & Lindenberger, U. (1997). Emergence of a powerful connection between sensory and cognitive functions across the adult life span: A new window to the study of cognitive aging? *Psychology and Aging, 12*(1), 12–21.

Baltes, P. B., & Willis, S. L. (1982). Plasticity and enhancement of intellectual functioning in old age. In F. I. M. Craik & S. Trehab (Eds.), *Advances in the study of communication and affect* (Vol. 8, pp. 353–389). New York: Plenum Press.

Botwinick, J. (1984). *Aging and behavior* (3rd ed.). New York: Springer.

Boxtel, M. P. J. van, Buntinx, F., Houx, P. J., Metsemakers, J. F. M., Knottnerus, A., & Jolles, J. (1998). The relation between morbidity and cognitive performance in a normal aging population. *Journal of Gerontology: Medical Sciences, 53A,* M147–M154.

Carpenito, L. J. (1997). *Nursing diagnosis: Application to clinical practice* (7th ed.). Philadelphia: J. B. Lippincott.

Clites, J. (1984). Maximizing memory retention in the aged. *Journal of Gerontological Nursing, 10*(8), 34–39.

Cutler, S. J., & Grams, A. E. (1988). Correlates of self-reported everyday memory problems. *Journal of Gerontology: Social Sciences, 43*(3), S82–S90.

Etnier, J. L., & Landers, D. M. (1997). The influence of age and fitness on performance and learning. *Journal of Aging and Physical Activity, 5,* 175–189.

Fisk, J. E., & Warr, P. B. (1998). Associative learning and short-term forgetting as a function of age, perceptual speed, and central executive functioning. *Journal of Gerontology: Psychological Sciences, 53B,* P112–P121.

Fogler, J., & Stern, L. (1994). *Teaching memory improvement to adults* (rev. ed.). Baltimore: The Johns Hopkins University Press.

Fozard, J. L., Vercruyssen, M., Reynolds, S. L., Hancock, P. A., & Quilter, R. E. (1994). Age differences and changes in reaction time: The Baltimore Longitudinal Study of Aging. *Journal of Gerontology: Psychological Sciences, 49*(4), P179–P189.

Goodwin, J. S., Goodwin, J. M., & Garry, P. J. (1983). Association between nutritional status and cognitive functioning in a healthy elderly population. *Journal of the American Medical Association, 249*(21), 2917–2921.

Hänninen, T., Reinikainen, K. J., Helkala, E-L., Koivisto, K., Mykkänen, L., Laakso, M. Pyörälä, K., & Reikkinen, P. J. (1994). Subjective memory complaints and personality traits in normal elderly subjects. *Journal of the American Geriatrics Society, 42,* 1–4.

Hasher, L., and Zacks, R. T. (1979). Automatic and effortful processes in memory. *Journal of Experimental Psychology: General, 108,* 356–388.

Horn, J. L. (1970). Organization of data on life-span development of human abilities. In L. R. Goulet and P. B. Baltes (Eds.), *Life-span developmental psychology: Research and theory* (pp. 424–466). New York: Academic Press.

Horn, J. L. (1982). The theory of fluid and crystallized intelligence in relation to concepts of cognitive psychology and aging in adulthood. In F. I. M. Craik and S. Trehab (Eds.), *Advances in the study of communication and affect* (Vol. 8, pp. 237–378). New York: Plenum Press.

Hultsch, D. F., & Dixon, R. A. (1990). Learning and memory in aging. In J. E. Birren & K. W. Schaie (Eds.), *Handbook of the psychology of aging* (3rd ed., pp. 258–274). New York: Academic Press.

Johansson, B., Allen-Burge, R., & Zarit, S. H. (1997). Self-reports on memory functioning in a longitudinal study of the oldest old: Relation to current, prospective, and retrospective performance. *Journal of Gerontology: Psychological Sciences, 52B*(3), P139–P146.

Katz, I. R., Sands, L. P., Bilker, W., DiFilippo, S., Boyce, A., & D'Angelo, K. D. (1998). Identification of medications that cause cognitive impairment in older people: The case of oxybutynin chloride. *Journal of the American Geriatrics Society, 46,* 8–13.

Labouvie-Vief, G., & Blanchard-Fields, F. (1982). Cognitive ageing and psychological growth. *Ageing and Society, 2,* 183–209.

Lachman, M. E., Weaver, S. L., Bandura, M., Elliott, E., & Lewkowicz, C. J. (1992). Improving memory and control beliefs through cognitive restructuring and self-generated strategies. *Journal of Gerontology: Psychological Sciences, 47*(5), P293–P299.

Luszcz, M. A., Bryan, J., & Kent, P. (1997). Predicting episodic memory performance of very old men and women: Contributions from age, depression, activity, cognitive ability, and speed. *Psychology and Aging, 12*(2), 340–351.

Lyness, S. A., Eaton, E. M., & Schneider, L. S. (1994). Cognitive performance in older and middle-aged depressed outpatients and controls. *Journal of Gerontology: Psychological Sciences, 49*(3), P129–P136.

Manheimer, R. J. (1996). Adult education. In J. E. Birren (Ed.), *Encyclopedia of gerontology: Age, aging, and the aged* (Vol. 1, pp. 61–69). San Diego: Academic Press, Inc.

Perlmutter, M., Adams, C., Berry, J., Kaplan, M., Persons, D., & Verdonik, F. (1987). Aging and memory. In K. W. Schaie & C. Eisdorfer (Eds.), *Annual review of gerontology and geriatrics* (pp. 57–92). New York: Springer Publishing Company.

Perlmutter, M., & Nyquist, L. (1990). Relationships between self-reported physical and mental health and intelligence performance across adulthood. *Journal of Gerontology: Psychological Sciences, 45*(4), P145–P155.

Perrig, W. J., Perrig, P., & Stähelin, H. B. (1997). The relation between antioxidants and memory performance in the old and very old. *Journal of the American Geriatrics Society, 45,* 718–724.

Poon, L. W. (1985). Differences in human memory with aging: Nature, causes, and clinical implications. In J. E. Birren & K. W. Schaie (Eds.), *Handbook of the psychology of aging* (pp. 427–462). New York: Van Nostrand Reinhold.

Ressler, L. E. (1991). Improving elderly recall with bimodal presentation: A natural experiment of discharge planning. *Gerontologist, 31*(3), 364–370.

Rohling, M. L., & Scogin, F. (1993). Automatic and effortful memory processes in depressed persons. *Journal of Gerontology: Psychological Sciences, 48*(2), P87–P95.

Ryan, E. B., & See, S. K. (1993). Age-based beliefs about memory changes for self and others across adulthood. *Journal of Gerontology: Psychological Sciences, 48*(4), P199–P201.

Ryan, M. C. (1998). The relationship between loneliness, social support, and decline in cognitive function in the hospitalized elderly. *Journal of Gerontological Nursing, 24*(3), 19–27.

Salthouse, T. A., & Coon, V. E. (1993). Influence of task-specific processing speed on age differences in memory. *Journal of Gerontology: Psychological Sciences, 48*(5), P245–P255.

Schaie, K. W. (1977–1978). Toward a stage theory of adult cognitive development. *Journal of Aging and Human Development, 8,* 129–138.

Schaie, K. W., & Willis, S. L. (1986). *Adult development and aging.* Boston: Little, Brown and Company.

Schaie, K. W., Willis, S. L., & O'Hanlon, A. M. (1994). Perceived intellectual performance change over seven years. *Journal of Gerontology: Psychological Sciences, 49*(3), P108–P118.

Sliwinski, M., Lipton, R. B., Buschke, H., & Stewart, W. (1996). The effects of preclinical dementia on estimates of normal cognitive functioning in aging. *Journal of Gerontology: Psychological Sciences, 51B*(4), P217–P225.

Smith, A. D. (1996). Memory. In J. E. Birren (Ed.), *Encyclopedia of gerontology: Age, aging, and the aged* (Vol. 2, pp. 107–117). San Diego: Academic Press.

Verhaeghen, P., Marcoen, A., & Goossens, L. (1993). Facts and fiction about memory aging: A quantitative integration of research findings. *Journal of Gerontology: Psychological Sciences, 48*(4), P157–P171.

Weinrich, S. P., & Boyd, M. (1992). Education in the elderly: Adapting and evaluating teaching tools. *Journal of Gerontological Nursing, 18*(1), 15–20.

Whitehouse, P. J., Juengst, E., Mehlman, M., & Murray, T. H. (1997). Enhancing cognition in the intellectually intact. *Hastings Center Report, 27*(3), 14–22.

Willis, S. L. (1987). Cognitive training and everyday competence. In K. W. Schaie & C. Eisdorfer (Eds.), *Annual review of gerontology and geriatrics* 159–188. New York: Springer.

Woodruff, D. S. (1983). A review of aging and cognitive processes. *Research on Aging, 5*(2), 139–153.

Psychosocial Assessment

Chapter

5

Learning Objectives	1. *Describe the goals of and the procedure for psychosocial assessment of older adults.*
	2. *Discuss barriers to communication as well as techniques that may be used to enhance communication with older adults, including strategies to promote effective cross-cultural communication.*
	3. *Critically analyze the influence of culture on the psychosocial assessment of older adults.*
	4. *Explain the criteria for assessing the following specific components of mental status: physical appearance, motor function, social skills, response to the interview, orientation, alertness, memory, speech characteristics, calculation and higher language skills, and decision making.*
	5. *Discuss guidelines for assessing affective function.*
	6. *Compare and contrast the characteristics of delusions, hallucinations, and illusions as they relate to underlying causes.*
	7. *Explain the criteria for assessing the following components of sociocultural supports: sociocultural network, barriers to services, economic resources, and spirituality and religious affiliation.*
	8. *Develop a list of interview questions for assessing sociocultural supports and identifying barriers to the use of those supports.*

*P*sychosocial assessment is the most complex and challenging part of a multidimensional assessment. Although impaired psychosocial function may often be attributed to factors relating to normal aging or to untreatable conditions, a careful psychosocial assessment can identify the underlying cause(s) of mental changes, many of which can then be reversed or addressed through interventions. Traditionally, many aspects of psychosocial function have been viewed as the exclusive purview of psychologists, psychiatrists, social workers, and other mental health professionals. However, when applying a holistic functional approach to the care of older adults, psychosocial assessment falls well within the scope of practice of gerontological nursing.

A psychosocial assessment includes consideration of the following parameters, each of which is reviewed in this chapter: cognitive function, affective function, contact with reality, and sociocultural supports. Like Chapter 17, this chapter focuses solely on assessment and does not address the other components of the nursing process. The information presented is intended to be used, in conjunction with that contained in chapters focusing on various aspects of function, as a basis for psychosocial assessment. The assessment information presented in this chapter is particularly relevant to the information provided in those chapters that address psychosocial function (Chapters 3, 4, and 19–21).

Goals of Psychosocial Assessment

The goals of psychosocial assessment, like those of physical assessment, are to detect asymptomatic or unacknowledged health problems at an early stage and to address any existing symptoms of illness. In addition, within the context of the functional approach to nursing care, one of the purposes of psychosocial assessment is to identify those risk factors (especially those that are amenable to intervention) that interfere with cognitive, emotional, or social function. Last, a good psychosocial assessment provides information about the person's usual personality, coping mechanisms, and cognitive abilities, as well as how those characteristics may have changed during older adulthood. This information can then be used to establish goals based on realistic expectations, an especially important consideration when the nurse's initial contact with the older adult occurs during a crisis situation, without an opportunity to observe the person's usual patterns of behavior.

When mental changes are identified during the nursing assessment, a multidisciplinary team approach is essential for further assessment and for implementation of effective interventions. A mistake that is frequently made is to label the changes as "normal for the person's age." This mistake is not only unfair to the older adult, it can also be detrimental, especially in cases in which a treatable underlying condition is overlooked or appropriate interventions to improve functional abilities are neglected. As should be clear from the previous discussion of cognitive function (see Chapter 4), age-related cognitive changes are only rarely brought to the attention of health care professionals. For example, it would be highly unlikely for an older adult to describe the following complaint: "I know I can learn new information, but I don't seem to be able to comprehend information as quickly as I used to." Mental changes that are noted by other people or brought to the attention of health care professionals are more likely to arise from a pathologic process than from age-related processes. Therefore, whenever changes in psychosocial function are identified, a concerted effort must be made to identify the underlying cause.

Procedure for Psychosocial Assessment

Unlike physical assessment procedures, which are viewed as routine methods for periodically evaluating a person's physical health, psychosocial assessment procedures usually are viewed as exceptional measures, involving mysterious batteries of tests aimed at identifying people who are in need of psychiatric treatment. Thus, physical assessment procedures generally are perceived as acceptable ways of either detecting illness in its early stages or identifying the underlying cause of troublesome symptoms for the purpose of alleviating them. By contrast, psychosocial assessment procedures do not enjoy the same level of acceptance and are not routinely incorporated into overall health assessments.

As a normal part of care of older adults, nurses often participate in physically intimate activities, such as bathing, when the need arises. These activities are accepted as a usual part of nursing care, and nurses generally feel comfortable providing such care, which would not be required by healthy, independent adults. Because some aspects of psychosocial assessment involve emotionally charged issues that would not normally be discussed with strangers, the establishment of a trusting relationship and the use of good communication skills are prerequisites for performing an accurate psychosocial assessment. Initially, both the nurse and the older adult may feel uncomfortable when psychosocial nursing care is provided. However, it is important for the nurse to become comfortable addressing psychosocial issues, which are essential components of nursing assessment and intervention, even though they may be considered to be private under usual circumstances. Display 5-1 presents a self-assessment tool that nurses can use to assess their awareness of and to increase their degree of comfort with the psychosocial and cultural aspects of gerontological nursing.

In performing psychosocial assessments, it is important to establish the right atmosphere to set the stage for obtaining emotionally charged information. In acute care settings, nurses perform an assessment at the time of admission to establish a baseline for planning the patient's nursing care. When patients are admitted for acute medical-surgical problems, the focus of the assessment is necessarily on physical care

related to their immediate needs. In such cases, it is not always appropriate to do a psychosocial assessment upon admission. However, this assessment should not be overlooked because it may provide clues to the causes of existing medical problems, in addition to providing a basis for discharge planning. As soon as the patient's condition is medically stable, the nurse should begin addressing psychosocial questions.

Nurses working in long-term care settings usually have more time to collect psychosocial assessment information than do those working in hospitals. Except in crisis situations, gerontological nurses in home and community settings also have sufficient time to perform a psychosocial assessment. In these settings, nurses may have the additional advantage of observing the person's environment and meeting the caregiv-

DISPLAY 5-1
Psychosocial and Cultural Self-Assessment

With what sociocultural and religious groups do I most closely identify? What does it mean to belong to these groups? Is there any stigma associated with any of these groups? What do I like and dislike about these groups and my sociocultural identity?

When I was growing up . . .

- How were older adults treated?
- How were people with mental or emotional disorders viewed?
- What language was used to describe aging, old age, and older adults with disturbed mental function?
- What words did my family use, and what was the *connotative meaning* of the words used, to describe older adults? Was it positive, negative, or mixed?

What experiences have I had with older adults . . .

- From different racial, ethnic, and religious backgrounds?
- With functional impairments or mental, psychological, or emotional disorders?

To what groups of older adults do I find it easy or difficult to relate? Why?

What is my attitude toward older adults . . .

- Who are immigrants?
- Who have difficulty with the English language?
- Who have difficulty communicating?

What do I do and how do I feel when I have trouble understanding people whose accents and primary language are different from my own?

How do I feel about older adults who are single, divorced, widowed, separated, or are living together in a same-sex or heterosexual but unmarried relationship?

How comfortable am I discussing emotional, cultural, spiritual, and psychosocial subjects? Are there certain topics with which I am uncomfortable (e.g., suicide, alcoholism, sexuality, spirituality, terminal illness, abusive relationships)?

What are (were) the health care practices of my parents, grandparents, great-grandparents (e.g., herbs, poultices, folk remedies)? Do (did) they consult with folk, indigenous, religious, or spiritual healers? How do I feel about alternative or complementary health care practices for myself and for older adults?

ers who are involved in the daily routines of the older adult's life. Observations of interactions between older adults and their environments and caregivers can provide valuable information for the psychosocial assessment.

In addition to interviewing and observing older adults, nurses can obtain psychosocial assessment information from other sources. In situations in which the older person's cognitive functions have declined, it is essential to obtain information from family and others who can provide a reliable history of the mental changes. In long-term care settings, nursing assistants usually are the health care workers who spend the most time with residents, and they can be an important source of psychosocial information. However, nursing assistants usually are not included in team conferences at which psychosocial problems are addressed. Nurses can either obtain information from them prior to these conferences or they can facilitate their participation in the conferences.

In summary, the procedure for collecting psychosocial assessment information involves interviewing older adults and their caregivers and observing older adults in their environments. The tools for an effective psychosocial assessment are a trusting relationship, a listening ear, an intuitive mind, and a sensitive heart. The following section addresses the communication skills that are essential for performing a thorough psychosocial assessment of older adults.

Communication: The Assessment Tool

Skillful use of communication techniques is an essential factor in psychosocial assessment, just as the skillful use of a stethoscope and sphygmomanometer is essential for an accurate determination of blood pressure. This text does not review basic physical assessment techniques, but rather addresses those aspects that are unique to gerontological nursing. Similarly, although this discussion of communication techniques re-

views communication skills in general, it focuses on those aspects that are unique to older adults.

Unique Aspects of Communication with Older Adults

Communication involves the following components: a sender, a message, verbal and nonverbal methods of sending the message, a receiver, and feedback. In terms of the psychosocial assessment interview, the sender of the message is the nurse, and the message is that information about the person's psychosocial function is important to planning care for that person. Verbal methods for sending the message include the posing of many open-ended questions. Nonverbal communication methods include the following, which convey both messages and attitudes: touch, clothing, grooming, gestures, physical distance, body language, eye contact, facial expressions, and the tone, rate, and volume of one's voice. A significant source of nonverbal messages is the interview environment, which can either facilitate or hinder the psychosocial assessment. Nonverbal messages must convey a nonjudgmental attitude, and the environment must be conducive to conducting the interview. The receiver is the older adult or a caregiver, either of whom may never have participated in this type of interview and thus may be uncomfortable discussing pertinent information. Feedback is important, not only in determining whether the question was understood, but also in determining the person's receptivity to further questions. Because much of the feedback will be subtle and nonverbal, excellent listening and observational skills are essential for the gerontological nurse.

Barriers to Communication with Older Adults

Gerontological nurses often encounter communication barriers that can be particularly challenging during the psychosocial assessment. For example, older adults may have sensory impairments that interfere with communication. For conversations about ordinary topics, the use of techniques for communicating with hearing-impaired people may be effective. However, these techniques often seem inadequate when the conversation is about sensitive issues. Visual impairments, too, can interfere with communication, compromising the person's ability to use visual cues to compensate for a hearing impairment and to perceive nonverbal messages.

Sensory overload is another barrier that may interfere with the psychosocial assessment. This may be particularly problematic for older adults, especially in the presence of any cognitive impairments. Sensory overload can be caused by certain circumstances, such as being asked to receive and process too much information at one time (e.g., have to respond to questions about social background, cognitive abilities, and emotional function during a single interview), or it may result from too many people trying to communicate at one time (e.g., family members, caregivers, or more than one professional). Sensory overload may also result from environmental noises. These may be particularly bothersome to older adults who use hearing aids, as background noises are magnified by the devices. Nurses usually become accustomed to background noise in their work environment, learning to "tune out" stimuli, like alarms and call systems, that do not pertain to them. People who are not used to an environment, however, may be distracted by such noises. In these situations, a simple measure like closing a door or drawing a bed curtain may reduce the sensory input, thereby improving communication.

Internal distractions arise from any physical discomfort that interferes with a person's ability to focus on a conversation. Pain, thirst, hunger, fatigue, bladder fullness, or uncomfortable temperatures all can interfere with a person's attention to psychosocial issues. Neurologic disorders can interfere with language and communication skills, as can adverse medication effects, like dry mouth, clouded mentation, and tardive dyskinesia. Cognitive deficits can interfere with a person's ability to listen, remember, and respond to interview questions. People who are actively delusional or hallucinatory, or who are not fully in touch with reality for any reason, may have difficulty attending to the interviewer.

It is important to assess the older adult for internal distractions early in the interview so that interventions can be implemented to enhance communication. Some interventions, such as the alleviation of thirst or hunger, are quite simple to implement. These considerations are especially important when interviewing older adults who depend on the nursing staff to meet their basic needs. Simply offering water, food, or assistance with toileting prior to the interview may markedly improve the person's ability to attend to questions. These simple interventions also may help to establish a trusting relationship because the older adult may then perceive the nurse as someone who understands essential needs.

In an effort to be reassuring, nursing staff and caregivers sometimes offer such remarks as "Why cry over spilled milk?" or "Everything's going to be OK." Although such remarks might be well-intentioned and effective in some circumstances, they may become barriers to communication in most situations. For example, people who are seriously depressed or coping with an untreatable illness might consider these remarks to be insensitive. In addition to trite responses and false reassurance, other verbal barriers include changing the subject, avoiding sensitive issues, jumping to conclusions, giving unwanted advice, or minimizing the person's feelings.

The way the older person is addressed also can be a barrier to communication. For example, many caregivers consider names like "dear," "honey," or "grandma" to be complimentary, and they habitually use them to address the older adults in their care. Some people, however, take offense when these names or phrases are used. Nurses must be aware of any tendency to use such trite or standard titles, because even if these terms are not objectionable, they usually do not enhance communication and they certainly do not affirm the older person's individuality. Nurses must also be cautious about addressing people by their first names because many older people interpret that as disrespectful.

Other sources of verbal barriers include inarticulate speech or obstructive mannerisms, such as covering one's mouth or turning one's head away while talking. In institutional settings, much verbal communication takes place while nurses are walking down the hall, pushing a wheelchair, assisting with personal care, or performing other activities. During these activities, nurses can listen to patients/residents and engage in social conversation, but these are not the best times for asking personal questions or giving important information. Not only are the activities a distraction, but they interfere with the face-to-face positioning that enhances communication and might even be essential for communication with people who are hearing impaired.

Cultural differences may also create communication barriers that are difficult, and some-

times impossible, to overcome. If either the older adult or the interviewer holds stereotypes or prejudices about the other person, it will be difficult to establish a trusting relationship. Foreign-born people who have a dementing illness or a physical illness that drains their energy may revert to their native language, even if they previously spoke English well. In these situations, family members may be able to facilitate communication. Display 5-2 summarizes the communication barriers that nurses may need to address before performing a psychosocial assessment interview.

Techniques to Enhance Communication with Older Adults

The manner in which conversations are initiated establishes the basis for further communication. The exchanging of names is an important but simple ritual that is often overlooked by nurses. Even in social settings, the exchange of proper names is a first step in establishing a mutual relationship. Nurses generally have access to information about the older person's name before the older person has information about the

---

DISPLAY 5-2
Barriers to Communication with Older Adults

Sociocultural Factors Relating to the Older Adult or the Interviewer

- Stereotypes
- Differences in age, language, or cultural background
- Biases with regard to differences in race, cultural background, sexual orientation, religious or spiritual beliefs, and the like

Barriers for Older Adults

- Sensory impairments
- Physical discomfort (e.g., pain, thirst, hunger)
- Medication effects or pathologic conditions
- Impaired psychosocial function secondary to dementia or depression
- Diminished contact with reality

Barriers Associated with the Interviewer

- Insensitivity
- Poor listening skills
- Use of trite remarks
- False reassurance
- Judgmental attitudes, expressed verbally or nonverbally
- Use of inappropriate or unacceptable names
- Inarticulate speech
- Obstructive mannerisms

Barriers in the Interview Environment

- Noise and distractions
- Presentation of too much information at one time
- Too many people speaking at the same time

nurse's name. In institutional settings, nurses can simply look at a wristband or a name card to find out the patient's/resident's name. Although this method may be an efficient and reliable one for identifying patients/residents, it does nothing to promote a sense of respect for the person as an individual. A more personal approach is to ask the person his or her name, using the wristband only as a means of confirming information when necessary.

Nurses do not always take the time to introduce themselves to patients/residents, especially when name tags are in standard use. A verbal exchange of names, however, can be an effective way of establishing rapport. People sometimes feel at a disadvantage if someone else knows their name when they do not know the other person's name. A simple exchange of names can remove this barrier, and is especially important for older adults who either cannot read name tags or cannot remember names. Such an exchange is also important for those who need assistance, as people generally feel more secure and more comfortable about asking for help when they can address someone by name. Therefore, the nurse should begin any initial contact by stating his or her own name and role, acknowledging the other person's name, and inquiring about the person's preference with regard to how he or she would like to be addressed. The following message is an example of this kind of introduction: "Good morning, my name is Carol Miller and I'm the charge nurse today. Are you Señor Juan Garcia? . . . You can call me Carol. What do you like to be called? . . . I have your morning pills for you to take. Do you mind if I check your wristband first?" This approach is more likely to foster a trusting relationship than a scenario in which the nurse walks into a patient's/resident's room, silently checks the wristband to confirm that the person is Juan Garcia, and says, "Here are your morning pills."

At the time of initial contact, a handshake can be used to facilitate communication and to promote the development of a positive relationship. Although older adults from some Near and Middle Eastern and other cultures may not be receptive to this form of nonverbal communication, no harm is done as long as a response has not been forced. In most instances, the handshake dispels some of the formality of the situation and the person may then be more receptive to discussing psychosocial issues. A handshake also provides physical assessment information about skin temperature, the presence or absence of tremors, and other characteristics of one upper extremity. It also can provide clues about the person's social skills and awareness of others.

Physical touch can be used purposefully during the course of the interview to enhance communication, provided the person is receptive to this approach. Older adults generally are quite receptive to touch, especially by a nurse whose responsibilities naturally entail much physical contact. However, the nurse should be aware of cultural variations, especially among older adults from some Asian American and Mexican American groups. Important gender issues also should be considered. In every culture there are rules, some unwritten, about who may touch whom, when, and where. The effectiveness of touch by nurses in their contacts with care recipients has been addressed in nursing research. Langland and Panicucci (1982) summarized their conclusions, derived from four studies, by stating that touch is an important way of developing more positive nurse-client relationships. In their study of the use of touch with elderly confused clients, they found an increase in nonverbal responses, specifically in attention and appropriate action, when the nurse combined touch with a verbal request. A more recent study found that a comforting touch to the arm of nursing home residents was an effective way of communicating love and belonging (Moore and Gilbert, 1995).

In beginning a psychosocial assessment interview, the nurse should explain the purpose of the questions with a statement like one of the following: (1) "I'd like to get to know you better so we can make the best plans for follow-up after you leave the hospital"; (2) "I'd like to ask you some questions about your interests so we can plan for your care while you're here at the nursing home"; or (3) "I'd like to ask some questions about how you manage from day to day so we can identify any community services that might be helpful to you." Starting with questions about events of the remote past, such as where the person was born or grew up, is a nonthreatening way of introducing psychosocial assessment questions. Nurses may believe that it is unprofessional to talk about themselves, but incorporating some personal information in conversations can facilitate the establishment of a trusting relationship. Offering a little information about their own pets or family, for instance, might encourage the older adult to share feelings that they might not mention otherwise, and may help to establish a framework of mutual interest. Be aware, however, that older adults from some Asian and African cultures may not approve of dogs, cats, and other domestic animals being kept as pets, particularly when they are allowed indoors. Culturally, it may be considered inappropriate to keep these animals in one's home because they are considered unclean carriers of fleas, ticks, rabies, and other disease-causing organisms. On the other hand, the nurse may find that these older adults consider birds or other types of pets to be entirely acceptable. Sharing information about ethnic background also can be an effective and nonthreatening way of obtaining information about possible cultural influences.

If formal mental status assessment questions are asked, they can be introduced toward the end of the assessment. Because questions about memory can be very threatening, the topic might be introduced as follows: "I notice you have a hard time remembering dates. Have you noticed any other problems with your memory? . . . Is it OK with you if I ask some questions about your memory?" If no evidence of cognitive impairment is noted during the interview, but other people have expressed concern about the person's memory, a statement such as the following might be used: "Your daughter is concerned that you don't remember to keep appointments. Have you noticed any problems with your memory? . . . Is it OK with you if I ask some questions about your memory?"

During a psychosocial interview, attentive listening is the most effective communication skill. Usually, the best interviews occur when the interviewer is verbally quiet and nonverbally responsive. Most important information can be obtained by asking open-ended questions and nonverbally responding to indicate your interest in what the person is saying. Nonverbal responses, like sustained eye contact, and short verbal responses like, "And then what happened?" will encourage the person to elaborate on the information that is considered most important.

During the early part of an interview, nurses can encourage older adults to talk about issues of their choice. Using this technique, the nurse can identify the issues that are least threatening and most dominant. Carefully listening as the older adult leads the conversation will help to identify appropriate questions. As an example, consider the case of Mrs. P who, during an admission interview, gave the following response to a question about where she lives:

I moved to Sunnybrook Retirement Village after my last stroke. I couldn't stay in my own home because the bedrooms were on the second floor. The doctor told me I had to live where I could get help, and my daughter didn't want me with her. Now that I've fallen and broken my wrist, I'm not sure what the doctor will tell me. My daughter doesn't want to be bothered with me."

The nurse who is listening carefully will be able to identify several issues in this response to a relatively simple question. In response, the nurse might ask any of the following questions: (1)

"What do you miss most since you moved?"; (2) "You mentioned that your daughter didn't want you living with her. Is that something you had hoped you could do?"; (3) "Do you worry that the doctor will suggest that you go to a nursing home?"; and (4) "Do you see your daughter as often as you'd like?" Each question may lead to a discussion of significant issues. Answers to these questions also will provide information that is helpful for discharge planning, and might uncover some concerns that can be addressed by the nurse.

During an interview about psychosocial issues, the nurse periodically clarifies the messages. One clarification technique is to repeat part of a prior answer when asking further questions. For example, saying to Mrs. P., "You mentioned that your daughter doesn't want you living with her . . ." gives feedback about what the nurse heard and also provides a basis for asking a question about the individual's underlying feelings. Feedback can also be helpful when discrepancies between verbal and nonverbal communication are observed. For example, Mrs. P. might begin to cry and clench her fists as she says, "My daughter has her own life to worry about; I can take care of myself. It doesn't bother me that I can't live with her." A statement like, "You look awfully sad. Are you sure it doesn't bother you?" might lead to an acknowledgment of feelings, such as anger, rejection, and loneliness.

During a psychosocial interview, nurses might hear information that is contrary to their own values or cultural expectations. The following are examples of such situations: (1) older people may express feelings of racial prejudice; (2) older women may express attitudes of extreme passivity about their role in decisions; (3) older people may be in situations in which they are exploited by friends, family, or others; and (4) older men may express attitudes about women that are not in accordance with the nurse's beliefs about women. Nurses deal with these differences in many care situations, but they are even more likely to encounter anxiety-producing attitudes or responses during psychosocial interviews with older adults. In any such situation, it is important to be aware of one's own feelings and to deal with these feelings in appropriate ways. During the interview, nurses must maintain a nonjudgmental attitude, but after the interview, they can share their feelings with colleagues. In some situations, however, it is appropriate for nurses to acknowledge their feelings or opinions during the interview. For instance, if the person describes an episode of extreme exploitation and expresses feelings of anger about the situation, the nurse can show empathy and understanding by a statement such as, "That sounds like a terrible situation to have been in."

Any communication between people who do not speak the same language or dialect is challenging. This challenge is magnified when the person also has dementia or sensory impairments. Examples of successful communication techniques to overcome language barriers for residents of long-term care facilities can be found in the gerontological literature (e.g., Camp et al., 1996). Emphasis is placed on finding simple and cost-effective audio and visual aids to teach staff essential foreign-language skills. Some nurses have found the AT&T Language Line Service to be a useful resource when interpreters are unavailable (see the list of Educational Resources at the end of this chapter). Display 5-3 summarizes guidelines for using interpreters in health care settings with older adults.

The Interview Environment

Because psychosocial interviews are very personal, as much privacy as possible must be provided the older adult. This may be difficult in institutional settings, especially when patients or residents share rooms with others. Even in these situations, however, closing the door and pulling the bed curtain will increase the percep-

---

DISPLAY 5-3
Guidelines for Using Interpreters

Before the Interview

- Allow sufficient time for the interview and expect that it will take longer than an assessment interview of an older adult for whom English is the primary language.
- Organize your thoughts and plan ahead to ensure that the most important topics are covered.
- Be aware of age, gender, and socioeconomic class considerations in selecting an interpreter. In general, it is best to use an interpreter who is the same gender and of the same approximate age and socioeconomic class as the older adult.
- Whenever possible, use the services of a professional interpreter. Avoid using visitors or staff from auxiliary services unless permission to do so has been obtained from both the older adult and the interpreter.
- Given that there are more than 140 languages spoken in North America, be certain that the correct language and dialect have been identified. For example, does the person speak Cantonese or Mandarin Chinese?
- If an interpreter for the primary language is unavailable, determine whether the older adult speaks other languages. For example, many older adults from Vietnam and some African nations are also fluent in French.

During the Interview

- Review the importance of confidentiality.
- Talk to the older adult, not the interpreter.
- Talk about one topic at a time.
- Use short sentences and simple vocabulary.
- Use the active voice. Avoid vague modifiers.
- Avoid professional jargon, idioms, and slang.
- Be aware that many words do not translate into another language. For instance, the English word *depression* has no equivalent in many Asian and other languages.

---

tion of privacy. In addition, nurses can take advantage of times that the roommate is out of the room, or it may be appropriate for the nurse to ask the roommate to allow private use of the room. Eliminating distracting noises is also essential for establishing a good interview environment. In institutional settings, closing the door to bedrooms not only increases privacy, but also eliminates noises from the hallway. Before closing a door or bed curtains, however, the nurse should ask permission from the older person. Asking permission shows respect for the person's territory and may be especially important when interviewing people who become anxious when they are in closed spaces. Likewise, if a radio or television is on, the nurse can ask permission to turn it off.

Face-to-face positioning facilitates verbal as well as nonverbal communication and is particularly important when any visual or hearing impairments interfere with communication.

Moreover, people feel more comfortable talking with others when they are at the same level. Therefore, if the person being interviewed is in a bed or wheelchair, the interviewer should sit in a chair. Any physical barrier that interferes with direct face-to-face contact should be removed, if possible. For example, putting side rails down when interviewing someone confined to bed, or moving a walker that is placed in the line of vision, can improve face-to-face contact. Before moving walkers or side rails, however, the nurse should ask the older person's permission to do so; this demonstrates respect for the wishes of the individual. Attention must also be paid to the possible influence of cultural differences between the interviewer and the older adult. Display 5-4 summarizes strategies for promoting cross-cultural communication and techniques and environmental modifications for enhancing communication with older adults.

DISPLAY 5-4
Strategies to Enhance Communication and Promote Cross-Cultural Communication with Older Adults

Culturally Sensitive Communication Strategies

- Use culturally appropriate titles of respect, such as Señor/Señora/Señorita, Mr., Mrs., Ms., Dr., Reverend, Elder, Bishop, and so forth.
- Before calling a person by his/her first name, obtain permission or wait until you have been invited to use this familiar form of address. In some cultures, it is considered inappropriate or disrespectful for anyone but family or close friends to use first names.
- Be sure to pronounce names correctly. When in doubt, ask the older adult to say his or her name. Names that are difficult to pronounce may be written phonetically on the chart for later reference.
- Be aware of subtle linguistic messages that may convey bias or inequality (e.g., using Mr. and the last name to call a White man but addressing a Black woman by her first name).
- Avoid slang expressions, such as "Pop," "Grandma," "dear," "chief," or similar terms, unless the older adult suggests that you do so.
- Never use slang, pejorative, or derogatory terms to refer to ethnic, racial, religious, or any other group (e.g., gays or lesbians).

Verbal and Nonverbal Communication

- Begin contacts with an exchange of names and, if appropriate, a handshake.

- Use touch purposefully to reinforce verbal messages and as a primary method of nonverbal communication.
- Explain the purpose of the interview in relation to a nursing goal.
- Begin with questions about remote, non-threatening topics.
- Use open-ended questions, and learn to use silence effectively and comfortably.
- Periodically clarify the messages.
- Maintain good eye contact, use attentive listening, and encourage the person to elaborate on information.
- Remain nonjudgmental in your responses, but show appropriate empathy.
- Ask formal mental status questions, or the most threatening questions, toward the end of the interview.
- Gain the person's permission before asking formal assessment questions regarding memory and other cognitive abilities.

The Interview Environment

- Sit in a face-to-face position.
- Ensure as much privacy as possible.
- Provide good lighting and avoid background glare.
- Eliminate as much background noise as possible.

All the environmental modifications discussed in Chapters 6 and 7 may be appropriate interventions for enhancing the interview environment. One particularly easy and important consideration is the avoidance of background glare. In hospital or long-term care settings, people often stand in front of a window when talking to a patient/resident in a bed near the window. When the sun is shining or lights are reflected in the window, the background glare may interfere with the older person's ability to see the person in front of the window. In these situations, simply closing the window curtains or standing on the other side of the bed may significantly improve communication. In home settings, lack of lighting is a more common problem than glare. Asking the person's permission to turn on lights can be a very effective and easy way of improving communication. At the end of an interview, the nurse must remember to ask whether the person wants the environment returned to its preinterview status. Turning on radios and televisions, replacing walkers and side rails, and leaving bed curtains and doors the way they were found shows respect for the person's preferences.

Cultural Considerations

The importance of addressing cultural considerations in the assessment of psychosocial function has been recognized by the National Institute of Mental Health and the American Psychiatric Association in the fourth edition of the *Diagnostic and Statistical Manual of Mental Disorders,* or *DSM-IV* (see Culture Box). The inclusion of this information in the *DSM-IV* is expected to promote sensitivity to the relevance of race, culture, and minority status to psychiatric assessment (Perone, 1997).

Culturally Based Perceptions of Psychosocial Function

In assessing psychosocial function, nurses must consider how a person's cultural background may influence the way a person defines and perceives mental health and mental illness. Every society labels some behavior as abnormal. For older adults from diverse backgrounds, culture determines all of the following factors: definition of mental health and mental illness; belief about the causes of mental health and illness; expression of symptoms or clinical manifestations; criteria for labeling or diagnosing someone as mentally ill; decisions concerning appropriate healer(s); choice of treatment(s) to cure mental illness; determination that mental health has been restored following an illness episode; and relative degree of tolerance for abnormal behavior by other members of society. The Culture Box on p. 136 summarizes some culturally determined perspectives on mental health and mental illness.

Culture-Bound Syndromes

In some instances, older adults from diverse cultures may perceive or interpret physical symptoms and their interconnected psychological or emotional components in a manner that is unfamiliar to the nurse. When a disorder is unique to a particular culture and unrecognized as a

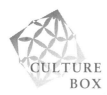

CULTURE
BOX

Cultural Perspectives and the *Diagnostic and Statistical Manual of Mental Disorders (DSM-IV)*

In a collaborative effort to ensure cultural validity and sensitivity of the diagnostic system, members of the National Institute of Mental Health and the American Psychiatric Association enhanced the *DSM-IV* to include information pertaining to culture and mental health in the following areas:

- discussion of cultural variations in the clinical manifestations of conditions listed in the DSM-IV
- description of culture-bound syndromes
- an outline for culture formation in which mental health providers describe the nature and extent of psychopathology from the vantage point of the patient's sociocultural reference group and personal experience.

Source: D. Perone (1997, September).

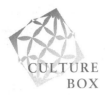

CULTURE
BOX

Cultural Perspectives and the Definitions and Causes of Mental Illness

Examples of Definitions of Mental Health Problems

- Hispanic older adults define mental health problems as alcohol and other drug abuse (American Association of Retired Persons, 1997).
- Filipino Americans consider forgetfulness and anger to be mental health problems (American Association of Retired Persons, 1997).

Examples of Beliefs About the Cause of Mental Disorders

- In traditional Chinese culture, many diseases are attributed to an imbalance of yin and yang, a concept of cosmic energy that few Western biomedical health care providers include in the assessment or treatment of older adults with mental disorders.
- Many Native American groups embrace a belief system in which balance and harmony are essential for mental and physical health.
- For some Hispanics, mental illness may be viewed as a punishment by a supreme being for past transgressions.
- Some African Americans, especially those of circum-Caribbean descent, may attribute the cause of mental illness to voodoo, sorcery, or other spiritual forces (Kavanagh, in press).
- Some European Americans believe that mental illness has physiologic origins related to chemical and/or genetic disturbances.

disease condition in the biomedical health care system, it is sometimes called a *culture-bound syndrome*. Culture-bound syndromes commonly are known to folk or indigenous healers who generally are knowledgeable about interventions and treatments aimed at curing the conditions. Older adults may be reluctant to discuss culture-bound syndromes or folk treatments during the course of a psychosocial assessment. The reasons for withholding such information are complex and may include fears that the nurse or other health care provider will disapprove, ridicule, or fail to understand their folk or indigenous healing system. It is sometimes reassuring to the older adult when the nurse interviewer asks permission to include folk or indigenous healers in the psychosocial assessment process. These healers frequently have considerable insight into the cultural and

psychosocial aspects of human behavior, and they may be remarkably successful in treating culture-bound syndromes and other disorders that have psychological and emotional clinical manifestations. Because herbal remedies that sometimes are used to treat culture-bound syndromes may interact with prescription or over-the-counter medications, nurses should make every effort to elicit information about such remedies during the assessment. In recognition of the relevance and importance of culture in the psychosocial and psychiatric assessment, the National Institute of Mental Health and the American Psychiatric Association have included information pertaining to culture-bound syndromes and cultural variations in clinical manifestations in *DSM-IV*. The Culture Box on p. 137 summarizes information about culture-bound syndromes.

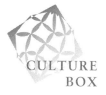

Culture-Bound Syndromes

Disorders that are restricted to a particular culture or group of cultures because of certain psychological characteristics are called *culture-bound syndromes.* Anthropologists have identified approximately 150 culture-bound syndromes.

Culture-bound syndromes are thought to be created by social, cultural, and personal reactions to malfunction in biologic or physiologic processes.

Examples of culture-bound syndromes include the following:

- Among some African Americans, a condition called *blackout* refers to collapse, dizziness, and an inability to move, usually after a person receives startling or unexpected news.
- Some European Americans, especially those from more affluent socioeconomic circumstances, experience *anorexia nervosa* (an excessive preoccupation with thinness and self-imposed starvation) or *bulimia* (gross overeating followed by vomiting or fasting).
- Some Native American groups experience *ghost,* a condition characterized by a sense of impending danger, terror, and hallucinations.

Source: M. M. Andrews, (1995), Transcultural nursing care, in M. M. Andrews & J. S. Boyle (Eds), *Transcultural concepts in nursing care* (pp. 79–81) (Philadelphia: J. B. Lippincott).

Mental Status Assessment

A mental status assessment is an organized approach to collecting data about a person's psychosocial function. This examination addresses the following indicators of psychosocial function: physical appearance, cognition, affect, perceptual-motor skills, insight and reasoning, contact with reality, and sociocultural supports. Mental status assessments are performed by various health care professionals, with each discipline specializing in various components. For example, psychiatrists are skilled in assessing affective and cognitive components, whereas social workers are skilled in assessing family relationship components. In the framework of this text, gerontological nurses assess various aspects of psychosocial function as they influence the day-to-day activities of older adults.

Although there are many formal assessment tools for geriatric use, a formal tool is not a requirement for a nursing psychosocial assessment. The forms that are widely used in geriatric settings, such as the Folstein Mini-Mental State Exam (also known as the MMSE), are limited in their scope, and their purpose is to screen for specific impairments, such as dementia, or to assess changes over time. Nurses may use these tools as a measure of some aspects of cognitive function, but they do not provide a broad perspective of psychosocial function. One discussion of the use of MMSE has emphasized the need for nursing assessment of related functional abilities when a cognitive impairment is detected through the use of this screening tool (Agostinelli et al., 1994).

In this text, the mental status assessment addresses all the aspects of psychosocial function that can be assessed by nurses and that are important to the overall assessment of older adults. This comprehensive overview can be likened to the emergency cart that is available in every hospital unit. The cart stands ready at all times and is equipped with any items that would be needed to handle medical emergencies. When a serious medical problem arises, the cart is quickly pulled to the patient's bedside and the health care professionals select the needed items. Similarly, gerontological nurses must have access to an array of skills for assessing psychosocial function as the need arises. In a few situations, their entire array of skills will be called into play, but in most situations, only a few of the examination tools will be necessary. Nurses can use the material in this chapter to "fill their mental status assessment carts" so they are prepared to select the appropriate tools for each situation.

Physical Appearance

Physical appearance is readily observed and reveals many aspects of psychosocial function. Clothing, grooming, cosmetics, and hygiene provide many clues to psychological function, but they are only clues, and questions must be asked before any conclusions can be drawn. For example, when assessing an older woman who has a body odor, poor hygiene, and tattered clothing, a nurse might ask questions about depression, incontinence, cognitive abilities, financial resources, overwhelming caregiving responsibilities, impaired vision or sense of smell, and access to and ability to use bathing facilities.

Other observations about personal appearance can precipitate a similar array of questions. For example, the person's weight, particularly a history of weight loss, may provide clues to depression, dementia, medical status, and environmental problems. Observations about how the person's clothing fits can provide clues to weight changes that might not be acknowledged by the person. For instance, nurses may gain important information about weight changes if they notice that many buckle holes have been punched in a belt to make it smaller. Of course, before any conclusions are drawn, it is important to find out if the belt originally belonged to that person. Observations such as this can

give the nurse a natural lead-in for a question such as "Your belt looks like it's pretty big for you now. Have you been losing weight?"

The nurse should note the person's apparent age, as well as cosmetic and grooming practices that influence the apparent age. Some questions that might arise from the observation that an 85-year-old woman dyes her hair include the following: Is this a reflection of positive or negative self-esteem? Does she want to appear younger than her age because she knows that old age is not as socially acceptable as youth? Does she want to deny her age because she associates old age with negative images? High-heeled shoes may also reflect a woman's self-image and her desire to avoid looking like an "old lady." This is an important assessment issue because high-heeled shoes may also be risk factors for falls and fractures.

Motor Function

Stooped posture may be a clue to depression, whereas erect posture may indicate positive self-esteem. If the gait is shuffling, staggering, or uncoordinated, this could indicate that the person has neurologic deficits secondary to a disease process or is experiencing adverse effects from alcohol or medications. Gait disturbances, as well as other abnormal movements, should be viewed as possible signs of tardive dyskinesia or extrapyramidal symptoms. Any evidence of tardive dyskinesia should raise the question of past or present use of psychotropic medications. This information is particularly useful in assessing people who deny having any psychiatric illness or who cannot give an accurate psychiatric history. In addition, observations about how the person navigates in the environment can provide clues to the individual's judgment and vision.

Body language and movement provide clues to affective illnesses and behavioral disturbances. Slouching and head-hanging, for example, are common manifestations of withdrawal and depression. Poor eye contact, especially looking at the floor, is indicative of either depression or the inability to answer questions. Cultural factors can influence the type and amount of eye contact that is considered to be appropriate. Depressed older adults frequently are very slow in their activities; if they are experiencing agitated depression, however, they may be excessively active. Repetitive body motions, especially of the extremities, could indicate anxiety, but these motions also can be manifestations of tardive dyskinesia. Agitation can be symptomatic of cognitive, affective, or other psychiatric disturbances, or it may be an adverse medication effect.

Social Skills

If the level of social skills is not considered, nurses may draw faulty conclusions about other aspects of psychosocial function. For example, friendly and cooperative people with good conversational skills may be able to hide their cognitive deficits, especially if they are motivated to perform well. By contrast, people with longstanding patterns of hostility, social isolation, inadequate social skills, and lack of ambition are less likely to be motivated to perform well and are more likely to be viewed as psychosocially impaired. Any of the following social skills may be used to obscure cognitive deficits: humor, evasiveness, leading the conversation, and making up answers to questions. Some older adults with dementia maintain very good social skills, even in the latter stages of dementia when other skills have declined long before. It is important to be aware of cultural differences in social skills and to consider the cultural context of the relationship between the interviewer and the interviewee.

Response to the Interview

The nurse should note the older adult's initial response to the interview, as well as changes in attitude that occur during the interview. In addition, nurses should assess the amount of effort expended in answering questions. Such observations are especially important when trying to differentiate between dementia and depressive pseudodementia, as cognitively impaired people may exert great effort in responding to questions. By contrast, depressed people often fail to answer correctly because they lack the energy or motivation. Two people may score the same on a formal mental status questionnaire, but one may miss the questions because of dementia and the other may miss them because of depression. When nurses suspect that lack of motivation is a reason for incorrect or missing answers, they might clarify this by asking, "Is it that you don't know the answers, or that you just don't feel like answering the questions?"

Confabulation, which involves making up information, can be used successfully when the interviewer does not know the correct information. For example, the accuracy of answers regarding one's place of birth or childhood experiences cannot always be determined. Therefore, these kinds of questions are not good indicators of mental status unless the accuracy of the answers can be confirmed. Circumstantiality, another cover-up technique, involves the use of excessive details and roundabout answers in responding to questions.

Hostility, resistance, and defensiveness also may be exhibited during an interview. Depressed people may be indifferent to the interview and may not want to expend the energy to answer the questions. Cognitively impaired people may be angry, hostile, or defensive, especially if they are trying to deny the deficits. People who have always been reclusive or suspicious may not be receptive to a mental status assessment and may refuse to answer the questions. Because any of these attitudes can interfere with responses to mental status questions, an accurate assessment of the underlying attitude is as important an indicator of psychological function as are the actual responses, or lack of responses, to questions.

Finally, the person's attitudes and responses must be considered in relation to their usual (baseline) personality traits. For example, highly sociable people might always use humor, whereas talkative people might naturally use circumstantiality. In people who are normally quiet and serious, the use of humor and circumstantiality might be indicative of a great effort to cover up cognitive deficits. On the other hand, people who are normally quiet and withdrawn may be perceived falsely as being depressed. Finding out about the usual personality of an individual is difficult; however, a question such as, "Would you describe what you were like when you were 40 years old?" might be asked. Information about lifelong personality characteristics also can be obtained from family members and caregivers who have known the person for a long time. Display 5-5 summarizes various considerations, relating to a person's general appearance and response to the interview, which may provide important clues to the individual's psychosocial function.

Orientation

Because orientation to person, place, and time is easy to measure, it is the indicator of mental status that is most frequently documented on patients'/residents' charts. Often it is inaccurately viewed as the primary indicator of cognitive function, rather than one small piece of a larger puzzle. This indicator, however, can be overused or used too simplistically to the point that more meaningful standards of mental status are ignored. For example, the following questions are considered to be the standards for determining orientation: "What is your name?"

DISPLAY 5-5
Guidelines for Assessing Some Indicators of Psychosocial Function

Observations to Assess Physical Appearance and Motor Function

- What is the person's apparent age in relation to his or her chronologic age?
- How do the following factors reflect psychological function: hygiene, grooming, clothing, cosmetics?
- Does the person's physical appearance provide clues to dementia or depression, or other impairments of psychosocial function?
- What do the person's gait, posture, and body language indicate about his or her psychological function?
- Is there any evidence of tardive dyskinesia or other adverse medication effects?
- How does the person maneuver in the environment, and what does this reflect regarding judgment, vision, and other skills?

Observations to Assess Social Skills and Response to the Interview

- What are the person's lifelong patterns of social skills, and how do these influence the assessment process?

- How do the person's social skills influence the interviewer's interpretation of other aspects of psychosocial function?
- Is the person motivated to answer questions?
- What is the person's attitude about the interview?
- If the person does not answer the questions, or gives incorrect answers, is it because of inability, cultural factors, or lack of motivation?
- Does the person use any of the following in an attempt to hide possible cognitive deficits: humor, sarcasm, avoidance, evasiveness, confabulation, circumstantiality, or leading the conversation?
- Does the person manifest any of the following characteristics: anger, hostility, resistance, defensiveness, or suspiciousness?
- Do the person's underlying attitudes reflect his or her usual personality, or are they manifestations of cognitive or affective disturbances?

"Where are you?" and "What time is it?" Based on whether each answer is correct or incorrect, the person is then labeled as "oriented times one," "oriented times two," or "oriented times three." The superficial use of orientation questions, especially in institutional settings, and the subsequent labeling of the patient/resident as oriented times one, two, or three, ignores several important considerations:

1. Are there cultural factors that influence orientation?
2. Does the person have medical problems that interfere with cognition?
3. Can the person name familiar people, such as a spouse or children?
4. Is the person taking medications that can influence mental function?
5. Are any environmental clues available to the person to orient them to the time or place?
6. How long has the person been at the institution (i.e., long enough to have learned the name of it)?
7. If the person cannot state the exact time, can they give the general time of day?
8. If the person cannot give specific names of other people, can they describe the correct role of the other person?
9. If the person cannot state the exact name of the facility, can they describe the type of facility it is or its general location?

A good assessment extends beyond the classical three questions and describes levels of orientation that are meaningful for the person in a particular setting. For example, the following description is far more useful than simply noting that the person is "oriented times one":

Mrs. S. could state her name, but she did not remember the name of this hospital. She could not give her daughter's name, but she was able to introduce her daughter to me, without stating her name. She thought the month was December because of the Chanukah decorations in her room. She could not state the time because she did not have her watch with her, but she thought it was afternoon because lunch had recently been served.

If the nurse had used only the standard questions of "What is your name?" "Where are you?" and "What time is it?" Mrs. S. would be judged to be "oriented times one." Most health care providers, after reading the results of that assessment, would have assumed that Mrs. S. had serious cognitive impairment, especially if she was 85 years of age or older. Mrs. S.'s actual responses, however, reflected various cognitive skills involved in organizing information, making associations, and using judgment. The more detailed description shows that Mrs. S. is probably a quite logical person who has not yet learned the name of the hospital and who might have some temporary memory impairment because of anxiety, medications, or acute medical problems.

Alertness

Along with orientation, level of alertness is the cognitive characteristic that is most frequently documented on patients'/residents' charts. Level of alertness is usually measured according to a continuum ranging from hyperalertness to stupor. The levels between these two extremes include drowsiness, somnolence, and intermittent alertness/drowsiness. One of the most important considerations in assessing alertness is the influence of medications, affective disorders, and pathologic conditions. Information about some of these influences might not be readily available, but the nurse should seek clues about probable underlying reasons for any alterations in alertness. For example, one of the possible adverse effects of a hypnotic with a long half-life might be daytime somnolence. Medications and chemical substances may be utilized primarily for their effects on alertness. For example, caffeine is a commonly used stimulant, and alcohol is sometimes used to diminish one's level of alertness. Undetected medical disturbances, such as electrolyte imbalances, may be manifested by drowsiness in their early stages, especially in older adults. As a practical consideration, people who are caregivers may be somnolent during the daytime because of nighttime caregiver responsibilities. Evidence of daytime somnolence raises many questions about potential causative factors. Therefore, if the person shows any sign of altered alertness, additional information must be obtained to identify potential causes, especially those that can be remedied through nursing measures.

Memory

Formal memory testing addresses memory from three perspectives: remote events, recent past events, and immediate memory, the last of which is further divided into retention, recall, and recognition. Examples of questions that can be used to assess each of these areas are listed in Display 5-6, which appears on page 143. Memory can be assessed during all conversations because all verbal communication depends to some degree on memory function. Using a functional approach, nurses assess memory by observing the person in daily activities and by interviewing older adults and their caregivers. The assessment is focused on activities that are important in daily life, such as remembering to pay bills, take medications, and shop for groceries. This assessment is made in relation to the expectations and demands of the person's usual environment. For example, if the person lives alone and manages finances independently, the ability to pay bills is quite important. By contrast, if the person lives with a daughter and her family, remembering the birth dates of grandchildren may be an important memory task.

Assessment of memory is especially challenging because although memory complaints are common among older adults, the complaints are not necessarily based on actual deficits in memory function. Thus, the question "Do you ever have trouble remembering things?" may elicit a positive response, but the response is likely to tell you more about the person's perception of memory than about his or her actual memory function. Although this question may be quite useful in identifying any concerns that the older adult might have, it is not very useful in assessing memory function. This is particularly true for older adults who deny the deficits or attempt to hide their memory difficulties.

In addition to assessing memory directly, the nurse can assess the person's use of memory aids by posing a question like, "Is there anything you do to help you remember appointments or other things?" Assessment of the extent to which the person depends on memory aids is useful in setting goals and planning for improved memory function. For example, if the person's memory function is barely adequate and is based heavily on memory aids, then the potential for further improvement is minimal. On the other hand, if the person has some memory deficits but does not use any memory aids, then the potential for improvement is increased. Observations about the use of memory aids may also provide clues to unacknowledged memory deficits. For example, if the person denies any problems with memory, but repeatedly refers to written notes during an interview, then it may be that their memory is quite impaired and they are compensating for the deficit. In this situation, the person is quite willing to use memory aids, but is unwilling to acknowledge the need for such aids. Display 5-6 summarizes guidelines for nursing assessment of orientation, alertness, and memory. Examples of direct questions are identified by quotation marks to distinguish them from other considerations.

Speech Characteristics

Speech patterns reflect the content and organization of thoughts and, therefore, provide important clues to psychological function. Because speech patterns can be assessed during any verbal interaction, formal assessment questions are not necessary as long as the nurse is alert to

DISPLAY 5-6
Guidelines for Assessing Orientation, Alertness, and Memory

Interview Questions to Assess Orientation

- *Person:* "What is your name?" "What is your wife's name?" If names can't be given, does the person understand roles?
- *Place:* "What is your address?" "What is the name of this place?" "What kind of place is this?" "What is the name of this city?" "What is the name of this state?"
- *Time:* "What time is it?" "What day of the week is today?" "What month and date is it today?" "What season is it?"

Observations to Assess Alertness

- What is the person's level of alertness on the following continuum: hyperalert, alert, drowsy, somnolent, stuporous?
- Does the person's level of alertness fluctuate? If so, is there any pattern to the fluctuations?
- Are there physiologic factors that might influence the person's level of alertness, such as medical conditions or effects of chemicals or medications?
- Are there psychosocial factors that might influence the person's level of alertness, such as anxiety, depression, nighttime caregiving responsibilities, or any other factor that might disrupt nighttime sleep?

Interview Questions to Assess Memory

- *Remote events:* "Where were you born?" "Where did you go to grade school?" "What was your first job?" "When were you married?"
- *Recent past events:* "Do you live with anyone?" "Do you have any grandchildren?" "What are the names of your grandchildren?" "When was the last time you went to the doctor?"
- *Immediate memory, retention:* State three unrelated facts and ask the person to repeat the information, both immediately and again after 5 minutes.
- *Immediate memory, general grasp and recall:* Ask the person to read a short story and then to summarize the information presented in the story.
- *Immediate memory, recognition:* Ask a multiple-choice question and then ask the person to choose the correct answer.

---

the information provided during conversations. Nurses should observe the following speech characteristics of the older adult: pace, quantity, quality, and coherency. Rapidly paced verbal communication may arise from anxiety, agitation, or mental illness. Slow-paced or excessively brief verbal communication may indicate depression, cognitive impairment, or simple cautiousness. Cultural factors also may influence speech characteristics.

The quality of a person's speech includes a variety of characteristics, such as tone, volume, and articulation. Tone of voice is one of the best indicators of indirectly expressed feelings, such as anger, hostility, and resentment. Abnormally low speech volume, called hypophonia, may be associated with depression, physical illness, low self-esteem, or long-standing speech habits. An abnormally loud volume may be indicative of

a hearing impairment or prolonged experience communicating with someone else who is hearing impaired. Poor articulation or slurred speech may be attributable to any of the following factors: ill-fitting dentures; lack of teeth or dentures; long-term hearing impairments; central nervous system impairments, including dementia; or the effects of alcohol or medications.

The ability to organize speech sounds into words and sentences requires many cognitive skills, and this ability may be impaired for a number of reasons. Errors in pronunciation, called phonemic errors, can arise from hearing impairments, cognitive deficits, or educational and cultural influences. Misinterpretation of the meaning of words, or semantic error, may result from cognitive deficits, but it may also be attributable to hearing impairments that interfere with the person's ability to hear words accurately. The use of neologisms, or self-created and meaningless words, usually occurs secondary to dementia or psychopathologic conditions; however, their use may be attributable to the repetition of a word that was not heard accurately in the first place. Some of the factors that can cause incoherent speech are dementia, aphasia, psychiatric disorders, and alcohol or medication effects.

Language skills are highly dependent on cultural, educational, and socioeconomic factors. Thus, it is important to consider these influences, especially when assessing foreign-born older adults. A good assessment of language skills not only provides clues to mental status, but it also helps the nurse identify words and language patterns that are most appropriate for use with the older person. In addition to being influenced by cognitive abilities, speech is influenced by physical factors, such as poorly fitting dentures or the lack of teeth or dentures. Other factors to consider as potential influences on verbal communication are dry mouth, impaired hearing, and neurologic disorders.

Perseveration and agnosia are manifestations of neurologic disturbances, such as dementia. *Perseveration* is a repetitive or stuttering pattern of verbal or written communication. For example, the affected person may begin speaking or writing a sentence and remain stuck on the first few words or letters. *Agnosia* refers to difficulty finding the correct words, or the inability to name objects accurately. People with only small deficits in word-finding ability may be able to give correct answers about familiar objects with simple names. The deficit may be more apparent, however, if the person is asked to name parts of an object, such as the buttonhole of a shirt.

Aphasia often is associated with strokes or vascular dementia, and it may be the only persistent neurologic deficit following a stroke. *Expressive aphasia* occurs when comprehension abilities are not affected but word retrieval or word-finding abilities are impaired. *Receptive aphasia* occurs when verbal and comprehension abilities are impaired but some language skills are retained. *Global aphasia*, or a combination of receptive and expressive aphasia, results from more extensive neurologic damage and is manifested in inconsistent and poorly controlled language skills.

Calculation and Higher Language Skills

Reading, writing, spelling, and arithmetic are calculation and higher language skills that are assessed as indicators of cognition. Psychometric tests rely heavily on measures of these skills to assess cognition. Nurses, however, have many opportunities to assess these skills informally to determine whether the older adult is able to perform daily activities. For an older adult who lives alone, an assessment of the ability to pay utility bills and use money to purchase groceries is more valuable than a measurement of mathematical skills using a psychometric test. Likewise, a person's ability to read a thermostat or the daily paper may be a more valid gauge of functional ability than a score on a formal reading test.

Written health education materials can be used to assess reading and comprehension skills informally, and they also have a practical purpose. For example, when collecting a clean voided urine sample from a patient/resident, the nurse can give the patient/resident a list of instructions and ask the person to read the instructions aloud. Observations of how well the person comprehends the instructions will provide an excellent assessment of the reading skills that are important in daily life. Another opportunity for assessing reading comprehension may arise if the nurse observes that an older adult has a newspaper nearby. A nonthreatening question, such as "What's new in the paper today?" can provide information about the person's interests in outside events and their ability to comprehend and remember written information.

Writing skills can be observed when older adults are asked to sign their names, such as on permission forms. A more complex task involves helping the older adult compile a written medication list or a list of questions to discuss with the primary care provider. Difficulty with writing skills is a common sign of early stages of dementia. Of all the higher language skills, spelling is the least important in terms of the daily function of most older adults, but it is a good indicator of changes in mental abilities. As with the assessment of other cognitive skills, the person's education, occupation, and other influencing factors must be considered.

With traditional psychometric testing, calculation is measured with the "serial sevens" test. That is, the person is asked to subtract seven from 100 and to continue subtracting sevens. This test depends on education, and it is not necessarily the most appropriate test for older adults. It may be more appropriate to ask the older person to add three plus three, and to continue adding threes. Older adults who are depressed may not answer correctly because they do not want to expend the energy to calculate serial sevens. Older adults who have a dementing illness may be able to perform well on this task if they try hard and if they previously had highly developed mathematical skills. From the point of view of the functional approach, performance on formal tests is not as important as performance in daily activities. If people can manage money to meet their daily needs, then their ability to subtract seven from one hundred is not important, except as one small indicator of cognitive abilities.

Decision Making

Decision making, one of the most important and complex of all cognitive abilities, involves insight, learning, memory, reasoning, judgment, problem solving, and abstract thinking. Abstract thinking is often one of the earliest skills to be affected by a dementing illness, but it is also one of the most difficult aspects to assess because it is strongly influenced by other factors, such as education and affective state. People who are very anxious or depressed may lack the attention or motivation required to respond to the questions typically used for the assessment of abstract thinking patterns. Similarity questions, such as "How are apples and oranges alike?" are used to assess the person's ability to think abstractly. Asking someone to explain the meaning of a saying, such as "People who live in glass houses shouldn't throw stones," is another way to assess the person's level of abstract thinking. In recent years, questions have been raised about the use of these traditional tests with older adults. Studies have found that older adults perform poorly when tests use highly abstract examples, but that their performance improves when tests use concrete examples (Botwinick, 1984).

During the course of an interview, opportunities for assessing abstract thinking may arise, and the nurse can listen for clues to the person's level of abstract, versus concrete, thinking. The following exchange is an example of an unsolicited opportunity this author had to assess one older adult's concrete thinking pattern:

> *Nurse:* How did you feel about having to move from your home in Texas to live with your daughter and her family here in Ohio?
> *Mr. L.:* I don't know, how would you feel?
> *Nurse:* I'm not sure how I'd feel, that's never happened to me. I'm not in your shoes.
> *Mr. L.:* Well, here, put them on [stated emphatically while taking off his shoes to give to the nurse].

One interpretation of Mr. L's response is that his thinking pattern is very concrete, rather than abstract.

Nurses can assess problem-solving abilities through observation. For instance, the nurse can observe the way older adults use call lights to meet their needs when confined to bed, or the way they engage in the complex decisions related to discharge planning. Within the functional approach framework, assessment of problem solving is based on the needs of an individual in a particular situation. For example, a most important problem-solving task for an older adult who lives alone may be meeting basic safety needs. Therefore, a question such as "What would you do if you woke up at night and smelled smoke?" might be an appropriate way of assessing judgment related to safety. For an older adult who lives in a nursing home, a most important but complex problem-solving task may involve dealing with a roommate who is disruptive. In this situation, the answer to a question such as "What would you do if your roommate started taking your belongings?" might provide the most pertinent information for assessing problem-solving skills.

Assessment of judgment can be based on various observations, such as the following: Does the person pay bills on time? Does the person have enough food in the house? What resources does the person use in dealing with illness? Are the person's clothing and grooming appropriate for the situation? Does the person use memory aids to compensate for any deficits? Does the person know how to find phone numbers when help is needed? Can the person prepare food, or use resources such as a home-delivered meals program, to meet nutritional needs?

Insight is the ability to understand the significance of the present situation. This skill is a component of the problem-solving process, as it establishes a basis for planning care. Perhaps more than any other cognitive skill, insight is influenced by feelings and other psychosocial factors. Denial is a defense mechanism that is often used to protect oneself from unpleasant realities; the stronger the denial, the more limited the insight. For example, if the person refuses to acknowledge that a condition exists, the person will not be able to plan interventions. The most important aspects of insight to be assessed by nurses are those areas of function that are the focus of the nurse's care plan and interventions. For example, in assessing the insight of an older adult who has been brought to the hospital for assessment of malnutrition and uncontrolled hypertension, the nurse may ask questions, such as the following: What's the reason your daughter brought you to the hospital? How do you manage with grocery shopping and getting your meals? Do you take any medications? What are the medications for? What kinds of things does your daughter do for you? Answers to questions such as these allow the nurse to assess the person's understanding of the present situation, and they provide a basis for planning care.

When answers to questions indicate that the person has little or no insight, the nurse should try to identify the factors that interfere with insight. In the example just described, insight may be absent or limited because of feelings of depression and hopelessness, lack of information about the medication regimen, denial of a reality that is too threatening, inability to remember information, or fear of losing independence. Before the nurse can begin discharge planning, both the level of insight and the factors that interfere with insight must be identified. In addition, the nurse must attempt to identify factors that may improve the insight. For example, if insight is lacking because of denial that stems from exaggerated fears, then alleviating the fears may facilitate insight. Display 5-7 summarizes the considerations that are important in assessing speech characteristics, calculation and higher language skills, and decision-making skills. Examples of direct questions are identified by quotation marks to distinguish these from other considerations and observations.

Affective Function

Affective function refers to a person's mood, emotions, and expressions of emotions. Happiness and sadness are the feelings most commonly associated with affective states, but all of the following have been identified as primary affects: joy, awe, fear, pain, rage, guilt, shame, anger, hatred, surprise, interest, confusion, jealousy, elation, depression, suspicion, anxiety, bewilderment, amorousness, and lack of feelings.

DISPLAY 5-7
Guidelines for Assessing Speech, Calculation and Higher Language Skills, and Decision-Making Skills

Observations to Assess Speech Characteristics

- Is the pace of speech normal, slow, or fast?
- Is the tone of voice suggestive of underlying feelings, such as anger, hostility, or resentment?
- Is the volume abnormally soft or loud?
- Do the sentences flow coherently and smoothly?
- Is there evidence of any problem with integrating speech sounds into words (e.g., neologisms, or phonemic or semantic errors)?
- Do any of the following factors affect the person's speech: dry mouth, poorly fitting dentures, absence of teeth or dentures, alcohol or medication effects, or neurologic or other pathologic processes?
- Does the person exhibit any of the following: agnosia; perseveration; or expressive, receptive, or global aphasia?

Observations to Assess Calculation and Higher Language Skills

- What is the person's ability to comprehend written materials encountered in the course of routine activities, such as the daily newspaper or instructions for medications?
- What is the quality of the person's handwriting (e.g., his or her signature)?
- Is the person able to perform mathematical computations necessary for daily activities?

Interview Questions to Assess Decision-Making Skills

- *Abstract versus concrete thinking:* "How are apples and oranges alike?"
- *Reasoning and judgment:* "What would you do if you woke up in the middle of the night and smelled smoke?" "If you received $100 as a gift, how would you spend it?"
- *Insight:* "What's the reason for your hospitalization?" "What kind of help do you think you might need when you leave the hospital?"

Self-esteem usually is not listed as a primary affect; rather, it is defined as the feelings one holds about oneself.

The components of affective state that are reviewed in this section are general mood, anxiety, self-esteem, depression, and happiness. These five aspects were selected for the following reasons:

1. An assessment of general mood assists the nurse in determining appropriate goals based on the person's usual affective state.
2. Anxiety is a common factor in older adults that can often be alleviated or minimized through nursing interventions.
3. Self-esteem is a major determinant of feelings, especially depression and happiness.
4. Self-esteem is a particularly important affective consideration for older adults because

old age and its accompanying problems can present many threats to self-esteem.
5. Depression and happiness are two primary affects that have been the target of much of the research regarding affective states in older people.
6. Nursing interventions can be directed toward all of these affective components to improve the quality of life of older adults.

Before discussing these five emotions in relation to older adults, a review of the general guidelines for assessing affective function is warranted.

Guidelines for Assessing Affective Function

Affect is assessed both quantitatively and qualitatively in relation to certain expectations. For example, people are expected to show some expression of sadness when talking about sad events. When the quality of expressed feelings is not consistent with the external event, the affect is considered to be inappropriate. The quantity of affect also is assessed in relation to the personal meaning and the nearness in time of an event. People are expected to show greater feelings of sadness in response to tragic news than in response to neutral events. Likewise, people are expected to show a deeper affective response soon after experiencing a sad event than they would years after the event occurred.

Therefore, in assessing affect, it is important to assess the meaning of events for the person. The depth and duration of affect, which are important considerations in differentiating between dementia and depressive pseudodementia in older adults, also are assessed. The affect of depressed people generally is sad and negativistic and is not influenced by external circumstances. By contrast, the affect of people who are demented fluctuates more, and it changes in response to distractions. Emotional lability is a characteristic of vascular dementia that is often seen in people who have had strokes.

Nonverbal behaviors provide a wealth of useful information about a person's affective state. Anxiety, happiness, and sadness are readily manifested in observable behaviors. During a mental status assessment, nonverbal behaviors provide information that might not be offered directly. For example, despite the fact that a person might deny feeling sad, he or she may exhibit the following nonverbal cues: crying, slouching over, looking at the ground, and having a mournful facial expression. The nurse can use this information as the basis for a leading comment, such as "You look like you're feeling sad."

Expressions of emotions are strongly determined by cultural norms and personality characteristics. In most Western societies, crying is more acceptable for women and children than for men and older boys, and showing anger and rage is more acceptable for men than for women.

Cultural expectations also influence the way a person expresses feelings in certain circumstances. For example, a person may be expected to cry and loudly proclaim mournful feelings at a funeral, but may be prohibited from expressing any feelings in front of strangers or in a public place, such as a hospital. Because certain emotions, such as anger or depression, are viewed as less acceptable than others, such as happiness, people learn to deny and hide some feelings. Older adults, especially, may have learned that certain feelings should not be expressed directly or verbally. Thus, it is especially important to observe for any indirect or nonverbal clues of anger, depression, and other less socially acceptable feelings.

In assessing the affective state of older adults, it is important to consider acceptable terminology. Many people will not admit to feeling depressed because they associate this term with a serious mental illness or with a socially unacceptable state. Likewise, feelings of anxiety often are considered to be socially unacceptable. Therefore, the nurse should begin the assessment of affective state by focusing on feelings that are viewed positively or neutrally. If the person initiates the topic of feeling anxious or depressed, the nurse can respond to those feelings and pursue a related line of questioning. In most circumstances, however, it is best to begin with open-ended questions. A simple question, such as "How are you feeling today?" when asked with sincerity, is a familiar and comfortable way of eliciting information.

Mood

Mood is closely associated with emotions, but mood can be distinguished from emotions in that it is more pervasive, less intense, and longer lasting. People are usually quite comfortable describing their mood as either bad or good, and they are more likely to refer to their mood than their emotions. Thus, during a mental status examination, a question, such as "How would you describe your usual mood?" may be perceived as less threatening than the question, "How do you feel most of the time?" Nonverbal behaviors provide many clues about a person's mood and may be more accurate than verbal responses as an indicator of affective state. Joy, anger, anxiety, sadness, happiness, and depression are examples of moods that are expressed in nonverbal behaviors in everyday life by most people.

Anxiety

Anxiety is defined as a feeling of distress, subjectively experienced as fear or worry and objectively expressed through autonomic and central nervous system responses. Anxiety is beneficial when it motivates protective behaviors, but it is detrimental when it channels personal energy into defensive behaviors. The degree of anxiety influences its effects, with extreme levels having detrimental effects and moderate levels having beneficial effects. Therefore, it is important to assess the degree of anxiety and the extent to which the anxiety is beneficial or detrimental.

In assessing anxiety, nurses must identify the terminology that is most acceptable to the older adult. Words like "worries" and "concerns" are readily understood and usually elicit responses about sources of anxiety. One study found that older people were more likely to define stressors in terms of "concern" rather than "problems" (Aldwin et al., 1996). Older adults often use the phrases "nerve trouble" or "trouble with my nerves" in reference to anxiety states. Asking questions, such as "Do you ever have nerve trouble?" or "What kinds of things give you trouble with your nerves?" may elicit a response filled with information about sources of anxiety.

Observations of nonverbal manifestations of anxiety can supplement the information obtained from verbal communication. In any adult, anxiety may be manifested in the following nonverbal ways: pacing, shakiness, restlessness, irritability, fidgeting, diaphoresis, tachycardia, hyperventilation, dry mouth, voice changes, smoking habits, urinary frequency, increased muscle tension, poor eye contact, poor attention span, inability to sit still, changes in eating patterns, rapid or disconnected speech, or repetitive motions of facial muscles or any extremities. Although any of these indicators may be observed in older adults, the presence of mobility limitations or pathologic conditions can interfere with some of the typical nonverbal signs. For example, older adults who are confined to bed cannot pace, but they may experience subtle changes in eating or sleeping patterns because of anxiety. Any of the following complaints about physical discomfort may be indirect indicators of anxiety: pain, fatigue, anorexia, insomnia, or stomach distress.

In addition to assessing the level of anxiety, the nurse should attempt to identify the sources of anxiety. Anxiety is considered to be a normal response to real or perceived threats in any of the following areas: health, assets, values, environment, self-concept, role function, needs fulfillment, goal achievement, personal relationships, and sense of security. Anxiety also can arise from unconscious conflicts, maturational crises, or developmental challenges. Also, older adults may experience anxiety because of fears of becoming a victim of crime or elder abuse (Thomae, 1991). When all of these potential sources of anxiety are considered, it would be logical to conclude that older adults tend to be more anxious than younger adults. Studies on anxiety and aging, however, have failed to show any age-related increase in anxiety (Blazer, 1998). Theories of stress, coping, and older adulthood suggest that older adults may be less anxious because they have acquired more effective coping mechanisms through experience.

Anxiety is always a response to real or perceived threats, but the source of anxiety is not always readily identified. Even when people recognize the source of anxiety, they are not always willing to talk about their fears, or they may refer to the threat only indirectly. The more threatening the fear, the more difficult it will be to identify or acknowledge the source of anxiety. For example, an older adult may have the perception that other people have the power to "put him away" in a nursing home simply because of a slight memory impairment. If the person knows other older adults who have been admitted unwillingly to a nursing home, this fear may be exacerbated. Further anxiety might arise from the person's fear of discussing the subject because of the perception that initiating the topic might precipitate actions leading to nursing home admission. Rather than directly talking about the fears, the person might provide vague clues, such as by stating, "I felt so sorry for Mildred when her son put her in the nursing home."

Fear of crime is a significant source of anxiety for about 25% of older adults. A recent nursing article emphasized the importance of including an assessment of the older adult's fear of crime as a component of comprehensive nursing care (Benson, 1997). Benson's review of the literature revealed that fear of crime was associated with the following factors: being female or a frail male, having a low socioeconomic status, and living alone in urban, high-crime areas. Social isolation, impaired function, and diminished quality of life are some of the potential health consequences for older adults who are fearful of becoming a victim of crime.

Interview questions aimed at identifying sources of anxiety must be phrased in the least threatening way. When older adults express feelings about other older people, the nurse can respond with questions aimed at determining whether they have the same worries about themselves. For example, in response to the statement "I felt so sorry for Mildred," the nurse might ask, "Do you ever worry that you'll have to go to a nursing home?" Open-ended questions that allow for a wide range of answers can be used to identify sources of anxiety that might not otherwise be revealed. For example, nurses in institutional settings can ask, "What is your biggest worry about going home?" or "Do you have any worries about how you'll manage at home after you leave here?" In home settings, the nurse might ask an even broader question, such as "Do you have any concerns about the future?" or "What kinds of things do you worry about?" Answers to these questions usually are filled with clues to sources of anxiety and provide a basis for many additional questions.

Anxiety can be precipitated or exacerbated by physiologic conditions arising from disease processes or adverse chemical effects. Therefore, obtaining information about medical conditions, as well as about the person's use of herbs, caffeine, and medications, is an essential component of the assessment of anxiety. Pathologic processes that diminish cerebral oxygen, such as pulmonary or cardiovascular diseases, can be manifested as anxiety. In older adults, endocrine disorders, such as hyperthyroidism, may be manifested primarily by anxiety or other psychosocial symptoms. People with dementia may show signs of excessive anxiety when they are experiencing pain or physical discomfort, especially if their verbal communication skills are impaired. Pacing is a commonly observed manifestation of anxiety in ambulatory older adults who have dementia.

Chemicals or medications that stimulate the central nervous system or act on the autonomic nervous system may precipitate or exacerbate anxiety. Akathisia is an extrapyramidal effect of some neuroleptic medications that may subjectively or objectively be interpreted as anxiety. *Akathisia* is defined as an inner sense of restlessness that is worsened by inactivity and is manifested by motor restlessness. It can occur early or late in the course of treatment with psychotropic medications. Akathisia is a frequently reported extrapyramidal symptom, and it is more common in women and older people. Therefore, if an older adult who is taking neuroleptic medications complains of certain feelings, such as "shaking on the inside," the possibility of adverse medication effects must be considered as a cause.

In addition to identifying sources and manifestations of anxiety, it is important to identify acceptable methods for reducing anxiety. Even if the sources of anxiety are not identified or cannot be changed, the experience of anxiety can be addressed. To this end, questions should be asked about usual coping methods. Questions, such as "What do you do when you have trouble with your nerves?" or "What do you find helpful when your nerves are bad?", may initiate a problem-solving process aimed at helping the person cope with the anxiety. If the person does not respond with concrete suggestions, the nurse can offer suggestions in a nonjudgmental way and assess the person's response to these suggestions. For example, any of the following questions can be asked: "Does it help to talk to someone about your worries?" "Have you ever tried any relaxation methods when you're nervous?" "Do you find that taking a walk outside helps you when your nerves are bad?" Incorporating questions such as these in the assessment sets the stage for planning interventions.

Self-Esteem

In much of the literature on mental health and aging, self-esteem is cited as one of the characteristics most highly associated with both depression and happiness. One landmark study refers to self-esteem as "the linchpin of quality of life for the aged" (Schwartz, 1975, p. 470). The nursing literature echoes this assertion, as evidenced by the following statement: "If we, as nurses, can enhance only one aspect of our clients' mental health, we should strive to enhance their self-esteem" (Whall, 1987).

Self-esteem is defined as the feelings one has about one's self, or the extent to which one perceives oneself to be worthy or significant. It is the emotional aspect of self-concept, and it is based on one's perceptions of other people's opinions about oneself. Because self-esteem depends on the opinions held by others, and because industrialized societies generally hold negative opinions about old age, it is logical to conclude that the self-esteem of older adults may be lower than that of younger adults. Rather than supporting this deduction, most studies have found that self-esteem increases throughout adulthood, beginning in adolescence (Giarrusso and Bengtson, 1996). One study found that subjects aged 65 years and older experienced heightened self-esteem compared to younger subjects (Dietz, 1996). This conclusion about the self-esteem of older adults is encouraging, but it does not negate the importance of assessing and enhancing self-esteem in older adults. It is cited to emphasize the underlying strength of older adults and the importance of interventions to maintain and promote self-esteem. A recent longitudinal study found that positive attitudes about aging emerged as the best predictor of maintained self-esteem over a 13-year period (Coleman et al., 1993). Thus, nursing interventions that promote positive attitudes about aging may enhance the self-esteem of older adults.

Nurses often make judgments about self-esteem, describing it as low or high, good or bad, positive or negative. Unlike high or low blood pressure, however, self-esteem cannot be measured numerically with standard equipment. Judgments about self-esteem are based on a compilation of verbal and nonverbal indicators of how a person views himself or herself. Verbal cues about self-esteem are revealed in self-initiated statements, such as "You're wasting your time on me, you have more important things to do." Nonverbal indicators of self-esteem include the way people dress, care for themselves, and present themselves to others.

Although caution must be employed in interpreting behaviors in relation to self-esteem, the following behaviors may be associated with low self-esteem: rigidity, procrastination, unnecessary apologies, lack of confidence, expectations of failure, exaggeration of deficits, disappointment in self, self-destructive behaviors, constant approval-seeking, overemphasis on weaknesses, inability to accept compliments, minimizing of one's abilities, disregard for one's own opinions, inability to form close relationships, inability to accept help from others, and inability to say no when appropriate. In most situations, nurses do not ask formal questions to assess self-esteem, but they note the many behaviors that may reflect self-esteem. It may be appropriate to ask some questions, however, especially about the person's perception of positive qualities. For example, a question, such as "What is the quality in yourself that other people admire the most?", is nonthreatening and is aimed at helping the person identify strengths. The answer can provide valuable information about self-esteem, especially if the person offers an answer such as, "I can't think of anything."

In addition to identifying whether the older adult has high or low self-esteem, the assessment of self-esteem is aimed at identifying actual and potential threats to self-esteem. This is especially important when older adults are admitted to institutional settings, as nurses may be able to identify environmental or other factors that can quickly and easily be modified to minimize or eliminate a threat to self-esteem. For example, in some institutional settings, staff members are accustomed to addressing residents or patients by their first names because they believe that this helps to establish a comfortable atmosphere. Some older people, however, may be insulted if they are addressed by any name other than their formal name. If, during the admission interview, the nurse asks the older adult about his or her preferences in this matter and explains the usual procedure in the institution, a potential threat to self-esteem may be averted.

Another potential threat to self-esteem that may be addressed during an admission interview concerns the issue of what the person needs to maintain independence. For example, for the person with mobility or sensory limitations, the provision of good lighting and the assurance that assistive devices will be accessible may be the most important means of preserving self-esteem. For other people, a factor as simple as having a choice about food might be important to self-esteem. The assessment of such factors can most readily be accomplished by asking open-ended questions, such as "Is there anything that we can do to help you manage better while you're here?" or "Is there anything you're worried about that I can help you with?" If the person has already identified potential threats to self-esteem, this question will provide an opportunity to discuss the threat and to plan interventions.

Because self-esteem is influenced by the person's perception of the opinions held by significant others, it is important to identify who the significant others are for any particular person. Studies have identified the following categories of significant others who influence the self-esteem of adults: spouse or partner; peers (especially for men); authority figures (especially for women); people with whom one lives; and people in the work, church, and social environments (Meisenhelder, 1985). Studies have also shown that the self-concept of nursing home residents gradually becomes increasingly similar to the views held by the staff (Kahana and Coe, 1969). For older adults, therefore, the nurse may assume several of the roles of a significant other, especially if the older adult has few or no significant others outside the facility. Culture often defines who is the significant other. Some Chinese American older adults, for example, expect their oldest son to look after their affairs and make key decisions about their health and well-being. Widows in some Middle Eastern and African cultures expect one of their husband's brothers to take care of them, a system that fosters social and economic security for women who have lost a spouse. Being cared for by a family member (rather than by strangers) enhances self-esteem for older adults from all cultural backgrounds and increases the likelihood that their needs will be met as they age.

In addition to the influence of significant others, self-esteem is affected by one's perceptions of the effect one exerts on the environment. Therefore, the environment also must be assessed for sources of threats to self-esteem, especially in long-term care settings in which older adults view the institution as their home but have little control over the environment. A study of various determinants of self-esteem in older people residing in a nursing home revealed that the environment had a more negative impact on residents who had comparatively few outside sources of self-esteem (Coleman, 1984). Environmental factors that can influence self-esteem include decor, social roles, perceived control, social interactions, architectural design, amount of space and privacy, and the extent to which the environment impedes or promotes an individual's ability to function. Health status, particularly with regard to functional abilities, is another factor that strongly correlates with self-esteem. The results of one study indicated that older adults with the lowest self-esteem are those who have poor health, the greatest degree of disability, and the greatest amount of daily pain (Hunter et al., 1981–1982).

For dependent older adults, the negative impact of disability and functional impairments on self-esteem is heightened by caregiver attitudes of infantalization. Such attitudes may be reflected in remarks by caregivers, such as "He acts just like a baby" or "Now, now, dear, let's be a good girl." Infantalization also may be reflected in the use of diapers for incontinence, especially when used solely for the caregiver's convenience. Another threat to self-esteem arises when caregivers promote unnecessary dependence for their own convenience. For example, telling a bedridden person to wet the bed because it is easier to change the disposable bed pad than to assist with toileting is a tremendous blow to the person's self-esteem.

Depression

Like other indicators of affective state, depression is assessed by examining both verbal and nonverbal cues. Blunt questions such as "Are you depressed?" are usually not effective in eliciting information because most people are reluctant to admit that they are depressed. Because depression is commonly associated with states of overwhelming grief, the use of more neutral terms, like "sad" or "blue," or a phrase such as "down in the dumps," to describe an older adult's affective state may meet with greater acceptance. Therefore, unless the older adult uses the term depressed to describe his or her feelings, other terminology is more likely to elicit an accurate response. As with other aspects of the mental status assessment, it is best to start with open-ended questions, such as "How are you feeling right now?" or "How do you feel most of the time?"

One of the purposes of an assessment of depression is to identify the person's usual patterns of coping with losses. For this reason, the nurse should encourage older adults to express their feelings about significant changes in their lives. For instance, if the older adult initiates a discussion of certain losses, the nurse might ask open-ended questions about the loss. Examples of nonthreatening questions that might lead to a discussion of feelings include: "What's it like to live alone after 50 years of being married?" "How is life different since your friend moved away?" "Are there people you miss seeing since you retired?" Questions like these can be asked easily once the person has given information about a change that might be experienced as a loss. If the open-ended questions do not elicit information about feelings, the nurse can comment on specific feelings that the person is likely to be experiencing. For example, a remark such as, "It seems like it would be pretty sad and lonely being here all by yourself after 55 years of marriage" allows the person to agree or disagree with, or offer an alternative to, the suggested feelings. Be aware that, for older adults from some Asian, Native American, and other cultures, it may be considered inappropriate to express one's emotions overtly or to discuss them with a stranger.

A psychosocial assessment considers the meaning of events for each person, even for events that occurred many years before the interview. A question such as "What kind of work did you do?" can easily lead to a discussion of feelings about retirement. Changes in living arrangements also can precipitate feelings of loss. A nonthreatening question, such as "How long have you lived here?" might lead to further discussion of the meaning of the living arrangement for that person. A question such as "Do you ever think about moving from this house?" encourages a discussion of concerns about living arrangements. People who have experienced the loss of a pet may be reluctant to acknowledge the depth of their feelings. When an older person asks the nurse a question, such as "Do you have a dog?", he or she may be indirectly testing the nurse's feelings about pets. The astute nurse will use this opportunity to explore the person's feelings about the subject, perhaps responding, "No, but I have a cat. Have you ever had any pets?" Pets may be especially significant for older adults, and, indeed, may be the only meaningful relationships that remain in their life. In planning for hospital admissions and long-term care arrangements, consideration also must be given to the person's responsibilities for and relationship with pets. Therefore, even if the person does not initiate the topic, at least one question about pets should be included in the psychosocial assessment of older adults.

Perhaps more than any other adjustment of older adulthood, the adjustment to medical problems and functional limitations is the most difficult. People usually are very receptive to discussing concerns about their health with a nurse because they view the nurse as someone who possesses knowledge about health problems and is committed to helping people deal with these problems. Nurses readily discuss identified medical problems, like diabetes and hypertension, and these problems cannot be overlooked in the assessment. For the purposes of the psychosocial assessment, however, it is important to assess the meaning of medical conditions for the person, as well as the meaning of more subtle changes that do not have a medical label but are often more significant to the person. For example, older adults with diabetes are probably less interested in knowing how the pancreas functions than they are about learning to cope with the attendant visual impairment or their fear of increasing dependence on others.

Therefore, rather than focusing the assessment on medically labeled problems, the nurse should begin with open-ended questions about the person's self-perceptions of health and function. Rather than asking specifically about the identified problem of diabetes, the nurse might begin with a question such as "If you had to rate your health on a scale of 0% to 100%, what rating would you give it today?" After the person responds to this question, the nurse might ask additional questions, such as "What would have to be changed for you to feel 100% healthy?" or "What rating would you have given yourself a year ago?" Answers to these questions can assist the nurse in establishing realistic goals for interventions.

Happiness and Life Satisfaction

In studies of happiness in relation to aging, happiness has been called morale, contentment, well-being, life satisfaction, successful aging, and "the good life." These terms are used interchangeably to describe subjective perceptions of one's quality of life. Happiness is distinguished from life satisfaction in that happiness is an affective quality, whereas satisfaction is a cognitive quality. These terms have also been differentiated in relation to time, with happiness being defined as a current and relatively temporary feeling, life satisfaction as contentment with life up to the present, and morale as a future-oriented optimism or pessimism (Mannell and Dupuis, 1996). Important components of happiness and life satisfaction include good health, positive self-evaluation, adequate external gratifications, and someone to be with and confide in.

Based on these definitions of happiness and well-being, it is clear that an assessment of the older person's functional abilities, personal relationships, and socioeconomic resources is an essential component of a psychosocial assessment. Psychologists sometimes use the following question to assess happiness: "Taking all things together, how would you say things are today—would you say you're very happy, pretty happy, or not too happy these days?" Asking the person to rate their happiness is an effective way of eliciting information, and the answer can provide a basis for further discussion. A question similar to the question about health can be used: "If you had to rate your present level of happiness on a scale of 0% to 100%, what rating would you give it?" Based on the response to this question, additional questions could be asked: "What would have to change to increase the rating by 10%?" "What kinds of things interfere with your happiness?" "If you could change one thing to be happier, what would it be?" Older adults usually will respond to these questions in a realistic manner, and their answers will provide information for establishing appropriate goals. Display 5-8 summarizes the considerations involved in assessing affective function in older adults. Questions that can be asked are indicated with quotation marks; other questions are observations and considerations.

Contact with Reality

Although a certain amount of fantasy is acceptable, people are expected to remain in contact with the world around them and to respond appropriately to the same realities that others perceive. People who deviate from this norm to a notable degree are labeled as "nuts" or "crazy" or are described as "off their rockers" or "a little bit touched in the head." People lose contact with reality for numerous reasons, ranging from serious schizophrenic disturbances to a transient denial of a threatening reality. Many causes of loss of contact with reality are amenable to interventions, and older adults are just as likely as younger adults to have a treatable reason for any disturbance in their contact with reality. It is important to recognize that perceptions of reality are highly influenced by cultural factors, as discussed in the next section.

When older people lose their contact with reality, however, a different set of labels may be applied to them. They may be viewed as "senile" or they may be faced with the attitude of "it's what you'd expect at the age of 84." Families may explain the behavior of an older person as "always a little eccentric, but a little more so now." Because of stereotypes about older people, as well as the broad array of potential causes for loss of contact with reality, the assessment of an older person's contact with reality is an especially challenging aspect of the psychosocial evaluation.

The primary goal of the nursing assessment of disturbances in contact with reality is to identify any underlying causes that can be alleviated. Another goal is to plan interventions for the management of disturbing behaviors that arise from untreatable conditions. Based on these assessment goals, this section on assessment addresses delusions and hallucinations in terms of the characteristics that are likely to be associated with specific underlying disorders. Before the

DISPLAY 5-8
Guidelines for Assessing Affective Function

General Affective Function

- Are the quantity and quality of emotions appropriate for the objective reality?
- What is the depth and duration of emotions regarding a particular event?
- What are the nonverbal cues to the person's affective state?
- How do sociocultural or environmental factors influence the person's expression of emotions?
- What terminology is acceptable to this person, especially with regard to feelings, such as anger, anxiety, and depression?
- Does the person have any pets, or have they lost any pets?

Observations/Questions to Assess Mood

- What is the person's usual affective state?
- What are the nonverbal indicators of the person's mood?

Observations/Questions to Assess Anxiety

- What are the nonverbal indicators of anxiety?
- What real or perceived threats are present that might be sources of anxiety for the person?
- Might any of the following factors be contributing to the person's anxiety: caffeine, pathologic conditions, medications, herbs, or interventions by folk or indigenous healers that act on the central or autonomic nervous systems?
- What methods of coping has the person tried, and what have been the effects of these interventions?
- "What kinds of things do you worry about?"
- "Do you have any worries that you'd be willing to discuss with me?"
- "Do you ever have trouble with your nerves?"

Observations/Questions to Assess Self-Esteem

- What verbal and nonverbal clues to self-esteem can be detected?
- What are the factors that influence self-esteem for this person?
- Does the environment present any real or potential threats to self-esteem?
- How are my actions as a nurse influencing the self-esteem of the older adults to whom I relate?
- Are caregiver attitudes, such as infantalization or the promotion of unnecessary dependence, influencing the person's self-esteem?

Observations/Questions to Assess Depression

- What are the verbal and nonverbal clues to depression?
- "Do you ever feel blue or down in the dumps?"
- "How has your life changed since your husband died?"
- "What do you miss the most since you moved from your family home?"

Observations/Questions to Assess Happiness and Life Satisfaction

- How is the person's happiness and life satisfaction influenced by the following: functional abilities, personal relationships, and socioeconomic resources?
- "On a scale of 0% to 100%, how happy would you say you are right now?"
- "If you could change one thing to increase your happiness rating, what would it be?"

discussion of delusions and hallucinations, however, denial of reality, in addition to the general principles of assessment of contact with reality, are discussed.

Cultural Considerations in the Expression of Symptoms

In assessing the mental status of older adults from diverse cultures, it is necessary to consider culturally influenced expressions of symptoms and the clinical manifestations of disease or illness that have psychological or emotional origins. This is particularly important and relevant when assessing contact with reality and perceptions of reality. The Culture Box below, which

summarizes some cultural considerations relating to the expression of symptoms, can be used in conjunction with the Displays in this section to assess contact with reality.

Denial of Reality

Denial of reality is a defense mechanism used, to some extent, by all people as protection from threats to the ego. In the early stages of dementia, denial of reality may be used to conceal memory deficits or avoid acknowledging an unpleasant reality. In a safe environment, denial is usually harmless as long as it does not interfere with obtaining needed assistance or an evaluation of treatable components. As the dementia

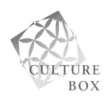

CULTURE BOX

Cultural Considerations in the Expression of Symptoms

- Psychotic disorders occur in every society and are characterized by similar primary symptoms, such as insomnia, delusions, mood changes, flat affect, visual and auditory hallucinations, physical or social withdrawal from others, and other manifestations.
- Secondary clinical manifestations of psychotic disorders are influenced by cultural factors (Kavanagh, in press). In some groups, symptoms are expressed physically or somatically rather than as psychological manifestations.
- Clinical manifestations, such as any of the following, may be viewed as normal or abnormal according to the settings and circumstances in which they occur: dreams, fainting, visions, trances, sorcery, delusions, hallucinations, intoxication, speaking in tongues, communication with spirits, the use of certain substances (e.g., alcohol, tobacco, peyote, marijuana, and other drugs), and even suicide. (Consider the World War II Japanese kamikaze pilots and the Muslims who sacrificed their lives in *jihads* or holy wars.)
- *Somatization* refers to a process by which a person expresses a mental condition in terms of disturbed body function. In older adults from Asian American or Hispanic backgrounds, symptoms may be expressed somatically. For instance, a Chinese American who recently lost a spouse may complain of chest pain rather than verbally expressing the feelings of sadness, loss, and grief.
- General malaise, headaches, abdominal discomfort, stomach aches, backaches, and muscle pains may also be cues that a differentiation between physical and psychological origins should be considered (Kavanagh, in press).

progresses, however, denial often increases to the point at which judgment is seriously impaired and the person is at risk for harm or self-neglect. Denial can progress to the point at which it may become a strongly held delusional system that interferes with safety and basic survival.

General Principles for Assessing Contact with Reality

Delusions, illusions, and hallucinations present a special assessment challenge for gerontological nurses for several reasons:

1. People may try to conceal delusions and hallucinations.
2. When delusions and hallucinations arise from social isolation, opportunities for assessment are extremely limited.
3. To determine whether a reported experience is delusional, the nurse needs information about the reality, which is difficult to obtain if a reliable and objective observer is not available.
4. Even after delusions or hallucinations are identified as such, the underlying factors may be difficult to identify.
5. Ethnocultural background may influence the nature of the delusion or hallucination. For example, older adults whose cultural identity is Irish Catholic are likely to include religious figures, such as Jesus, a saint, or the Virgin Mary, in their delusions and hallucinations. By contrast, delusions or hallucinations of Muslims with African, Near Eastern, or Middle Eastern cultural heritage may include the Prophet Mohammed.

Delusions usually are more readily acknowledged than hallucinations, and the most effective way of detecting delusions is to listen carefully. Especially if a trusting relationship has been established, most older adults will confide their delusions to a nurse whom they perceive as interested, sympathetic, and nonjudgmental. Difficulty can arise, however, when nurses hear information that may be interpreted as delusional, but that is partially or wholly founded on reality. Financial exploitation, violation of rights, and other aspects of elder abuse are not uncommon, especially in older adults who are cognitively impaired or who live with family members who are psychosocially impaired. When older adults who have cognitive impairments or a lifelong suspicious personality describe abusive or exploitative situations, they are likely to be considered delusional or not to be taken seriously. In these situations, the assessment challenge is to find out what is real, what is distorted, and what is not based at all in reality.

A person's contact with reality is influenced by environmental and interpersonal factors. As a general principle, the more severe the cognitive impairment, the more the environment will influence the person's contact with and interpretation of reality. In addition, the more severe the cognitive impairment, the more likely it is that the resulting behaviors will be attributed, perhaps inaccurately, to the dementing process, rather than to reversible factors. Finally, in identifying factors that influence a person's contact with reality, it is important to assess whether a lack of assistive devices, such as eyeglasses and hearing aids, is contributing to the perceptual alteration. If someone usually depends on eyeglasses, contact lenses, or a hearing aid for visual or auditory function, the absence of these items may be the cause of illusions or hallucinations. The effects of lighting also should be considered as a potential influence. For example, in an institutional setting, the reflection of fluorescent lights on a highly polished floor can produce the illusion of water on the floor, and an older adult might be seen walking around the reflection. Display 5-9 summarizes guidelines for assessing an individual's contact with reality.

DISPLAY 5-9
Guidelines for Assessing Contact with Reality

General Principles

- In assessing any loss of contact with reality, the effects of alcohol, medications, and physiologic disturbances must always be considered as potential causative influences.
- People who are not demented are usually more reluctant to talk about delusions and hallucinations than people who are demented.
- When people talk about things that might be delusional, it is important to determine, through information provided by a reliable and objective observer, whether their perceptions have any basis in reality.
- When delusions are initially identified, it is important to determine whether they are of recent onset or whether they have been long-standing but only recently discovered.
- When delusions are identified in someone who is demented, it is especially important to consider the influence of treatable causative factors, such as depression or physiologic disturbances.
- People who are demented are likely to have illusions rather than hallucinations.
- People who are socially isolated are usually quite successful in concealing hallucinations.

- In assessing hallucinations and illusions, it is especially important to consider the influence of the environment.

Interview Questions to Assess Delusions, Hallucinations, and Illusions

- "Do you have any thoughts that you can't seem to get rid of?"
- "People sometimes have thoughts that they're afraid to talk about because they believe others will think they're 'crazy.' Do you ever have thoughts like that?"
- "Do you sometimes hear voices when you're all alone?"
- "Do you sometimes think you see things that other people don't see?"

Nonverbal Clues to Hallucinations

- Extreme withdrawal and isolation
- Contentment with social isolation, especially if the person previously had many social contacts
- Gestures and other actions that normally occur in response to perceived stimuli

Delusions and Paranoia

Delusions are defined as fixed false beliefs that have little or no basis in reality and cannot be corrected by appealing to reason. Delusions arise from the need to preserve one's ego and maintain one's sense of power and control in threatening situations. Delusions serve as a means of organizing information that is difficult to process, even though they may be bizarre and implausible to others (Blazer, 1998). Just as a fever is one manifestation of a physical illness, delusions are one manifestation of a psychiatric illness. In older adults, delusions are associated most often with dementia, depression, delirium,

a paranoid disorder, or sensory impairments. Delusions arising from each of these disorders are characterized in particular ways and are seen in combination with other clues to the specific underlying disorder.

Paranoia, one of the most common forms of delusions, can be described as an extreme degree of suspiciousness. In older adults, paranoia is so closely associated with delusions that the terms are sometimes used interchangeably, but inaccurately, in the geriatric literature. Typical paranoid complaints or behaviors of older adults include the accusation that others are stealing their money or belongings; the perception that they are being cheated, observed, attacked, persecuted, or sexually harassed; the accusation that others are coming in and taking things, or messing up their belongings; and the belief that they have been injured by medical interventions, such as pills or radiation. When paranoia begins in older adulthood, it is usually associated with dementia, delirium, or persistent persecutory states.

Delusions Arising from Delirium and Physiologic Disturbances

Delusions arising from delirium are only one manifestation of a complex pathologic process that is further characterized by physiologic disturbances, diminished attention, a clouded state of consciousness, and possibly, hallucinations. Assessment of such delusions is relatively easy because they are commonly accompanied by the usual manifestations of delirium and will disappear once the delirium is resolved. Another characteristic of delusions associated with delirium is that they are likely to be poorly organized and persecutory in nature. Delusions as a manifestation of delirium are not unique to older adults, and they often accompany delirium in people of any age. Older adults, however, are more susceptible to delirium because the aged brain is less able to adapt to metabolic disturbances, and the older person is more likely to have precipitating conditions, such as physiologic disturbances and adverse medication reactions. Some of the factors that are likely to cause delirium in older adults are listed in Table 5-1.

In addition to the delusions associated with delirium, delusions that are the sole manifestation of a central nervous system dysfunction have been the subject of studies presented in the geropsychiatric literature (Cummings, 1985). This is an important consideration for gerontological nurses because delusions may be a subtle manifestation of a treatable condition, disappearing once the condition is treated. The gerontological nurse may be the only health professional who identifies or is informed of delusions in an older adult, especially in the absence of serious cognitive impairment or obvious physiologic disturbances. Cummings (1985) cited more than 70 physiologic disorders that have been identified as producing delusions, sometimes without other overt manifestations of a pathologic condition. Some of the delusion-producing disorders cited by Cummings that are most likely to occur in older adults are listed in Table 5-1.

Delusions Arising from Dementia

Delusions associated with dementia may be caused by impaired memory and an inability to integrate information. The psychiatric literature usually does not differentiate between delusions that are typical of people with dementia and those that are characteristic of nondemented people with psychotic disorders. Despite the lack of published studies, however, gerontological nurses and other professionals who care for people who are demented can describe many

TABLE 5-1
Physiologic Disorders Causing Delusions

Type of Disorder	Specific Examples
Metabolic disorders	Uremia, dehydration, electrolyte imbalance
Endocrine disorders	Hypoglycemia, hypothyroidism, hyperthyroidism
Neurologic disorders	Stroke, cerebral trauma
Deficiency states	Vitamin deficiencies (B_{12}, folate, niacin, thiamine)
Infections	Septicemia, pneumonia, urinary tract infections, subacute bacterial endocarditis
Adverse medication effects	Anticholinergics, anticonvulsants, antidepressants, antiparkinsonian agents, benzodiazepines, cimetidine, clonidine, corticosteroids, digitalis toxicity, propranolol

examples of delusions that are not typical psychotic delusions. In contrast to delusions arising from psychotic states, delusions arising from dementia are not as fixed and not as well organized, and they are readily changed or forgotten. Common themes of these delusions are fearfulness, theft of property, and concern about deprivation. Nurses may be reluctant to label these behaviors as delusions because they are probably misinterpretations of reality, rather than fixed false beliefs. Until the geropsychiatric literature suggests a better term, however, delusion is the most accurate label that can be used.

In one of the few studies that has specifically addressed delusions associated with dementia, Cummings (1985) identified four distinct categories of delusions. In addition to the so-called grandiose delusions and delusions related to specific neurologic deficits, Cummings (1985, p. 190) described the categories of complex delusions and simple persecutory delusions:

> Simple persecutory delusions consisted of elementary, loosely structured, usually transient beliefs, such as believing that possessions or money were being stolen or that one's spouse was unfaithful. Complex delusions were characterized by a more complicated and intricate structure, rigidity, and stability and were supported by substantial, though distorted, "confirmatory" observations.

The terms *simple delusion* and *complex delusion* are not widely used, but they could be used to distinguish delusions associated with dementia from those that are associated with psychosis. This distinction could be quite helpful because different interventions are effective for dealing with demented and psychotic people. For example, a typical psychiatric nursing approach for dealing with delusions includes discussions with the client about the delusional thoughts as a problem in their life. Although such an intervention is appropriate for the nondemented person with complex delusions, it usually is not appropriate or effective for people with simple delusions associated with a dementing process.

Delusions regarding theft of personal belongings are one of the most common behavioral manifestations of dementia, and they are particularly problematic in home and long-term care settings. The explanation for these delusions is that the person with dementia forgets where an article is kept or was placed. In an attempt to deny the memory impairment, or as a defense against acknowledging the deficit to others, the person comes to believe that the article has been stolen and accuses someone else of stealing it. Caregivers, roommates, and family members are often the targets of such accusations for those who live with others. For people living alone, the accusations may be directed toward "strangers who come in when I'm gone." Assessment of this type of delusion is not difficult for the nurse, who often deals not only with the delusional person but also with the family, caregivers, and nursing staff who are the target of the accusations.

Nurses who work with demented people frequently deal with delusions that stem from an inability to recognize or remember significant others. This "delusional misidentification of persons" results from the dementia-related inability to match perceptions with memories of a once-familiar person (Mendez, 1992). In home settings, this behavior is especially problematic when the target of the delusion is the spouse or other devoted caregiver, who may be accused of being a stranger intent on harming the person.

People who are demented may be delusional because of their inability to recognize and remember familiar environments. These delusions may be accompanied by troublesome behaviors, such as wandering and agitation, with the person insisting on going out "to find my home." Another delusion associated with dementia is the belief that close relatives who have died, such as parents, are still alive. Delusions such as this precipitate agitation and searching behavior, typified by the person who insists that "I have to go take care of my mother." Another specific type of delusion associated with dementia is a false belief about spousal infidelity.

The assessment of delusions associated with dementia is facilitated by the comparative ease with which information generally is offered, which contrasts with the secretiveness and withholding of information that is typical of nondemented people. In many cases, the nurse is given more information than is desired! The challenge in assessing these delusions, however, is to identify the possible reality of the situation. Just because people have serious cognitive impairments, it should not be assumed that all accusations are unfounded. Before labeling the thoughts as delusional, the nurse must be sure that there is no basis in reality. Even the most bizarre-sounding delusions may be based partially or entirely on reality.

Delusions Arising from Depression

Persecutory and other delusions can be one manifestation of a major depression, such as that commonly seen in patients admitted to psychiatric settings. When these manifestations are seen in older adults living in community or long-term care settings, however, they are often overlooked or attributed to other factors. For example, when dementia and depression coexist, the delusions may be attributed to the dementia, rather than considered as possible indicators of a treatable affective disorder. Likewise, when a person with a paranoid personality becomes depressed, the delusions may be falsely attributed to the personality, rather than to the affective disorder, especially if the delusions are persecutory in nature.

When delusions arise from depression, other manifestations of depression usually can be identified in a thorough assessment. All the considerations discussed in Chapter 20 with regard to depression can be applied to the assessment of delusions that may arise from depression. Delusional themes may provide clues to an affective disorder, especially if the focus is on a recent loss. Therefore, carefully listening to the content of the delusions is essential to an accurate assessment.

In depressed older adults, delusional themes often revolve around an exaggerated emphasis on guilt, money, illnesses, self-reproach, foreboding of gloom, diminished self-esteem, or feelings of worthlessness. Although there may be some basis in reality, the feelings of being persecuted and deserving of punishment are grossly exaggerated. The following are some examples of delusions arising from depression:

- *Mrs. N. believes she is responsible for her husband's death; therefore, she believes she does not deserve help for her own illness.*

- *Mr. A. believes that his Medicare insurance has been cancelled as punishment for his not cashing his Social Security check, and he insists that he cannot go to a doctor because of his lack of insurance.*

- *Ms. K. has an unshakable belief that she has undiagnosed cancer, and she begins to plan for her funeral even though numerous doctors have not found any disease process.*

- *Mr. M., who recently had surgery for prostate cancer, is convinced that his house is going to explode from a gas leak, and he repeatedly calls the gas company to come check it.*

Persistent Persecutory Delusions

Paraphrenia, also called late-life paraphrenia, is a term that was first used in Germany in 1919 and is now being used by some geropsychiatrists in the United States (Blazer, 1998). It describes a disorder of late life that is characterized primarily by persecutory delusions and by the absence of any cognitive impairments or affective manifestations. Paraphrenia usually develops after the age of 60 years and affects women more often than men (Raskind, 1982, p. 184). Raskind (p. 185) describes the typical manifestations of paraphrenia as follows:

These symptoms are usually bizarre, and frequently include primary delusions, delusions of influence and passivity, and hallucinations of voices communicating about the patient in the third person. . . . They may be convinced that they are being spied upon, that persons repeatedly enter their living quarters by mysterious means at night, that lethal gases are pumped into their homes, or that food and water are poisoned. . . . The variety of delusions and hallucinations is endless, but frequent themes are plots involving sexual molestation, poisoning, and other bodily harm.

Post (1980, p. 596) describes similar manifestations but uses the phrase "simple paranoid psychosis." Post's description is based on his study of almost 100 patients older than 60 years of age whose symptoms were not associated with dementia or depression, but who experienced persistent persecutory states commencing after the age of 50 years. Post emphasizes that many people having this disorder are likely to function well in the community, with the exception of one or two functional areas that are influenced by the delusions. Delusional content often focuses on noises, threats, obscenities, stolen belongings, or sexual infidelity. The delusions may be associated with social isolation, and they may be present only when the person is in a particular environment, such as the home. If the person takes action based on the delusions, such as moving to another apartment or living with a family member, the delusions may subside temporarily (Post, 1980, pp. 596–597).

The importance of identifying this type of disorder in the assessment is that the disturbing symptoms can be alleviated with appropriate interventions. When left unattended or written off as eccentricities, these disorders can cause much anxiety and may progress to a point at which they seriously disrupt functional abilities. Sometimes, a delusional state that was previously well hidden will be discovered by nurses upon making a home visit or interviewing an older person who has been admitted to the hospital. If the person also suffers from dementia, the delusions may mistakenly be attributed to the dementia or be interpreted as evidence of advancing dementia. When this occurs, a recommendation for long-term institutional care may be made when other recommendations might be more appropriate. In other situations, delusions may surface when someone is admitted to a long-term care facility, and the staff may think that the problem is new, rather than just newly discovered.

When delusions and cognitive impairments coexist, therefore, it is essential, as part of the assessment, to determine whether the delusions existed before the dementia, and to what extent, if any, they interfered with daily activities. If the delusions are part of a long-term pattern that has not interfered with the person's ability to function in daily life, the person may be able to remain in the community with support services directed toward the cognitive impairment and without medical interventions for the delusions. If delusions do interfere with daily activities, however, medical intervention for the person in the community may be necessary and effective in eliminating the delusions or minimizing their effects. With interventions directed toward both the delusions and the cognitive impairment, the older person's functional abilities may prove to be adequate for community living.

Paranoid Delusions Associated with Sensory Impairments

In the mid-1950s, mental health professionals began theorizing about a relationship between hearing impairment and paranoid symptoms. According to this theory, people who are deaf doubt their auditory images and memories, and they misinterpret auditory messages. These doubts and misinterpretations lead to feelings of inferiority that are projected onto the environment in ideas of reference. Persecutory delusions eventually develop, and if the person is unstable, a psychotic illness ensues. Prior to the 1990s, this assumption remained unchallenged, but questions are currently being raised about conclusions based on cross-sectional studies (Prager and Jeste, 1993). A recent longitudinal study did not find any relationship between baseline hearing impairment and paranoid symptoms, but it did indicate a weak positive relationship between baseline visual impairment and paranoid symptoms (Blazer et al., 1996). Another recent study showed that when subjects with mild hearing impairment wore bilateral, functional hearing aids, their performance on mental status tests improved, and they were less likely to be diagnosed as having a psychopathologic condition (Kreeger et al., 1995). In assessing delusions, therefore, nurses must consider the possibility that sensory impairments may cause or contribute to the delusional state. Also, it is important to make sure that any sensory deficits are compensated for to the extent that this is feasible.

Hallucinations and Illusions

Hallucinations are sensory experiences that have no basis in an external stimulus. Visual and auditory hallucinations are most common, but tactile, olfactory, and gustatory hallucinations also occur. Illusions are misperceptions of an external stimulus. They may be mistaken as hallucinations, but they are different in that they have some basis in reality, whereas hallucinations do not. Therefore, in assessing any abnormal sensory experience, it is essential to consider the effect of the environment on sensory perception and to look for any external stimuli before determining that someone is hallucinating. In older adults, hallucinations and illusions are associated most often with dementia, depression, sensory deprivation, and physiologic disturbances, including adverse medication effects. Dementia and delirium are the most common causes of predominantly visual hallucinations, whereas paraphrenia and depression are the most common causes of predominantly auditory hallucinations (Wattis and Church, 1986, p. 111).

Gerontological nurses deal less frequently with hallucinations than with delusions, but this is partially because hallucinations are more easily overlooked or hidden. People experiencing hallucinations may know that their behavior is not socially acceptable. They may not offer information about hallucinations; in fact, they may try to hide their hallucinatory experiences. Older adults who are socially isolated can be especially successful in hiding hallucinatory experiences. As with delusions, it is important to identify the underlying cause of hallucinations and illusions, because the selection of appropriate interventions depends on an accurate assessment.

Hallucinations and Illusions Arising from Delirium and Physiologic Disturbances

As with delusions associated with delirium, hallucinations and illusions arising from delirium are relatively easy to assess because they are only one manifestation of a complex process. These hallucinations are characteristically vivid, visual, colorful, threatening, and accompanied by other signs of delirium. When illusions arise from a delirium, they are usually brief and poorly organized. Occasionally, hallucinations or illusions arise from altered physiologic states or adverse medication effects, and they may not be accompanied by overt signs of delirium in the early stages. When hallucinations or illusions are caused by adverse medication effects, they are likely to be overlooked, underreported, or attributed to some other cause. One study found that when patients treated with propranolol were asked direct questions about symptoms, the reported incidence of recurrent visual perceptual disorders was 17.5% (Fleminger, 1978). Hallucinations arising from withdrawal from drugs or alcohol may be seen during the first days of admission to an acute care setting, or in any circumstance in which the person suddenly does not have access to their usual drugs or alcohol. The auditory hallucinations arising from alcohol-induced delirium are characterized as accusatory and threatening, and they are sometimes organized into a complete paranoid system. Table 5-2 summarizes the physiologic

TABLE 5-2
Physiologic Disorders Causing Hallucinations

Type of Disorder	Specific Examples
Adverse medication effects	Alcohol, anticholinergics, clonidine, corticosteroids, digitalis toxicity, levodopa, propranolol
Endocrine disorders	Thyrotoxicosis
Neurologic disease	Brain tumor or cortical ischemia
Deficiency state	Niacin deficiency
Drug or alcohol withdrawal	Alcohol, barbiturates, meprobamate

disorders, including some adverse medication effects, that are most likely to cause hallucinations.

The detection of alcohol-induced delirium is especially important in acute care settings because people who are dependent on alcohol are more likely to acknowledge the problem and agree to appropriate interventions when they are in a crisis situation. The following case example is typical of such a situation.

Mr. K. is 73 years old and has been caring for his wife, who has Alzheimer's disease. He is a very proud man who has difficulty accepting help. One morning, Mr. K. begins vomiting coffee-ground emesis and is admitted to an acute care setting with the diagnosis of gastrointestinal bleeding. On admission, Mr. K. is very pleasant and expresses concern about his wife's care. The next morning, Mr. K. complains angrily to the nurses about the bars on the windows and is very belligerent about the fact that he has been put in jail. He develops additional manifestations of delirium and is treated for alcohol withdrawal.

When the delirium has subsided, the nurse initiates a conversation about the care of his wife and asks him how he copes with the responsibility. Mr. K. admits that he has difficulty coping with his and his wife's declining health and his increasing loneliness and re-sponsibilities. He has always been a "social drinker," but he has gradually increased his consumption of alcohol to three six-packs of beer a day. As part of the discharge plan, Mr. K. agrees to talk with a sponsor from Alcoholics Anonymous.

Visual hallucinations may occur in older adults who are visually impaired and have no additional functional or cognitive impairments (Teunisse et al., 1995). One review of the literature on visual hallucinations found that eye disease was the most common cause of visual hallucinations for people of all ages, and that one third of the people who underwent surgery for cataracts reported no further experience with visual hallucinations (Beck and Harris, 1994). Another finding of this review was that visual hallucinations were most prevalent among people 71 years of age or older.

Hallucinations and Illusions Arising from Dementia

Hallucinations and illusions may occur during a transient ischemic attack or at any time in the course of a dementing illness. When illusions occur, they often are related to environmental conditions that can easily be modified. For example, visual illusions may be caused by poor lighting or reflections from glass or mirrors, and auditory illusions may be caused by background noises. Especially for people with hearing aids, background noises may contribute to auditory illusions.

The psychiatric literature usually addresses illusions only with regard to misperceptions of visual or auditory stimuli, but the definition of an illusion is a misinterpretation of any external stimulus. Nurses who care for people with dementia can cite numerous examples of behaviors that fit this broader definition of an illusion: (1) mistaking the identity of caregivers, family members, or other familiar people; (2) perceiving an object as something other than what it really is; (3) taking an object under the mistaken belief that it belongs to them; and (4) refusing to believe that they are in their home when they really are. These experiences might be labeled as delusions or disorientation, but they are more accurately defined as illusions because they involve a misinterpretation of reality.

Hallucinations Arising from Paranoia or Depression

Along with paranoid delusions, hallucinations can arise from persistent persecutory states, and their focus may be closely related to the theme of the delusions. The following examples are characteristic of hallucinations arising from paranoid states:

- *Mr. F. says that he hears people in the next apartment talking about him. These are the same people whom he believes will come in and steal things when he leaves the apartment.*

- *Ms. J. reports seeing men observing her when she undresses or takes a bath. Moreover, when she goes to the grocery store, the man at the checkout always offers her money in exchange for sexual favors.*

In affective disorders, delusions are more common than hallucinations, but people who are severely depressed may experience hallucinations. For example, visual and auditory hallucinations of deceased loved ones are experiences commonly associated with bereavement. When hallucinations occur, they are likely to be auditory and derogatory, or they may involve visual perceptions of dead people. The following examples are typical of hallucinatory experiences arising from depression:

- *Ms. C. reports that, at night, she hears the people in the next apartment saying that she has cancer.*

- *Mr. T. reports hearing younger men say that he is sexually impotent and that he was not a good provider to his wife (who died within the past year).*

- *Ms. F. looks down from her second-floor window and sees a man, dressed in black, lying injured on the sidewalk.*

Olfactory hallucinations are less common than other hallucinations associated with depressive states, but they can occur. When olfactory hallucinations accompany depression, they are likely to be associated with rotten smells, such as pervasive pollution, or with impending danger, such as a gas leak. Table 5-3 summarizes the characteristics that distinguish delusions, hallucinations, and illusions according to their underlying causes.

Sociocultural Supports

Gerontologists variously define social supports as follows: (1) the types of actions or services that are considered supportive; (2) the person's perception of social supports; and (3) the positive or negative outcomes of a supportive interaction (Antonucci, 1985). Social supports affect one's ability to cope with stressful life experiences, and their influence increases in direct relation to the degree of functional impairment of the older adult. The more dependent the older person, the more important are his or her social supports. The purpose of a nursing assessment of sociocultural supports is to identify resources that can help older adults function at their highest level. Based on a nursing assessment of overall function, the nurse then addresses those areas of function with which the older adult needs support or assistance and assesses the available resources for providing the needed care. For nurses in hospitals and nursing homes, the assessment of sociocultural supports is the basis for discharge planning; for nurses in home and community settings, it is the basis for planning long-term care.

Assessment of sociocultural supports generally is viewed as the responsibility of social workers. In the provision of health care to older

TABLE 5-3
Distinguishing Features of Delusions, Hallucinations, and Illusions

Underlying Cause	Accompanying Manifestations	Characteristics
Delirium	Diminished attention, a clouded state of consciousness, and other typical manifestations of delirium; metabolic disturbance, adverse medication effect, or other underlying cause	*Delusions:* poorly organized, persecutory. *Hallucinations:* vivid, visual, colorful, threatening; accusatory auditory hallucinations induced by alcohol withdrawal. *Illusions:* brief, poorly organized.
Dementia	Cognitive impairment (especially memory deficits); alert level of consciousness. Agitation, anxiety, or wandering may be associated with a loss of contact with reality. Neurologic manifestations may accompany hallucinations, particularly when the underlying cause is vascular dementia.	*Delusions:* not fixed, loosely organized, readily changed or forgotten. Themes may include theft, fears, misidentification of places or people, and spousal infidelity. *Illusions:* occur more commonly than hallucinations; may be partially attributable to environmental factors. *Hallucinations:* more often visual than auditory; may be partially attributable to environmental factors.
Depression	Typical depressive symptoms, including anorexia, lack of energy, sleep disturbances, and weight loss	*Delusions:* Themes may include death, guilt, money, illnesses, self-reproach, foreboding of gloom, diminished self-esteem, and feelings of worthlessness. There may be some basis in reality, but perceptions are exaggerated. *Hallucinations:* typically auditory and derogatory.
Paranoid disorder	Absence of cognitive deficits or affective disorders; long-term social isolation or suspicious personality; may be well hidden for years	*Delusions:* fixed and well organized; may subside temporarily in different environments. Themes usually involve plots, noises, threats, obscenities, or sexual assaults. *Hallucinations:* If present, these are related to the delusional themes.

adults, however, it is most often the nurse who assesses sociocultural supports. When older adults are discharged from hospitals or nursing homes, the nurse is the professional person who reviews the discharge plan, which usually includes at least one social support. In institutional settings, nurses are the professionals who are most available to observe and meet with visitors, and they are the professionals who are most likely to be approached when family members have questions or wish to discuss an issue. In home care settings, nurses have many opportunities to assess sociocultural supports, and they often observe relationships and environmental conditions that would not be discussed or discovered outside the home setting.

Social Network

A method commonly used for assessing sociocultural supports is to ask the person to identify people who assist with specific tasks, defining these resources as the social network. Another method, which renders less information, is to ask the person a question, such as "Whom do you rely on for help?" Although the latter method may be a good opening for the identification of sociocultural supports, more specific questions must then be asked. Using the functional approach, the nurse can identify the areas that are most important for day-to-day function and then inquire how the person accomplishes these tasks. For example, in discussing a follow-up appointment for medical care, the nurse might ask, "How do you get to your doctor appointments?" Other questions that can help to identify sociocultural supports are listed in Display 5-10.

In addition to assessing the sociocultural supports that are available for and essential to the older person's daily functioning, it is important also to identify those supports that influence the person's quality of life. Because a relationship with a confidant(e) is a significant predictor of quality of life for older adults, at least one question relating to this factor, such as "Is there anyone you can talk to about your worries?", should be posed. The answer to this question may also be important if the nurse or health care team is assisting the older adult with a decision about long-term care, as the older adult may want the confidant(e) to be involved in the decision-making process. In addition, the response to this question may provide important information as to whether the older person has recently experienced a loss of or change in the availability of a confidant(e).

Once existing resources are identified, the nurse can then identify additional resources that might be helpful in addressing unmet needs. Such questions as "Do you have any grandchildren or neighbors who could help with shoveling the snow?" are aimed at identifying informal supports that may be available but are not currently being used. A question such as "Are you aware that the senior center has a van that takes people to doctor appointments?" is aimed at

identifying the person's awareness of formal supports that might not be in use. Examples of questions designed to identify potential resources are listed in Display 5-10.

Barriers to Sociocultural Supports

In addition to assessing the number and types of sociocultural supports available, the older person's attitudes toward sociocultural supports must be assessed. In the United States and most western European countries, self-sufficiency is highly valued as an indicator of maturity and ego integrity. Social gerontologists have theorized that older people cope with increasing dependence by perceiving the informal network of family and friends as a natural extension of themselves. This perspective serves to minimize any damage to ego systems based on norms of self-sufficiency and self-reliance (Cantor and Little, 1985). In the absence of adequate informal supports, or when conflicts exist between older adults and their informal supports, an increase in dependence can trigger less effective coping mechanisms. The following case example is typical of such a situation:

Mr. and Mrs. S. always expected their children to care for them, but the children have moved to other cities and only visit several times a year. Mr. and Mrs. S. refuse to accept any of the formal services that are available because of their cost, and also because they expect their children to provide the services out of filial responsibility. Furthermore, Mrs. S. cared for her parents when they were old, so she expects her daughter to do the same for her.

Mr. and Mrs. S. frequently call their daughter and son-in-law to complain about their inability to get groceries and go to doctors' appointments. Rather than making use of transportation or other services available from the community, they neglect themselves. During the children's visit over the Christmas holiday, they find that their parents have not been eating adequately and are not taking their prescribed medications. When they mention these observations to their parents, Mr. and Mrs. S. tell their children, "If you loved us, you'd be taking care of us, and this wouldn't be happening."

In addition to some older people's preference for obtaining services from families rather than outside agencies, there are many other barriers to the use of formal services. Fears about outsiders coming into the home rank high among the barriers to the provision of in-home services. Financial barriers also often exist, either because of an inability or an unwillingness to pay for services. The identification of these barriers is essential because counseling and educational interventions can address many of these issues. Issues that are not amenable to intervention may represent impenetrable barriers to the provision of sociocultural supports.

The assessment of barriers to support services is particularly challenging because direct questions about these issues often are inappropriate and usually are very threatening. Rather, identification of these barriers is best accomplished by carefully listening to older people and their caregivers and by asking nonthreatening questions. For example, a caregiver might talk about a friend who had a home health aide "who did nothing but watch television all day and got paid 12 dollars an hour." In response to this, the nurse might ask, "Do you think that might happen if we arrange for a home health aide to care for your father?" Other attitudinal barriers, such as prejudices, may be identified through statements made by the caregiver about prior experiences. Display 5-10 summarizes the many barriers that can thwart the use of formal support services.

Economic Resources

Financial issues are generally within the purview of social workers, and nurses usually prefer to avoid discussing money with older adults or their families. In planning for formal services for older adults, however, some assessment of financial assets is necessary, and the nurse is often the health care professional who obtains this information, especially in home or other community settings. If no long-term care or community-based services are needed, the nurse can forego the financial assessment.

Many older adults are shocked to find out that the costs of long-term care, with the exception of skilled care, are not covered by Medicare. In addition, people are often appalled by the restrictive definition of skilled care, as well as many other restrictions, that are applied to determine eligibility for services. Even if a social worker has explained these facts, it is usually the nurse who deals with the related anxiety and other emotional reactions of the older adult and their families. Because gerontological nurses are in a position of helping older adults and their families address and cope with the financial issues of long-term care, they frequently become involved in assessing the financial resources of the person and family.

It is not necessary to ask details about monthly income or the exact amount of savings and assets, but questions must be asked about the resources available for the purchase of services. Asking a question such as "Do you have any money worries?" might reveal some anxieties that can be dealt with or allayed through counseling or the provision of accurate information. When the nurse reviews with the older adult or caregiver the services that are available, information can also be provided about the cost of these services, at which time a question such as "Do you think you could afford this kind of help?" can be posed. Display 5-10 lists questions that can be asked to assess financial resources for the planning of long-term care of older adults.

Religious Affiliation

Another component of the psychosocial assessment is the identification of the older person's spiritual needs, which are universal, and his or her religious affiliation, if any. As discussed in Chapter 3, religion and spirituality increase in importance with age, and they are resources that should be identified as a part of a comprehensive psychosocial assessment. The person's religious affiliation is assessed as a component of his or her sociocultural supports, whereas spirituality is assessed as a separate component of the psychosocial assessment.

Identification of religious affiliation is a simple but important part of the psychosocial assessment because available religion-based programs for older adults may be perceived as more acceptable than those provided by a public or nonreligious agency. For example, an older Jewish person might be willing to go to the Jewish Community Center for a senior meal program, and an older Roman Catholic adult might be willing to accept mental health services from Catholic Social Services, but these people might refuse to avail themselves of the same kinds of services when they are offered by another organization. Often, religion-based services are viewed by the older adult as services that they deserve as a reward for years of attendance at or service to a church or synagogue. Although most religion-based programs serve older adults regardless of their religious affiliations, the programs often are perceived as more acceptable if the person is of the same faith.

In addition to being perceived as more acceptable, some religion-based services are not available elsewhere, and they often are provided by trained volunteers free of charge. Examples of programs or services that may be available to members of a particular church or synagogue include transportation, respite care, peer counseling, chore assistance, friendly visiting, and telephone reassurance. Older adults also can take advantage of any church- or synagogue-based program that is available for people of all ages. The Stephen Ministries, founded in 1975, is an example of a volunteer program that is available in many Christian denominations throughout the United States. This program offers peer counseling and other services, provided by volunteers with special training in ministering to older, depressed, shut-in, and grieving persons.

Identification of any specific place of worship is also important because attendance at religious services may be a significant factor in the older adult's social life. For many older adults, especially those with limited mobility or those who have full-time caregiving responsibilities, attendance at religious services is their only opportunity for social interaction and personal support. Most people who are unable to attend religious services can arrange for home visits by a clergy person or lay minister; indeed, these visits may be the only source of outside contact and emotional support that is acceptable to a homebound older adult. Moreover, for people who are socially isolated, a visitor from their place of worship may be the only person monitoring the home situation. In these situations, health professionals who are concerned about homebound older adults may be able to monitor their status through these visitors, as in the following example:

Mr. S. was admitted to the hospital after a syncopal episode that resulted in a minor car accident. On admission, Mr. S. was slightly unkempt and showed some memory deficits, but his self-care abilities improved during his 2-day hospitalization. The nurse suggested that Mr. S. consider home-delivered meals and the use of other community resources, but he refused these services. His situation did not warrant a report to a protective services agency.

The nurse was concerned because Mr. S. lived alone and had no outside contacts other than Ms. C., a lay minister who had visited weekly for 2 years. The nurse asked for and received permission from Mr. S. to contact Ms. C. to inform her of available community services. Ms. C. was grateful for the information and said she would contact the appro-

priate agencies if Mr. S.'s condition declined or if he agreed to accept help.

In this situation, information about the church affiliation enabled the nurse to implement a discharge plan that otherwise would not have been possible. Display 5-10 summarizes important questions and considerations involved in assessing sociocultural supports, including religious affiliation.

Spirituality

Nursing assessment of spiritual needs, like nursing assessment of sexual needs, is not routinely included in an assessment because it is not always relevant to the health issues being addressed. There are times, however, when a nursing assessment of the spiritual needs of older adults is warranted. When an older person provides clues about spiritual distress or discomfort, the nurse must be willing to respond to the older

---

DISPLAY 5-10
Guidelines for Assessing Sociocultural Supports

Interview Questions to Assess Sociocultural Supports

- "On whom do you rely for help?"
- "Is there anyone who helps you with grocery shopping? Getting to doctor appointments? Getting prescriptions filled? Managing your money and paying bills?"
- "Is there anyone you can talk to when you have worries or difficulties?"
- "Is there anything you would like help with that you don't have help with now?"
- "Is there anyone in the family who could help with grocery shopping?"
- "Have you ever received information about the transportation services (or meals, or other services) that are available through the senior center?"

Potential Barriers to the Use of Formal Supports

- Unwillingness to acknowledge, or lack of insight to recognize, the need for services
- Expectation that family members will provide the needed care
- Unwillingness to admit that family members cannot or will not provide the needed care
- Lack of financial resources to purchase services, or unwillingness to spend money for services
- Perceived correlation between formal services and "welfare"
- Lack of transportation to access services
- Mistrust of service providers, or an unwillingness to allow outsiders into the home

- Bad experiences with service providers, or hearsay about the bad experiences of others
- Fear that the home situation will be judged as socially unacceptable, or embarrassment because it is socially unacceptable
- Fear that having outsiders in the house will lead to admission to a nursing home
- Lack of time, energy, or problem-solving ability to obtain information about and select the appropriate services
- Fear that the service will be provided by someone about whom the care recipient holds prejudices
- Language and cultural barriers

Interview Questions to Assess Financial Resources

- "Do you have any money worries?"
- "Do you have any concerns about paying for services that you might need?"
- "Would you like to talk to someone about any financial concerns?"
- "Do you think you can afford the kind of help that your doctor recommended?"
- "Have you received any advice about financial planning for nursing home care?"

Interview Questions to Assess Religious Affiliation

- "Do you belong to any particular church or synagogue?"
- "Are you aware of any programs available at your church or synagogue that might be helpful to you?"

DISPLAY 5-11
Guidelines for Assessing Spiritual Needs

Guidelines for Nursing Assessment

- Be aware of your own feelings about spirituality so you can recognize and respond to the spiritual needs of others.
- Recognize that spiritual needs are a universal human phenomenon. Although not all people experience spiritual distress, all people have spiritual needs and the potential for spiritual growth.
- Recognize that it is within the realm of holistic nursing care to identify and plan interventions for spiritual growth, as well as for spiritual distress.
- Convey a nonjudgmental, open-minded attitude when eliciting information about a person's spirituality and religious beliefs.

Questions to Spiritual Health

- "What in your life is meaningful and important?"
- "What do you hope to accomplish in your life?"
- "What do you do that gives you pleasure and satisfaction?"
- "Who are the people you can turn to when you need someone to listen to you or to help you?"
- "Do you believe in a higher being?" (examples: God, Goddess, Divinity) "How do you describe this being?"
- "Do you participate in any activities (rituals) that foster a connection with a higher being?" (examples: prayer or other religious activities)
- "What activities are helpful in bringing you inner peace and relieving stress?" (examples: meditation, walking in the woods)
- "What are your beliefs about death?"
- "Do you see a connection between your body, your mind, your emotions, and your soul?"

- "Is there anything you need or would like to have to support your beliefs and your spiritual needs?" (example: Bible, sacred or revered object)
- "Would you like to arrange a visit from a spiritual leader?"
- "Are there any health practices that you would like to consider, even though our society may not consider them to be conventional?" (examples: therapeutic touch, guided imagery)

Observations/Questions to Assess Spiritual Distress

- During the psychosocial interview, listen for clues to spiritual distress, such as the following: suicidal ideation; anger toward God; inability to forgive others; feelings of hopelessness, uselessness, or abandonment; questions about the meaning of life, losses, or suffering.
- "Are there any conflicts between your beliefs or values and actions that you feel you should be taking?" (example: feeling entitled to some time to oneself, which may be in conflict with the demands of caregiving for a spouse)
- "Are there any conflicts between what you believe in and what society or health care professionals are encouraging or suggesting you do?" (example: questioning the wisdom of using a feeding tube for a spouse who is chronically and severely impaired and unable to participate in the decision)
- "Do you have any special religious considerations that are not being addressed?" (examples: dietary practices, observance of religious holidays)
- *For people in institutional settings:* "Is there anything here that interferes with your spiritual needs?" (examples: noisy environment, lack of privacy).

person, rather than simply ignoring the clues. (A few examples of situations in which older adults are likely to express spiritual needs were previously discussed in Chapter 3.) Moreover, when a nurse is addressing quality-of-life issues, it is important to include questions about spirituality. For example, when long-term care is being planned, it is especially important to assess and address spiritual needs.

Nurses, like many people, may not be comfortable discussing spirituality, but they can increase their comfort level by recognizing their own feelings and acknowledging that spirituality is a universal human need. Nurses might avoid discussion of spiritual needs because they believe they are not skilled in meeting these needs. However, nurses routinely identify many needs they are not trained to meet directly. If nurses can view the assessment of spiritual needs as one aspect of overall health, they may become comfortable addressing the spiritual needs of the older adults to whom they provide care. Like many health problems, nurses can address the nursing aspects of those problems, referring the person to the appropriate resource for interventions that may resolve other non-nursing aspects. In addition to providing direct nursing interventions to address spiritual needs, nurses can suggest referrals to appropriate clergy or spiritual practitioners. Involvement with support groups can also be effective in dealing with spiritual distress when it arises from feelings of guilt, anger, or inadequacy. Display 5-11 presents guidelines for assessing spiritual needs. It is important to recognize that the assessment of spiritual needs should include, not only the factors that cause spiritual distress, but also the factors that are essential to spiritual growth, even in the absence of spiritual distress.

Chapter Summary

Assessment of psychosocial function is a very complex process that requires a high degree of skillful communication and awareness of socio-cultural considerations. Nurses must be able to establish a comfortable interview environment and identify and address barriers to communication with older adults. A psychosocial and cultural self-assessment may be a useful means of increasing one's comfort level in performing a psychosocial assessment of older adults. Culturally specific aspects of the psychosocial assessment include the use of interpreters, information about culture-bound syndromes, cultural considerations in the expression of symptoms, and an awareness of culturally based perceptions of psychosocial function.

An assessment of mental status involves an assessment of all of the following: physical appearance, motor function, social skills, response to the interview, orientation, alertness, memory, speech characteristics, calculation and higher language skills, and decision making. An assessment of effective function should include consideration of mood, anxiety, self-esteem, depression, and happiness and life satisfaction. Assessment of a person's contact with reality is a most complex aspect of psychosocial function, and emphasis must be placed on identifying potential underlying causes of any loss of contact with reality. An assessment of sociocultural supports addresses all of the following: social network, barriers to sociocultural supports, economic resources, religious affiliation, and spirituality.

Critical Thinking Exercises

1. Complete the psychosocial and cultural self-assessment in Display 5.1.
2. Think of several different situations in the past few weeks in which you communicated with older adults. What actual or potential barriers to communication may have affected these exchanges? What factors hindered or enhanced interaction with these older adults? Are there verbal or nonverbal communication techniques that might have improved the interactions?

3. Think of the various settings in which you work with older adults. Describe what you would do or whom you would call if you needed to communicate with an older adult who did not speak English.

4. Describe your definition of and beliefs about mental health and mental illness. How are your perceptions influenced by sociocultural factors?

5. Name at least three things you would observe or determine in order to assess *each* of the following: physical appearance, social skills, orientation, alertness, memory, speech characteristics, calculation and higher language skills, decision-making skills, anxiety, self-esteem, depression, and contact with reality.

6. What questions would you ask an older adult to identify social supports and barriers to the use of services?

7. What approach would you use to assess an older adult's spiritual health and identify spiritual distress?

Educational Resource

AT&T Language Line
(800) 752–6096
• Fee-for-service translation in nearly 150 languages available around the clock

References

Agostinelli, B., Demers, K., Garrigan, D., & Waszynski, C. (1994). Targeted interventions: Use of the Mini-Mental State Exam. *Journal of Gerontological Nursing, 20*(8), 15–23.

Aldwin, C. M., Sutton, K. J., Chiara, G., & Spiro, A., III. (1996). Age differences in stress, coping, and appraisal: Findings from the normative aging study. *Journal of Gerontology: Psychological Sciences, 51B*(4), P179–P188.

American Association of Retired Persons (AARP). (1997). *Mental health issues for minority seniors.* Washington, DC: AARP.

Antonucci, T. C. (1985). Personal characteristics, social support, and social behavior. In R. H. Binstock & E. Shanas (Eds.), *Handbook of aging and the social sciences* (pp. 94–128). New York: Van Nostrand Reinhold.

Beck, J., & Harris, M. J. (1994). Visual hallucinosis in non-delusional elderly. *International Journal of Geriatric Psychiatry, 9,* 531–536.

Benson, S. (1997). The older adult and fear of crime. *Journal of Gerontological Nursing, 23*(10), 24–31.

Blazer, D. (1998). *Emotional problems in later life: Intervention strategies for professional caregivers* (2nd ed.). New York: Springer.

Blazer, D. G., Hays, J. C., & Salive, M. E. (1996). Factors associated with paranoid symptoms in a community sample of older adults. *The Gerontologist, 36*(1), 70–75.

Botwinick, J. (1984). *Aging and behavior.* New York: Springer.

Camp, C. J., Burant, C. J., & Graham, G. C. (1996). The InterpreCare System™: Overcoming language barriers in long-term care. *The Gerontologist, 36*(6), 821–823.

Cantor, M., & Little, V. (1985). Aging and social care. In R. H. Binstock & E. Shanas (Eds.), *Handbook of aging and the social sciences* (pp. 745–781). New York: Van Nostrand Reinhold.

Coleman, P. G. (1984). Assessing self-esteem and its sources in elderly people. *Ageing and Society, 4,* 117–135.

Coleman, P. G., Aubin, A., Robinson, M., Ivani-Chalian, C., & Briggs, R. (1993). Predictors of depressive symptoms and low self-esteem in a follow-up study of elderly people over 10 years. *International Journal of Geriatric Psychiatry, 8,* 343–349.

Cummings, J. L. (1985). Organic delusions: Phenomenology, anatomical correlations, and review. *British Journal of Psychiatry, 146,* 184–197.

Dietz, B. E. (1996). The relationship of aging to self-esteem: The relative effects of maturation and role accumulation. *International Journal of Aging and Human Development, 43*(3), 249–266.

Fleminger, R. (1978). Visual hallucinations and illusions with propranolol. *British Medical Journal, 1,* 1182.

Giarrusso, R., & Bengtson, V. L. (1996). Self-esteem. In J. E. Birren (Ed.), *Encyclopedia of gerontology: Age, aging, and the aged, Vol. 2.* (pp. 459–466). San Diego: Academic Press.

Hunter, K., Linn, M., & Harris, R. (1981–1982). Characteristics of high and low self-esteem in the elderly. *International Journal of Aging and Human Development, 14,* 117–126.

Kahana, E., & Coe, R. (1969). Self and staff conceptions of institutionalized aged. *The Gerontologist, 9*(4), 264–267.

Kavanagh, K. H. (in press). Transcultural perspectives in mental health. In M. M. Andrews & J. S. Boyle (Eds.), *Transcultural concepts in nursing care.* Philadelphia: Lippincott-Raven.

Kreeger, J. L., Raulin, M. L., Grace, J., & Priest, B. L. (1995). Effect of hearing enhancement on mental status ratings in geriatric psychiatric patients. *American Journal of Psychiatry, 152,* 629–631.

Langland, R. M., & Panicucci, C. L. (1982). Effects of touch on communication with elderly confused clients. *Journal of Gerontological Nursing, 8*(3), 152–155.

Mannell, R. C., & Dupuis, S. (1996). Life satisfaction. In J. E. Birren (Ed.), *Encyclopedia of gerontology: Age, aging, and the aged, Vol. 2* (pp. 59–64). San Diego: Academic Press.

Meisenhelder, J. B. (1985). Self-esteem: A closer look at clinical interventions. *International Journal of Nursing Studies*, 22(2), 127–135.

Mendez, M. F. (1992). Delusional misidentification of persons in dementia. *British Journal of Psychiatry*, *160*, 414–416.

Moore, J. R., & Gilbert, D. A. (1995). Elderly residents: Perceptions of nurses' comforting touch. *Journal of Gerontological Nursing*, 21(1), 6–13.

Perone, D. (1997, September). Culture and mental health. *Closing the Gap* (p. 3). Washington, DC: Office of Minority Health.

Post, F. (1980). Paranoid, schizophrenia-like, and schizophrenic states in the aged. In J. E. Birren & R. B. Sloane (Eds.), *Handbook of mental health and aging* (pp. 591–615). Englewood Cliffs, NJ: Prentice-Hall.

Prager, S., & Jeste, D. V. (1993). Sensory impairment in late-life schizophrenia (review). *Schizophrenia Bulletin*, *19*, 755–772.

Raskind, M. (1982). Paranoid syndromes in the elderly. In C. Eisdorfer & W. E. Fann (Eds.), *Treatment of psychopathology in the aging* (pp. 184–191). New York: Springer.

Schwartz, A. N. (1975). An observation of self-esteem as the linchpin of quality of life for the aged. *The Gerontologist*, *15*, 470–472.

Teunisse, R. J., Cruysberg, J. R. M., Verbeek, A., & Zitman, F. G. (1995). The Charles Bonnet syndrome: A large prospective study in the Netherlands. *British Journal of Psychiatry*, *166*, 254–257.

Thomae, H. (1991). Emotion and personality. In J. E. Birren, R. B. Sloane, & G. D. Cohen (Eds.), *Handbook of mental health and aging* (pp. 355–375). San Diego: Academic Press/Harcourt Brace Jovanovich.

Walls, C. T., & Zarit, S. H. (1991). Informal support from black churches and the well-being of elderly blacks. *Gerontologist*, *31*(4), 490–495.

Wattis, J., & Church, M. (1986). *Practical psychiatry of old age.* New York: New York University Press.

Whall, A. L. (1987). Self-esteem and the mental health of older adults. *Journal of Gerontological Nursing*, *13*(4), 41–42.

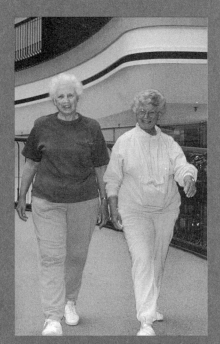

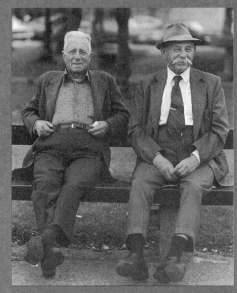

Changes, Consequences, and Care Related to Physiologic Function

Hearing

Chapter

1. *Delineate age-related changes that affect the ability of older adults to hear.*
2. *Examine risk factors that influence the ability of older adults to hear.*
3. *Discuss the functional consequences of age-related changes and risk factors that affect hearing.*
4. *Describe interview questions, behavioral cues, and hearing tests that may be used to assess the hearing ability of older adults.*
5. *Identify interventions to enhance the auditory abilities of older adults and address risk factors that interfere with hearing.*

The auditory system receives and interprets verbal communications by converting sound waves into neural impulses. Auditory function influences the performance of many daily activities, particularly those that depend on understanding verbal instructions. In addition, safe maneuvering in one's environment is highly dependent on the accurate perception of auditory cues. Also, one's quality of life is influenced significantly by the ability to hear sounds, such as voices, music, and sounds of nature.

Age-Related Changes

Auditory function takes place in the three compartments of the ear and the auditory cortex of the brain. Interpretation of sounds entails the coding of sounds according to intensity and frequency. Intensity, or amplitude, reflects the loudness or softness of the sound and is measured in decibels. Frequency, which is measured in cycles per second or hertz, determines whether the pitch is high or low. Age-related changes that occur in the ear and the auditory nervous system affect the ability of older adults to per-

ceive accurately the pitch of sounds. Perception of sound intensity is not significantly affected by age-related changes, but it can be impaired as a consequence of risk factors that are likely to occur in older adults. Thus, hearing impairments are a very common functional consequence for older adults.

External Ear

Hearing begins in the outer ear, which consists of the pinna and the external auditory canal. These cartilaginous structures control the discernment of resonance and provide the basis for sound localization, especially for higher-frequency sounds. This function enables a person to identify the source of a sound. Although the pinna undergoes changes in size, shape, flexibility, and hair growth with increasing age, there is no evidence that the conduction of sound waves is altered in healthy older adults. The auditory canal is covered by skin and lined with hair follicles and cerumen-producing glands. Cerumen is a natural protective substance that is categorized as either dry (thick, gray, flaky) or wet (moist, dark brown). Whites and Blacks are likely to have wet cerumen, whereas Asians and Native Americans are likely to have dry cerumen. Cerumen normally is expelled through natural processes. Age-related changes, however, such as an increased concentration of keratin, the growth of longer and thicker hair (especially in men), and thinning and drying of the skin lining the canal, predispose the older adult to a build-up of cerumen. An age-related diminution in sweat gland activity further increases the potential for cerumen accumulation by making the wax increasingly dry and difficult to remove. A prolapsed or collapsed ear canal is another age-related change that may occur. This structural alteration of the canal may affect the localization and perception of sounds, particularly those in the highest frequency ranges.

Middle Ear

From the auditory canal, sound vibrations pass through the tympanic membrane to the three auditory ossicles: the malleus, incus, and stapes. These bones transmit vibrations across the air-filled middle ear, through the oval window, and to the fluid-filled inner ear. Transmission of sounds is influenced by the frequency of each sound and is most effective in the frequency range of normal voices and least effective at the lowest and highest frequencies.

The tympanic membrane is a transparent, pearl-gray, slightly cone-shaped layer of flexible tissue that protects the inner ear and assists in transmission of sound energy. With increased age, collagenous tissue replaces the elastic tissue, resulting in a thinner and less resilient eardrum. Degenerative changes in the surrounding muscles and ligaments further compromise the resiliency of the tympanic membrane.

The three bones of the ossicular chain are connected to each other but move independently, acting as a lever to amplify sound. With advanced age, these bones become calcified and hardened, possibly interfering with the transfer of sound vibrations from the tympanic membrane to the oval window.

The middle ear muscles and ligaments contract in response to loud noises, stimulating the acoustic reflex. This reflex protects the delicate inner ear and filters out auditory distractions originating from one's own voice and body movements. With increased age, the middle ear muscles and ligaments become weaker and stiffer, which may have a detrimental effect on the acoustic reflex.

Although it seems logical that these age-related middle ear changes would cause a conductive hearing impairment, the results of research on the effects of middle ear changes are as yet inconclusive. Functionally, changes in the tympanic membrane may interfere with the transformation of sounds between the ear canal and the ossicular chain, and calcification of the ossicles may interfere with sound conduction. Studies on the impact of these changes have been inconclusive, and there is no current evidence that they contribute to significant conductive hearing loss.

Inner Ear

In the inner ear, vibrations are transmitted to the cochlea, where they are converted to nerve impulses and coded for intensity and frequency. Nerve impulses stimulate fibers of the eighth cranial nerve and send the auditory message to the brain. This process transpires primarily in the sensory hair cells of the organ of Corti in the cochlea.

Age-related changes of the inner ear structures include loss of hair cells, reduction of blood supply, diminution of endolymph production, decreased basilar membrane flexibility, degeneration of spiral ganglion cells, and loss of neurons in the cochlear nuclei. These inner ear changes result in the degenerative hearing impairment termed *presbycusis*.

One commonly used classification system for presbycusis is based on the specific structural source of the impairment, and can be delineated as follows:

1. *Sensory presbycusis,* which is associated with degenerative changes of the hair cells and the organ of Corti, is characterized by a sharp hearing loss at high frequencies, with little effect on speech understanding.
2. *Neural presbycusis* is related to widespread degeneration of nerve fibers in the cochlea and spiral ganglion; it is characterized by reduced speech discrimination.
3. *Metabolic or strial presbycusis* is caused by degenerative changes in the stria vascularis and a subsequent interruption in essential nutrient supply. Initially, these changes reduce the sensitivity to all sound frequencies; eventually, they interfere with speech discrimination.
4. *Mechanical presbycusis* results from mechanical changes in the inner ear structures and is characterized by a hearing loss that gradually increases from low to high frequencies. When sensitivity to the higher frequencies becomes impaired, speech discrimination is diminished.

As useful as this classification may be for analyzing the physiologic basis for various types of presbycusis, its application to older people is limited by the fact that presbycusis usually involves not one, but several, age-related processes.

Auditory Nervous System

From the inner ear, the auditory nerve fibers pass through the internal auditory meatus and enter the brain. Functions of the auditory nerve pathway include localizing sound direction, fine-tuning auditory stimuli, and transferring information from the primary auditory cortex to the auditory association area.

With increased age, the entire auditory nerve pathway undergoes atrophic changes and is further influenced by degenerative changes in related structures. Hair cell atrophy in the organ of Corti, narrowing of the auditory meatus from bone apposition, and degeneration of the arterial blood vessels that supply the auditory nerve are age-related changes that affect the auditory nervous system. Age-related changes in the central nervous system, particularly those that affect speech-specific cognitive abilities, interfere with auditory processing. These changes occur independently of the peripheral auditory changes and contribute to hearing deficits in older adults (Neils et al., 1991). Recent studies of the relationship between sensory and cognitive function suggest that age-related central nervous system changes are the common factors contributing to both the sensory and the cognitive deficits that affect older adults (Baltes and Lindenberger, 1997). Indeed, age-related changes in cognitive abilities may be responsible for much of the increased difficulty that older adults experience with speech perception in noisy environments (Sommers, 1997).

Risk Factors

In addition to the age-related changes that interfere with hearing, other factors, such as lifestyle, heredity, environment, and disease processes, also may have a negative impact on hearing. Most would agree that the risk factors for hearing impairment include exposure to excessive noise, systemic and auditory disease processes, and the use of ototoxic medications. Potential risk factors that are still under investigation include stress, diet, exercise, metabolism, cigarette smoking, genetic factors, serum cholesterol levels, and arteriosclerotic vascular disease.

Disease Processes

Ossicular function may be impaired by otosclerosis, which affects 10% to 12% of the population. This hereditary disease causes ankylosis of the footplate of the stapes to the oval window.

Although otosclerosis usually begins in youth or early adulthood, detection of the symptoms may be delayed until middle or later adulthood, when age-related middle ear changes compound the disease-related changes.

Ménière's disease and acoustic neuromas are examples of diseases that affect the auditory system and that may cause or contribute to hearing impairment. Examples of systemic diseases that cause or contribute to hearing impairment are syphilis, myxedema, diabetes, hypothyroidism, and Paget's disease. Other disorders that may cause hearing deficits are meningitis, head trauma, high fevers, and viral infections (e.g., measles and mumps).

Ototoxic Medications

Medications can cause or contribute to hearing impairments by damaging the ear structures, particularly the cochlear and vestibular divisions of the auditory nerve. Despite the fact that quinine and salicylate ototoxicities were first observed more than a century ago, the ototoxic effects of medication have received little attention in clinical settings. Although age alone does not increase the risk of ototoxicity, older adults are more likely to be taking ototoxic medications, such as aspirin and furosemide. Other

contributing factors that frequently affect older adults include renal failure, long-term use of ototoxic medications, and potentiation between two ototoxic medications, such as furosemide and aminoglycoside antibiotics.

Salicylates, furosemide, and mycin antibiotics have all been found to cause temporary or permanent hearing loss, which is often dose-related. Although ototoxicity is potentially reversible, both professionals and nonprofessionals often ascribe the hearing deficit to inevitable and irreversible degenerative changes. Display 6-1 presents a list of medications that may be ototoxic.

Environmental Influences

Prolonged exposure to noise in occupational or avocational environments may cause permanent damage to the auditory system. This may be especially true for older adults who may have worked in settings where recommendations that are now enforced by the National Institute of Occupational Safety and Health were not implemented. For instance, older people who were once employed as weavers or textile workers are likely to have been exposed to detrimentally noisy environments during their work years. Activities that are likely to cause neurosensory damage unless protective mechanisms are used

---

DISPLAY 6-1
Medications with Potential Ototoxicity

Aspirin	Diuretics
Aminoglycosides	Bumetanide
Amikacin	Ethacrynic acid
Gentamicin	Furosemide
Kanamycin	Erythromycin
Neomycin	Indomethacin
Netilmicin	Quinine
Streptomycin	Quinidine
Tobramycin	*Rauwolfia* derivatives
Cisplatin	

include the following: listening to loud music; riding motorcycles, airplanes, or snow mobiles; operating tractors, chain saws, and jackhammers; and shooting firearms while hunting or during target practice. People taking ototoxic drugs are even more susceptible to the damaging effects of noise exposure (National Institutes of Health Consensus Conference, 1990).

Functional Consequences

It is not uncommon for older adults to experience several age-related changes, as well as contributing factors, that influence hearing ability. Despite the limited knowledge about specific relationships between structural changes and functional consequences, distinguishing characteristics of age-related hearing impairments can be identified.

Speech Comprehension

Accurate comprehension of speech depends on speech pace, sound frequencies, environmental noise, and internal auditory function. Structural changes in the ear and nervous system influence different sound frequencies. Consequently, older adults typically experience changes in their ability to code sound frequencies precisely. Between the ages of 50 and 80 years, speech comprehension declines by 25% (Berg and Cassells, 1990, p. 105). Older adults with cognitive impairments will have increased difficulty with speech comprehension.

Speech comprehension is most directly influenced by the frequency of phonemes, the smallest units of sound. Each phoneme in a word has a different frequency, with vowels generally having lower frequencies and consonants usually having higher frequencies. Although most word phonemes have lower-range frequencies, the sibilant consonants (those that have a whistling quality) have higher-range frequencies. Because the earliest and most universal age-related changes affect one's ability to code higher-

frequency sounds, words rich in sibilants will be most affected by age-related changes of the auditory system.

Along with the pace of the verbal messages, the ability to understand speech is also influenced by environmental conditions. For older adults, any adverse environmental condition, especially the presence of background noise, may compound the negative influences of age-related changes. Research has consistently demonstrated that, in adverse listening situations, the speech comprehension of older people is disproportionately more impaired than that of younger subjects. Studies also have consistently shown that competitive background noises and increased rates of presentation have detrimental effects on speech comprehension in older adults. The results of one study of self-reported hearing problems revealed that difficulties in comprehending speech when it is distorted, or when adverse listening conditions are present, contributes more to age-related hearing disability than do other auditory problems (Slawinski et al., 1993).

Types and Prevalence of Hearing Impairments

Hearing losses are categorized according to the site of the impairment. Abnormalities of the external and middle ear impair the sound conduction mechanism and are classified as *conductive* hearing losses. Abnormalities of the inner ear interfere with the sensory and neural structures and are classified as *sensorineural* hearing losses. Hearing losses that involve both conductive and sensorineural impairments are called *mixed losses*.

Estimates of the prevalence of age-related hearing impairments among healthy older adults range from 10% to 30% for those aged 65 years and older, and from 25% to 52% for those aged 85 years and older (LaForge et al., 1992). A national survey of noninstitutionalized older people revealed that 58% of men and 44% of women aged 85 years and older reported hearing impairments (National Center for Health Statistics, 1985). Data from studies of the ill elderly suggest that hearing impairments affect as many as 96% of older people residing in nursing homes (Mahoney, 1993). Hearing impairment is most likely to occur in men, people of low economic status, and people exposed to prolonged job-related or recreational noise. The probability of hearing impairment also increases with a family history of otosclerosis. Whites are twice as likely as Blacks and Hispanics to be deaf or hard-of-hearing. The Culture Box summarizes additional variations.

Conductive Hearing Loss

Age-related changes in the external ear predispose older adults to wax accumulation and occlusion of the auditory canal. Impacted cerumen is the most common cause of conductive hearing deficit in older adults. About one third of community-living and hospitalized older adults, and up to 42% of older adults in nursing homes, have been found to have severe to complete cerumen impaction (Mahoney, 1996). The functional consequences of conductive deficits are an inability to hear low-pitched tones and a reduction in intensity of sound. Cerumen accumulation is the most easily preventable and treatable cause of hearing deficits; most importantly, it is readily amenable to nursing interventions. One study found that hearing was improved in 75% of the ears of hospitalized older adults with impacted cerumen once the wax was removed (Lewis-Cullinan and Janken, 1990).

Presbycusis

Presbycusis is the term applied to the sensorineural hearing loss associated with age-related changes. Studies indicate that presbycusis involves a sensorineural hearing loss and an age-related degeneration of central processing systems (Stein and Bienenfeld, 1992). An early functional consequence of presbycusis is the loss of ability to hear high-pitched sounds and sibilant consonants, such as *ch, f, g, s, sh, t, th,* and *z*. With the filtering out of high-pitched sounds, words become distorted and jumbled, and sentences become incoherent. A sentence like "I think she should go to the store" might be interpreted by a listener with presbycusis as "I wish we could go to the show." This characteristic is known as diminished speech discrimination and is influenced by the speaker's rate of speech. Rapid, slow, or slurred speech patterns make it increasingly difficult for the older person to discern words. As the hearing loss progresses, explosive consonants, such as *b, d, k, p,* and *t*, also become distorted.

Older people with presbycusis have even greater difficulty with speech discrimination when background noises are present, or when they are in a room with poor acoustics or echoing. The older adult in a hospital or long-term care facility may be particularly sensitive to background noises to which the staff may have become accustomed. Many hearing-impaired older adults experience hypersensitivity to high-intensity sounds, which makes these sounds disproportionately loud. This may cause amplified sound to feel unpleasantly harsh and difficult to

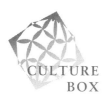

CULTURE
BOX

Cultural Variations in Hearing Acuity

- Approximately 51% of American Indians and approximately 48% of older Hispanic Americans have impaired hearing; less than 10% of the people in these groups who have impaired hearing have hearing aids (Bassford, 1995; Rousseau, 1995).
- Compared with Whites, Blacks are less susceptible to noise-induced hearing loss and have better hearing at high and low frequencies (Overfield, 1995).

TABLE 6-1
Age-Related Changes Affecting Hearing

	Change	Consequence
External Canal	Longer, thicker hair Thinner, drier skin Increased keratin	Potential for impacted cerumen with impaired sound conduction
Middle Ear	Diminished resiliency of tympanic membrane Calcified, hardened ossicles Weakened and stiff muscles and ligaments	Impaired sound conduction
Inner Ear and Nervous System	Diminished neurons, endolymph, hair cells, and blood supply Degeneration of spiral ganglion and arterial blood vessels Decreased flexibility of basilar membrane Narrowing of auditory meatus Degeneration of central processing systems	Presbycusis: diminished ability to hear high-pitched sounds, especially in the presence of background noise

tolerate. Table 6-1 summarizes the age-related changes affecting hearing, as well as the functional consequences of these changes.

Psychosocial Consequences

Hearing is a primary component of communication for daily living in society. Through the ears, one enjoys humor, appreciates music, obtains information, and relates to others. Hearing deficits inevitably affect these and many other activities of daily life. Communication impairments caused by an inability to understand spoken words often have a profoundly negative effect on self-confidence. People who are unable to discriminate words are afraid to respond to questions, and they may choose not to answer rather than risk feeling foolish. Performance on mental status examinations may be influenced negatively by a person's fear of not hearing the questions accurately, as well as by the concomitant reduction of sensory stimuli.

Studies on the relationship between auditory acuity and performance on mental status tests consistently show that hearing deficits have a negative impact on the results of cognitive function tests, with a greater impact being documented on verbal than on nonverbal measures. Poor performance on tests of cognitive abilities may mistakenly lead to the labeling of older people as demented when, in fact, they simply have a hearing loss.

Hearing deficits may lead to fear, boredom, apathy, depression, social isolation, and feelings of low self-esteem. A recent study of the effects of hearing impairments on nursing home residents revealed a strong association between hearing impairments and low levels of social engagement and little or no time spent in activities (Resnick et al., 1997). The ability to test reality may also be impaired, leading to suspiciousness, paranoia, and psychosis (Butler et al., 1991, p. 216; Stein and Thienhaus, 1993). When only parts of conversations are heard, one may come to believe that the conversation is about oneself, and persecutory delusions may develop. Additionally, hearing deficits may have a negative impact on the ability of the older person to negotiate the environment safely when warning signals are sounded for fires, ambulances, and other emergency situations. In addition to creating actual safety hazards, the hearing deficit may lead to fear and anxiety.

Negative societal attitudes about aging and hearing deficits may result in a doubly negative effect on the person who is old as well as hard of hearing. The older person may be reluctant to acknowledge a hearing deficit, choosing to limit opportunities for communication rather than face the stigma associated with hearing impairments. These attitudes and accompanying behaviors may contribute to further social isolation and other psychosocial consequences of loneliness and isolation.

Figure 6-1 summarizes age-related changes, risk factors, and negative functional consequences that influence the ability to hear.

Nursing Assessment

Nursing assessment of hearing is aimed at identifying: (1) past and present risk factors, especially those that are amenable to interventions; (2) the presence of a hearing deficit; (3) psychosocial consequences of any hearing deficit; and (4) outcomes of prior diagnostic tests and interventions. Each of these factors is important in helping older adults and their caregivers compensate for hearing deficits. Assessment is accomplished through interview questions, observation of behavioral cues, and administration of hearing tests.

Interview Questions

Interview questions are used to acquire information about: (1) present and past risk factors; (2) the person's awareness and acknowledgment of a hearing impairment; (3) the psychosocial impact of any hearing deficit; and (4) attitudes that might influence the use of assistive devices. The hearing assessment interview begins with questions about family history of hearing impairments or a personal history of prolonged exposure to loud noises. Identification of ototoxic medications as a risk factor can be included as part of the hearing assessment or as part of the medication history. Questions about risk factors may prompt the older person to discuss a hearing problem.

If the older adult does not initiate a discussion of hearing problems, the nurse should ask direct questions about the person's discernment of any hearing deficit. If the older adult denies having a hearing problem but shows behavioral cues indicative of a hearing deficit, the nurse should try to elicit further information. This may be accomplished by asking a leading question like "I notice you turn your left ear toward me. Is your hearing better in that ear?" Hearing impairments that interfere with meaningful communication may result in psychosocial consequences and lifestyle changes. Questions about any changes in the social activities of the older adult may reveal psychosocial consequences that can be alleviated through interventions aimed at improving communication.

The psychosocial consequences of hearing impairment are influenced by the lifestyle of the person affected. For example, hearing impairments are relatively more detrimental for people whose occupations or avocations are highly dependent on good hearing. By contrast, hearing impairments may be less detrimental for people who have few social relationships and who do not depend on hearing for occupational or leisure activities. If no hearing impairment is present, questions about lifestyle do not necessarily have to be included as part of the hearing assessment. When a person acknowledges the existence of a hearing impairment, however, the nurse should ask about any associated changes in social and occupational activities.

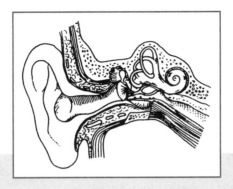

AGE-RELATED CHANGES

Inner Ear
- Decreased neurons, blood supply, endolymph, and hair cells
- Less flexible basilar membrane
- Narrowing of auditory meatus

Middle Ear
- Less resilient tympanic membrane
- Calcified ossicles
- Stiffer muscles and ligaments

External Ear
- Thicker hair
- Thinner skin
- Increased keratin

NEGATIVE FUNCTIONAL CONSEQUENCES
- Predisposition to impacted cerumen
- *Presbycusis*: Diminished ability to hear high-pitched sounds, especially in the presence of background noise

RISK FACTORS
- Impacted cerumen
- Ototoxic medications
- Prolonged exposure to noise
- Background noise
- Systemic diseases (e.g., diabetes)
- Auditory diseases (e.g., Ménière's disease)

FIGURE 6-1. Hearing in older adults.

The nurse must assess the older person's attitudes toward assistive hearing devices, as these will influence his or her acceptance of interventions. Older adults may believe that hearing aids are too costly or of little use, or they may be embarrassed to use a device that is visible to others. Resistance toward hearing aids may also arise from lack of money, transportation, or motivation to communicate. One study of nursing home residents found that 21% of the subjects wished to try a hearing aid. When asked about barriers to trying such a device, the residents cited cost, the fact that such a device was not needed before entering the nursing home, and lack of knowledge about how to arrange for an evaluation (Garahan et al., 1992). A careful assessment of attitudes about hearing aids may identify barriers that can be addressed through nursing interventions. Display 6-2 provides guidelines for nursing assessment of hearing.

DISPLAY 6-2
Guidelines for Assessing Hearing

Interview Questions to Assess Risk Factors for Hearing Loss

- Do you have a family history of hearing loss or deafness?
- Have you been exposed to loud noises in your job or leisure activities?
- Do you have a history of any of the following: diabetes, hypothyroidism, Ménière's disease, or Paget's disease?
- What medications do you take? (Refer to Display 6-1 to identify potentially ototoxic medications.)

Interview Questions to Assess Awareness of Hearing Deficit

- Do you have any trouble with your hearing?
- Have you noticed any change in your ability to understand conversations or hear words?
- Are you bothered by any noises in your ears, such as ringing or buzzing?

Additional Questions If Hearing Loss Is Acknowledged

- How long have you noticed a hearing loss?
- Has there been a progressive loss, or did the hearing problem begin suddenly?
- Describe your hearing difficulty.
- Are there any conditions, such as noisy environments or particular voices or sounds, that especially interfere with your hearing?
- Do you notice differences in hearing between your left and right ears?
- Does your hearing loss interfere with your ability to communicate with others, either individually or in groups?

- Are there any activities that you would like to do, but feel you cannot do because of hearing problems?
- Have you ever had, or thought about having, an evaluation for a hearing aid?
- Have you ever tried using a hearing aid?

Observations If a Hearing Loss Is Noted

- What are the person's attitudes about hearing loss? Is it considered normal and untreatable? Is a hearing aid considered to be a stigma?
- If the person is resistant to an audiologic evaluation, what are the barriers? (For example, are there financial or transportation limitations that interfere with obtaining a hearing aid?)
- Does the hearing loss contribute to a sense of isolation, depression, paranoia, or low self-esteem?
- What are the person's usual communication opportunities, and how does the hearing loss influence these usual patterns? (For instance, does the person live in an environment where it is important to be able to use the phone? Does the person live in a noisy environment and find relief in the hearing impairment? If the person lives in an environment where group activities are a large part of daily activities, does the person want to participate in these activities?)

Behavioral Cues

Behavioral cues related to hearing loss provide important information about the presence of a hearing impairment, the psychosocial consequences of any such impairment, and the person's attitudes about assistive devices. If the older adult denies a hearing deficit that has been noticed by others, behavioral cues may be the primary source of assessment information. Denial of a hearing deficit may result from lack of awareness of the impairment because of gradual onset or, if the older person is socially isolated, it may result from a paucity of opportunities for communication. Feelings of embarrassment or misconceptions that the hearing loss is an inevitable and untreatable consequence of aging may also contribute to denial. Display 6-3 lists behavioral cues that should be observed by the nurse as part of the hearing assessment.

Hearing Tests

The nursing assessment of hearing includes the use of a tuning fork to check hearing and examination of the external ear and tympanic membrane with an otoscope. The purpose of the tuning fork test is to detect hearing impairments and to differentiate between conductive and sensorineural losses. The purpose of the otoscopic examination is to identify factors, such as cerumen accumulation, that might interfere with hearing. Display 6-4 describes the procedure for performing a nursing assessment of hearing using the otoscope and tuning fork. If any hearing deficits are reported by the older adult or identified as a result of this examination, the nurse should recommend that a further evaluation be conducted at a speech and hearing center or by a specialized physician, such as an otolaryngologist.

Nursing Diagnosis

Based on the focused nursing assessment, the nurse may identify an actual hearing deficit or risk factors for impaired hearing. The hearing impairment may or may not have psychosocial

---

DISPLAY 6-3
Guidelines for Assessing Behavioral Cues to Hearing

Behavioral Cues to a Hearing Deficit

- Inappropriate or no response to questions, especially in the absence of opportunities for lipreading
- Inability to follow verbal directions without cues
- Short attention span, easy distractibility
- Frequent requests for repetition or clarification of verbal communication
- Intense observation of the speaker
- Mouthing of words spoken by the speaker
- Turning of one ear toward the speaker
- Unusual physical proximity to the speaker
- Lack of response to loud environmental noises
- Too loud or inarticulate speech
- Abnormal voice characteristics, such as monotony

- Perception that others are talking about him or her

Behavioral Cues About Psychosocial Consequences

- Uncharacteristic avoidance of group settings
- Lack of interest in social activities, especially those requiring verbal communication or those that the person enjoyed in the past (e.g., bingo, card games)

Behavioral Cues About Assistive Devices

- Lack of use of a hearing aid that has been purchased
- Failure to obtain batteries for a hearing aid
- Expression of embarrassment about using assistive devices

DISPLAY 6-4
Guidelines for Otoscopic and Tuning Fork Assessment

Guidelines for Otoscopic Examination

- Use the largest speculum available.
- Hold the otoscope upside down, resting your hand on the person's head to stabilize the instrument.
- Before inserting the speculum, pull the pinna upward and backward, while tilting the person's head slightly back and toward the opposite shoulder.
- If cerumen has accumulated to the point of interfering with the examination or occluding the canal, follow the procedure described in the section on Nursing Interventions.
- Normal otoscopic findings in older adults include the following:
    Small amount of cerumen
    Pinkish-white epithelial lining, no redness or lesions
    Pearl-gray tympanic membrane, which is less translucent than in younger adults
    Light reflex anteroinferiorly from the umbo
    Visible landmarks

Use of Tuning Forks for Hearing Tests

- Use a tuning fork with frequencies of 512 to 1024 cps (Hz).
- Hold the tuning fork firmly at the stem.
- Strike the fork against the palm of your hand, or strike the fork with a rubber reflex hammer, to set it in motion.

Weber Test
Procedure: Place the tip of a vibrating tuning fork at the center of the person's forehead. Ask where they hear the sound and whether it is louder in one ear than in the other.
Normal finding: The tuning fork is heard equally in both ears.
Abnormal finding: The tuning fork is heard better in one ear, indicating a possible hearing loss.

Rinne Test
Procedure: Mask one ear, then place a vibrating tuning fork on the mastoid process of the opposite ear until the person indicates that it can no longer be heard. Then, quickly place the tuning fork in front of the ear canal with the top near the ear canal.
Normal finding: The length of time the tuning fork can be heard over the ear canal is about twice as long as the time it can be heard over the mastoid bone.
Abnormal finding: The length of time the tuning fork is heard in front of the ear is not twice as long (or longer) as the time it can be heard when placed on the mastoid process. In such a case, the person should undergo further tests for impaired hearing.

---

consequences, such as social isolation. An appropriate nursing diagnosis for an older adult with a hearing impairment would be Impaired Communication. The definition of this nursing diagnosis is "the state in which the individual experiences, or is at high risk to experience, a decreased ability to send or receive messages (i.e., has difficulty exchanging thoughts, ideas, or desire)" (Carpenito, 1997, p. 209). Related factors that are common in older adults are hearing loss, auditory nerve damage, ototoxic medications, and environmental conditions, such as background noise.

If psychosocial consequences are identified,

other pertinent nursing diagnoses might include Anxiety, Impaired Adjustment, Impaired Social Interaction, and Ineffective Individual Coping. When the hearing impairment is severe and uncompensated to the point that the person does not function safely, then High Risk for Injury might be an applicable nursing diagnosis. If paranoia or denial are consequences of the hearing deficit, then the nursing diagnosis of Sensory-Perceptual Alterations might be applied. The care plan at the end of this chapter is based on a nursing diagnosis of Impaired Social Interaction related to the effects of hearing loss.

Nursing Goals

One goal of nursing care for hearing-impaired older adults is the elimination of reversible risk factors. For example, cerumen accumulation can be addressed through the nursing measures discussed in the next section. Another goal is the facilitation of optimal communication for people with irreversible hearing loss. This is accomplished through the use of appropriate sound amplification devices, the use of compensatory communication techniques, and the education of families and other caregivers about these techniques. A third goal would be maintaining quality of life, which would be achieved through interventions that address psychosocial consequences, such as impaired social interaction.

Nursing Interventions

Eliminating Risk Factors

Heredity, disease processes, exposure to noise, and use of ototoxic medication are common risk factors for hearing impairment. Although the effects of most of these risk factors are irreversible, the use of ototoxic medication is one factor that can be addressed. Nurses should teach older adults and their professional and family caregivers about the potential ototoxicity of the medications listed in Display 6-1. When effective alternatives are available, or when the older adult is experiencing hearing difficulties, efforts should be made to avoid the use of these medications. As with other questions about medication, older adults and their caregivers should be advised to discuss their concerns about ototoxic medications with the prescribing health care practitioner.

Conductive hearing impairment caused by impacted wax can be prevented by educating older adults and their caregivers, and can be alleviated through nursing interventions. Over-the-counter otic solutions containing ingredients such as glycerin, hydrogen peroxide, mineral oil, carbamide peroxide, and propylene glycol, when periodically instilled in the ear canal, will prevent cerumen accumulation. The schedule for instillation of otic drops may vary from semi-weekly to monthly, depending on the person.

When an ear canal is impacted with cerumen, the nurse must determine whether there is a possible ruptured tympanic membrane or any other contraindication to irrigation. If any contraindications, such as pain or a recent ear infection, are identified, the person should be instructed to seek medical care from a qualified professional, such as an otolaryngologist.

If there are no contraindications, the following procedure should clear the canal of cerumen:

1. Soften the cerumen with 3% hydrogen peroxide or an over-the-counter otic preparation.
2. Irrigate the canal with body-temperature tap water using a syringe or dental irrigation device and gentle pressure.
3. Aim water at the sides of the canal, and allow drainage from the ear to collect in a basin.
4. Drain excessive fluid from the ear by tilting the head toward the affected side.
5. Instill a drying agent, such as an otic solution or 70% isopropyl alcohol.
6. If the cerumen is difficult to remove, a softening preparation can be instilled twice daily for several days, followed by the irrigation procedure.

After the wax build-up has been removed, teach the person to prevent the recurrence of impacted cerumen by using otic drops, as discussed earlier in this section.

Facilitating Optimal Communication Through Sound Amplification

Sound amplification should be considered only after completion of an audiologic examination and identification of any treatable causes for the hearing deficit. People with irreversible hearing deficits who are interested in corrective measures may participate in an aural rehabilitation program. These programs are available at speech and hearing centers, which are often affiliated with hospitals, medical centers, or universities. The National Association for Hearing and Speech Action is an excellent source of information about professional services for the evaluation and treatment of hearing disorders. (Consult the Educational Resources section at the end of this chapter.)

Individualized aural rehabilitation programs consist of counseling, together with any or all of the following services: amplification devices, auditory training, lipreading, and speech conservation. Although nurses usually are not involved with these programs, they may have opportunities to suggest referrals for aural rehabilitation and to facilitate the use of recommended sound amplification devices.

Sound amplification generally is achieved by using hearing aids or assistive hearing devices. Hearing aids are individually prescribed and require audiology services, whereas assistive hearing devices are not individualized and are available without professional assistance or recommendation.

Hearing Aids

A hearing aid is a battery-operated amplifier consisting of a microphone, a conductive cord, and a receiver. Most hearing aids amplify sounds without correcting distortions, but some hearing aids developed in recent years do have the ability to amplify sounds selectively. Because of their limited ability to amplify sounds at selected frequencies, traditional hearing aids are more beneficial to people with impairments at multiple frequencies than to those with impairments only at the highest frequencies.

Hearing aids have many drawbacks, including their cost, which is not covered by Medicare and usually ranges from $500 to several thousand dollars. Additional limitations may be

identified, particularly if the person has difficulty with manual dexterity or fine motor movements. Despite these limitations, older adults using hearing aids have reported significant improvements in communication ability and in social, cognitive, and emotional function (Gordon-Salant, 1996; Tesch-Römer, 1997). People with presbycusis may find that a conventional hearing aid does not improve their ability to understand words because it does not selectively enhance high-frequency sounds. In recent years, digitally programmable hearing aids have been developed. These aids are selectively programmed to meet the needs of the hearing-impaired person in various listening conditions. A major advantage of these newer hearing aids is that they are acoustically superior to conventional models and can be adjusted for different listening situations. Disadvantages include high cost and the need for considerable training and frequent adjustments on the part of the hearing-impaired person. More than 500 models of hearing aids—and four general types—are available, each of which has certain advantages and disadvantages. The advantages and disadvantages of each type of hearing aid are summarized in Table 6-2.

Older adults and their families should be encouraged to obtain initial information about hearing aids from consumer and professional organizations, rather than directly from hearing aid dealers. The International Hearing Society distributes a Hearing Aid Helpline consumer kit free of charge, and the Better Business Bureau provides information about local hearing aid dispensers. (See the Educational Resources section at the end of this chapter.)

If the nursing assessment identified barriers to obtaining an evaluation, attempts should be made to address these issues. For example, when misinformation or lack of information creates barriers, the nurse can suggest that the older person obtain accurate information from one of the organizations listed in the Educational Resources section. If financial or transportation

TABLE 6-2
Advantages and Disadvantages of Four Types of Hearing Aid

Type	Advantages	Disadvantages
Body-worn	Most powerful, with best sound quality	Clothing and movement produce noise
	Best for severe loss	Cord gets tangled
	Easiest to manipulate	Most visible
Behind-the-ear	More powerful than in-the-ear types	Very visible
Eyeglass style	More powerful than in-the-ear types	Must wear eyeglasses all the time
In-the-ear	Least conspicuous	Requires very good manual dexterity

limitations are problematic for an older person who is otherwise receptive to obtaining a hearing aid, interventions can be aimed at identifying community resources to address these concerns.

Assistive Hearing Devices

Any device that amplifies or replaces sounds for individual or group communication without being individualized is categorized as an assistive hearing device. A stethoscope is an example of an assistive hearing device commonly used by health care workers. Megaphones and microphones are examples of amplification devices used for group communication. Closed-captioned television is an example of an assistive device that substitutes visual cues for auditory cues.

The advantages of assistive hearing devices over hearing aids are the ready availability of the former and their lower cost, which may be shared by several users in some settings. In addition, most of these devices do not require as much manual dexterity as hearing aids, and some of them are more effective than hearing aids in filtering out background noise. Assistive hearing devices can be used in conjunction with hearing aids, or they can be used by people who do not use hearing aids.

Assistive hearing devices, which consist of a small, battery-powered amplifier and headphones, can be used easily in any setting to improve communication temporarily. Nurses in a general hospital tested one such product and found that the positive outcomes of this device included increased privacy, improved patient education, increased patient cooperation, and improved nurse-patient communication (DeBlase and Kucler, 1985). Similarly, nurses in a residential care facility identified the following benefits from using a small portable amplifier for nurse-resident communication: improved communication, fewer misunderstandings, fewer disruptions to conversation, and considerably less effort required for communication (Erber, 1994).

Assistive hearing devices are available for home use to amplify specific sounds, such as those from the radio, television, or telephone. Other devices serve as substitutes for sound when amplification is impractical or ineffective. Flashing lights for doorbells or doormats, and alarm clocks that vibrate the pillow or flash a light, are examples of such substitution devices. People with more serious hearing impairments but with adequate vision may benefit from closed-captioned television, which provides subscripts for many programs. Since 1990, all televisions with screens 13 inches or larger must feature a closed-captioned option.

Portable assistive hearing devices are available for use in public places. Small, hand-sized amplifiers can be attached temporarily to pay phones and other telephones. Churches, theaters, and government buildings sometimes equip their facilities with assistive devices to amplify sound.

Catalogues describing various assistive hearing devices are available, and an international nonprofit organization called Self Help for Hard of Hearing People (SHHH) provides consumer information about assistive hearing devices. Local chapters of this organization distribute information about public buildings equipped with assistive hearing devices. (See the Educational Resource section.)

Teaching Related to Hearing Aids

Nurses must be familiar enough with hearing aids to assist older adults and their caregivers with the hearing aid's use and care. Although nurses can expect that hearing aid dispensers will provide initial instructions regarding the use and care of the hearing aid, these instructions may have to be reviewed or revamped as dependency needs and caregiver roles change. Older adults who normally depend on family members for assistance with hearing aids may not be able to use and care for a hearing aid properly when they are in a hospital or nursing home. Likewise, nurses in home settings may have to teach caregivers about hearing aids if the older adult needs assistance that was not previously provided by that caregiver. This is likely to occur if the caregiver changes, or if the older adult becomes more dependent because of increased functional impairment. Display 6-5 summarizes the teaching points related to the use and care of hearing aids.

DISPLAY 6-5
Use and Care of Hearing Aids

Guidelines for Insertion and Use

- With the volume of the device turned off and the canal portion pointing into the ear, insert the hearing aid.
- Make sure the aid fits snugly in the ear canal.
- M, T, and O designate "microphone," "telephone," and "off," respectively.
- Turn the M-T-O switch to M.
- Turn the volume up slowly, beginning at one third to one half volume, until a comfortable level is reached.
- If whistling (feedback) is heard, check the position of the device in the ear and the volume. (The aid may not fit snugly enough, or the volume may be too high.)
- Begin wearing the aid for short periods, in a familiar and quiet environment, and in one-to-one conversations.
- Gradually increase the length of time the aid is worn, the variety of environments, and the number of people included in conversations.
- Allow several months before expecting to feel totally comfortable with a hearing aid.
- Avoid noisy environments and eliminate background noise when possible (e.g., turn off TVs and radios; close doors to rooms).
- Use the appropriate switch (T) for telephone calls.

- Understand that hearing aids do not restore hearing to normal, but rather amplify sound, including all environmental noises.

Guidelines for Care and Maintenance

- Keep a fresh battery available (batteries can be expected to last for 70 to 85 hours), but do not purchase batteries more than 1 month in advance.
- Turn off the hearing aid before changing the battery.
- Remove the battery or turn off the aid when not in use.
- Clean the aid weekly, using warm, soapy water for the earmold and a toothpick or pipe cleaner for the channel.
- Never use alcohol on the earmold because this will cause drying and cracking.
- Check the earmold for cracks or scratches.
- Avoid extreme heat, cold, or moisture (e.g., do not leave the hearing aid near the stove, do not wear it while using a hair dryer, and do not wear it outside, unless it is protected well in rainy or extremely cold weather).
- Avoid exposure to chemicals, such as hair spray or permanent solutions.
- Avoid dropping the aid on a hard surface; when handling it, keep it over a soft or padded surface.

Techniques for Facilitating Optimal Communication

Good communication techniques are essential in assisting the older adult to compensate for hearing deficits. The primary functional consequence of presbycusis is a diminished acuity for high-frequency sounds, which is exacerbated by fast speech pace and environmental noise. Therefore, communication interventions must be aimed at improving the clarity of words, slowing the rate of speech, and eliminating environmental noise and distractions. Techniques that directly enhance auditory communication should be augmented by effective use of nonverbal and written communication techniques. Display 6-6 summarizes the communication techniques that should be used to enhance the hearing abilities of older adults with impaired hearing. Nurses should use these techniques and should teach professional and family caregivers to use them.

In recent years, increased attention has been directed toward planning or modifying environments to diminish background noise and to improve the ability of people to hear. Some noise control modifications, such as using window draperies, are relatively simple and can be applied to many settings. Other noise control measures, such as selection of building materials, need to be implemented while environments are being designed. References on noise control measures are now available, and these can serve as helpful resources in planning environments for people with hearing impairments (e.g., Brawley, 1997).

Maintaining Quality of Life

Interventions that improve communication with hearing-impaired older adults can also improve their quality of life. As discussed earlier, many negative psychosocial consequences are associated with impaired hearing. For example, older adults may withdraw from social interactions, particularly in large groups, if they cannot readily participate in conversations. The case example at the end of this chapter illustrates a

---

DISPLAY 6-6
Communicating with Hearing-Impaired People

- Stand or sit directly in front of, and close to, the person.
- Talk toward the better ear, but make sure your lips can be seen.
- Make sure the person pays attention and looks at your face.
- Address the person by name, pause, and then begin talking.
- Speak distinctly, slowly, and directly to the person.
- Do not exaggerate lip movements because this will interfere with lipreading.
- Avoid chewing gum, covering your mouth, or turning your head away.
- If the person does not understand, repeat the message using different words.
- Avoid or eliminate any background noise.
- Do not raise the volume of your voice; rather, try to lower the tone while still speaking in a moderately loud voice.

- Keep all instructions simple, and ask for feedback to assess what the person heard.
- Avoid questions that elicit simple yes or no answers.
- Keep sentences short.
- Use body language that is congruent with what you are trying to communicate.
- Demonstrate what you are saying.
- Use large-print written communication and pictures to supplement verbal communication.
- Make sure only one person talks at a time; arrange for one-on-one communication whenever possible.
- If eyeglasses normally are worn to improve vision, make sure they are clean.
- Provide adequate lighting so that the person can see your lips; avoid settings in which there is glare behind or around you.

ALTERNATIVE
AND
PREVENTIVE
HEALTH
CARE
PRACTICES

Preventing or Alleviating Tinnitus and Hearing Problems

Herbs
- For tinnitus: ginkgo, sesame, goldenseal, black cohosh
- To improve circulation to the ear: ginger, ginkgo

Homeopathic Remedies
- Tinnitus: Salicyclic, Carbonium sul, China sul, Kali iod, Kali carb, 2 drops of almond oil in each ear weekly
- To reduce earwax: Causticum

Nutritional Considerations
- Zinc, magnesium, vitamins A, D, and E

Preventive Measures and Additional Approaches
- For tinnitus: acupuncture; avoid aspirin, cinchona, meadowsweet, wintergreen, black haw, willow bark, birch bark, uva ursi
- For ear wax: warm German camomile oil in 5 drops of olive oil in the ear

care plan that addresses the goal of maintaining quality of life. Alternative and preventive health care practices, as summarized in the box above, may improve quality of life with regard to tinnitus and hearing problems.

Evaluating Nursing Care

Nursing care for the hearing-impaired older adult is evaluated by measuring the extent to which goals have been achieved. A common short-term goal would be that the person will communicate effectively with others. Display 6-6 summarizes some of the communication techniques that nurses can use to achieve this goal. A subjective measurement of this goal would be the older adult's report of improved satisfaction with exchanges of verbal information. Objective measurements include observations that the person uses a hearing aid effectively in one-to-one conversations and follows through accurately when given verbal directions. The nursing care plan at the end of this chapter includes evaluation criteria that can be applied to these kinds of short-term goals.

Long-term goals for older adults with impaired hearing address the need for ongoing management of hearing deficits. For example, one goal might be for the older adult to obtain an evaluation for a hearing aid. Nurses in short-term institutional settings would address such a goal through a discharge plan that includes information about resources for hearing evaluations and other relevant community services. Educational resources that might be used to achieve this goal are listed at the end of this chapter. Evaluation of this goal would be based on the patient's positive response to the nurse's suggestions. In home, community, and long-term care settings, nurses may have opportunities to address long-term goals more directly by assisting older adults and their caregivers in using additional services. In these settings, the evaluation of long-term goals might be based on the actual use of additional resources that improve the person's verbal communication abilities.

Another issue that might be addressed through long-term goals would be the psychosocial effects of impaired hearing. For example, if social isolation is a consequence of a hearing deficit, the first priority would be to ensure that the person's hearing deficit is addressed through direct interventions (e.g, sound amplification, effective communication techniques, and control of environmental noise). A second priority would be to identify activities that the person would find satisfying, despite the hearing deficit. For example, in long-term care facilities, hearing-impaired residents might enjoy participating in card games that take place in small, quiet rooms, but they might dislike activities that are held in large, noisy rooms. This kind of long-term goal is evaluated in the nursing care plan at the end of this chapter.

Chapter Summary

Older adults experience an age-related hearing impairment called presbycusis. In the early stage of presbycusis, high-pitched sounds, as well as words with sibilants, become distorted. Eventually, speech comprehension becomes more impaired, and the older person has difficulty understanding verbal communication. This hearing deficit is exacerbated by the presence of background noise and by rapid-paced speech. Besides the age-related changes that can impair hearing, risk factors, such as impacted wax and ototoxic medications, are common causes of hearing problems in older adults.

Nursing assessment of hearing focuses on identifying any hearing deficits and treatable risk factors. Also, it is important to assess any barriers to the use of hearing aids. Pertinent nursing diagnoses would be Impaired Verbal Communication or Impaired Social Interaction. Nursing care plans are directed toward addressing risk factors and improving communica-

tion. Nursing responsibilities regarding risk factors include raising questions about ototoxic medications and preventing and alleviating impacted cerumen. Nursing responsibilities regarding communication include addressing the need for a hearing evaluation and sound amplification, using techniques to enhance communication, and controlling or eliminating background noise. Nursing care is evaluated based on the improved ability of the older adult to understand verbal communication.

Critical Thinking Exercises

1. Describe presbycusis and explain the functional consequences of this condition as it affects the everyday life of an older adult.
2. What risk factors would you consider in an 83-year-old person who complains of recent problems with hearing?
3. What advice would you give to someone who asks you about a brochure they received describing a new high-powered hearing aid provided by a company that provides free hearing tests? The person has trouble hearing but has never had an evaluation.
4. Describe at least 10 ways in which you can adapt your communication for a hearing-impaired person.
5. Find at least one resource (*not* a hearing aid dealer) in your community that you could recommend to an older adult who needs a hearing evaluation.

Case Example and Nursing Care Plan

Pertinent Case Information

Mr. H. is an 87-year-old widower who was diagnosed as having Parkinson's disease 23 years ago. Presbycusis is listed as an additional diagnosis on his medical record. He is being admitted to a nursing home because his condition has declined to the point that his daughter, Ms. D., can no longer manage his care in her home. He is medically stable but needs assistance in all activities of daily living.

Nursing Assessment

During the admission interview, you notice that Mr. H. has difficulty hearing your questions and that he frequently asks his daughter to give the requested information. He shows no significant cognitive deficits, but he seems to have difficulty understanding verbal communication. When you ask about any hearing impairment, Ms. D. tells you that her father has used hearing aids for 10 years and has been reevaluated periodically at a speech and hearing center. Two months ago, he obtained new hearing aids, but he wears them only for one-to-one conversations with her. Because of Mr. H.'s tremors and difficulty with fine motor movements, Ms. D. cares for his hearing aids and assists with their insertion and removal.

Ms. D. has encouraged her father to wear his hearing aids during family gatherings, but he says the noise from the small children is too annoying. Except for family gatherings, Mr. H. has very few opportunities for social interaction, and he has become more and more withdrawn. He used to enjoy playing poker, but he has not played in several years because all of his friends have died. Now he spends much of his time watching closed-captioned television programs. Ms. D. hopes that her father will respond to the opportunities for socialization provided at the nursing home and that his depression will improve.

Nursing Diagnosis

In addition to nursing diagnoses related to Mr. H.'s chronic illness and self-care deficits, you identify a nursing diagnosis of Impaired Social Interaction related to the effects of hearing loss. You select this, rather than Impaired Verbal Communication, as a nursing diagnosis because Mr. H.'s hearing impairment has already been evaluated and sound amplification devices are available to him. In your care plan, you will address the psychosocial consequences of his hearing impairment. Your nursing care is directed toward improving his social interaction through the use of available devices and through other communication techniques that will enhance his social interaction skills.

Goals	Nursing Interventions	Evaluation Criteria
To develop effective verbal communication techniques for resident-staff interactions	During the initial interview, talk with Mr. H. and Ms. D. about the importance of good verbal communication with staff; emphasize the need for the staff to get to know Mr. H. so his needs can be addressed.	Mr. H. will wear his hearing aids during all one-to-one conversations with staff members.
	Ask Mr. H. to wear his hearing aids during all one-to-one interactions with staff.	Mr. H. will report satisfactory verbal interactions with the staff.
	Use good communication techniques when talking with Mr. H.	Mr. H.'s hearing aids will be maintained in good operating condition.

	(e.g., sit face-to-face, eliminate as much background noise as possible). Make sure all staff members provide appropriate assistance with insertion and removal of Mr. H.'s hearing aids. Include hearing aid maintenance as part of the daily responsibilities of the nursing aide.	
To engage in social interactions with one other resident	During the admission team meeting, identify several other residents who might converse with Mr. H. Ask the staff to encourage one-on-one social interaction between Mr. H. and selected resident(s) (e.g., suggest that they watch closed-captioned television programs together). Ask Mr. H. to wear his hearing aids during one-on-one interactions with residents. Provide assistance with inserting and removing hearing aids as needed. Provide a quiet environment for one-on-one conversations with other residents.	Mr. H. will wear his hearing aids at least once daily for a conversation with one other resident.
To engage in small group activities with other residents	During the first monthly review conference, ask the activities staff to invite Mr. H. to a poker game with three other residents in the small group room. Make sure that environmental noise is controlled as much as possible.	By the second month in this facility, Mr. H. will participate in weekly poker games with three other residents.

Educational Resources

Better Hearing Institute
P.O. Box 1840, Washington, DC 20013
(703) 642-0580; (800) 327-9355
www.betterhearing.org
• Lists of specialists in hearing problems and aids
• *Your Guide to Better Hearing* (free brochure)

International Hearing Society (IHS)
20361 Middlebelt, Livonia, MI 48152
(248) 478-2610; (800) 521-5247
• Referral to qualified hearing instrument specialists
• *The World of Sound: Facts about Hearing and Hearing Aids* (free booklet)

National Association for Hearing and Speech Action (NAHSA)
10801 Rockville Pike, Rockville, MD 20852-3279
(301) 897-8682; (800) 638-8255
www.asha.org
•Professional referrals
•Products catalogue
•Free brochures about adult aphasia, tinnitus, assistive listening devices, communication disorders and aging
•*How to Buy a Hearing Aid* (free booklet)

Self Help for Hard of Hearing People, Inc. (SHHH)
7910 Woodmont Avenue, Suite 1200, Bethesda, MD 20814
(301) 657-2248
www.shhh.org
•Journal and newsletter for members
•Publications catalogue listing educational brochures, audiotapes, videotapes, and other resources
•Network of self-help groups

References

Baltes, P. B., & Lindenberger, U. (1997). Emergence of a powerful connection between sensory and cognitive functions across the adult life span: A new window to the study of cognitive aging? *Psychology and Aging, 12*(1), 12–21.

Bassford, T. L. (1995). Health status of Hispanic elders. *Clinics in Geriatric Medicine, 11*(1), 25–38.

Berg, R. L., & Cassells, J. S. (Eds.). (1990). *The second fifty years: Promoting health and preventing disability.* Washington, DC: National Academy Press.

Brawley, E. C. (1997). Designing for Alzheimer's disease: Strategies for creating better care environments. New York: John Wiley & Sons.

Butler, R. N., Lewis, M. I., & Sunderland, T. (1991). *Aging and mental health: Positive psychosocial and biomedical approaches* (4th ed.). New York: Merrill.

Carpenito, L. J. (1997). *Nursing diagnosis: Application to clinical practice* (7th ed.). Philadelphia: J. B. Lippincott.

DeBlase, R., & Kucler, M. (1985). Assistive hearing device aids patient-staff communication. *Geriatric Nursing, 6,* 223–224.

Erber, N. P. (1994). Communicating with elders: Effects of amplification. *Journal of Gerontological Nursing, 20*(10), 6–10.

Garahan, M. B., Waller, J. A., Houghton, M., Tisdale, W. A., & Runge, C. F. (1992). Hearing loss prevalence and management in nursing home residents. *Journal of the American Geriatrics Society, 40,* 130–134.

Gordon-Salant, S. (1996). Hearing. In J. E. Birren (Ed.), *Encyclopedia of gerontology: Age, aging, and the aged* (Vol. 1, pp. 643–653). San Diego: Academic Press.

LaForge, R. G., Spector, W. D., & Sternberg, J. (1992). The relationship of vision and hearing impairment to one-year mortality and functional decline. *Journal of Aging and Health, 4,* 126–147.

Lewis-Cullinan, C., & Janken, J. (1990). Effect of cerumen removal on the hearing ability of geriatric patients. *Journal of Advanced Nursing, 15,* 594–600.

Mahoney, D. F. (1993). Cerumen impaction: Prevalence and detection in nursing homes. *Journal of Gerontological Nursing, 19*(4), 23–30.

Mahoney, D. F. (1996). Cerumen impaction and hearing impairment among nursing home residents: Nursing implications. In V. Burggraf & R. Barry (Eds.), *Gerontological nursing: Current practice and research* (pp. 159–168). Thorofare, NJ: SLACK.

National Center for Health Statistics. (1985, September). *Current estimates from the National Health Interview Survey, United States, 1982.* (DHHS Publication No. PHS 85-1578). Washington, DC: U.S. Government Printing Office. (*Vital and Health Statistics,* Series 10, No. 150.)

National Institutes of Health Consensus Conference. (1990). Noise and hearing loss. *Journal of the American Medical Association, 263*(23), 3185–3190.

Neils, J., Newman, C. W., Hill, M., & Weiler, E. (1991). The effects of rate, sequencing, and memory on auditory processing in the elderly. *Journal of Gerontology, 46,* P71–P75.

Overfield, T. (1995). *Biologic variation in health and illness: Race, age, and sex differences.* Boca Raton, FL: CRC Press.

Resnick, H. E., Fries, B. E., & Verbrugge, L. M. (1997). Windows to their world: The effect of sensory impairments on social engagement and activity time in nursing home residents. *Journal of Gerontology: Social Sciences, 52B*(3), S135–S144.

Rousseau, P. (1995). Native-American elders: Health care status. *Clinics in Geriatric Medicine, 11*(1), 83–95.

Slawinski, E. B., Hartel, D. M., & Kline, D. W. (1993). Self-reported hearing problems in daily life throughout adulthood. *Psychology and Aging, 8*(4), 552–561.

Sommers, M. S. (1997). Speech perception in older adults: The importance of speech-specific cognitive abilities. *Journal of the American Geriatrics Society, 45,* 633–637.

Stein, L. M., & Bienenfeld, D. (1992). Hearing impairment and its impact on elderly patients with cognitive, behavioral, or psychiatric disorders: A literature review. *Journal of Geriatric Psychiatry, 25,* 145–156.

Stein, L. M., & Thienhaus, O. J. (1993). Hearing impairment and psychosis. *International Psychogeriatrics, 5,* 49–56.

Tesch-Römer, C. (1997). Psychological effects of hearing aid use in older adults. *Journal of Gerontology: Psychological Sciences, 52B*(3), P127–P138.

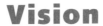

Vision

Chapter

7

Learning Objectives	1. *Delineate age-related changes that affect the visual abilities of older adults.*
	2. *Examine risk factors that influence the visual abilities of older adults.*
	3. *Discuss the functional consequences of age-related changes and risk factors that affect vision.*
	4. *Describe interview questions, behavioral cues, and tests of visual skills that can be used to assess vision in older adults.*
	5. *Identify environmental modifications and other interventions designed to assist older adults attain and maintain optimal visual performance.*

*I*mportant daily activities, such as communicating, enjoying visual images, and maneuvering in the environment, are influenced by one's ability to see. Thus, visual impairments can affect safety, performance of daily activities, and quality of life. Age-related changes, as well as risk factors, such as environmental conditions, cause some degree of visual impairment for most older adults. Rather than focusing on pathologic processes that may be addressed through medical interventions, this chapter emphasizes the age-related changes and risk factors relating to vision that can be addressed through nursing interventions. Much of the focus is on environmental modifications (e.g., providing adequate illumination) that can improve the older person's ability to perform activities of daily living (ADL).

Age-Related Changes

Visual function depends on a sequence of processes, beginning with the visual perception of an external stimulus and ending with the processing of neural impulses in the cerebral cortex. Age-related changes affect all of the structures involved in visual function and alter visual perception for the older adult. In the absence of disease processes, these gradual changes have only a subtle impact on the daily activities of the older person. Unless compensatory actions are taken, however, age-related vision changes may interfere with the older person's quality of life and influence the enjoyment and safe performance of many activities.

General Appearance and Tear Production

Although age-related changes in the appearance of the eye do not affect visual performance, these changes may be a source of anxiety and discomfort. Education about age-related changes may alleviate anxiety, and interventions aimed at eye comfort may relieve bothersome symptoms. Thus, changes in eye appearance and tear production are briefly reviewed in this section on age-related changes.

As the eye ages, lipids accumulate in the outer part of the cornea, and a white or yellowish ring develops between the iris and the sclera. This phenomenon, termed arcus senilis, can be observed in most eyes by the 9th decade. Other changes in the eye's appearance include a loss of translucency of the cornea, a yellowing of the sclera, and fading of the pigment in the iris.

Changes in the eyelids and surrounding skin also affect the appearance of the eye, but they have little or no impact on visual function. Certain changes, such as loss of orbital fat, development of wrinkles, decreased elasticity of the eyelid muscles, and accumulation of dark pigment around the eyes, contribute to the overall appearance of sunken eyes, called enophthalmos. If the loss of orbital fat and muscle elasticity progresses to the point that a lid fold develops, vision may be impaired. This condition, termed blepharochalasis, can be surgically treated.

Relaxation of the lower lid muscles to an extreme degree may result in the age-related conditions of ectropion or entropion. In ectropion, the lower lid falls away from the conjunctiva, causing a blockage of tears through the lower punctum and decreased lubrication of the conjunctiva. In entropion, the lower lid becomes inverted and the eyelashes may irritate the cornea, eventually leading to infection.

Age-related diminution in tear production may lead to chronic dry eye syndrome. The older adult may complain of dryness, burning, or photosensitivity. Subsequent irritation and rubbing of the cornea may lead to infections.

Cornea and Sclera

The cornea is a translucent covering over the eye that refracts light rays and provides 65% to 75% of the focusing power of the eye. As the eye ages, the cornea becomes more opaque and yellowed, interfering with the passage of light, especially ultraviolet rays, to the retina. Other corneal changes, such as the accumulation of lipid deposits, cause an increased scattering of light rays and may have a blurring effect on vision. In younger adults, the cornea is more highly curved and, therefore, has greater refractive power on the horizontal plane than on the vertical plane. As the cornea ages, the curvature

changes, causing a reversal in this pattern and influencing the refractive ability.

Lens

The lens consists of concentric and avascular layers of clear, crystalline protein. Because it lacks a blood supply, the lens depends on the aqueous humor for all metabolic and support functions. The transparent lens fibers are continually forming new layers without shedding old layers. As new layers form peripherally, the old layers are compressed inward toward the center, where they eventually become absorbed into the nucleus. This process gradually increases the size and density of the lens, causing a tripling of its mass by the age of 70 years. Thus, the lens gradually becomes stiffer, denser, and more opaque.

Because of these age-related changes, the lens moves forward in the eye and responds less effectively to the ciliary muscle. These changes also interfere with the transmission of light rays, resulting in a scattering of the rays that pass through the lens and a reduction in the amount of light reaching the retina. These changes do not affect all wavelengths equally; rather, the most detrimental effect occurs in the shorter blue and violet wavelengths.

Extreme opacification of the lens leads to the formation of cataracts. In their early stages, cataracts do not necessarily affect visual acuity, but as they progress, they can lead to complaints of glare, blurred vision, and decreased night vision. Cataract formation is attributable to a combination of age-related changes and risk factors, such as medications, pathologic factors, and environmental conditions.

Iris and Pupil

The iris is a pigmented sphincter muscle that dilates and contracts to control pupillary size and to regulate the amount of light reaching the retina. With increasing age, the iris becomes more sclerotic and rigid, reducing the size of the pupil and interfering with its ability to respond to changes in light. The pupillary size begins to diminish during the 3rd decade and levels off during the 7th decade. This condition, called senile miosis, causes a marked diminution in the amount of light reaching the retina.

Ciliary Muscle and Body

The ciliary body is a mass of muscles, connective tissue, and blood vessels surrounding the lens. These muscles regulate the passage of light rays through the lens by changing the shape of the lens. Near vision and accommodation are the functions controlled by the ciliary body. In addition, the ciliary body is responsible for the production of aqueous fluid. Beginning in the 4th decade, the ciliary muscle gradually atrophies, and muscle cells are replaced with connective tissue. By the 6th decade, the ciliary muscle is smaller, stiffer, and less functional. With advanced age, less aqueous humor is secreted, interfering with the ability to nourish and cleanse the cornea and lens.

Vitreous

The vitreous is a clear, gelatinous mass that forms the inner substance and maintains the spherical shape of the eye. During the 5th decade, this gelatinous substance begins to shrink and the proportion of liquid increases. These age-related changes may cause the vitreous body to pull away from the retina, causing the older person to experience any of the following symptoms: floaters, blurred vision, distorted images, or light flashes without any external stimuli. Additionally, these changes may scatter light more diffusely through the vitreous, reducing the amount of light reaching the retina.

Retina

The transformation of visual stimuli into neural impulses begins in the rods and cones of the retina. Rods and cones are photoreceptor cells that produce pigments and perform specific visual functions. Cones are responsible for acuity and color perception, and they require high levels of light to function effectively. Rods are responsible for vision under low light conditions, and they have no ability to perceive color. Cones are concentrated in the central and most sensitive part of the macula, called the fovea, whereas rods are distributed over the peripheral retina.

Age-related changes affect the photoreceptor cells, particularly the cones, beginning around the age of 20 years when the number of cones begins to decrease. There is only a minimal loss of cones in the fovea, where they are most highly concentrated, with most of the loss occurring in the peripheral part of the retina. Although the number of rods declines in the central retina, the remaining rods increase in size and are able to maintain their ability to capture light.

Additional retinal structures that undergo age-related changes include the pigment epithelium and the blood vessels, which become thinner and more sclerotic. Lipofuscin accumulates in the retinal pigment epithelium, and the choroid protrudes through it. Research on the effect of these changes on visual function is sparse. It is generally agreed, however, that these retinal changes do have functional consequences, as discussed later in this chapter.

Retinal-Neural Pathway

Photoreceptor cells converge in the ganglion cells that form the optic nerve. Neurosensory information is passed from the optic nerve, through the thalamus, to the visual cortex. Neurons in the visual cortex decline in quantity and quality with increased age. Age-related changes in the retinal-neural pathway affect the speed of processing visual information, particularly in conditions of low illumination. Age-related central nervous system changes that affect cognitive function may be associated with declines in visual function, although the common mechanism of these functional consequences has not been identified (Baltes and Lindenberger, 1997).

Risk Factors

Extraocular and environmental factors exacerbate age-related vision changes in the lens and retina. Exposure to ultraviolet sun rays has been associated with the development of cataracts and the loss of photoreceptor cells, particularly the cones. Warmer environmental temperatures have been associated with an earlier age of onset for presbyopia. People with Alzheimer's disease, even in the early stages, may have impaired contrast sensitivity and other visual impairments. Medications are another extraocular factor that may adversely affect visual function. Some of the medications that have been cited as having detrimental ocular effects are haloperidol, indomethacin, tricyclic antidepressants, anticholinergics, and corticosteroids (Morse and Rosenthal, 1996).

The development of cataracts has been associated with the following conditions: malnutrition; alcohol consumption; cigarette smoking; low socioeconomic status; infections, such as rubella; exposure to ultraviolet B or microwave radiation; congenital abnormalities, such as Down's syndrome; chronic diseases, such as diabetes and renal failure; and the use of certain drugs, including steroids, benzodiazepines, gout medications, and major tranquilizers. Age-related macular degeneration has been associated with the following risk factors: family history, cigarette smoking, cardiovascular disease, and high serum cholesterol levels. Also, preliminary evidence suggests that low serum levels of zinc, riboflavin, and the antioxidant vitamins A, C, and E may be associated with cataracts and age-related macular degeneration (Tumosa, 1995). Similarly, there is evidence that antioxidants, particularly those in beta-carotene and vitamins C and E, may reduce the risk

of cataracts and macular degeneration (Johnson, 1995). Despite these associations, very little is known about the exact causative relationships between risk factors and the vision changes that are universally present with advanced age.

Risk factors for dry eyes include vitamin A deficiency; certain diseases, such as collagen disorders; and medication effects. Some medications that can cause or contribute to dry eyes are atropine, estrogen, antihistamines, phenothiazines, beta-blockers, and antiparkinsonian medications. Environmental conditions that can exacerbate dry eyes include wind, sunlight, low humidity, and cigarette smoke.

Functional Consequences

All adults, regardless of race, gender, ethnicity, or socioeconomic status, experience some evidence of visual impairment during their 5th decade. Even the rare person who has 20/20 visual acuity at the age of 90 years experiences subtle changes in overall vision. Despite the universal prevalence of age-related vision changes, however, most older adults can perform the usual ADL if they use low-vision aids and modify their environment. The most serious visual impairments that affect older adults are generally caused by pathologic conditions, such as glaucoma, retinopathy, or macular degeneration, all of which are increasingly likely to occur with increased age.

Prevalence of Visual Impairments

In the 1984 National Health Interview Survey of almost 6000 community-living older adults, the prevalence of self-reported visual impairments ranged from 9.5% of people aged 65 to 74 years, to 26.8% of those aged 85 years and older. Thirty-one percent of Americans older than 65 years of age reported "little trouble" (25.6%) or "a lot of trouble" (5.4%) seeing with glasses. More than 50% of Americans aged

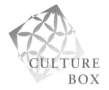

Variations in Prevalence of Eye Conditions

- Cataracts more common in women than in men.
- Blacks have a higher prevalence of blindness and visual impairment than do Whites; they also have an earlier age of onset of glaucoma.

85 years and older, however, reported some trouble with vision. With the exception of an increased frequency of cataracts reported in older women, the occurrence of visual impairments in men and women was found to be similar (National Center for Health Statistics [NCHS], 1986). A recent survey found that age-adjusted prevalence rates for primary open-angle glaucoma were 4 to 5 times higher for Blacks as compared with Whites, but no different for men or women (Tielsch et al., 1991). Additional cultural variations in the prevalence of eye conditions are summarized in the Culture Box.

Impact of Vision Changes on Activities of Daily Living

National Health Interview Survey statistics indicate that limitations in ADL are more likely to occur in older people with sensory impairments than in those without any sensory loss. Visually impaired participants reported more difficulty with walking, getting outside, and getting in and out of bed or a chair than did participants of the same age who reported no visual impairment. The percentage of participants aged 65 to 74 years with visual impairments who reported difficulties with these activities was more than double that for those who reported no visual impairments (NCHS, 1986). Visual impairment has been found to be an independent risk factor for mobility restrictions and increased disability in performing ADL (Maino, 1996; Rudberg et al., 1993).

A study of the everyday visual problems of healthy adults aged 18 to 100 years identified some ADL that were influenced by age-related changes in visual performance (Kosnik et al., 1988). Kosnik and colleagues identified five visual performance tasks that were likely to be problematic for older adults: visual processing speed (e.g., reading speed), light sensitivity (e.g., seeing in dim light), dynamic vision (e.g., reading a moving scroll on television), near vision (e.g., reading small print), and visual search (e.g., locating a sign). Also, an association has been found between lower scores on mental status tests and loss of vision in older people.

Visual impairments have been found to have a negative influence on the safety of older adults. Visual impairments and age-related vision changes may contribute to falls and fractures in a number of ways. Age-related vision changes and risk factors may predispose older people to postural instability and gait and balance problems. Visual impairments can interfere with the perception of environmental hazards. Delayed processing of visual information may interfere with the quick responses necessary for preventing falls. Visual impairment may also increase the risk of serious injury secondary to falling. One study found that visually impaired women have a fivefold increase in the odds of experiencing a hip fracture (Grisso et al., 1991). Another recent study found that visual impairment is strongly associated with two or more falls in older adults (Ivers et al., 1998). Ivers and colleagues suggested that poor visual acuity, reduced visual field, impaired contrast sensitivity, and the presence of cataracts may explain the increased risk for falls.

Studies have examined the relationship between age-related visual changes and driving skills of older adults. Visual dimensions that influence driving abilities are near vision, visual search, dynamic vision, light sensitivity, and visual processing speed. With regard to driving, older adults have increased difficulty reading signs, seeing dim displays, accurately determining vehicle speed, perceiving and responding to unexpected vehicles, and adjusting to glare.

Accommodation

Loss of accommodation, or the ability to focus clearly and quickly on objects at various distances, is usually the earliest age-related vision change. Presbyopia, or loss of near vision, usually begins during the 5th decade. This vision change is caused primarily by age-related changes in the lens, which controls the adjustment of the eye's focus for different distances. Degenerative changes of the ciliary muscle may play a minor role in the development of presbyopia. Functionally, accommodative changes cause a gradual increase in the near point of vision, the closest point at which a small object can be seen clearly. Consequently, the person with presbyopia will hold reading materials farther from the eye to focus clearly on the print.

Acuity

Acuity is the ability to detect details and discern objects. This visual skill is customarily assessed using a Snellen chart, and it is measured against a normal value of 20/20. Visual acuity is best around the age of 30 years, after which it gradually declines with increasing age. Diminished acuity results from the following age-related ocular changes: decreased pupillary size, scatter in the cornea and lens, opacification of the lens and vitreous, and loss of photoreceptor cells in the retina. These changes interfere with the passage of light to the retina, contributing to the threefold reduction in retinal illumination that occurs between the ages of 20 and 60 years.

Acuity is also influenced by extraocular factors, such as the size and movement of an object and the amount of light reflected off an object.

Conditions of low or poor illumination compound the effects of age-related ocular changes. Visual acuity for moving objects is more impaired than acuity for static objects, and acuity becomes more impaired as the speed of the object increases. This combination of age-related changes and external factors hinders the older person's ability to see moving objects and to perform tasks in low illumination. Consequently, older people require a relatively greater degree of illumination and may experience a marked decline in night driving competence.

Dark and Light Adaptation

The ability to respond to dim light is gauged by the level of vision achieved and the length of time needed to reach maximum visual perception. This visual capacity, called dark adaptation, begins to decline around the age of 20 years and diminishes more markedly after the age of 60 years. This decline is associated with decreased retinal illumination as well as age-related changes in retinal metabolism and retinal-neural pathways. The functional impact of these changes is that the older adult will need more time to adapt to decreased illumination when moving from a brighter to a darker environment. For instance, when entering a darkened movie theater, the older person will need extra time to adapt to the dim environment before proceeding down the aisle to find a seat.

The ability to respond to high levels of illumination is also affected by age-related changes in the lens and pupils, which reduce the amount of light reaching the retina. Functionally, this means that the older person requires increased time to recover from exposure to glare and bright lights, such as flashbulbs, and has a decreased ability to respond to bright lights, such as the headlights of oncoming cars.

Glare

Glare occurs when a scattering of light in the optic media reduces the clarity of visual images. Glare is experienced when light is reflected from shiny surfaces, when it is excessively bright or inappropriately focused, or when bright light originates from several sources at once. Glare is classified according to three types: veiling, dazzling, and scotomatic. *Veiling glare* is caused by the scattering of light over the retinal surface and results in diminished contrast of the viewed object. Veiling glare may occur, for example, when bright fluorescent lights in a grocery store reflect on the clear plastic covering over meat products in a white case. *Dazzling glare,* which is caused by bright visual displays, interferes with the ability to discern details. Glass-covered directories in brightly lit shopping malls may produce a dazzling glare that interferes with a person's ability to read the words in the directory, particularly if there is poor contrast between the letters and the background. *Scotomatic glare* is a blinding glare caused by loss of retinal sensitivity and overstimulation of retinal pigments after exposure to bright lights. On sunny or snowy days, scotomatic glare may be noted when driving toward the sun.

Beginning in the 5th decade, age-related changes increase a person's sensitivity to glare and the time required to recover from glare. Glare sensitivity is influenced primarily by opacification of the lens; it also may be affected by age-related changes in the pupil and vitreous. Functionally, these changes may have a significant impact on night driving, as well as on a person's ability to read signs, see objects, and maneuver safely in bright environments. In many modern buildings and shopping malls, the bright lights, large windows, and highly reflective floors generate glare that can lead to accidents and inaccurate perceptions.

Visual Field

A visual field is an oval-shaped area containing the total view that the person can perceive while keeping the eye fixed on a constant point straight ahead. The scope of the visual field narrows slightly between the ages of 40 and 50 years and then declines steadily. Functionally, the visual field is important in the performance of tasks requiring a broad perception of the environment and moving objects. Walking in crowded places and driving a vehicle are examples of activities that depend on the field of vision.

Depth Perception

Depth perception is the visual skill responsible for localizing objects in three-dimensional space, for judging differences in the depth of objects, and for observing relationships among objects in space. As with many other visual skills, depth perception depends on interactions between ocular and extraocular factors. Stereopsis, or the disparity between retinal images that is caused by the separation of the two eyes, is the primary ocular characteristic that affects depth perception. Extraocular factors that influence depth perception include prior perceptual experiences of the observer; movement of the observer's head or body; and characteristics of the object, such as size, height, distance, texture, brightness, and shading.

Information about age-related changes in depth perception is limited by the complexity of the ocular and extraocular factors involved and by the fact that stereopsis has been the only factor studied. Researchers generally agree, however, that there is a decline in depth perception in older people, but the origins of these changes have not been identified. Functionally, depth perception enables people to use objects effectively and to maneuver safely in the environment. Thus, alterations in depth perception may lead to falls and tripping because of miscalculations about the distance and height of objects.

Color Vision

Pigments in three types of cones are responsible for the detection of the primary colors of red, blue, and green. As with many other visual functions, color perception is influenced by the type and quantity of light waves reaching the retina. Consequently, any age-related changes that interfere with retinal illumination, such as lens opacification and pupillary miosis, can interfere with accurate color perception. Opacification and yellowing of the lens interfere most directly with shorter wavelengths, causing an altered perception of blues, greens, and violets. Age-related retinal or retinal-neural changes may also affect color perception, as will such extraocular influences as low levels of illumination.

Functionally, altered color perception is manifested as a relative darkening of blue-colored objects and a yellowed perception of white light. Color perception is increasingly impaired in conditions of poor illumination. Accurate color perception is not essential in all daily activities, but it is important, for instance, in differentiating between medications that are similar in color or tone, especially those in the blue-green range and the yellow-white range. In addition, altered color perception may interfere with the detection of spoiled food.

Critical Flicker Fusion

Critical flicker fusion is the point at which an intermittent light source is perceived as a continuous, rather than flashing, light. The ability to perceive flashing lights accurately is a function of the retinal receptors and is influenced by extraocular factors, such as the size, color, and luminance of the object. Age-related changes in the retina and retinal-neural pathway, as well as the changes that decrease retinal illumination, interfere with the critical flicker fusion. Low levels of illumination further exacerbate the effects of these changes.

Functionally, diminished critical flicker fusion distorts the perception of a flashing light, making it appear to be a continuous light. Thus, diminished critical flicker fusion may interfere with the discernment of emergency vehicles and road construction lights, especially at night.

Visual Information Processing

The retinal-neural pathway is responsible for processing visual information accurately and efficiently. Older adults need additional time to process visual information and to search their visual memory in the performance of everyday tasks, but age-related differences are minimal or negligible when the tasks are familiar or well practiced. Table 7-1 summarizes age-related vision changes and their functional consequences.

Overall Functional Consequences Relating to Activities of Daily Living

Studies have found a strong link between vision impairments and increased dependency in performing ADL (Horowitz, 1994). The daily activities most directly influenced by age-related vision changes include driving a vehicle; shopping for groceries; going up and down stairs; maneuvering safely in dark or unfamiliar environments; seeing markings on clocks, radios, thermostats, appliances, and televisions; and reading newspapers, small-print signs, posters, or directories, and labels on food items and medication containers. Most of these daily activities are affected by alterations in several visual skills. In addition, performance of these activities is influenced significantly by environmental factors. Visual impairments also are associated with an increased risk of falls in older adults. Some of the age-related vision changes that increase one's risk for falls and unstable mobility are diminished acuity, narrowing of the visual field, and increased sensitivity to glare.

Examination of the impact of age-related changes on the ability to drive safely illustrates the complex functional consequences of altered visual skills for performing daily activities. Slower dark and light adaptation creates problems when driving in and out of tunnels and when driving at night on streets with inconsistent lighting. Decreased peripheral vision interferes with the wide visual field that is important in avoiding collisions. Decreased acuity inter-

TABLE 7-1
Age-Related Changes Affecting Vision

Change	Consequence
Appearance and Comfort	
• Decreased elasticity of the eyelid muscles	Potential for ectropion, entropion, blepharo-chalasis
• Enophthalmos	
• Decreased tears	Potential for dry eye syndrome
Structures	
• Yellowing and increased opacity of cornea	**Presbyopia:** diminished ability to focus on near objects
• Changes in the corneal curvature	
• Increase in lens size and density	Diminished accommodation
• Sclerosis and rigidity of the iris	Diminished acuity
• Decrease in pupillary size	Slower response to changes in illumination
• Atrophy of the ciliary muscle	Increased sensitivity to glare
• Shrinkage of gelatinous substance in the vitreous	Narrowing of the visual field
• Atrophy of photoreceptor cells	Diminished depth perception
• Thinning and sclerosis of retinal blood vessels	Altered color perception
• Degeneration of neurons in the visual cortex	Distorted perception of flashing lights
	Slower processing of visual information

feres with the perception of moving objects, especially vehicles moving at fast speeds. Diminished accommodation and acuity create problems when the older adult tries to read the speedometer or other dashboard instruments after focusing on the road. If the car has tinted windows, the diminished illumination further interferes with visual skills. Glare interferes with the perception of objects and is heightened by rainy, snowy, or sunny conditions. Bright sunlight shortly after sunrise or before sunset may totally interfere with the perception of red and green traffic lights because of the older adult's increased sensitivity to glare.

Psychosocial Consequences

Age-related vision changes develop gradually and often go unnoticed for many years. As the changes progress to the point of interfering with ADL, the older adult may withdraw from usual activities rather than acknowledge a vision problem or adjust to the changes. A recent study of the effects of sensory impairments on nursing home residents found a strong association between visual impairments and low levels of social engagement and little or no time involved in activities (Resnick et al., 1997). Another recent study found that impaired vision was a significant independent contributor to disruptive behaviors among long-term care residents (Horowitz, 1995).

Of course, a person's usual lifestyle influences the extent of any psychosocial impact related to vision changes. If the leisure activities chosen by the older adult require good visual skills, such as with reading, sewing, or needlework, the older adult may become bored and even depressed when vision changes interfere with these endeavors. If artistic pursuits and entertainment events are important activities for the older adult, diminished visual function may interfere with the

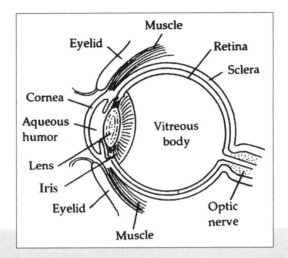

AGE-RELATED CHANGES

- Yellowing and opacity of cornea
- Changes in corneal curvature
- Increase in size and density of lens
- Sclerosis of the iris
- Decrease in pupillary size
- Atrophy of ciliary muscle
- Decrease in blood supply and neurons in the retina
- Loss of neurons in the visual cortex

NEGATIVE FUNCTIONAL CONSEQUENCES

- *Presbyopia*: Decreased ability to focus on near objects
- Increased sensitivity to glare
- Need for greater illumination
- Slower response to changes in illumination
- Narrowing of visual field
- Diminished depth perception
- Altered color perception
- Slower processing of visual information
- Difficulty with night driving

RISK FACTORS

- Poor lighting
- Environmental glare
- Diseases of the eye (e.g., cataracts, macular degeneration)
- Systemic diseases (e.g., diabetes)
- Exposure to ultraviolet rays

FIGURE 7-1. Vision in older adults.

person's quality of life. By contrast, if the person prefers music or other activities that are less dependent on visual skills, the effect on the adult's usual lifestyle may be minimal.

One's living environment and support systems are other determinants of the psychosocial consequences of vision changes. Good visual skills are more important for people who live alone or who provide care for others than for people who live with or have frequent contact with others who have good vision. Also, if visually impaired people can modify their living environment to compensate for the impairments, the psychosocial consequences will be minimized. By contrast, people who live in institutional settings may experience relatively greater negative consequences because of unalterable environmental conditions.

Older adults who notice declines in their vision may mistakenly fear going blind because they think they have a serious and progressive disease. Fear of blindness may be based on myths, inaccurate information, or experiences of friends who have serious visual impairments. Negative or hopeless attitudes about vision changes may deter the older person from acknowledging the problem or seeking help.

Fear of falling is a serious concern for many older adults who notice visual changes. Inaccurate depth perception may lead to frequent bumping into objects, and the older adult may feel insecure and unsafe, even in familiar environments. If the person has experienced falls or tripping, or knows someone who suffered a fracture as a result of falling, the fears may be magnified.

Figure 7.1 summarizes some of the important age-related changes, risk factors, and negative functional consequences that may affect vision in older adults.

Nursing Assessment

Nursing assessment of vision is aimed at identifying (1) risk factors that might be amenable to

interventions, (2) the functional consequences of any vision changes, (3) the psychosocial consequences of visual impairments, and (4) any negative attitudes about interventions for visual disorders. Nursing assessment of visual function is not a substitute for an examination by an eye doctor. Whereas the purpose of an eye examination is to detect and initiate appropriate treatment of vision problems, the goal of the nursing assessment is to assist the older adult in minimizing the negative consequences of vision changes. Nursing assessment of visual performance is accomplished by interviewing the older adult, testing visual skills, and observing the older adult's ability to perform ADL.

Interview Questions

Interview questions are used to elicit the following information: past and present risk factors, the person's awareness of any vision changes, the impact of these changes on daily activities and quality of life, and the person's attitudes about interventions. The interview begins with direct questions about the person's awareness of any changes in vision. If a visual impairment is acknowledged, additional details about the onset and progression of vision changes should be elicited. Questions about symptoms that cause discomfort or that indicate the possible presence of disease processes also should be asked.

Subsequent questions focus on the person's awareness of any differences in his or her usual activities that might be associated with vision changes. If the person has acknowledged vision changes, specific questions may be asked about how these changes have influenced everyday activities. If the person has denied that any vision changes have occurred, the nurse should inquire about any changes in the performance of complex ADL, such as driving, shopping, and meal preparation.

Questions about leisure interests should be incorporated into the interview to obtain additional information about the psychosocial consequences of vision impairments. Although the older adult may not associate lifestyle changes with vision impairments, questions about changes in hobbies and leisure activities may reveal a need for interventions to improve visual function.

Responses to questions about the source, frequency, and last date of eye examinations will provide information about the use of and attitudes toward eye care. If visual impairment has been acknowledged, questions should be asked to ascertain the person's attitude toward eye examinations. If a visual impairment has been denied, questions should be directed toward identifying attitudes about early detection of problems, such as glaucoma.

Last, if the older person is likely to spend time outdoors in sunny climates, an inquiry should be made about exposure to sunlight. By placing this question toward the end of the interview, the nurse will set the stage for educating the older adult about protective measures, such as the use of sunglasses. The nurse can then proceed with additional advice about corrective and adaptive measures. Questions that should be included in a nursing assessment of visual function are listed in Display 7-1.

Behavioral Cues

Reliable information can be obtained by observing an older person's performance of usual activities and noting evidence of visual skills, especially if these observations can be made in the

---

DISPLAY 7-1
Guidelines for Assessing Vision

Interview Questions to Assess Awareness and Presence of Vision Impairment

- Have you noticed any changes in your vision during the past few years?
- Do you experience any uncomfortable symptoms, such as dry eyes?
- Do you have difficulty managing any of your usual activities because you have trouble seeing? (Specifically, ask about the following: sewing, reading, driving, grooming, preparing meals, watching television, managing money, writing letters, using the telephone, using dials on appliances, shopping for groceries, and going up and down stairs.)
- Have you ever tripped or fallen because you had trouble seeing?
- Have you stopped doing any activities because of vision problems? (For example, have you stopped driving at night because of difficulty seeing?)
- Are there things you'd like to do if you could see better?

Interview Questions If Vision Loss Is Acknowledged

- When did you first notice the problem? Have the changes been gradual, or did you notice sudden changes at any particular time?

- How would you describe the changes in your ability to see?
- Have you noticed any of the following symptoms: pain, blurred vision, burning or itching, halos around lights, intolerance to bright light, difference in day and night vision, or spots or flashing lights in front of your eyes?
- What kind of medical evaluation and care, if any, have you had for this problem?

Interview Questions to Assess the Use of and Attitudes Toward Eye Care Practitioners

- When was the last time you had your eyes checked?
- Where do you go for eye care?
- Have you ever had your eyes checked for glaucoma?
- What do you think about going for regular check-ups for glaucoma and other eye problems?

Interview Questions to Assess Risk Factors for Vision Loss

- When you spend time outdoors in the sun, do you use sunglasses or a hat to protect your eyes from bright light?
- Have you taken any steroid medications over a long period of time?

person's normal environment. Observations about ADL should be judged in relation to the person's usual patterns of personal care and daily activities. For example, observation of spots and soiled marks on the person's clothing would be interpreted differently for someone known to be meticulous about their clothing than for an individual who had never showed much concern about their personal appearance.

When observing older people who are not in their usual environment, any circumstances that might influence their visual performance, either positively or negatively, should be noted. An example of a positive influence might be the presence of good overhead lighting and good color contrast. Negative influences, such as glare from fluorescent lights reflecting on highly polished floors, are more likely to exist in an institutional setting than a home setting.

Observations of the person's visual performance outside the home setting also must take into account the influences of factors such as illness, medication effects, psychological stress, changes in routines, and unavailability of corrective lenses. These influences are of particular concern in institutional settings and are likely to have a negative impact on the older person's performance of daily activities. In these settings, nurses can ask the older person and caregivers for information about the person's abilities in the home setting. Suggestions for observing behavioral cues related to visual function are listed in Display 7-2. Finally, the nurse also should examine the older person's eyes to detect any abnormalities, such as serious lid lag, that might interfere with visual function.

Tests of Visual Skills

Peripheral vision and acuity for near and distant objects can be measured using both formal and informal tests. These tests are not a substitute for a complete eye examination, but they can provide objective information that will assist the nurse in planning care and identifying the need for further evaluation. Some tests, such as check-

---

DISPLAY 7-2
Guidelines for Assessing Behavioral and Environmental Cues to Visual Performance

- Is clothing spotted, soiled, or mismatched, in contrast to a former pattern of neatness and sense of style?
- Is makeup applied in heavy quantities, in contrast to the usual manner of application?
- Does the person rely heavily on nonvisual cues, such as the use of their hands for probing, in performing usual activities, especially maneuvering in the environment?
- What kind of lighting is used for various tasks?
- Does the person try to economize at home by using dim lights or no lights at all? Does this interfere with visual abilities?
- Where does the person usually sit in relation to light sources? Does glare from a facing window interfere with vision? Do shadows from lamps interfere with vision? Do overhead lights cause glare? Are light bulbs of sufficient wattage?

- What are the sources of light on stairways and hallways?
- Is there sufficient color contrast in the following areas: walls and floors; stairs and landings; furniture, walls, and floors; eating utensils and place settings; cooking utensils and counter tops; markings and background on appliance dials?
- Are night-lights used in hallways and bathrooms?

ing distance vision with the Snellen chart, assessing visual fields with the confrontation test, and evaluating near vision by asking the person to read small-print text, require minimal equipment. Nursing assessment of these three parameters will provide information about visual functions that often are affected by age-related changes and that influence the safe performance of daily activities.

For accurate assessment of visual skills, a good light source should be placed above the person's head to provide lighting and to avoid shadows. If the person normally wears corrective lenses, these should be clean and in place. Each eye should be tested separately, using an appropriate eye cover; avoid using a hand as a cover.

To assess near acuity, the nurse can ask the person to read a newspaper or other printed material of various type sizes. An informal assessment of near acuity can also be made in cases in which the signature of an older person is required on a form. The nurse can ask the person to read a line or two of the form, subsequently observing his or her ability to find the signature line. Other opportunities for assessment may be created by providing written educational materials and asking the older person to read a specific part, such as a phone number to call.

The Snellen chart, described in Display 7-3, is a standard test for measuring distance acuity. An informal assessment of distance acuity, however, can also be accomplished by asking the older person to look out a window or down a hallway and to describe certain details, such as the words on a sign. This test is based on the assumption that the nurse's distance acuity is normal. When performing any distance vision tests in older adults, the nurse should remember to eliminate all sources of glare and make sure that color contrast for the viewed object is adequate.

A standard confrontation test provides a gross estimate of the peripheral visual fields of the examinee, as measured against the examiner's peripheral vision. As with informal distance acuity tests, the results of the confrontation test are based on a comparison with the examiner's visual skill, which must be normal for an accurate comparison to be made. Instructions for performing the confrontation test are given in Display 7-3.

Nursing Diagnosis

The nursing assessment is designed to identify both actual visual impairments and risk factors for poor visual function (e.g., a dimly lit environment). In addition, the nurse may be able to identify functional consequences relating to visual impairments that interfere with safety, self-care, or quality of life. A suitable nursing diagnosis for visually impaired older adults would be Sensory-Perceptual Alterations, defined as "a state in which the individual/group experiences or is at risk of experiencing a change in the amount, pattern, or interpretation of incoming stimuli" (Carpenito, 1997, p. 803). Related factors that commonly affect older adults include age-related vision changes (e.g., presbyopia), sensory organ alterations (e.g., glaucoma), and environmental factors (e.g., glare, dim lighting, or poor color contrast). The care plan at the end of this chapter is based on a nursing diagnosis of Sensory-Perceptual Alterations: Visual, related to age-related changes, sensory organ alterations, and environmental factors.

Other nursing diagnoses might be addressed if the visual impairment interferes with the older adult's safety, quality of life, or performance of ADL. Possible diagnoses to address these functional consequences include Anxiety, Activity Intolerance, Self-Care Deficit, Impaired Social Interaction, Impaired Physical Mobility, and High Risk for Injury.

Nursing Goals

Nursing care plans for older adults with age-related vision changes are directed toward at-

DISPLAY 7-3
Guidelines for Using Vision Screening Tests

Guidelines for Testing Distance Acuity Using the Snellen Chart

- Position the chart 20 feet away from the person, at eye level.
- If space does not permit a 20-foot distance, the distance between the person and the chart should be either 15 or 10 feet, with final measurements adjusted for distance. Alternatively, a scaled-down Snellen card can be used, if available.
- Test only the corrected vision if the person usually wears corrective lenses.
- Ask the person to start reciting the letters in the line that can be read most easily; then ask them to read as many letters as possible in the lines directly below that line.
- Document the findings for each eye by noting the figure at the end of the last line on which at least half of the letters were read correctly.
- The upper figure denotes the distance of the person from the chart, whereas the lower figure denotes the distance from the chart at which a person with normal vision would be able to read the line. (That is, a vision measurement of 20/50 indicates that the person being tested can see things at a distance of 20 feet that a person with normal vision would be able to see at a distance of 50 feet.)

Normal Snellen Chart Test Results for Older Adults

- A corrected vision of 20/20 is considered to be normal.

- If a distance of 10 feet is used, the corrected vision should be 10/10.
- The average corrected vision for older adults ranges from 20/20 to 20/50.

Guidelines for Performing the Confrontation Test for Peripheral Vision

- Sit directly across from the older person, approximately 2 feet away.
- Cover your left eye and the examinee's right eye.
- Instruct the examinee to focus on your right eye while you focus on the examinee's left eye.
- Fully extend your right arm midway between you and the examinee.
- Slowly move your right hand, with the fingers wiggling, from the outer periphery toward the center, testing visual fields from top to bottom.
- While maintaining continuous eye contact, ask the examinee to report the point at which your fingers are visualized.
- Repeat these steps, covering your right eye and the examinee's left eye and using your left arm.

Normal Findings

- Your wiggling fingers should be seen simultaneously by both you and the older person in all quadrants.

taining and maintaining optimal visual function and compensating for any visual impairments. The goal of attaining and maintaining optimal visual function is addressed by educating the older adult about eye comfort and protection measures, as well as the correction, treatment, and early detection of vision disorders. The goal of compensating for deficits in visual skills is addressed through education about the use of low-vision aids and modifications of the living environment. Another goal is to maintain and improve the quality of life of older adults. This is accomplished through nursing interventions

that foster increased safety and independent performance of ADL and other desirable activities. The next section of this chapter discusses the interventions that are appropriate for addressing these goals.

Nursing Interventions

Attaining and Maintaining Optimal Visual Function

Prolonged exposure to ultraviolet (UV) light (especially UVB light) is one environmental risk that may lead to visual impairment. Broad-rimmed hats and close-fitting sunglasses with UVB-absorbing lenses have the long-range effect of protecting the eyes from harmful rays; they also have the immediate benefit of screening out sun glare that can interfere with visual function. Nurses should educate older adults, as well as their caregivers, about the benefits of these simple measures.

Nurses also should educate older adults and their caregivers about the importance of early detection of glaucoma and about treatments available for cataracts and other eye disorders. People aged 35 years and older should undergo biannual measurements of intraocular pressure to detect glaucoma. People 65 years of age or older should undergo such measurements annually. Nurses can encourage older adults to take advantage of glaucoma screening tests that might be available in the community through nonprofit organizations like the International Lions Club.

If cataracts interfere with visual function, the older person should be encouraged to obtain information about surgical treatment from an ophthalmologist. When discussing interventions for cataracts, nurses need not be thoroughly familiar with the various surgical techniques; rather, they can emphasize that highly successful techniques for cataract surgery are now available. Older people should be persuaded to undergo an eye evaluation and to obtain information from a qualified professional rather than relying on hearsay from friends. Educational brochures on cataracts and glaucoma can be used to dispel myths and misunderstandings and to reinforce the nurse's teaching.

In providing health education about vision care, it may be helpful to review the differences between opticians, optometrists, and ophthalmologists (see Display 7-4). Educational materials describing the scope of services of these eye care providers are distributed by some of the organizations listed in the Educational Resources section. Do-it-yourself eye test kits are available from Prevent Blindness America, listed at the end of this chapter. This kit enables people to determine whether they are seeing as well as they should and provides guidelines for obtaining further evaluation.

Many educational materials are available on the subjects of eye diseases, common vision problems, low-vision aids, and age-related eye changes. Nurses can use these publications to supplement and reinforce the health education components of their care plans. Local sight centers, or the organizations listed in the Educational Resources section of this chapter, provide these materials at little or no cost, and some brochures are available in Spanish and other languages. The National Association for the Visually Handicapped (NAVH) is an excellent resource for information about interventions for older adults with visual impairments. In contrast to publications from organizations that focus primarily on blindness, materials from the NAVH are written for people with gradual and partial visual losses. The American Academy of Ophthalmology and the American Optometric Association also are good sources of free pamphlets about eye problems that commonly affect older adults.

If pertinent, simple measures to relieve dry eyes can be discussed. Use of over-the-counter artificial tears or ocular lubricants, especially before reading or other activities that require frequent eye movements, usually will afford symptomatic relief. People who use eye drops more frequently than every 3 hours should be advised to use preservative-free solutions to prevent any adverse effects from the preservatives. Other comfort measures, such as applying cold compresses or wearing wraparound glasses, are designed to prevent evaporation of tears. Maintenance of adequate environmental humidity, especially during the winter months or in dry climates, also decreases evaporation of eye moisture and adds to eye comfort. People who experience discomfort from dry eyes should avoid irritants, such as smoke and hair sprays, as well as adverse environmental conditions, such as hot rooms and high wind.

DISPLAY 7-4
Eye Care Practitioners

Ophthalmologists

Ophthalmologists are licensed doctors of medicine (M.D.) or osteopathy (D.O.) who are trained to diagnose and treat diseases and conditions of the eye.

Ophthalmologic services include:
- Comprehensive eye examinations
- Diagnosis of eye diseases and disorders of the eye
- Prescription medications for eye problems (e.g., glaucoma)
- Eye surgery and postoperative care (e.g., cataracts)
- Laser treatments (e.g., retinopathy)
- Prescriptions for eyeglasses and contact lenses
- Prescriptions for low-vision aids
- Referrals for low-vision aids and training
- Medical referrals for diseases of the body that affect the eyes

Optometrists

An optometrist is a licensed doctor of optometry (O.D.), not a physician, who is trained to examine eyes, screen for common eye problems, and prescribe eye exercises or corrective lenses. Optometrists use diagnostic medications, and in more than half the states in America, they can prescribe certain therapeutic drugs for eye diseases.

Optometric services include:
- Comprehensive eye examinations
- Eye refractions to determine the need for corrective lenses
- Prescriptions for eyeglasses, contact lenses, and low-vision aids
- Vision therapy to improve certain skills, such as tracking and focusing the eyes
- Referrals for low-vision aids and training
- Referrals to physicians for surgery, medication, or further evaluation
- Diagnosis of eye disorders (in some states)
- Postoperative care (in some states)

Opticians

Opticians are eye care practitioners who are trained to fit, adjust, and dispense eyeglasses and contact lenses that have been prescribed by an optometrist or ophthalmologist. In many states, opticians are licensed. They do not perform eye examinations or refractions, and they cannot prescribe corrective lenses or medications.

Medicare Coverage

Medicare covers many optometric and ophthalmologic services for the diagnosis and treatment of eye diseases, but it does not pay for routine eye examinations or corrective lenses. Eyeglasses and contact lenses are not covered by Medicare, except after cataract surgery. Optician services are not covered by Medicare.

Prescription and over-the-counter medications may contribute to or cause dry eyes. People who are bothered by dry eyes and are taking a medication that might exacerbate the discomfort should be encouraged to discuss the problem with their primary care practitioner. Categories of medications that are likely to cause dry eyes include diuretics, antihistamines, anticholinergics, and adrenergic agents.

Compensating for Visual Deficits Through Low-Vision Aids

People with visual impairments can improve their functional abilities through the use of low-vision aids that affect focus, contrast, magnification, or illumination. Low-vision aids are most beneficial when used in conjunction with environmental modifications. For example, magnifiers are most effective when combined with measures that improve illumination and control glare.

Although special low-vision aids must be ordered through catalogues or obtained at sight centers, everyday items, if used advantageously, can serve as low-vision aids. An example of a low-vision aid that may be available to nurses in their workplace is a photocopy machine that can be used to convert regular-print materials into large-print materials. Likewise, household lamps, placed in the correct position and equipped with the right wattage bulb, can also serve as low-vision aids. A free brochure describing and illustrating guidelines for designing printed materials for improved legibility is available from The Lighthouse, Inc. (see the appropriate listing in the Educational Resources at the end of this chapter).

Reading glasses and other optical aids that magnify an image for visual tasks are available with or without a prescription. Nonoptical aids are devices that enhance contrast, reduce glare, improve lighting, or enlarge the image. Catalogues of low-vision aids are available through several organizations (see Educational Resources). Also, local sight centers are good sources of low-vision aids, as well as training related to their use. Display 7-5 lists a number of low-vision aids, categorized according to their primary purposes.

Training in the use of low-vision aids should be provided to maximize the beneficial effects on visual performance. For example, the likelihood that an illumination aid is placed in the most effective position may be increased if the person understands that halving the distance of a light source increases the illumination fourfold. As an illustration of this principle, a light bulb that is 1 foot away from someone will provide four times as much illumination as one that is 2 feet away. To teach others how to adapt to visual limitations, nurses should be familiar with the basic principles of magnification and illumination, listed in Displays 7-6 and 7-7. Local sight centers provide detailed training in the use of low-vision aids, and the NAVH publishes a helpful guide regarding their use.

DISPLAY 7-5
Aids for Improving Visual Performance

Enlarged Images and Objects

- Microscopic spectacles
- Hand-held or standing magnifiers
- Binoculars and hand-held or spectacle-mounted telescopes
- Magnifying sheets
- Field expanders for diminished peripheral vision
- Large-print books, magazines, and newspapers
- Photocopy machines or laser printers (when used to enlarge print)
- Telephones with enlarged letters and numbers, or a pad with enlarged letters and numbers designed to fit over rotary-dial or push button phones
- Large numbers on rulers, playing cards, and other items
- Thermometers with good color coding and enlarged numbers
- Large-eye needles

Illumination Aids

- High-intensity lights
- Gooseneck lamps
- Floor or table lamps with three-way light bulbs

Contrast Aids

- Use of broad-tipped felt markers in dark, yet bright colors and colored construction paper for making signs
- Red print on a yellow background or white letters on a green background
- Reading and signature guides (typoscopes)
- Clip-on yellow lenses

Glare Control Aids

- Sunglasses with ultraviolet-absorbing lenses
- Sun visors and broad-rimmed hats
- Nonglare (antireflective) coating on eyeglasses
- Yellow and pink acetate sheets
- Pinhole occluders

DISPLAY 7-6
Guidelines for Using Magnifying Aids

Using a Hand-Held Magnifier
- Begin with the magnifier close to the reading material.
- Slowly move the magnifier toward the face until the image totally fills the lens.
- For optimal focus, move the magnifier back toward the print about a distance of 2 cm.

Using a Stand Magnifier
- Rest the stand flat against the reading material.
- Do not move the stand.

Using a Spectacle-Mounted Magnifier
- Begin with the reading material close to the nose.
- Slowly move the material away until it becomes clear.

Compensating for Visual Deficits Through Environmental Adaptations

Simple environmental modifications can improve the older person's safe performance of ADL. Architectural designs and institutional constraints may limit the extent of environmental adaptations that nurses can implement in hospitals and nursing homes. In any setting, however, nurses can improve the visual abilities of older adults by using appropriate colors to enhance contrast, by using curtains to control light and glare, and by placing chairs in positions that enhance illumination and avoid glare. Nurses have many opportunities to teach older adults and their caregivers about the environmental influences most conducive to optimal visual function. References on environmental adaptations aimed at improving visual function

---

DISPLAY 7-7
Considerations for Optimal Illumination

- Older adults need at least three times as much light as younger people do.
- Older adults function best in environments with bright, broad-spectrum, nonglaring, indirect sources of light.
- Sources of illumination should be placed 1 to 2 feet away from the object to be viewed.
- Flickering light, such as that generated by a single fluorescent tube, will cause fatigue and decreased visual performance.
- Light bulbs should be dusted periodically.
- Light bulbs should be changed when they become dim, rather than waiting for them to burn out.
- The amount of light decreases fourfold when the distance is doubled.
- Increased illumination has a greater positive effect on impaired vision than it does on normal vision.
- A gradual decrease in illumination from foreground to background is preferred over sharp contrasts.
- Moderate overhead lighting can be used to enhance brighter foreground lighting and prevent sharp contrasts.
- To reduce glare from reading material, place the light source to the left side of right-handed readers, and to the right side of left-handed readers.
- Avoid glossy paper for reading materials.

are now available and can serve as helpful resources for planning environments for people who have visual impairments (e.g., Brawley, 1997). Display 7-8 describes some environmental adaptations that may compensate for deficits in visual skills.

Because many functional consequences result from the age-related reduction in retinal illumination, proper lighting is the single most important intervention in improving the vision of older people. Increased illumination is one of the easiest and least costly modifications that can be made in any setting. Both the quality and quantity of light should be considered in

providing illumination for optimal visual performance. Studies suggest that broad-spectrum fluorescent lights and daylight-simulating lamps may be particularly beneficial in compensating for age-related vision changes (Kolanowski, 1992). Display 7-7 summarizes the principles that should be considered in providing illumination.

A second important consideration in adapting the environment for optimal visual function is color contrast. Appliances and other items, such as ovens, irons, radios, thermostats, and televisions, may be difficult to use because of poor color contrast around the control mecha-

---

DISPLAY 7-8
Environmental Adaptations for Improving Visual Performance

Illumination, Glare Control, and Dark/Light Adaptation

- Position a 60- or 75-watt soft-white light bulb above and close to the head of the older person.
- Use a clear plastic shower curtain, rather than solid colors or printed curtains, for the tub or shower.
- Use light-colored, sheer curtains to eliminate glare from windows.
- Place night-lights in hallways and bathrooms, or keep a high-intensity flashlight at the bedside.
- Use illuminated light switches.
- Provide adequate lighting in stairways and hallways.
- Use illuminated or magnified mirrors.

Color Contrast

- Use brightly colored tape or paint on the edges of stairs, especially on the top and bottom steps.
- Use light-colored and dark-colored cutting boards to contrast with dark and light foods.
- Use contrasting, rather than matching, colors for china, placemats, and napkins.
- Use a toilet seat that contrasts with the bathroom walls and floor.
- Use colored bars of soap on white sinks and tubs.

- Use utensils with brightly colored handles.
- Place pillows of contrasting colors on stuffed furniture.
- Use decorative or lighted plates over light switches and wall sockets; avoid light switch plates that blend in with the wallpaper or paint.
- Place decorative items of contrasting colors, such as plants and ceramics, on tables to provide clues to depth, especially on light-colored furniture that is in a room with light-colored walls.
- Use brightly colored grooming utensils, such as combs, brushes, and razors.
- Use pens with black ink rather than blue ink.

General Adaptive Measures and Environmental Modifications

- Do not rearrange furniture without informing or showing the older person.
- Advise older adults to pause in doorways when going from light to dark rooms (or vice versa) to allow time for their eyes to adjust to the light change.
- Teach older people to use their feet and hands as probes to feel for curbs, steps, edges of chairs, and the like.
- When walking with an older person, stop when necessary to allow a change in focus from near to far and from light to dark.

nisms. Modifications can easily be made to improve the older person's ability to use these items safely and accurately. For example, two dots of red nail polish can be used to mark the most commonly used temperature settings, and the older adult can be instructed to turn the dial above or below the dots for different settings. Additional environmental adaptations aimed at improving color contrast are listed in Display 7-8. A free brochure, describing guidelines for and illustrating examples of effective color contrast, is available from The Lighthouse, Inc. (see the list of Educational Resources).

Maintaining and Improving Quality of Life

As discussed earlier, the psychosocial consequences of impaired vision can be quite significant for older adults. Many of the interventions that help older adults compensate for visual deficits and function at their highest level also will improve their quality of life and address the psychosocial consequences of impaired vision. For example, the use of appropriate reading glasses and good environmental lighting may enable the older adult to read books, newspapers, and magazines. Subsequently, they may experience an improvement in their quality of life because they have more satisfying social interactions and increased intellectual stimulation. Certain alternative and preventive health care practices, as summarized in the box below, may also improve the older adult's quality of life with regard to vision.

Evaluating Nursing Care

Nursing care for older adults with visual impairments is evaluated by measuring the extent to which identified goals have been achieved. A common short-term goal that might be addressed in a nursing care plan would be that the older adult perform his or her daily activities safely and independently. Interventions could be based on the suggestions in Displays 7-7 and 7-8. The goal would be measured according to the older adult's improved ability to perform tasks, such as reading, dressing, personal care, using appliances, and managing medications. Another measurement of goal achievement

ALTERNATIVE
AND
PREVENTIVE
HEALTH
CARE
PRACTICES

Improving Vision

Herbs
- For prevention of cataracts: catnip, bilberry, rosemary, turmeric, ginger, purslane

Homeopathic Remedies
- For prevention of catarcts: silica, calcarea, phosphorus

Nutritional Considerations
- Nutritional supplements: selenium, magnesium, manganese, and vitamins A, B-complex, C, and E
- Avoidance of coffee, alcohol, cigarettes, black tea, artificial sweeteners, and excessive doses of riboflavin (i.e., more than 10 mg/day)

Preventive Measures and Additional Approaches
- Reflexology
- Avoidance of exposure to sunlight
- Annual eye examinations for glaucoma, cataracts, and vision problems

would be that the person remains free of injury secondary to falling, tripping, or bumping into objects. The nursing care plan at the end of this chapter includes evaluation criteria for these kinds of short-term goals.

Long-term goals for older adults with visual impairments would address the need for further evaluation and ongoing management. Nurses in institutional settings would address these goals through a discharge plan that includes information about local resources for further evaluation. Also, the discharge plan might include suggestions for obtaining educational materials from a local sight center or one of the resources listed at the end of this chapter. Evaluation of this goal would be based on the person's indication of his or her intent to follow through with the recommended course of action. In home, community, and nursing home settings, nurses may be able to address long-term goals by facilitating referrals for additional services. In these settings, the evaluation of long-term goals may be based on feedback from the older adults or their caregivers about the actual use of suggested resources. Evaluation criteria for this type of goal are identified in the nursing care plan at the end of this chapter.

Chapter Summary

Beginning around the age of 40 years, adults experience the earliest effects of age-related vision changes when they notice they need reading glasses for small print. Additional age-related vision changes include diminished depth perception, a narrower visual field, difficulty seeing objects clearly, an increased sensitivity to glare, and delayed adaptation to dark and light. As a result of these changes, older adults may have problems performing activities, such as reading, shopping, walking safely, and seeing markings on objects such as clocks and appli-

ances. Also, they are at increased risk for falls and injuries because of difficulty maneuvering safely in stairways and unfamiliar or dimly lit environments.

Nursing assessment of vision focuses on identifying risk factors (e.g., dimly lit environments), problems with visual skills (e.g., increased glare sensitivity), and the psychosocial consequences of impaired vision (e.g., impaired social interaction). Relevant nursing diagnoses would include Sensory-Perceptual Alteration: Vision, Activity Intolerance, Self-Care Deficit, and High Risk for Injury. Nursing care is directed toward assisting the older adult attain and maintain optimal visual function and compensate for any visual limitations. Interventions focus on environmental modifications, use of low-vision aids, and education about resources. Nursing care is evaluated according to the degree of improvement in level of function, the use of low-vision aids, the effectiveness of environmental modifications, and the response of the older adult to the suggested resources.

Critical Thinking Exercises

1. Describe presbyopia and explain the functional consequences of this condition in the everyday life of an older adult.
2. What environmental factors are likely to interfere with the visual function of older adults?
3. How would you assess the visual abilities of an older adult?
4. Explain the differences between opticians, optometrists, and ophthalmologists.
5. List at least 10 adaptations that might be implemented to improve the visual function of older adults.
6. Identify at least one resource in your community that might provide help or information to a person who is visually impaired.

Case Example and Nursing Care Plan

Pertinent Case Information

Mrs. V. is an 82-year-old woman who is staying at her daughter's house while she recovers from a recent bout with congestive heart failure. She normally lives alone in her own home, but she began needing help with her ADL after she was hospitalized for an acute episode of congestive heart failure. Additional medical diagnoses include arthritis, right-eye cataract, hypertension, and history of fractured hip. Current medications are furosemide, 20 mg q.d.; digoxin, 0.125 mg q.d.; and enalapril, 2.5 mg t.i.d. A 2-g sodium diet has been prescribed, and she can self-administer oxygen per nasal cannula at a rate of 2 L/min as needed. After a recent 7-day hospitalization, she was referred to a home care agency for assessment and monitoring of her cardiovascular status, teaching about her medication and treatment regimen, and evaluation of her ability to manage at home.

Nursing Assessment

During your initial nursing assessment, you determine that Mrs. V. is motivated to learn about her condition and follow through with her treatment plan, but she has difficulty reading small-print instructions because of poor vision. When you review her medications, you observe that she cannot read the labels on the bottles. You also observe that Mrs. V. keeps her medicines on the shelf above the kitchen counter, where the lighting is very dim. When you review the proper use of the oxygen, you note that she has difficulty seeing the markings on the flowmeter. Her daughter has been helping her with these regimens, but Mrs. V. hopes to perform these activities independently so she can return to her own home.

Mrs. V. tells you that she has never stayed overnight in her daughter's home before and is concerned about falling when she gets up during the night to go to the bathroom. You observe that the hallway between the bedroom and bathroom is dark, and that the bedroom has an overhead light, but no bedside lamp. You assess the home for safety and determine that the pathways are clear and there is good lighting on the stairway and in the living areas. You identify no additional risks (e.g., throw rugs) to Mrs. V.'s safe mobility.

When questioned about her vision problems, Mrs. V. states that, 2 years ago, her family doctor told her she had a cataract developing in her right eye. She has not had this evaluated by an eye doctor because she can still see out of her left eye. She has not had a complete eye examination in 5 years. She says she gets large-print books from the library and is not interested in reading the newspaper because she watches the news on television. She hasn't seen an eye doctor because she doesn't want to have cataract surgery until her vision is bad in both eyes. She acknowledged that she is fearful of the procedure because a friend had complications from cataract surgery 10 years ago. Also, she's concerned about the cost of the surgery because she has no supplemental insurance.

Nursing Diagnosis

In addition to the nursing diagnoses related to Mrs. V.'s medical condition, you identify a nursing diagnosis of Sensory-Perceptual Alteration: Visual, related to age-related changes, sensory organ alterations, and environmental factors. Supporting evidence for this diagnosis can be found in her inability to read labels, instructions, or the flowmeter markings; her dependency on her daughter for help with instrumental ADL; and the poorly lit environment.

The nursing diagnoses of Anxiety, Self-Care Deficit, and High Risk for Injury might also be applicable. The diagnosis of Sensory-Perceptual Alteration, however, addresses the source of Mrs. V.'s anxiety, high risk for injury, and inability to perform her instrumental ADL. Also, this diagnosis prompts the nurse to include a long-term goal of encouraging further evaluation and management of the cataract and other visual impairments.

Goals	Nursing Interventions	Evaluation Criteria
To manage medication regimen independently	Print simplified medication instructions on large index cards using a black felt-tip marker. Use colored dots to match pill bottles with instruction cards. Establish a medication management system using pill organizer boxes with markings that are bold and have good color contrast. Teach Mrs. V. how to fill the pill boxes weekly, using the directions on the cards. Suggest that Mrs. V. fill the pill boxes at the kitchen table during daylight hours while using the overhead light.	Mrs. V. will demonstrate that she can accurately fill the pill boxes. Mrs. V. will take her medications correctly. Mrs. V.'s daughter will observe that her mother follows the prescribed regimen.
To manage oxygen treatments independently	Use a copy machine to enlarge the small-print instructions for the oxygen machine. Place a colored dot at the 2-L mark on the flowmeter. Keep the oxygen tank in a well-lit location and suggest using a flashlight to help visualize the flowmeter setting.	Mrs. V. will demonstrate the safe and independent operation of the oxygen equipment. Mrs. V.'s daughter will observe that her mother administers her oxygen correctly.
To prevent injury when walking to the bathroom at night	Place a lamp on the night stand; make sure Mrs. V. can turn it on easily while in bed.	The bedroom-to-bathroom pathway will be lit at night. Mrs. V. will demonstrate that she

To obtain a medical evaluation of Mrs. V.'s visual impairment

Teach Mrs. V. to turn the bedside lamp on and sit at the edge of her bed a few minutes before getting up at night.

Position night-lights in the hallway and bathroom.

Educate Mrs. V. and her daughter about the importance of annual eye examinations for glaucoma, cataract, and other visual problems.

Allow Mrs. V. to verbalize her fears; provide health education brochure to correct any myths.

Emphasize that, in recent years, many advances have been made in cataract surgical procedures.

Explain that there are many low-cost, low-vision aids that can improve vision.

Give Mrs. V. and her daughter the phone number for the National Eyecare Project (800-222-3937) and encourage them to obtain the name of a local eye doctor who treats older patients without them incurring out-of-pocket expenses.

can turn the light on from her bed.

Mrs. V. will state that she feels safe when walking to the bathroom at night.

Mrs. V. will be free of injury.

Mrs. V. will make and keep an appointment for an eye examination.

Mrs. V. will use low-vision aids to improve visual function.

Educational Resources

American Academy of Ophthalmology
655 Beach Street, P.O. Box 7424, San Francisco, CA 94120-7424
(415) 561-8500
www.eyenet.org
• Free brochures and fact sheets about eye diseases and conditions

American Foundation for the Blind
11 Penn Plaza, Suite 300, New York, NY 10001
(800) 232-5463
www.afb.org
• Catalogue of publications and audiovisuals

American Optometric Association
243 North Lindbergh Boulevard, St. Louis, MO 63141
(314) 991-4100; (888) 396-3937
www.aoanet.org

• Free single copies of brochures
• Referrals to state optometric associations, which have lists of local doctors who provide needed services in their offices or in nursing homes

The Lighthouse Inc.
111 East 59th Street, New York, NY 10022
(212) 821-9200; (800) 829-0500
www.lighthouse.org
• Catalogue of products for people with impaired vision
• Educational publications, videos, newsletters, and inservice training materials for consumers and professionals

National Association for Visually Handicapped (NAVH)
22 West 21st Street, New York, NY 10010
(212) 889-3141
www.navh.org

- Large-print pamphlets, newsletters, and health education materials (some materials are available in Spanish or Russian)
- Catalogue of visual aids
- Free large-print library
- Information about various household items and appliances that have been modified for people with low vision

National Eye Care Project
P.O. Box 429098, San Francisco, CA 94142-9098
(800) 222-3937
www.eyenet.org/public/pi/service/necp.html
- Referral and information for citizens or legal residents of the United States who are financially in need of the medical and surgical eye care services of a volunteer ophthalmologist (this is not an eyeglass program)

National Eye Institute (NEI)
31 Center Drive MSC 2510, Building 31, Room 6A32, Bethesda, MD 20892–2510
(301) 496–5248
www.nei.nih.gov
- Information about current research on specific eye diseases

Prevent Blindness America
500 East Remington Road, Schaumburg, IL 60173
(800) 331–2020
www.preventblindness.org
- Support groups, special screenings, community programs
- Catalogue of videos and publications (some materials available in Spanish)

References

Baltes, P. B., & Lindenberger, U. (1997). Emergence of a powerful connection between sensory and cognitive functions across the adult life span: A new window to the study of cognitive aging? *Psychology and Aging, 12*(1), 12–21.

Brawley, E. C. (1997). Designing for Alzheimer's disease: Strategies for creating better care environments. New York: John Wiley & Sons.

Carpenito, L. J. (1997). *Nursing diagnosis: Application to clinical practice* (7th ed.). Philadelphia: J. B. Lippincott.

Grisso, J. A., Kelsey, J. L., Strom, B. L., Chiu, G. Y., Maislin, G., O'Brien, L. A., Hoffman, S., Kaplan, F., & Northeast Hip Fracture Group. (1991). Risk factors for falls as a cause of hip fracture in women. *New England Journal of Medicine, 324,* 1326–1331.

Horowitz, A. (1994). Vision impairment and functional disability among nursing home residents. *The Gerontologist, 34*(3), 316–323.

Horowitz, A. (1997). The relationship between vision impairment and the assessment of disruptive behaviors among nursing home residents. *The Gerontologist, 37*(5), 620–628.

Ivers, R. Q., Cumming, R. G., Mitchell, P., & Attebo, K. (1998). Visual impairment and falls in older adults: The Blue Mountains Eye Study. *Journal of the American Geriatrics Society, 46,* 58–64.

Johnson, L. E. (1995). Vitamin nutrition in the elderly. In J. E. Morley, Z. Glick, & L. Z. Rubenstein (Eds.), *Geriatric Nutrition,* (2nd ed., pp. 79–105). New York: Raven Press.

Kolanowski, A. M. (1992). The clinical importance of environmental lighting to the elderly. *Journal of Gerontological Nursing, 18*(1), 10–14.

Kosnik, W., Winslow, L., Kline, D., Rasinski, K., & Sekuler, R. (1988). Visual changes in daily life throughout adulthood. *Journal of Gerontology: Psychological Sciences, 43,* P63–P70.

Maino, J. H. (1996). Visual deficits and mobility: Evaluation and management. *Clinics in Geriatric Medicine, 12*(4), 803–823.

Morse, A. R., & Rosenthal, B. P. (1996). Vision and vision assessment. *Journal of Mental Health and Aging, 2*(3), 197–212.

National Center for Health Statistics (R. J. Havlik). (1986). *Aging in the eighties. Impaired senses for sound and light in persons age 65 years and over. Preliminary data from the Supplement on Aging to the National Health Interview Survey, U.S., January–June 1984.* (DHHS Publication no. 86–1250.) Hyattsville, MD: Public Health Service. (Advance Data from *Vital and Health Statistics,* no. 125.)

Resnick, H. E., Fries, B. E., & Verbrugge, L. M. (1997). Windows to their world: The effect of sensory impairments on social engagement and activity time in nursing home residents. *Journal of Gerontology: Social Sciences, 52B*(3), S135–S144.

Rudberg, M. A., Furner, S. E., Dunn, J. E., & Cassel, C. K. (1993). The relationship of visual and hearing impairments to disability: An analysis using the longitudinal study of aging. *Journal of Gerontology: Medical Sciences, 48*(6), M261–M265.

Tielsch, J. M., Sommer, A., Katz, J., Royall, R. M., Quigley, H. A., & Javitt, J. (1991). Racial variations in the prevalence of primary open-angle glaucoma. *Journal of the American Medical Association, 266*(3), 369–374.

Tumosa, N. (1995). Nutrition and the aging eye. In J. E. Morley, A. Glick, & L. Z. Rubenstein (Eds.), *Geriatric Nutrition* (2nd ed., pp. 283–288). New York: Raven Press.

Digestion and Nutrition

Chapter

8

Learning Objectives	1. *Delineate age-related changes that affect eating patterns and digestive processes.* 2. *Identify age-related changes in nutritional requirements.* 3. *Examine risk factors that affect the digestion and nutrition of older adults.* 4. *Discuss the functional consequences of age-related changes and risk factors affecting digestion and nutrition.* 5. *Describe interview questions, behavioral cues, and objective data that may be useful in assessing digestion and nutrition in older adults.* 6. *Identify interventions to assist older adults attain and maintain optimal nutrition.*

*D*igestion of food and maintenance of nutrition are influenced to a small degree by age-related gastrointestinal changes, to a moderate degree by the functional consequences of other age-related changes, and to a large degree by risk factors that commonly occur in older adulthood. Any functional consequences of age-related changes in the digestive tract can be compensated for by adjusting eating patterns and food selection. More significant consequences result from other age-related changes, such as impaired vision, that interfere with the older person's ability to obtain and prepare food, and from psychosocial circumstances, like a change in living situation, that alter established eating patterns. Because of the numerous influences on digestion and nutrition, age-related changes are addressed in this chapter according to changes in digestion, changes in nutritional requirements, and changes that influence eating patterns.

Age-Related Changes in Digestion

Age-related changes affect all the structures of the digestive tract. Although these changes have very few functional consequences for healthy, nonmedicated, older adults, they increase the vulnerability of older adults to risk factors. It is important for nurses to distinguish between age-related changes and risk factors so that appropriate interventions can be planned.

Oral Cavity

Digestion begins when food enters the mouth and is acted on by the teeth, saliva, and neuromuscular structures responsible for mastication. Age-related changes in the teeth and support structures influence digestive processes and food enjoyment. Additionally, tooth loss and other commonly occurring pathologic conditions interfere with oral digestion.

Age-related changes affect the tooth enamel, which becomes harder and more brittle, and the dentin (the layer underlying tooth enamel), which becomes more fibrous and less conductive of pain with increasing age. Because of these changes, as well as decades of abrasive and erosive action, the chewing cusps are gradually flattened.

The supporting structures for the teeth of older adults are affected both by age-related changes and by commonly occurring pathologic conditions, such as periodontal disease. As a result of degenerative processes, the bones supporting the teeth diminish in height and density, and teeth may loosen or fall out. Degenerative changes also affect the periodontal membrane, making it more susceptible to infection.

Age-related changes of the oral mucosa include loss of elasticity, atrophy of epithelial cells, and diminished blood supply to the connective tissue. Pathologic conditions may further compromise the function of the oral mucosa. Dry mouth and vitamin deficiencies, which are common conditions in older adults, compound the age-related changes, making the oral mucosa more friable and susceptible to infection and ulceration.

Saliva is secreted in response to food being broken into pieces by the act of chewing. Saliva facilitates digestion through the following mechanisms: provision of digestive enzymes, cleansing of the taste buds, lubrication of the soft tissue, remineralization of the teeth, regulation of oral flora, and preparation of food for chewing. Altered composition, increased viscosity, and diminished quantity of saliva have been attributed to age-related changes. Current evidence suggests that saliva reduction in healthy, nonmedicated, older adults is not attributable to age-related changes; however, older adults are likely to develop salivary dysfunction as a result of risk factors, such as medications, dehydration, or radiation therapy (Ship et al., 1995; Wu et al., 1995; Ship and Fischer, 1997). Thus, it is not age-related changes, but the common occurrence of diseases, medication effects, and other risk factors, that is likely to cause decreased saliva production in older adults (Atkinson and Fox, 1992; Wu et al., 1993).

Oral digestion is further influenced by the function of the neuromuscular structures involved in mastication and swallowing. Age-related changes affecting muscular tension and speed of responses have been identified, but these changes do not significantly affect the mechanisms involved in chewing or swallowing. Swallowing problems and complaints in older adults are generally attributable to risk factors, not to age-related changes alone. For example, tooth loss and altered dentition may be associated with prolonged chewing time, increased size of bolus, and a preference for softer foods (Sonies, 1992).

Esophagus

The second phase of digestion occurs when a combination of propulsive and nonpropulsive waves propels food through the pharynx and esophagus into the stomach. In older adults, the intensity of propulsive waves decreases and the frequency of nonpropulsive waves increases. This condition is called *presbyesophagus*. Researchers disagree about whether presbyesophagus is caused by age-related or pathologic processes, and whether it slows the transit time or affects the esophageal sphincter. They do agree, however, that the functional impact of presbyesophagus is minimal, and that most esophageal dysfunction is attributable to pathologic conditions, such as hiatal hernia.

Stomach

After passing through the esophageal sphincter, food enters the stomach, where it is liquefied by gastric juices and transformed into chyme by gastric action. As with esophageal changes, researchers disagree about the cause, extent, and consequences of gastric changes, particularly motility. Studies about age-related changes in gastric emptying have yielded contradictory results, with some studies indicating that there is delayed emptying and others indicating that there is little or no significant change.

Although some studies of age-related changes in gastric juice secretion point to a decrease in gastric secretions beginning during the 5th decade, this assumption is now being challenged. One recent study concluded that the prevalence of decreased levels of gastric acid secretions is no more than 11% in older adults—a prevalence similar to that found in younger adult populations (Hurwitz, 1997). Hurwitz and colleagues point out that most of the studies that have demonstrated impaired acid secretion in the elderly have focused on people with gastrointestinal symptoms. Although pernicious anemia, peptic ulcers, and stomach cancer occur more often in older adults, they are not necessarily associated with age-related gastric changes.

Small Intestine

After the chyme passes into the small intestine, digestive enzymes from the small intestine, liver, and pancreas convert the food substances into usable nutrients. A process of segmentation moves the chyme backward and forward, facilitating the digestion of food and the absorption of nutrients through the villi in the walls of the small intestine.

Although the available research on age-related structural changes affecting the small intestine is scant, most studies suggest that the following changes occur with increased age: atrophy of muscle fibers and mucosal surfaces; reduction in the number of lymphatic follicles; gradual reduction in the weight of the small intestine; and shortening and widening of the villi, which gradually form parallel ridges rather than finger-like projections. Research studies have not yet differentiated between the age-related and disease-related factors that cause or contribute to these changes. Functionally, there is no significant difference in mean small bowel transit time between younger and older subjects.

Studies of the effects of small intestine changes on the absorption of certain nutrients are inconclusive. Researchers generally agree that fat absorption is slowed with increased age, but they disagree about whether this is attributable to age-related changes or to pathologic conditions. Also, they disagree about whether the causative mechanism is pancreatic deficiency, delayed stomach emptying, changes in the small intestine, or a combination of these factors. The

results of studies of protein and carbohydrate absorption are also contradictory and inconclusive.

In contrast, there is general agreement about an age-related decline in the absorption of calcium and vitamin D. The mechanisms that influence calcium and vitamin D absorption are complex, with changes in the small intestine only partially accounting for malabsorption. Absorption of these nutrients in older adults may be further compromised by inadequate intake of calcium, which is a common dietary deficiency of older adults.

Liver and Pancreas

The liver assists in digestion by producing and secreting bile, which is essential for the utilization of fats. The liver undergoes structural changes with increasing age; however, the extent to which these changes are age-related or pathologic in origin is unclear. Despite any age-related or pathologic changes, the liver has an enormous regenerative and reserve capacity, which allows it to compensate for such changes without affecting digestive function.

The function of the pancreas in the digestive process is to produce the secretions essential for the breakdown of fats, proteins, and carbohydrates in the small intestine. As with the liver, the pancreas undergoes degenerative changes. However, with the possible exception of decreased enzymatic activity in the digestion of fats, these changes have little or no functional consequences.

Large Intestine

After nutrients are absorbed in the small intestine, the chyme passes into the large intestine, where water and electrolytes are absorbed and waste products are expelled. Age-related changes in the large intestine include a reduction in mucous secretion and a decreased elasticity of the rectal wall. Despite the emphasis on constipation as a common problem of older adulthood, the age-related changes that affect the large intestine have little or no impact on motility of feces through the bowel.

Age-Related Changes in Nutritional Requirements

Accurate information about the nutrient requirements of older adults is limited by a lack of research specifically addressing the nutritional impact of age-related changes. For example, age-related reductions in renal, cardiac, hepatic, and respiratory function may influence the nutritional needs of healthy, nonmedicated, older adults. Moreover, age-related changes in body composition and homeostasis regulation may also affect the nutritional needs of older people. The reliability of available data is further limited by the complex interactions between various age-related changes and the impact of these changes on nutrient requirements. For example, if iron absorption is impaired because of age-related gastric changes, any resultant detrimental effects may be offset by the age-related increase in iron stores.

In recent years, there has been a proliferation of recommendations concerning ideal nutritional intake for various conditions. The primary focus of many of these guidelines is the prevention of diseases, such as cancer and heart disease. Some of the guidelines emphasize the inclusion of foods containing antioxidants and other nutrients that may play a protective and preventive role. With the burgeoning availability and variety of nutritional supplements on the market, it is becoming increasingly difficult to determine minimum daily nutritional needs, and it is even more difficult to determine daily nutritional needs for the prevention of diseases and other unwanted conditions. In the late 1990s, the National Academy of Sciences began emphasizing "dietary reference intakes" rather than continuing to emphasize "recommended dietary allowances." Emphasis also is currently being placed on adequate intake and tolerable upper intake levels. Because most guidelines address the needs of healthy, nonmedicated, adults, they should be adjusted for medical conditions, age-related changes, and other factors that might affect nutritional needs. Also, adjustments for food and drug interactions may be necessary for people who take one or more medications. Because information about the role of nutrition in the prevention of unwanted conditions is rapidly evolving, it is important to keep abreast of scientifically based research and resources relating to this topic. The Educational Resources section at the end of this chapter lists a variety of sources for nutritional information, including Internet addresses.

Calories

The energy-producing potential of food is measured in units called calories. Caloric requirements are determined by various factors, including gender, usual level of physical activity, health-illness state, and height, weight, and body build. Energy requirements gradually decrease throughout adulthood, primarily as a result of reductions in activity and metabolism. Additional changes in the older body, such as decreases in muscular efficiency and lean body tissue, further reduce the need for calories. Nutritional guidelines generally recommend a gradual reduction in calories beginning around the age of 40 to 50 years.

Surveys of the nutritional status of older adults indicate that caloric intake is often deficient, especially in older women. One study found that 37% of men and 40% of women aged 65 to 98 years reported a caloric intake of less than two thirds the Recommended Dietary Allowance (Ryan et al., 1992). Moreover, older adults require higher-quality calories to meet their nutrient needs. Thus, nutritional deficiencies will occur unless a reduced caloric intake is accompanied by an increased intake of foods with a high nutritional value and a concomitant decrease in the intake of foods containing little or no nutrients.

Protein

Protein provides the essential components for new tissue growth in the human body. Research on the impact of age-related changes in protein requirements is inconclusive. However, researchers have identified certain age-related changes that may influence protein requirements, including (1) decreased lean body mass, muscle tissue, and total body protein; (2) decreased plasma albumin and total body albumin levels; and (3) decreased glomerular filtration rates with a concomitant decrease in protein tolerance. Further research is needed to determine the specific impact, if any, of these age-related changes on protein requirements. Older adults should consume a minimum daily protein intake of about 1 g/kg of body weight (Bidlack and Wang, 1995). The protein needs of older adults will usually be met if approximately 12% to 15% of the daily caloric intake is derived from protein.

Carbohydrates and Fiber

Carbohydrates provide an essential source of energy and fiber. Without an adequate intake of carbohydrates, energy will be derived from fat and protein, causing an increase in serum cholesterol and triglyceride levels and a depletion of water, electrolytes, and amino acids. In recent years, fiber has received much attention, primarily for its role in disease prevention, as an essential food component. Soluble fibers, found in oats and pectin, are beneficial in lowering serum cholesterol levels and improving glucose tolerance in diabetics. Insoluble fibers, found in most grains and many vegetables, are important for maintaining good bowel function and for preventing constipation. Display 8-4 (p. 253) identifies some of the foods that aid in preventing constipation. For the average American, intake of fiber is 10 to 20 g/day, which is less than half the amount recommended by the National Cancer Institute. Dietary guidelines suggest a daily intake of five or more servings of fruits and vegetables, with at least 55% of the total calories consumed derived from complex carbohydrates.

Fats

The primary functions of fat are to assist in temperature regulation, to provide a reserve source of energy, to facilitate the absorption of fat-soluble vitamins, and to reduce acid secretion and muscular activity of the stomach. Fats are also useful in providing a feeling of satiety and improving the taste of foods. Fats are categorized according to their source. Saturated fats are derived from animals, whereas unsaturated fats are found in vegetables. Although either type of fat can meet nutritional needs, only the saturated fats are associated with the detrimental accumulation of serum cholesterol.

Adults in most industrialized societies consume far more calories in fats than is healthy or necessary. Because excessive fat intake is associated with harmful effects, such as hyperlipidemia, fat should constitute no more than 10% to 30% of a person's daily caloric intake. Those fats that are consumed should be polyunsaturated and monounsaturated fatty acids, rather than cholesterol and saturated fats.

Vitamins

Vitamins are essential for almost all metabolic processes. Vitamin deficiencies in older adults are associated with many factors. Because older adults need fewer calories, if the quantity of calories is reduced without a corresponding increase in the quality of the food consumed, a deficiency of essential nutrients will occur. Additionally, older adults are more likely to have vitamin deficiencies because of other conditions, such as medication effects and alcohol use, that interfere with absorption and utilization. The vitamins most commonly found to be deficient, based on blood level measurements in older adults, are niacin, thiamine, riboflavin, and vitamins B_6, C, and D. Details about the causes and consequences of vitamin deficiencies in older adults are presented in Table 8-1.

TABLE 8-1
Causes and Consequences of Nutrient Deficiencies

Nutrient	Results of Deficiency	Possible Causes of Deficiency
Calories	Weight loss, lethargy, edema, anemia	Anorexia, depression, mental or physical impairments
Protein	Poor tissue healing, hypoalbuminemia, reduced protein binding of drugs	Lack of teeth or dentures, anorexia, depression, dementia, high alcohol or carbohydrate consumption
Fat	Inability to absorb vitamins A, D, E, and K	Neomycin, phenytoin, laxatives, alcohol, colchicine, cholestyramine
Vitamin A	Dry skin and eyes, photophobia, night blindness, hyperkeratoses	Mineral oil, neomycin, alcohol, cholestyramine
Thiamine	Neuropathy, muscle weakness, heart disease, dementia, anorexia	High consumption of alcohol or caffeinated tea, pernicious anemia
Riboflavin	Cheilitis, glossitis, photophobia, blepharitis, conjunctivitis	Malabsorption syndromes, chronic diarrhea, laxative abuse
Niacin	Dermatitis, stomatitis, diarrhea, dementia, depression	Poor dietary habits
Folate	Macrocytic anemia, dermatitis, stomatitis, diarrhea, dementia, depression	Anticonvulsants, triamterene, phenolphthalein, alcohol
Vitamin B_{12}	Pernicious anemia, weakness, dyspnea, glossitis, numbness, dementia, depression	Malabsorption syndrome, cimetidine, colchicine, oral hypoglycemics, potassium supplements, vegetarian diet
Vitamin C	Lassitude, irritability, anemia, ecchymosis	Aspirin, tetracycline, lack of fruits and vegetables in diet
Vitamin D	Muscle weakness and atrophy, osteoporosis	Phenytoin, mineral oil, phenobarbital, sunlight deprivation
Vitamin K	Ecchymosis; hemorrhage involving the gastrointestinal, urinary, or central nervous system	Mineral oil, coumadin, antibiotics, cholestyramine
Calcium	Osteoporosis, fractures, low back pain	Phenytoin, aluminum-based antacids, laxatives, tetracycline, corticosteroids, furosemide, high intake of fiber or caffeine
Iron	Anemia, weakness, lassitude, pallor	Achlorhydria; neomycin; aspirin; antacids; low intake of animal protein; high consumption of fiber, caffeine, or tannic acid (contained in some teas)
Magnesium	Cardiac arrhythmias, neuromuscular and central nervous system irritability, disorientation	Alcohol, diuretics, diarrhea, bulk-forming laxatives
Zinc	Poor wound healing, hair loss	Aluminum-based antacids, bulk-forming laxatives, high consumption of fiber
Potassium	Weakness, cardiac arrhythmias, digitalis toxicity	Laxatives, furosemide, antibiotics, corticosteroids, diarrhea
Water	Dry skin and mouth, dehydration, constipation	Diuretics, laxatives, immobility, incontinence, diarrhea
Fiber	Constipation, hemorrhoids	Poor dietary habits

Minerals

Minerals, like vitamins, are required for all metabolic processes. With the exception of zinc and calcium, healthy, nonmedicated, older adults derive adequate amounts of most minerals from food. However, many factors, such as diseases and adverse medication effects, may contribute to mineral deficiencies in older adults. For example, older adults who take potassium-wasting diuretics may develop hypokalemia. Medications may also contribute to zinc deficiency, especially if the older adult takes penicillamine, which is used to treat rheumatoid arthritis. For a summary of causes and consequences of mineral deficiencies that are common in older adults, refer to Table 8.1.

Although iron deficiency is cited as a common nutritional problem of older adults, studies of iron intake have failed to support any widespread dietary deficiencies. Certain high-risk groups have been identified, however, and these include people of low socioeconomic status, particularly older Black women. Iron deficiency anemia in older adults is more often related to chronic disease and blood loss from pathologic conditions than to low dietary intake of iron (Cohen and Crawford, 1992). Additional factors that may contribute to iron deficiency anemia are listed in Table 8.1.

In recent years, much attention has been focused on the calcium requirements of older adults, especially women, and the role of calcium in age-related bone loss. Both the absorption and excretion of calcium are affected by dietary intake of salt, fiber, sugar, protein, fluoride, phosphorus, magnesium, and vitamin D. Nondietary factors, such as stress, estrogen, cigarette smoking, and physical activity, further influence the calcium balance in the human body (Todd, 1989).

Much of the literature suggests that older adults, particularly older women, should consume 1200 to 1600 mg of calcium per day. Support for this recommendation is based on the following evidence:

1. Calcium deficiency is one of the most common nutrient deficiencies among older people, and it is more pronounced in older women than older men.
2. Calcium absorption gradually decreases with increasing age; in women, this is compounded by postmenopausal estrogen deficiency.
3. In older adults, regulation of calcium balance is less efficient, and adaptation to lower calcium intake is impaired.
4. Increased calcium intake is an important preventive measure for age-related conditions, such as osteoporosis and hypertension.

In 1997, the National Academy of Sciences began recommending 1200 mg calcium for adults aged 51 years and older (National Academy of Sciences, 1997).

Although there is much support for calcium supplementation, increased calcium intake is not without risks, and the ingestion of more than 2500 mg of calcium per day may be detrimental. In particular, risks are linked to the use of calcium supplements (Yen, 1997). Hypercalcemia, impaired renal function, and an increased risk of kidney stones have been associated with calcium carbonate. Additionally, the ingestion of calcium carbonate with meals may interfere with the absorption of iron, zinc, magnesium, and phosphorus.

Water

Water is such a commonly available and tasteless substance that it is often overlooked as a nutritional requirement. However, it is essential for all metabolic activities and must be consumed in adequate amounts for proper physiologic performance. The functions of water include regulating body temperature, maintaining a suitable metabolic environment, diluting water-soluble medications, and facilitating renal and bowel excretion. Potential consequences of reduced body water include decreased efficiency of thermoregulation, increased susceptibility to dehydration, and increased concentrations of water-soluble medications in the body.

Throughout life, the proportion of total body water as a percentage of body weight gradually decreases. Whereas water constitutes about 80% of a newborn infant's weight, it represents 60% of a younger adult's weight, and about 50% or less of an older adult's weight. This decrease in total body water is associated with a loss of lean body mass and is influenced by gender and degree of leanness, with women and obese people having a lower percentage of body water than men and lean, muscular people. In older adults, total body water may be further diminished by poor fluid intake secondary to age-related factors, such as diminished thirst sensation. It is recommended that older adults consume 1500 to 2000 mL of noncaffeinated fluid daily to maintain adequate hydration.

Age-Related Factors That Influence Eating Patterns

Eating patterns depend on a variety of factors, such as food appeal, physical health, economic status, activity level, functional abilities, and psychosocial, cultural, and environmental influences. Changes in any one of these factors will affect the nutritional status of older adults. Conditions that affect eating patterns most directly are sensory changes, psychosocial factors, and cultural, socioeconomic, and environmental influences. Additionally, lifelong economic and cultural influences are important determinants of eating patterns and attitudes toward food and nutrition.

Sensory Changes

Food appeal for people of all ages is significantly influenced by the odor, color, flavor, texture, temperature, and appearance of food. Age-related sensory declines, particularly in taste and smell, may negatively affect food appeal. The ability to taste depends primarily on the receptor cells in the taste buds, which are located on the tongue, palate, and tonsils. Unlike other neural cells, taste cells have the ability to regenerate and are replaced every few days. Although some studies have shown an age-related decline in the number of taste buds, recent reviews question this conclusion (Schiffman, 1996). Even if the number of taste buds does decline in older adulthood, this loss does not necessarily impair one's ability to taste.

Early studies consistently identified age-related declines in one or more of the taste thresholds (sweet, sour, salty, and bitter). However, many questions have been raised about the effects of these changes. A recent commentary concludes that there are small age-related declines in taste sensitivity, but that these declines do not necessarily impact the day-to-day taste experience of older persons (Weiffenbach and Bartoshuk, 1992). Recent studies conclude that taste, particularly the sweetness of sugar, is well preserved in older adults, but that there may be subtle variations with age (Bartoshuk and Weiffenbach, 1990). Although taste impairments may occur more commonly in older adults, they probably result from poor oral health, poor overall health, and adverse medication effects (Rolls and Drewnowski, 1996).

One's ability to smell depends on the perception of odorants by the sensory cells in the olfactory mucosa and on central nervous system processing of that information. Olfactory skills improve gradually until they reach peak performance around the age of 30 years. A recent literature review concluded that older adults demonstrate increased olfactory detection thresholds and an impaired ability to identify and discriminate odors (Ship and Weiffenbach, 1993). These deficits are found in healthy older adults, and their occurrence is independent of risk factors, such as medical conditions and adverse medication effects (Ship et al., 1996). Researchers now agree that olfactory ability diminishes to a greater extent than does gustatory function. Because the perception of food flavor is highly associated with olfactory stimulation, the diminished ability to discern flavors or identify foods in the mouth is probably associated with age-related declines in the sense of smell (Ship and Weiffenbach, 1993).

Risk factors that may further impair the age-related diminution in smell sensation include medications (e.g., antihistamines), periodontal and upper respiratory diseases, systemic diseases (e.g., dementia, diabetes), and environmental conditions (e.g., factory workplace) (Ship and Weiffenbach, 1993; Corwin et al., 1995; Nordin et al., 1995; Schiffman, 1997). In addition to being affected by risk and age-related factors, olfactory sensation can be influenced by gender and smoking habits, with women and nonsmokers exhibiting relatively better olfactory function. A recent cross-cultural survey of adults in America and Africa found that African respondents reported higher levels of olfactory function than did American respondents (Barber, 1997).

Psychosocial Factors

Stress and anxiety affect digestive processes through their influence on the autonomic nervous system. Although stress-related effects on digestion are not unique to older adults, any alteration of the autonomic nervous system may compound age-related effects that would otherwise remain unnoticed. For example, increased stress may inhibit salivary and gastric juice secretion. In younger people, these reductions may be insignificant, but in older adults, a further reduction in secretions that have already diminished may have a marked impact on digestion.

Studies have found that the psychosocial events that are likely to occur in older adulthood, such as widowhood or a change in living environment, may influence eating patterns and food enjoyment (Rosenbloom and Whittington, 1993). Living alone has been found to be associated with decreased caloric intake and a poor-quality diet, particularly in men aged 75 years and older (Rolls and Drewnowski, 1996). De-

pression and loneliness are common in older adults and are typically accompanied by anorexia and loss of interest in food. In long-term care facilities, the group mealtime atmosphere and the limited selection of foods can have a detrimental effect on the eating patterns of the residents. Based on individual nutritional assessments, the incidence of malnutrition among nursing home residents ranges from 40% to 85% (Coulston, 1995).

Cultural Considerations

Cultural factors influence the way food is defined, selected, prepared, and eaten. For instance, eating patterns of older adults may be influenced by ethnic background or religious beliefs. Cultural factors can also influence selection of food in relation to one's health status. For example, Asian and Hispanic people may classify foods, beverages, and medicines as hot or cold, and they may select a particular food based on their belief that their illness would respond to warm, hot, cool, or cold types of remedies. According to this health belief model, illnesses are caused by an imbalance between hot and cold, and so they must be treated with substances that have the opposite characteristics. Similarly, Chinese people may select foods to maintain a balance between yin and yang properties.

Dietary customs are usually not detrimental for healthy older adults, as long as essential nutrients are included in the diet and extremes are avoided. However, for the older adult with a medical condition that requires diet modification (e.g., diabetes or hypertension), cultural food patterns may aggravate the condition and create barriers to nutritional therapy. For example, the use of large amounts of soy sauce may contribute to hypertension. The Culture Box on p. 239 summarizes some of the food habits that are associated with major cultural and religious groups in the United States. It is usually not necessary to try to change culturally influenced eating patterns, but it is important to recognize

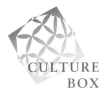

CULTURE
BOX

Cultural Influences on Eating Patterns

African Americans

- "Soul food" is common, particularly in the southern United States.
- Common main courses: wild game, fried fish and poultry, pork and all parts of the pig
- Common vegetables and side dishes: corn, rice, okra, greens, legumes, tomatoes, hot breads, sweet potatoes
- Methods of food preparation: stewing, barbecuing, and frying with lard or saltpork
- Low consumption of milk (possibly owing to lactose intolerance)
- Low calcium dietary intake

Asian Americans

- Common foods: rice, wheat, pork, eggs, chicken, soybean products, and a variety of vegetables
- Methods of food preparation: stir-frying with lard, peanut oil, or sesame oil; seasoning with ginger, soy sauce, sesame seeds, and monosodium glutamate
- Beverages: green tea; rare use of milk products because lactose intolerance is common

Hispanic Americans

- Common main courses: eggs, tacos, chicken, corn tortillas, pinto or calico beans
- Common vegetables and side dishes: rice, corn, squash, bread, tomatoes
- Methods of food preparation: frying with lard; seasoning with garlic, onions, and chili powder
- Beverages: herbal teas, carbonated soda, milk in hot beverages

Native Americans

- May obtain foods from their natural environment (e.g., fish, roots, fruits, berries, wild greens, and wild game)
- May rely on nonperishable foods because of lack of refrigeration
- May depend on commodity foods provided by the U.S. Department of Agriculture
- May be influenced by tribal culture

Religious Influences

- Orthodox Jews follow prescribed rules for preparing and serving foods (e.g., they eat only kosher meat and poultry and do not eat shellfish or any pork products).
- Mormons do not drink tea, coffee, or alcohol.
- Hindus are vegetarians.
- Seventh Day Adventists are lacto-ovovegetarians.
- Roman Catholics do not eat meat on Ash Wednesday or Good Friday.

any cultural factors that may affect an older adult's nutritional status.

Socioeconomic and Environmental Influences

A person's present and past economic status also influences food choices. If nutrient intake has been inadequate because of long-standing financial limitations, the progressive effects of poor nutrition may precipitate new problems in older adults, especially when combined with age-related changes in nutrient intake and utilization. People of low socioeconomic status usually have a narrower selection of foods than do people of higher socioeconomic status. Education may also affect nutritional status, with education beyond high school having a positive impact on nutrient intake (Rolls and Drewnowski, 1996). Nutritional deficits are likely to arise when these factors combine with other influences, such as limited food selection in institutional settings.

Environmental influences are most likely to affect older adults who are less able to compensate for inclement weather conditions. For example, an older person who usually walks to the store or who depends on public transportation may be unable or unwilling to obtain groceries in snowy or rainy weather. Likewise, the older adult may not be able to tolerate hot or sultry conditions, especially if car transportation is not readily available. Environmental conditions and packaging trends in the grocery store may create additional difficulties for older people. For example, the combined glare of fluorescent lights, highly polished floors, cellophane wrappers, and white freezer cases often make it extremely difficult, if not impossible, for the older adult with vision changes to read labels, especially when the print is small and faded.

Risk Factors

In addition to age-related changes, certain behaviors and common pathologic conditions are likely to interfere with nutrition and digestion in older adults. Pathologic conditions of the teeth and mouth affect oral function and food selection, and medications and alcohol affect nutrition and digestion in numerous ways. One study identified poor oral health as a potentially reversible contributor to significant involuntary weight loss in frail elderly people (Sullivan et al., 1993). Behaviors that are detrimental to nutrition and digestion, such as limited fluid intake, may be based on myths and misconceptions. Although these conditions can occur at any age, they are more typical in older adults, and the potential for harm is much greater than in other age groups because of the collective effects of risk factors and age-related changes.

Risks to Oral Health

Several decades ago, tooth loss was so common among older people that it was considered a normal consequence of aging. Several recent national surveys point toward a definite improvement in the oral health of older people. In 1960, more than 60% of older adults were edentulous (without teeth); this number has now declined to about 40%. It is predicted that, by the year 2024, only 10% of Americans between the ages of 65 and 74 years will be edentulous (Weintraub and Burt, 1985).

Tooth loss in older adulthood is often attributable to periodontal disease and other pathologic conditions that occur with increasing frequency in later years. Various factors that present barriers to obtaining dental care may contribute to tooth loss in older adults. These factors include lack of transportation, lack of dental insurance, the high cost of dental services, and inaccessibility of services as a result of distance or environmental barriers, such as stairs to dental offices. Xerostomia, a common medication side effect, also increases the risk for dental caries and tooth loss.

Negative attitudes on the part of dentists or older adults also may interfere with the provision of dental services. Because many older adults and some dentists view tooth loss as an inevitable concomitant of old age, restorative dental services may not be sought or provided. Additionally, many older adults have been fully or partially edentulous since the 1930s and 1940s because of the dental practices of that era, which espoused the removal, rather than the preservation, of teeth. Preventive dental care is a recent trend, and older adults may believe that the only time to go to a dentist is when a toothache does not respond to home remedies.

Behaviors That Interfere with Digestion and Nutrition

Myths and misunderstandings may cause or contribute to constipation by influencing food intake and behaviors related to bowel function. For example, during the l950s and 1960s, a widely held belief was that roughage and raw fruits or vegetables were harmful to the older person. On the contrary, elimination of roughage from the diet and the consumption of only cooked fruits and vegetables are eating patterns that contribute to constipation by slowing the transit time of feces through the large intestine. Another belief, which was widely promoted in the early 1900s, is that a daily bowel movement is the norm for good digestive function. Rigid adherence to this standard may, in fact, lead to the unnecessary and detrimental use of laxatives. This false belief has been further reinforced by advertisements implying that daily bowel movements should be attained through medication. Although recent advertising trends emphasize the achievement of healthy bowel patterns through the ingestion of high-fiber food items, the negative impact of long-term beliefs may be difficult to overcome.

Misunderstandings about fluid intake may also interfere with digestion and nutrition. Many older adults reduce the amount of liquids they consume with the expectation that this practice will decrease the incidence of urinary incontinence. Fluid intake may also be restricted if functional limitations, such as impaired mobility or manual dexterity, interfere with either the ability to obtain liquids or the ease of urinary elimination. Reduced fluid intake can have a number of detrimental consequences, such as constipation, dry mouth, and diminished food enjoyment.

Medication-Nutrient Interactions

Medications can directly influence the absorption and excretion of nutrients. Nutrient synthesis, for example, may be impaired by alterations in the intestinal flora caused by broad-spectrum antibiotics. Medications and vitamins that are similar in chemical structure may compete at sites of action, altering their excretion pattern. Other medications, such as tetracycline, bind to particular ions, such as iron and calcium, to form compounds that cannot be absorbed. Diuretics can interfere with the transport of water, sodium, glucose, and amino acids. With the increasing use of nutritional supplements and herbal preparations, attention should be paid to potential detrimental effects from these products. For example, the long-term use of beta-carotene supplements may cause a vitamin E deficiency. Nurses should keep in mind that little scientific information is available about the effects of nutritional supplments and herbal preparations on medications, but these substances are generally considered to be relatively safe. Additional examples of medication effects on specific nutrients are listed in Table 8-2. Food, herb, and medication interactions are further discussed in Chapter 18.

Even before any age-related changes occur, long-term patterns of alcohol consumption may alter an older person's nutritional status. Alcohol has a high caloric content but low nutrient value, so it provides empty calories. In addition, it interferes with the absorption of the B-complex vitamins.

TABLE 8-2
Effects of Some Medications on Nutrition

Medication	Effect on Nutrients
Mineral oil	Decreased absorption of vitamins A, D, E, and K
Anticonvulsants	Decreased storage of vitamin K, decreased absorption of calcium
Antacids containing aluminum	Decreased absorption of phosphorus and fluoride, increased excretion of calcium
Antacids containing aluminum or magnesium	Decreased absorption and increased intestinal elimination of phosphate
Antacids containing sodium bicarbonate	Sodium overload, water retention
Gentamicin	Increased potassium and magnesium excretion
Penicillin	Increased potassium excretion
Tetracyclines	Decreased absorption of zinc, iron, calcium, and magnesium
Aspirin	Decreased serum levels of folate and vitamin C, iron deficiency anemia
Corticosteroids	Decreased calcium and phosphorus absorption; increased need for folate, pyridoxine, vitamin C, and vitamin D
Potassium supplements	Decreased absorption of vitamin B_{12} secondary to diminished acidity in the ileum
Laxatives	Hypokalemia, hypoalbuminemia, decreased calcium absorption, malabsorption with steatorrhea
Cholestyramine	Decreased absorption of folate, calcium, and fat-soluble vitamins
Cimetidine	Decreased absorption of vitamin B_{12} as a result of hypochlorhydria
Neomycin	Decreased absorption of fat, iron, lactose, nitrogen, calcium, potassium, and vitamin B_{12}
NSAIDs	Iron deficiency anemia

NSAIDs, nonsteroidal anti-inflammatory drugs.

Medication Effects on Nutrition and Digestion

Medications may also have adverse effects that interfere with food intake and digestion. Although these medication effects are not uniquely age-related, they are more likely to occur in older adults because of the increased use of prescription and over-the-counter medications in this population. Moreover, medication effects tend to have an increased detrimental effect on older adults because they can exacerbate age-related changes and risk factors.

Medications may indirectly interfere with nutrition by causing such symptoms as anorexia, xerostomia (dry mouth), early satiety, and impaired smell and taste perception. In fact, medications have been cited as the most common cause of decreased saliva production and complaints of dry mouth in older people (Atkinson and Fox, 1992). Medications can also alter chemosensory perceptions through their action at peripheral receptors, neural pathways, and the brain; more than 250 medications have been identified as potentially interfering with the senses of smell or taste (Schiffman, 1996). Medications may also affect the oral tissue, causing eating or chewing discomfort. For example, gum hyperplasia is associated with phenytoin, nifedipine, diltiazem, and cyclosporine. Constipation is a common adverse effect of many medications, especially laxatives and agents that act on the central nervous system. Paralytic ileus, which has a serious impact on digestive function, may arise from anticholinergic medications or from hypokalemia caused by potassium-wasting diuretics. Table 8-3 identifies specific medications that can adversely affect food intake and digestion.

Postural hypotension, extrapyramidal symptoms, and tardive dyskinesia are examples of adverse medication effects that interfere with the functional skills involved in food procurement, preparation, consumption, and appreciation. Lastly, medications may indirectly impair nutrition by causing mental changes, such as dementia and depression, that interfere with appetite and functional abilities. These medication effects could compromise the nutritional status of some older adults, particularly if they live in independent settings and are responsible for their own meal preparation.

Functional Consequences

Functional consequences affect digestion and nutrition of older adults in the following areas: (1) procurement, preparation, and enjoyment of food; (2) mastication and digestion of food; (3) elimination of digestive wastes; and (4) psychosocial function. Negative functional consequences occur in these areas primarily because of risk factors, rather than because of age-related changes alone. In the following sections, each of these areas of functional consequences is examined.

Obtaining, Preparing, and Enjoying Food

Activities involved in procuring, preparing, consuming, and enjoying food depend on the skills of cognition, balance, mobility, manual dexterity, and all five senses. Age-related changes affecting any of these skills will influence one's

TABLE 8-3
Adverse Medication Reactions That Can Influence Nutrition

Medications	Possible Adverse Reaction
Digoxin, theophylline, antihistamines, over-the-counter cold or sleep preparations	Anorexia
Anticholinergics, narcotics, iron sulfate, psychotropic medications, aluminum- and calcium-based antacids, tricyclic antidepressants	Constipation
Cimetidine, laxatives, antibiotics, analgesics, iron sulfate, cardiovascular drugs, antacids containing magnesium hydroxide	Diarrhea
Diuretics, ibuprofen, hypnotics, antipsychotics, antidepressants, antihistamines, decongestants, anticholinergics, antiadrenergic agents (e.g., clonidine)	Dry mouth
Ibuprofen, phenylbutazone, indomethacin, aspirin, phenobarbital, corticosteroids	Increased gastric irritation
Anticholinergics, furosemide and other potassium-depleting medications, anticholinergics	Paralytic ileus
Bulk-forming agents taken before meals	Early satiety
Diuretics, vasodilators, hypoglycemics, antihistamines, antimicrobials, antilipidemics, antihypertensives, psychoactive agents	Interference with smell and taste sensations

eating patterns, as will any chronic illnesses or other risk factors. Despite the many factors that impact on food intake, however, adaptations can be made to compensate for age-related changes and risk factors.

Food procurement depends on getting to the grocery store, pushing a shopping cart, reaching for food items on high shelves, reading the small print on shelves and food packages for cost and nutrition information, and coping with the glare of bright lights, especially in the white-coated frozen food sections. Age-related changes and conditions that may interfere with these activities include vision impairments and any illness, such as arthritis, that limits mobility, balance, or manual dexterity.

Food procurement may also be influenced by environmental conditions and transportation resources. People who depend on others for transportation or who have difficulty maneuvering in adverse weather conditions are likely to shop for groceries less frequently and to purchase their groceries at smaller convenience stores, where prices are higher and selection is limited. The additional cost and limited selection may interfere with food intake and lead to nutrient deficiencies. Moreover, people living alone often have difficulty finding fresh foods that are packaged in small quantities. This discourages the purchase of fresh foods and encourages the purchase of prepared foods, which are likely to have a higher sodium content.

Food preparation activities that are likely to be more difficult for older adults include cutting food items, measuring ingredients accurately, carrying food and liquid without spilling, standing for long periods in the kitchen, reaching for items on high shelves and in cupboards, safely using the oven or stove, and reading the temperature controls correctly. Impairments of vision, balance, mobility, or manual dexterity are likely to cause difficulties in the performance of these tasks.

Food enjoyment is likely to be affected by sensory changes, which may interfere with the accurate perception of color, taste, or smell. Diminished gustatory and olfactory skills may lead to excessive use of condiments and seasonings, such as salt and sugar. Visual and olfactory impairments may make it difficult to detect spoiled food. Moreover, food choices are influenced by the condition of the oral cavity and teeth, as well as by the quantity and quality of natural or replacement teeth.

In addition to physical and environmental influences on food intake, psychosocial factors are likely to affect an older person's appetite and eating patterns. Any changes in mealtime companionship, as may occur through loss or disability of a spouse, are likely to have a negative impact on eating patterns. When a long-term pattern of preparing meals for family and spouse has been established, it may be especially difficult for the older adult to adjust to purchasing, preparing, and eating food for just one person. Similarly, older adults who have never participated in the purchase or preparation of foods may have great difficulty assuming these tasks after the loss of a spouse or other person who performed these tasks. If the older adult depended on others for assistance in procuring food, any factors that limit the availability of support resources may affect the older adult's ability to obtain food.

Changes in the living situation of the older adult can affect eating patterns and nutritional intake. For example, an older adult living in congregate housing or a long-term care facility may encounter difficulties adjusting to new and sometimes undesired opportunities for mealtime social interaction. A noisy or crowded dining room may have a negative impact on food enjoyment and consumption. Such an environment may be particularly stressful for an older adult who uses a hearing aid or who is accustomed to eating alone. An older adult who moves in with family members may have to accept new mealtime patterns that are determined by the needs of other family members. The potential outcomes of these changes include loss of interest in eating and poor nutrition, particularly during the initial adjustment period. Many times, however, a group meal setting has positive effects, such as more nutritious meals and no responsibility for food preparation. Also, the social interaction at group meals in pleasant surroundings may enhance food enjoyment.

Mastication and Digestion of Food

Xerostomia is a common disorder in older adults and may interfere with comfort as well as digestion. With diminished saliva production, food may be more difficult to chew, and the teeth and tongue become more susceptible to bacterial action. When xerostomia interferes with oral comfort and taste sensitivity, food is less enjoyable.

Although digestive processes are not significantly affected by age-related physiologic changes, digestive complaints are one of the most common symptoms for which older adults seek medical care. Additionally, older adults frequently use over-the-counter medications or home remedies for digestive complaints, such as gas, "heartburn," constipation, and stomach distress.

The functional consequences of being edentulous or using dentures include decreased masticatory efficiency, avoidance of certain foods, increased effort needed to pulverize foods, and increased susceptibility to accidental choking from improper mastication (Martin, 1995). The psychosocial consequences of edentulism include a negative impact on one's appearance and self-image. One study compared the nutrient intake of and feelings of satisfaction reported by 23 people aged 60 to 82 years before and after being fitted with full dentures. Pretreatment and posttreatment diets differed in several respects, with both positive and negative outcomes being derived from dentures. One positive effect was that calories and carbohydrates were deficient in the pretreatment group and adequate in the posttreatment group. One negative effect was

that sodium and cholesterol were normal in the pretreatment group but increased in the posttreatment group. An important finding of the study was that dentures were beneficial in improving the subjects' perceived chewing efficiency and sense of well-being concerning their appearance (Baxter, 1981).

Elimination of Digestive Wastes

The normal range of frequency for bowel movements, which shows significant individual variation, is three times daily to once or twice weekly. Constipation occurs when the stool is excessively hard and difficult to pass and the person's normal frequency pattern has decreased. Although constipation is a common complaint of older adults, it is not a functional consequence of age-related changes (Harari et al., 1993). Rather, constipation commonly occurs in older adults because of various conditions, such as diminished activity and mobility; lack of dietary fiber, bulk, and fluid; and adverse medication effects, including long-term laxative abuse.

Frequently, the complaint of constipation is based on a false definition of constipation (i.e., the lack of a daily bowel movement). One study of constipation in community-living older adults found that symptoms of constipation were common, but reported bowel frequency was similar to that of younger people. True constipation was present in less than half of the subjects who complained of it, and when it occurred, it was most often associated with depression and poor mobility (Donald et al., 1985).

Psychosocial Consequences

Many activities related to obtaining, preparing, and eating food are psychosocially significant. For example, in certain circumstances, food is a focal point of celebrations, religious rituals, or gatherings to share significant events. In day-to-day life, mealtime activities are often associated with caring, nurturing, and social interac-

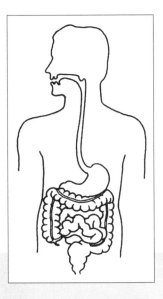

AGE-RELATED CHANGES
- Less efficient chewing
- Loss of elasticity in intestinal wall
- Slower motility throughout GI tract
- Decreased blood flow to intestines

NEGATIVE FUNCTIONAL CONSEQUENCES
- Decreased absorption of iron, calcium, folate, and vitamin B_{12}
- Malnutrition and dehydration
- Constipation
- Decreased ability to obtain, prepare, consume, and enjoy food

RISK FACTORS
- Absence of teeth
- Diminished smell and taste sensations
- Use of alcohol or medications
- Any factor that interferes with the ability to obtain, prepare, consume, or enjoy food (e.g., immobility, dementia)
- Psychosocial factors (e.g., isolation, depression)

FIGURE 8-1. Digestive function in older adults.

tion. Thus, when mealtime enjoyment is affected in any way, the psychosocial aspects of eating are also affected. Older adults who enjoyed participating in family meals or eating in restaurants may withdraw from these activities if food is no longer enjoyable. Consequently, they may lose the social interaction that occurs in these settings.

Perhaps even more detrimental than the psychosocial consequences of diminished food enjoyment are the psychosocial consequences of inadequate nutrition. When fluid or nutrient intake is inadequate, older adults are likely to develop malnutrition and dehydration because of impaired homeostatic mechanisms. Changes in mental status, including memory impairment, are among the early signs of malnutrition, dehydration, and electrolyte imbalance in older adults. Often, these mental changes are attributed to irreversible dementia rather than to a very treatable and reversible metabolic imbalance. For example, folate and vitamin B_{12} deficiencies are two of the most common nutritional causes of dementia. Vitamin B_{12} therapy has successfully reversed cognitive impairments in patients who had dementia but no other signs or symptoms of vitamin B_{12} deficiency (Gray, 1989).

Figure 8-1 illustrates some of the age-related changes, risk factors, and negative functional consequences that can influence digestion and nutrition.

Nursing Assessment

Nursing assessment of digestion and nutrition is aimed at identifying (1) the effects of age-related changes on digestion, nutrition, and eating patterns; (2) the presence of risk factors that interfere with optimal nutrition; (3) cultural factors that influence eating patterns; (4) the nutritional status and usual eating patterns of the older adult; and (5) any negative functional consequences of altered digestion or inadequate

nutrition. Nursing assessment of digestion and nutrition is accomplished through interview questions, behavioral cues related to eating and nutrition, and physical examination and laboratory data.

Interview Questions

Interview questions are used to acquire the following information: usual eating patterns and nutrient intake; age-related changes and risk factors that affect nutritional needs or digestive processes; environmental or social support factors that affect the procurement, preparation, and enjoyment of food; and symptoms of gastrointestinal dysfunction. A dietary history is important in assessing the adequacy of nutrient intake. If the assessment does not need to be completed during the initial visit, the older adult or caregiver can be asked to keep a 3-day diary of nutrient intake and eating patterns. If time does not allow for this, the person can be asked to describe foods and beverages consumed during an average day.

A logical sequence for assessment questions is to begin with information about the oral cavity and end with information about bowel elimination. If the older person is unable to convey this information accurately, the nurse can obtain the information from caregivers. Display 8-1 summarizes the interview questions that may be used to assess nutrition and digestion in older adults. The Culture Box on p. 249 summarizes cultural considerations that are important in assessing nutritional factors and eating patterns.

Behavioral Cues

Behavioral cues to digestion and nutrition can be observed directly in institutional settings by the staff. For community-living older adults, behavioral cues to digestion and nutrition may be obtained from caregivers or through a home visit assessment. Display 8-2 identifies the be-

---

DISPLAY 8-1
Guidelines for Assessing Digestion and Nutrition

Interview Questions to Assess Oral Comfort and Chewing Ability

- Do you have any difficulty with soreness or bleeding in your mouth?
- Do you have any teeth that hurt, or are loose, or are sensitive to hot or cold temperatures?
- Do your gums bleed?
- Do you have any problems chewing or swallowing food?
- Are there foods you avoid because of problems with chewing or swallowing?
- Does your mouth or tongue ever feel uncomfortably dry?

Interview Questions to Assess Dental Habits and Attitudes Toward Dental Care

- How often do you see a dentist?
- When is the last time you had dental care?
- Where do you go for dental care?
- (If the person does not seek dental care at least once per year): What prevents you from seeing the dentist?
- How do you care for your teeth? Do you use dental floss? (If yes): How often? (If no): Have you ever been taught to use dental floss?

Interview Questions to Assess Nutrient Needs

- Do you have diabetes, heart disease, or any condition that requires dietary modifications?
- Do you have any food allergies?

- What medications do you take?
- How would you describe your usual daily activity pattern?

Interview Questions to Assess Food Procurement Patterns

- How do you get your grocery shopping done?
- Do you have any help getting to the store?
- Where and how often do you do your grocery shopping?
- What is your usual food budget?
- Do you have any difficulty getting food because of problems with vision, walking, or transportation?

Interview Questions to Assess Food Preparation and Consumption Patterns

- Where do you eat your meals?
- With whom do you eat?
- Does anyone help you prepare your meals?
- Do you have any trouble fixing your meals (e.g., difficulty opening containers)?
- Do you have any difficulties getting around your kitchen, using appliances, or reaching the cupboards?
- Have there been recent changes in your eating or food preparation patterns (e.g., loss of eating companion or change in caregiver situation)?

---

havioral cues that should be considered in assessing nutrition and digestion.

Physical Examination and Laboratory Data

Important information for a nursing assessment of digestion and nutrition can be obtained from a complete physical examination and a review of any laboratory data available. Height, weight, and body build also should be assessed.

Information about changes in weight should be obtained because patterns of weight loss and gain are important indicators of the older person's overall health condition. In institutional settings, observations of bowel elimination should be made by the nursing staff if the person is unable to provide accurate information in this regard. In community settings, caregivers of dependent older adults should be asked to observe bowel elimination patterns if the older adult cannot reliably provide information. Physical

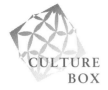

CULTURE
BOX

Cultural Considerations in Assessing Nutritional Factors and Eating Patterns

- What are the usual patterns of meals eaten (e.g., content, frequency, timing)?
- What is the usual social context of meals?
- Are there any culturally influenced food taboos or preferences? (Refer to "Cultural Influences on Eating Patterns," p. 239.)
- Does the older adult have access to special foods that are important because of religious or cultural factors?
- Are certain foods or beverages avoided or preferred in relation to an illness or chronic condition (e.g., foods or beverages that are considered yin and yang foods)?
- Is there a preference for the temperature of beverages (e.g., use of iced or heated beverages)?
- Is the person's ethnic background likely to increase his or her chance of being lactose intolerant? (Ninety percent of Asians and African Blacks, 75% to 80% of American Indians and American Blacks, 50% of Mexican Americans, and 15% of American Whites are lactose intolerant [Overfield, 1996].)

signs and symptoms of nutrient deficiencies that may be observed by nurses are summarized in Display 8-3 and Table 8-1.

Laboratory data are especially useful components of the nutritional assessment of older adults because abnormal biochemical blood values often offer the first clues to nutritional deficiencies, even before any clinical signs are evident. Additionally, nutritional deficits may be masked by illness states, and age-related changes may mimic the typical signs of fluid and nutritional deficits. Questions have been raised about the effect of age-related changes on the range of normal laboratory values, particularly regard-

DISPLAY 8-2
Behavioral Cues to Nutrition and Digestion

Observations to Assess Eating Patterns

- Does the person seem to enjoy eating meals with others, or does the presence of other people seem to interfere with mealtime enjoyment?
- If the person has dentures, are they worn at meals? If not, why not?
- What are the person's between-meal food and fluid consumption patterns?
- Are enjoyable decaffeinated liquids readily available for between-meal fluid intake?
- What cultural influences affect the person's food preferences and preparation?

Observations to Assess the Eating Environment

- What are the environmental or social influences that negatively affect mealtime enjoyment (e.g., a noisy dining room or disruptive mealtime companions)?
- If the person eats alone, is this the best arrangement, or should consideration be given to providing mealtime social interaction?

DISPLAY 8-3
Guidelines for Assessing Digestion and Nutrition on the Basis of Physical Examination and Laboratory Data

---

Examination of the Oral Cavity

- Inspect the oral cavity using a tongue depressor and a light.
- Observe for evidence of oral disease, including pain, lumps, soreness, bleeding, swelling, loose teeth, and abraded areas.
- Note the presence or absence of teeth, dentures, and partial bridges.

Normal Findings

- Lips: pink, moist, symmetrical, without cracks or fissures
- Teeth: intact, without cavities or tartar
- Gums: pink, no bleeding
- Mucous membranes: pink, moist, without ulcers, lumps, sores, inflammation, bleeding, lesions, or patches
- Tongue: pink, moist; presence of numerous varicosities on undersurface
- Pharynx: soft palate rises slightly when "Ahh" is vocalized.

Examination of the Abdomen

- Examine the abdomen with the person lying comfortably in a supine position.
- Perform a rectal examination with the person in side-lying position.

Abdomen: Normal Findings

- Symmetrical, soft abdomen that moves with respirations
- Audible bowel sounds (heard through the diaphragm of a stethoscope) occurring at irregular intervals (5 to 15 seconds apart)

Rectum and Stool: Normal Findings

- Smooth skin around anus; no evidence of hemorrhoids, fissures, inflammation, or rectal prolapse
- Soft, brown, stool that tests negative for occult blood

Laboratory Data for Nutritional Assessment

- The following biochemical data will provide information about nutritional status: serum ferritin; serum or red blood cell folate and B$_{12}$; complete lipid profile; and serum albumin, glucose, sodium, and potassium levels
- Total serum protein levels are not affected by age-related changes, but serum albumin concentrations decline equally in older men and women.
- With the exception of an age-related decline in the white blood cell count, the results of a complete blood count and differential should be within normal range.
- Serum B$_{12}$ and, possibly, serum folate levels may decline in healthy older adults.
- With the exception of a slight decline in serum magnesium levels, electrolyte test results should be within normal range.
- Slight increases in fasting and postprandial blood glucose levels are considered to be normal in older adults.
- Urinalysis results should be within the normal adult range, except for a slight decrease in the upper limit for specific gravity.

---

ing some of the indicators used to assess nutritional status. For example, despite the common finding of anemia in older adults, hemoglobin and hematocrit levels should still be within the normal range for healthy older adults. When results of laboratory data are evaluated, they should be considered in relation to the person's overall health status. For instance, hematology results may be falsely elevated in the presence of dehydration. Display 8-3 reviews the laboratory

values that are especially important in assessing the nutritional status of older adults.

Assessment of hydration in older adults is particularly challenging because typical manifestations of dehydration may either be caused by or masked by age-related changes or pathologic conditions. For example, in younger adults, the typical signs of dehydration include thirst, xerostomia, and loss of skin turgor. In older adults, assessment of skin turgor may be more accurate on the forehead and over the anterior chest wall because these areas are less affected by age-related skin changes. A study of dehydrated patients between the ages of 61 and 98 years identified the following signs and symptoms as significant clinical indicators of dehydration: confusion, tongue dryness, tongue furrows, dry mucous membranes, speech difficulty, upper body muscle weakness, and eyes that appear recessed. Factors that were not strongly associated with dehydration included skin turgor, thirst sensation, orthostatic changes, and lack of axillary moisture (Gross et al., 1992). Urinalysis provides clues to a person's hydration status, with highly concentrated urine being an indicator of dehydration. Blood values that may be altered in dehydration include high hematocrit and hemoglobin concentrations and elevations in sodium, osmolality, and blood urea nitrogen. Also, a sudden loss of body weight also might accurately reflect dehydration.

Nursing Diagnosis

The nursing assessment may identify problems related to nutrition, digestion, or oral health. If nutritional deficits are identified, a pertinent nursing diagnosis is Altered Nutrition: Less than Body Requirements. This is defined as "the state in which an individual who is not NPO experiences or is at risk of experiencing reduced weight related to inadequate intake or metabolism of nutrients for metabolic needs" (Carpenito, 1997, p. 581). Related factors that may affect older adults include medications, anorexia, depression, chewing difficulties, social isolation, and inability to procure or prepare food. The nursing care plan at the end of this chapter addresses this nursing diagnosis.

If the nursing assessment identifies actual or perceived constipation, or risk factors for constipation, the appropriate nursing diagnosis is Altered Bowel Elimination: Constipation. The nursing assessment may also identify certain oral

health problems that are common in older adults. These include xerostomia, medication effects, chewing difficulties, periodontal disease, diminished taste sensation, ill-fitting dentures, inadequate oral hygiene, and broken or missing teeth. A relevant nursing diagnosis to address these problems would be Altered Oral Mucous Membrane.

Nursing Goals

One goal that might be addressed is to alleviate the factors that interfere with food procurement, preparation, and enjoyment. This goal is achieved in part through interventions that relieve dry mouth, improve oral and dental care, and compensate for diminished smell and taste sensations. Interventions may also address the factors that interfere with the ability of older adults to obtain, prepare, and enjoy food. For example, interventions for community-living older adults might include the use of resources, such as home-delivered meals. For older adults in institutional settings, interventions might address individual food preferences and environmental factors that interfere with food enjoyment.

Another goal is to assist the older adult to attain and maintain the highest possible level of nutrition and digestive function. The outcome criteria used to measure attainment of this goal would be that the older adult: (1) consumes food and fluids that meet his or her daily nutritional needs; (2) maintains stable body weight; (3) establishes a bowel routine that achieves bowel movements at least three times weekly; and (4) maintains moist oral mucous membranes. This goal is addressed through education of independent older adults and caregivers of dependent older adults.

The quality of life of older adults can be significantly compromised by their inability to enjoy food. As discussed in the section on psychosocial consequences, many detrimental effects can occur when the ability of an older adult to obtain, prepare, consume, or enjoy food is compromised. For example, older adults who are dehydrated or malnourished are particularly susceptible to memory impairment and other manifestations of diminished mental function. A nursing goal for older adults with psychosocial consequences might be to maintain their quality of life. This is achieved through all the interventions that are discussed in the following sections.

Nursing Interventions

Alleviating Risk Factors That Interfere with Food Procurement, Enjoyment, and Consumption

Oral and dental problems that interfere with food enjoyment and consumption may be alleviated through dental services. If the older adult has avoided dental care because of resignation to poor oral health or a poor understanding of the need for preventive dental care, the nurse may attempt to change these attitudes through education. For homebound older adults, home dental services are often available, especially in large urban communities. In addition, low-cost dental services and dentures may be available through schools of dentistry. Nurses should be familiar with local resources so they can teach older adults and their caregivers about the dental services that are available in their community. Display 8-4 summarizes health education about oral and dental care.

When the older adult seems misinformed about constipation, nursing interventions should be directed toward education. Examples of effective programs for the prevention and management of constipation are found in nursing and medical literature (e.g., Gibson et al., 1995; Abyad and Mourad, 1996; Benton et al., 1997; Sheehy and Hall, 1998). When consumption of alcohol interferes with nutrition, interventions might address the potential problem of alcoholism or they may be aimed at compensat-

ing for the detrimental effects on nutrition. Vitamin supplementation for people with a history of alcoholism should be recommended only after a medical evaluation has been performed and any underlying conditions, such as pernicious anemia, have been identified. If medications affect nutrition and digestion, the prescribing health care practitioner should be involved in addressing this problem. If over-the-counter medications have a detrimental effect on nutrition or digestion, the nurse should educate the older adult about medication-nutrient interactions and discuss ways of addressing the negative effects. Pharmacists may be helpful in suggesting interventions that will compensate for, or minimize, the effects of both prescription and over-the-counter medications on nutrition and digestion.

If xerostomia interferes with digestion or nutrition, the nurse should emphasize the importance of undergoing a medical evaluation, as it may be caused by disease processes or by medication effects. In addition to being uncomfortable and interfering with nutrition and digestion, xerostomia is a major cause of excessive plaque build-up, periodontal disease, and dental caries. Many interventions are effective in alleviating xerostomia, and nurses should discuss these with affected older adults. Display 8-4 summarizes the information that should be presented in health education about xerostomia and other risk factors that contribute to nutrient deficits and digestive problems.

When nutrition and digestion are affected by the activities involved in procuring, preparing, and enjoying food, interventions must be focused on compensating for any underlying functional limitations. For the community-living older adult, this may involve identifying resources that offer assistance in obtaining food. Local offices on aging may provide assistance with transportation or grocery shopping, and home-delivered meal programs may be available to older adults at minimal cost. Group meal programs are available in almost every commu-

DISPLAY 8-4
Education Related to Nutrition and Digestion

Health Education Regarding Oral and Dental Care

- Oral care should include daily use of dental floss, as well as twice-daily brushing of all tooth surfaces.
- Use a soft-bristled toothbrush and a fluoride-containing toothpaste.
- Avoid alcohol-containing mouthwashes because of their drying effect.
- Because sugar is a major contributing factor to tooth decay, it is important to limit the intake of sugary substances, especially ones like gum and hard candy that may be kept in the mouth for long periods.
- After eating sugar-containing foods, rinse your mouth or brush your teeth.
- Visit a dentist every 6 to 12 months for regular oral care.
- If partial or complete dentures are worn, remove them at night, keep them in water, and clean them before placing them back in your mouth.

Health Education Regarding Constipation

- A bowel movement every day is not necessarily the norm for every adult.
- Each adult has an individual pattern of bowel regularity, with the normal range varying from 3 times a day to 3 times a week.
- Include several portions of the following high-fiber foods in your daily diet: fresh, uncooked fruits and vegetables; bran and other cereal products made from whole grains.

- Drink 8 to 10 glasses of noncaffeinated liquid, including fruit juices, every day.
- Avoid laxatives and enemas.
- If medication is needed to promote bowel regularity, a bulk-forming agent is least likely to have detrimental effects, especially if fluid intake is adequate.
- Do not ignore the urge to defecate; try to respond as soon as you feel the urge.
- Exercise regularly.

Health Education Regarding Dry Mouth

- Excessive dry mouth may be caused by medical conditions or medication effects and should be evaluated before symptomatic treatment is initiated.
- Chew sugar-free gum or suck on sugar-free sour hard candies to stimulate saliva production.
- Drink at least 10 to 12 glasses of noncaffeinated fluid during the day, and drink sips of water at frequent intervals.
- Avoid alcohol and highly acidic drinks, such as orange or grapefruit juice.
- Avoid mouthwashes that contain alcohol, as these tend to exacerbate the condition.
- Try using one of the many brands of saliva substitutes available at drugstores.
- Smoking will exacerbate the symptoms and further irritate the oral mucous membranes.
- Pay particular attention to oral hygiene because a dry mouth increases the risk of gum and dental diseases.

nity through the federally funded National Nutrition Program for the Elderly, established under the Older Americans Act. In addition to providing inexpensive and nutritionally balanced meals, these programs provide excellent opportunities for social interaction. When environmental barriers, such as high cupboards, interfere with the older adult's ability to prepare meals safely, environmental modifications can be made. Many of the environmental adapta-

tions suggested in the chapters on vision (Chapter 7) and mobility (Chapter 12) can be applied to improve the ability of the older person to prepare meals.

In institutional settings, environmental factors may interfere with food enjoyment. Although it is often difficult or impossible to modify large institutional environments, nurses may be able to identify simple interventions that will increase food enjoyment, particularly in nursing

Improving Digestion and Nutrition

Herbs
- For constipation (see Special Precautions, below): flax, aloe, senna, fennel, rhubarb, buckthorn, cascara, psyllium, fenugreek, licorice

Homepathic Remedies
- For constipation: graphites, bryonia, alumina, nux vomica, natrum muriaticum

Nutritional Considerations
- To improve taste and smell senses: zinc
- For constipation: vitamin C and magnesium

Preventive Measures and Additional Approaches
- For food allergies and poor digestive function: acupuncture
- For lactose intolerance: yogurt, buttermilk, and hard cheeses (Swiss, extra-sharp cheddar), cocoa added to milk
- For constipation: yoga, acupuncture, acupressure, reflexology, gentle massage of the abdomen, hot compresses to the abdomen
- For dry mouth: yohimbine

Special Precautions
- Avoidance of large amounts of herbal laxatives (including teas) containing aloe, senna, buckthorn, cascara, rhubarb root, and castor oil, as these have been associated with nausea, vomiting, diarrhea, stomach cramps, and other more serious adverse effects

homes. For example, the seating arrangement in a dining room might be planned to improve social interaction and to minimize the negative effects of disruptive people. In some long-term care settings, two mealtimes are scheduled for each meal to allow increased flexibility in seating arrangements.

When diminished smell and taste interfere with food enjoyment, food additives can significantly enhance a person's enjoyment of food. However, older adults should be cautioned about using food additives that are high in sodium, such as monosodium glutamate, and should be taught to check the sodium content of foods, as well as food additives. Good oral hygiene, especially prior to meals, will also enhance food enjoyment. Older adults who smoke should be encouraged to abstain from smoking for 1 hour prior to meals. If food intake is limited because of early satiety during meals, the older

adult may benefit from eating five smaller meals a day, rather than the customary three meals a day. Finally, older adults can be encouraged to maintain a sitting or upright position during eating and for 1/2 to 1 hour after eating to compensate for any effects of presbyesophagus. The box listing alternative and health care practices summarizes measures that can be used to address risk factors that interfere with optimal digestive function.

Attaining and Maintaining Optimal Nutrition

Nursing interventions to assist older adults attain and maintain optimal nutrition are focused on education about basic nutritional needs. Nutrition education can be provided on an individual basis or in group settings, perhaps in conjunction with dietitians. In acute care settings, registered dietitians are usually available, but their services are often limited to people who have special dietary needs or an identified nutritional problem. In long-term care settings, a registered dietitian should assess the nutritional needs and usual eating patterns of older adults and should establish a plan of care aimed at attaining and maintaining optimal nutrition. In community settings, nutrition education is more likely to be self-motivated, and might be obtained through group education programs. Nurses making home visits should include nutrition education in their health teaching and should use available community resources to supplement these educational interventions.

Healthy, nonmedicated, older adults should be able to maintain optimal nutritional status through the daily intake of the foods listed in Display 8-5. If the older adult has any illness or takes any medications or chemicals that interfere with homeostasis, digestion, or nutrition, the daily diet will have to be modified to compensate for these effects. If, for any reason, the food intake is inadequate to meet daily nutritional requirements, the older adult can be en-

couraged to use a broad-spectrum vitamin and mineral supplement.

Evaluating Nursing Care

Evaluation of nursing care is based on the nursing goals. Short-term goals that address altered nutrition are evaluated by determining whether the older adult has a daily nutrient intake that corresponds with metabolic needs. Long-term goals that address altered nutrition are often evaluated by the achievement of a body weight that is within 110% of the ideal body weight for that individual. For older adults with actual or perceived constipation, or risk factors for constipation, evaluation criteria for the short-term goals would hinge on the older adult verbalizing accurate information about constipation and the identification of the factors contributing to the constipation. Successful achievement of a long-term goal would be evaluated according to whether the older adult reports passing soft stools on a regular basis without any straining or discomfort.

DISPLAY 8-5
Daily Food Guide for Older Adults

- Nutrient requirements do not diminish with age, but caloric needs decrease gradually in older adulthood. Therefore, it is important to select a variety of high-quality foods.
- Use salt, sugar, and sodium only in moderation.
- The daily diet of older adults should include at least the minimum number of servings from each food group.
- The amount of each type of food will vary according to the caloric needs of each older person, with men generally needing a greater number of servings than women.
- Minimum nutrient requirements will be met if older adults follow the guidelines listed below and include complex carbohydrates and high-fiber foods in their diets.

Guidelines for Daily Food Intake

Servings	Food Item
6–9	Bread, rice, pasta, and cereal
3–4	Vegetables
2–3	Fruits
2–3	Meat, fish, poultry, or legumes (dried peas and beans, lentils, nut butters, soy products)
2–3	Milk, cheese, yogurt, and dairy desserts
≥8	8-ounce glasses of noncaffeinated liquid

Chapter Summary

Digestion and nutrition in older adults is often affected by risk factors, such as tooth loss, medication effects, diminished smell and taste, impaired cognitive and physical function, and socioeconomic, cultural, and environmental factors. Risk factors can directly affect digestion and nutrition, and they can also interfere with the activities involved with obtaining, preparing, and enjoying food. In the absence of risk factors, the primary consequence of age-related changes is a reduction in caloric requirements. Thus, older adults need to consume higher-quality foods and beverages to achieve adequate nutrient intake with fewer calories. Nursing assessment focuses on identifying risk factors that interfere with optimal nutrition and bowel elimination, determining the nutritional status and usual eating patterns of the older adult, and recognizing any detrimental effects associated with risk factors. Relevant nursing diagnoses include Altered Nutrition, Altered Bowel Elimination, and Altered Oral Mucous Membrane. Nursing interventions focus on addressing any risk factors that interfere with nutrition, digestion, and bowel elimination. Nursing goals may be evaluated by the degree of improvement in the older adult's eating patterns, nutritional status, or bowel elimination.

Critical Thinking Exercises

1. Describe how each of the following conditions might influence the eating patterns of older adults: depression, medications, sensory changes, cognitive impairments, functional impairments, economic factors, social circumstances, and oral health factors.
2. Describe at least three characteristics of eating patterns for each of the following cultural groups: Native Americans, Hispanic Americans, African Americans, and Asian Americans.
3. How would you assess digestion and nutrition for an older adult in each of the following settings: home, nursing home, and acute care facility?
4. Outline a health education plan for teaching older adults about constipation. Include the following points: definition of constipation, risk factors for constipation, and interventions to prevent and address constipation.
5. Outline a health education plan for teaching older adults about oral and dental care.

Case Example and Nursing Care Plan

Pertinent Case Information

Mr. D. is an 85-year-old widower who is being discharged to home after being hospitalized for prostatic surgery. He has recovered well from the surgery and is fully ambulatory but weak. Additional diagnoses are arthritis and malnutrition. Before this hospitalization, Mr. D.'s only medication was ibuprofen, 200 mg t.i.d. after meals. He is being discharged on the same medication with the addition of a multiple vitamin preparation.

Nursing Assessment

Mr. D. lives in a senior high-rise apartment, where he participates in social activities and takes advantage of van transportation to get to medical appointments and the grocery store. He prepares his own meals, eats alone in his apartment, and shops for his groceries once a week. Typical meals are toast and coffee for breakfast; soup, sandwich, and cookies for lunch; and a "Budget Gourmet" entree for supper. Mr. D. says he never really learned to cook very well, but he gets along "well enough for a man my age." He says he doesn't particularly enjoy the convenience foods that he eats, but states, "It sure is easy to shop for and fix for myself." Mr. D. acknowledges that he's thought about going to the daily noon meal offered at a nearby church, but he hasn't followed through because "the senior van doesn't go there, but it does go to the grocery store." Also, he is reluctant to go to the meal program because his wife was such a good cook and the meals wouldn't compare to her good Hungarian meals.

Mr. D. reports a gradual weight loss of about 50 pounds since his wife died 2 years ago. He says he was too heavy when his wife used to do the cooking, so he's not concerned about his weight loss. Mr. D. is 5'10" and weighs 130 pounds, which is 85% of his ideal body weight of 155 pounds. He has full dentures but hasn't used them for the past year because they don't fit well anymore. He hasn't done anything about his dentures because he manages to chew the kinds of food he buys. Abnormal laboratory values include hemoglobin level, 11%; hematocrit, 35%; and serum albumin level, 3.5 g/dL.

Nursing Diagnosis

One of the nursing diagnoses that you address during Mr. D.'s hospitalization is Altered Nutrition: Less than Body Requirements, related to social isolation, ill-fitting dentures, and lack of enjoyment of food. Evidence is derived from his low body weight, laboratory data consistent with poor nutritional status, and his descriptions of his eating and food preparation patterns.

Goals	Nursing Interventions	Evaluation Criteria
Mr. D. will describe has basic daily nutrient requirements.	Give Mr. D. a copy of Display 8-5 and use this as a basis for discussing daily nutrient requirements.	Mr. D. will describe an eating pattern that meets his daily nutritional needs.
Mr. D. will identify a method for meeting his nutrient needs without depending on a multiple vitamin.	Explore with Mr. D. various options for improving his nutritional intake (e.g., including dairy products and more fruits and vegetables).	Mr. D. will describe an acceptable plan for meeting his nutritional needs. Mr. D. will weigh between 140 and 155 pounds.
	Ask Mr. D. to identify prepared foods that he enjoys and that could be included in his meals but that are not currently part of his diet. Discuss the nutritional value of these foods and suggest that he add new food items in each of the food group categories in which he is deficient.	

Mr. D. will have his dentures evaluated and modified or replaced.

Suggest that Mr. D. use the transportation provided by the church-sponsored meal program to participate in that program three times weekly. Ask the social worker to provide the name of a contact person for these services.

Discuss with Mr. D. the importance of dentures in chewing efficiency and food enjoyment.

Discuss the potential relationship between weight loss and poorly fitting dentures.

Discuss the long-term detrimental effects of lack of dentures.

Explore ways of obtaining a dental evaluation.

Mr. D. will chew his food with dentures that fit properly.

Educational Resources

American Dietetic Association
216 West Jackson Boulevard, Chicago, IL 60606-6995
(800) 366-1655
www.eatright.org

Consumer Information Center
Pueblo, CO 81009
(888) 878–3256
www.pueblo.gsa.gov
• Brochures and booklets about nutrition and food preparation

Food and Drug Administration
5600 Fishers Lane, HFE-88, Rockville, MD 20857
www.fda.gov

Food and Nutrition Information Center
National Agriculture Library Building, Room 304, Beltsville, MD 20705-2351
(301) 504-6409
www.nal.usda.gov/fnic
• Bibliographies and resource guides on topics such as heart disease, vegetarianism, and nutrition and older people
• Library of printed and audiovisual materials about nutrition

National Dairy Council
10255 West Higgins Road, Suite 900, Rosemont, IL 60018-5616
(800) 426-8271

www.dairyinfo.com
• Brochures, booklets, and audiovisual materials about nutrition and health promotion (some materials are available in Spanish)

National Oral Health Information Clearinghouse
1 NOHIC Way, Bethesda, MD 20892-3500
(301) 402-7364
www.aerie.com/nohicweb/special.html

References

Abyad, A., & Mourad, F. (1996). Constipation: Commonsense care of the older patient. *Geriatrics, 51*(12), 28–36.

Atkinson, J. C., & Fox, P. C. (1992). Salivary gland dysfunction. *Clinics in Geriatric Medicine, 8,* 499–511.

Barber, C. E. (1997). Olfactory acuity as a function of age and gender: A comparison of African and American samples. *International Journal of Aging and Human Development, 44*(4), 317–334.

Bartoshuk, L. M., & Weiffenbach, J. M. (1990). Chemical senses and aging. In E. L. Schneider & J. W. Rowe (Eds.), *Handbook of the biology of aging* (pp. 429–443). New York: Academic Press.

Baxter, J. C. (1981). Nutrition and the geriatric edentulous patient. *Special Care in Dentistry, 1,* 259–261.

Benton, J. M., O'Hara, P. A., Chen, H., Harper, D. W., & Johnston, S. F. (1997). Changing bowel hygiene practice successfully: A program to reduce laxative use in a chronic care hospital. *Geriatric Nursing, 18,* 12–17.

Bidlack, W. R., & Wang, W. (1995). Nutrition requirements of the elderly. In J. E. Morley, Z. Glick, & L. Z. Rubenstein (Eds.), *Geriatric nutrition* (2nd ed., pp. 25–49). New York: Raven Press.

Carpenito, L. J. (1997). *Nursing diagnosis: Application to clinical practice* (7th ed.). Philadelphia: J. B. Lippincott.

Cohen, H. J., & Crawford, J. (1992). Hematologic problems in the elderly. In E. Chalkins, A. B. Ford, & P. R. Katz (Eds.), *The practice of geriatrics* (pp. 541–553). Philadelphia: W. B. Saunders.

Corwin, J., Loury M., & Gilbert, A. N. (1995). Workplace, age, and sex as mediators of olfactory function: Data from the National Geographic Smell Survey. *Journal of Gerontology: Psychological Sciences, 50B*(4), P179–P186.

Coulston, A. M. (1995). Nutrition management in nursing homes. In J. E. Morley, Z. Glick, & L. Z. Rubenstein (Eds.), *Geriatric nutrition* (2nd ed., pp. 295–302). New York: Raven Press.

Donald, I. P., Smith, R. G., Cruikshank, J. G., Elton, R. A., & Stoddart, M. E. (1985). A study of constipation in the elderly living at home. *Gerontology, 31,* 112–118.

Gibson, C. J., Opalka, P. C., Moore, C. A., Brady, R. S., & Mion, L. C. (1995). Effectiveness of bran supplement on the bowel management of elderly rehabilitation patients. *Journal of Gerontological Nursing, 21*(10), 21–30.

Gray, G. E. (1989). Nutrition and dementia. *Journal of the American Dietetic Association, 89,* 1795–1802.

Gross, C. R., Lindquist, R. D., Woolley, A. C., Granieri, R., Allard, K., & Webster, B. (1992). Clinical indicators of dehydration severity in elderly patients. *The Journal of Emergency Medicine, 10,* 267–274.

Harari, D., Gurwitz, J. H., & Minaker, K. L. (1993). Constipation in the elderly. *Journal of the American Geriatrics Society, 41,* 1130–1140.

Hurwitz, A., Brady, D. A., Schaal, S. E., Samloff, I. M., Dedon, J., & Ruhl, C. E. (1997). Gastric acidity in older adults. *Journal of the American Medical Association, 278*(8), 659–662.

Martin, W. E. (1995). The oral cavity and nutrition. In J. E. Morley, Z. Glick, & L. Z. Rubenstein (Eds.), *Geriatric nutrition* (2nd ed., pp. 169–181). New York: Raven Press.

National Academy of Sciences. (1997). *Dietary reference intakes—calcium, phosphorus, magnesium, vitamin D, and fluoride.* Washington, DC: National Academy of Sciences.

Nordin, S., Monsch, A. U., & Murphy, C. (1995). Unawareness of smell loss in normal aging and Alzheimer's disease: Discrepancy between self-reported and diagnosed smell sensitivity. *Journal of Gerontology: Psychological Sciences, 50B*(4), P187–P192.

Overfield, T. (1996). *Biologic variation in health and illness: Race, age, and sex differences.* Boca Raton, FL: CRC Press.

Rolls, B. J., & Drewnowski, A. (1996). Diet and nutrition. In J. E. Birren (Ed.), *Encyclopedia of gerontology: Age, aging, and the aged* (Vol. 1, pp. 429–440). San Diego: Academic Press.

Rosenbloom, C. A., & Whittington, F. J. (1993). The effects of bereavement on eating behaviors and nutrient intakes in elderly widowed persons. *Journal of Gerontology: Social Sciences, 48*(4), S223–S229.

Ryan, A. S., Craig, L. D., & Finn, S. C. (1992). Nutrient intakes and dietary patterns of older Americans: A national study. *Journal of Gerontology: Medical Sciences, 47,* M145–M150.

Schiffman, S. S. (1996). Smell and taste. In J. E. Birren (Ed.), *Encyclopedia of gerontology: Age, aging, and the aged* (Vol. 2, pp. 497–504). San Diego: Academic Press.

Schiffman, S. S. (1997). Taste and smell losses in normal aging and disease. *Journal of the American Medical Association, 278*(16), 1357–1362.

Sheehy, C., & Hall, G. R. (1998). Rethinking the obvious: A model for preventing constipation. *Journal of Gerontological Nursing, 24*(3), 38–44.

Ship, J. A., & Fischer, D. J. (1997). The relationhsip between dehydration and parotid salivary gland function in young and older healthy adults. *Journal of Gerontology: Medical Sciences, 52A*(5), M310–M319.

Ship, J. A., & Weiffenbach, J. M. (1993). Age, gender, medical treatment, and medication effects on smell identification. *Journal of Gerontology: Medical Sciences, 48,* M26–M32.

Ship, J. A., Nolan, N. E., & Puckett, S. A. (1995). Longitudinal analysis of parotid and submandibular salivary flow rates in healthy, different-aged adults. *Journal of Gerontology: Medical Sciences, 50A*(5), M285–M289.

Ship, J. A., Pearson, J. D., Cruise, L. J., Brant, L. J., & Metter, E. J. (1996). Longitudinal changes in smell identification. *Journal of Gerontology: Medical Sciences, 51A*(2), M86–M91.

Sonies, B. C. (1992). Oropharyngeal dysphagia in the elderly. *Clinics in Geriatric Medicine, 8,* 569–577.

Sullivan, D. H., Martin, W., Flaxman, N., & Hagen, J. E. (1993). Oral health problems and involuntary weight loss in a population of frail elderly. *Journal of the American Geriatrics Society, 41,* 725–731.

Todd, B. (1989). Calcium: Should we supplement? *Geriatric Nursing, 10,* 96–98.

Weiffenbach, J. M., & Bartoshuk, L. M. (1992). Taste and smell. *Clinics in Geriatric Medicine, 8,* 543–555.

Weintraub, J. A., & Burt, B. A. (1985). Tooth loss in the United States. *Journal of Dental Education, 49,* 368–376.

Wu, A. J., Atkinson, J. C., Fox, P. C., Baum, B. J., & Ship, J. A. (1993). Cross-sectional and longitudinal analyses of stimulated parotid salivary constituents in healthy, different-aged subjects. *Journal of Gerontology: Medical Sciences, 48*(5), M219–M224.

Wu, A. J., Baum, B. J., & Ship, J. A. (1995). Extended stimulated parotid and submandibular secretion in a healthy young and old population. *Journal of Gerontology: Medical Sciences, 50A*(5), M45–M48.

Yen, P. K. (1997). Elders need more calcium and vitamin D. *Geriatric Nursing, 18,* 280–281.

Urinary Elimination

Chapter

9

Learning Objectives

1. *Delineate age-related changes that affect the complex processes involved in urinary elimination.*

2. *Examine risk factors that influence kidney function and urinary elimination.*

3. *Discuss the following functional consequences of age-related changes and risk factors: incontinence; medication excretion; metabolism, homeostasis, and elimination of metabolic wastes in the kidneys; and the psychosocial consequences of incontinence.*

4. *Describe interview questions, behavioral cues, environmental observations, and laboratory data that may be used in the assessment of urinary function in older adults.*

5. *Identify interventions for addressing risk factors that influence urinary elimination, and for controlling and managing incontinence.*

*U*rinary elimination has as its primary function the excretion of water and chemical wastes, such as metabolic and pharmacologic by-products, that would become toxic if allowed to accumulate. Efficient urinary excretion depends on renal blood flow, filtering activities within the kidneys, performance of the urinary tract muscles, and nervous system control over voluntary and involuntary mechanisms of elimination. Control of urinary elimination depends on ambulatory and sensory abilities and on environmental, social, emotional, cognitive, and nervous system factors.

In the absence of risk factors, healthy, non-medicated, older adults experience very few negative functional consequences affecting urinary elimination. In the presence of risk factors, however, negative functional consequences, such as urinary incontinence, can readily occur. Perhaps the most important risk factor, which can be alleviated through nursing interventions, is belief in the myth that urinary incontinence is an inevitable part of old age. Other risk factors, such as environmental conditions, can also be remedied through nursing interventions. Be-

cause the impact of urinary incontinence is so serious, nursing interventions directed toward eliminating risk factors can be quite effective in improving the quality of life for older adults. In addition, urinary elimination problems are clearly within the realm of nursing and can often be addressed through nursing, rather than medical, interventions.

Age-Related Changes

Age-related changes in the kidneys, bladder, urethra, and nervous system affect the physiologic processes related to urinary elimination. In addition, any age-related factor that alters the skills involved in socially appropriate urinary elimination may interfere with urinary control, contributing to the development of incontinence, and will have far-reaching consequences. The next two sections discuss the age-related changes that affect the physiologic processes of urinary elimination and the skills involved in socially appropriate urinary elimination.

Physiologic Processes Related to Urinary Elimination

Urinary excretion is a complex process that begins in the kidneys with the filtering and removal of chemical wastes from the blood. Specifically, blood circulates through glomeruli, where liquid wastes, collectively termed the glomerular filtrate, pass through Bowman's capsule and the renal tubules to the collecting ducts. During this process, substances needed by the body (such as water, glucose, and sodium) are retained, whereas waste products are excreted in the urine. Excretory function is measured by the glomerular filtration rate (GFR) and depends on the number and efficiency of nephrons, as well as the amount and rate of renal blood flow.

The kidney increases in weight and mass from birth until early adulthood, when the number of functioning nephrons begins to decline, particularly in the cortex, where the glomeruli are located. This decline continues throughout life, resulting in approximately a 25% decrease in kidney mass by the age of 80 years. The remaining glomeruli undergo various age-related changes, such as increased size, diminished lobulation, and thickened basement membrane. The proportion of sclerotic glomeruli also increases from fewer than 5% at the age of 40 years to 35% by the age of 80 years. Beginning in the 4th decade, renal blood flow gradually diminishes, particularly in the cortex, at a rate of 10% per decade.

An average decline in renal function of 1% per year has been widely accepted as an age-related change that begins between the ages of 30 and 40 years. This conclusion was supported by initial data from the Baltimore Longitudinal Study of Aging (BLSA), which revealed a highly significant decline in creatinine clearance in healthy older men (Rowe et al., 1976). Analysis of additional data, however, has suggested that there is a great deal of individual variation in renal function among healthy older adults. One third of the BLSA subjects whose urinary function was monitored for up to 24 years experienced no decrease in renal function, and in a small group, creatinine clearance rates actually improved. These findings suggest that a decline in renal function is probably associated with common pathologic conditions rather than being attributable to age-related changes alone (Lindeman, 1996). Based on these findings, the medical literature now suggests that an older person's renal function be assessed according to the Crockcroft-Gault formula for predicting creatinine clearances from serum creatinine concentrations (Lindeman, 1992). This formula, which uses a person's age and weight to calculate creatinine clearance, is as follows (for men):

Creatinine clearance

$$= \frac{(140 - \text{age}) \times \text{weight (kg)}}{72 \times \text{serum creatinine (mg/100 mL)}}$$

The same calculation applies to women, except that the resulting value must be multiplied by 0.85.

Dilution and concentration of urine, and subsequent excretion of water from the body, are regulated in the renal tubules and have a diurnal rhythm. The physiologic processes responsible for urine concentration and water excretion are influenced by the following factors:

1. The amount of fluid in the body;
2. Resorption of water through, and transport of substances across, the tubular membrane;
3. Osmoreceptors in the hypothalamus, which regulate the level of circulating antidiuretic hormone (ADH) according to plasma water concentration;
4. Substances and activities that influence ADH secretion, such as caffeine, medications, alcohol, pain, stress, and exercise; and
5. The concentration of sodium in the glomerular filtrate.

Normally, production of ADH is stimulated by hemorrhage, dehydration, and other conditions that affect plasma volume or osmolality. This protective mechanism, along with other physiologic mechanisms, assists in conserving fluid and sodium and maintaining plasma volume under conditions of water or sodium deprivation.

Age-related changes that affect the renal tubules include fatty degeneration, the presence of diverticuli, a loss of convoluted cells, and alterations in the composition of the basement membranes. Although the exact mechanism of action is unclear, several age-related changes in renal tubular function have been identified. In the older adult, the kidney is less efficient in the tubular exchange of substances, the conservation of water and sodium, and the suppression of ADH secretion in the presence of hypoosmolality. Under normal conditions, these age-related changes may predispose a person to nocturia and hyponatremia, but they do not affect urine concentration or water excretion to any significant extent. However, in the presence of any condition that alters renal circulation, water or sodium balance, or plasma volume or osmolality, the kidney's ability to concentrate urine and excrete water will be compromised by such age-related changes.

After being filtered by the kidneys, liquid wastes pass through the ureters into the bladder. The bladder is a balloon-like structure, composed of collagen, smooth muscle, and elastic tissue, which serves as a temporary reservoir. Elimination of the liquid wastes from the bladder is accomplished through a complex physiologic process that depends on the following mechanisms:

1. The ability of the bladder to expand for adequate storage and to contract for complete expulsion of liquid wastes;
2. The maintenance of higher intraurethral pressure relative to intravesical pressure;
3. Regulation of the lower urinary tract through autonomic and somatic nerves; and
4. Voluntary control of urination through the cerebral centers.

Age-related changes alter each of these mechanisms, affecting the process of micturition in older adults.

The normal adult bladder is able to store about 200 mL of urine before there is a sensation of the need to void. The accumulation of 350 to 400 mL of urine is accompanied by sensations of fullness and discomfort. With increasing age, hypertrophy of the bladder muscle and thickening of the bladder wall interfere with the bladder's ability to expand, decreasing the amount of urine that can be stored comfortably to about 250 to 300 mL.

As urine flows into the bladder, the smooth muscle expands without increasing intravesical pressure. At the same time, the intraurethral pressure increases to a slightly higher level. As long as the volume of urine does not rise above 500 to 600 mL, this balance can be maintained, and micturition can be controlled voluntarily. If the volume rises above this level, however, the bladder pressure will exceed the urethral pressure, and incontinence may occur.

In addition to being influenced by the amount of urine in the bladder, the balance between intravesical and intraurethral pressure is influenced by the following factors: intra-abdominal pressure; tone of the pelvic, detrusor, urethral, and bladder neck muscles; and thickness of the urethral mucosa, which is affected by estrogen levels in women. With increasing age, some of the smooth muscle in the bladder and urethra is replaced by connective tissue. This age-related change alters the balance between the intravesical and intraurethral pressures and contributes to urinary incontinence.

Internal and external sphincters regulate urine storage and bladder emptying. The internal sphincter is part of the base of the bladder and is controlled by autonomic nerves. The external sphincter is part of the pelvic floor musculature and is controlled by the pudendal nerve. When micturition takes place, the detrusor and intra-abdominal muscles contract, and the perineal and external sphincter muscles relax. When necessary, the external sphincter contracts to inhibit or interrupt voiding and to compensate for sudden surges in intra-abdominal pressure. Age-related changes, such as loss of smooth muscle in the urethra and relaxation of the pelvic floor muscles, reduce the urethral resistance and alter the function of the sphincters.

Cerebral centers are responsible for detecting the sensation of bladder fullness, for inhibiting bladder emptying when necessary, and for stimulating bladder contractions for complete emptying. In healthy older adults, degenerative changes in the cerebral cortex may alter both the sensation of bladder fullness and the ability to empty the bladder completely. In younger adults, a sensation of fullness begins when the bladder is about half full. This sensation occurs at a later point for older adults, and it may not occur at all. Consequently, in the older adult, the interval between the initial perception of the urge to void and the actual need to empty the bladder is shortened, which may trigger an episode of incontinence. Also, age-related changes may precipitate bladder contractions during filling. In addition, when voiding occurs, the neurologic control of bladder emptying may be inefficient. This results in retention of up to 50 mL of residual urine. Age-related changes in the cortical control of micturition also may contribute to the increased occurrence of nocturia in the absence of any pathologic causes. Older adults with dementia or another condition that affects the cerebral cortex will have additional problems with voluntary control of urination.

Skills Related to Socially Appropriate Urinary Elimination

Standards for socially appropriate urinary elimination vary according to different social environments. For example, an independent, community-living older adult is expected to remain free of urinary odors or wetness and to perform urinary elimination in private, desig-

nated places. A dependent or institutionalized older adult may not be expected to adhere so strictly to these standards. In acute or long-term care settings, for example, staff attitudes and nursing procedures strongly influence the standards for urinary elimination. The use of absorbent pads or indwelling catheters might be encouraged because of patient illness, staff convenience, or lack of knowledge about other interventions. One study revealed that less than 50% of the nursing staff in 16 long-term care facilities reported receiving formal clinical instruction in managing urinary incontinence (Freundl and Dugan, 1992). Likewise, in home settings, the attitudes and behaviors of caregivers may influence expectations regarding urinary elimination for dependent older adults. Medicare policies also may influence the caregiver's approach to urinary management, as reimbursement for skilled home care services is provided for people with indwelling catheters, but not for those who manage incontinence by other methods.

In social settings, acceptable urinary elimination is influenced by the following factors:

1. Identification of a designated receptacle in a private area;
2. Accessibility and acceptability of toilet facilities;
3. Ability to get to and use a suitable receptacle;
4. The interval between the perception of the urge to void and the actual need to empty the bladder; and
5. Voluntary control over the urge to void from the time of its perception until an appropriate receptacle is reached.

These factors are influenced by age-related changes that directly affect urinary elimination, as well as by those changes that affect the ability to identify and reach appropriate toileting facilities. Thus, balance, mobility, visual impairments, manual dexterity, and age-related vision changes are some of the factors that may influence urinary control. In addition, factors associated with the caregivers or the environment may pose barriers to socially appropriate urinary elimination. For example, physical or chemical restraints can interfere with the physical and cognitive skills that are necessary for urinary control.

Older adults often experience an increase in postural sway, an age-related change that can interfere with one's ability to stand still. With increasing postural sway, older men may find it more difficult to maintain a standing position for urination. If urinary incontinence does occur, a diminished ability to smell may interfere with the older adult's perception of offensive odors. Although this does not have a functional impact on urinary elimination, the presence of urinary odors is viewed as socially inappropriate and may lead to isolation and rejection of the older adult.

Risk Factors

Although age-related changes create risks for the development of urinary incontinence in older adults, incontinence should not be considered a normal age-related change. If urinary incontinence develops, causes and risk factors usually can be identified through a comprehensive assessment. Risk factors include medications, lifestyle factors, pathologic conditions, psychosocial influences, and cognitive and functional impairments. Recent nursing articles emphasize the importance of identifying and addressing the risk factors that are modifiable (Luft and Vriheas-Nichols, 1998).

Common Pathologic Influences

Some pathologic conditions that cause negative functional consequences affecting urinary elimination are systemic, whereas others originate in the genitourinary tract. The following discussion addresses some of the common pathologic changes that affect male and female genitouri-

nary function, as well as some of the acute and chronic systemic conditions than can interfere with urinary elimination.

In women, postmenopausal estrogen depletion leads to weakening of the pelvic floor muscles. Obesity, and trauma secondary to pregnancy and childbirth, are additional factors that contribute to weakening of the pelvic floor muscles in some older women. With relaxation of the pelvic muscles, any sudden increase in intra-abdominal pressure may cause the involuntary expulsion of small amounts of urine. Pelvic muscle weakness also interferes with complete emptying of the bladder, resulting in residual urine and increased risk of bacteriuria.

In addition to causing degenerative changes in the pelvic floor muscles, decreased estrogen levels cause atrophy of the vaginal and trigonal tissue. With progressive atrophy, the resistance of those tissues to pathogens is diminished. Vaginitis and trigonitis may develop and may be accompanied by urinary urgency, frequency, and incontinence. A cystocele, rectocele, or urethrocele may develop as a result of extreme pelvic muscle stretching or relaxation. These disorders frequently coexist with uterovaginal prolapse, and they are often identified as causes of urinary incontinence.

Twenty-five percent of men aged 55 years and 55% of men aged 75 years experience dysuria as a result of benign prostatic hyperplasia. In its early stage, prostatic hyperplasia obstructs the vesical neck and compresses the urethra, causing a compensatory hypertrophy of the detrusor muscle and subsequent outlet obstruction. With progressive hypertrophy, the bladder wall loses its elasticity and becomes thinner. Subsequently, urinary retention occurs, increasing the risk of bacteriuria and infection. Eventually, the ureter and kidney are affected, and hydroureter, hydronephrosis, diminished GFR, and uremia may develop. Men with prostatic hyperplasia may experience nocturia, decreased urine flow, incomplete bladder emptying, and urinary urgency and frequency.

Another cause of decreased urethral resistance in men is the residual effect of transurethral surgery or radical prostatectomy. Other disease-related conditions that may cause or contribute to urinary incontinence include bladder calculi and prostatic carcinoma.

Urinary incontinence may also result from impaired neurologic function secondary to illnesses that affect either the central or peripheral nervous system. Examples of such conditions are dementia, diabetes, alcoholism, Parkinson's disease, multiple sclerosis, vitamin B_{12} deficiency, and cerebrovascular accident. Incontinence also can be the outcome of any condition that causes chronic urinary retention. Moreover, conditions such as arthritis or Parkinson's disease may slow the ambulation of older adults, increasing the time needed to reach a toilet. In the presence of age-related changes that shorten the interval between the perception of the urge to void and the actual need to empty the bladder, any delay in reaching an appropriate receptacle may result in incontinence.

Urinary incontinence may be the earliest or only sign of urinary tract infections in older adults. Other acute illnesses, such as delirium or gastroenteritis, may also be manifested or accompanied by urinary incontinence. Metabolic disturbances that induce diuresis, such as diabetes and hypercalcemia, also may contribute to incontinence. Any acute illness or surgical intervention that temporarily limits mobility or compromises mental abilities also represents a risk factor for urinary incontinence.

Fecal impaction and chronic constipation are very common physical causes of incontinence in older adults. In one study of urinary incontinence in female nursing home residents, 73% of the subjects had fecal impactions (Creason et al., 1992). The mass of stool diminishes the storage capacity of the bladder and obstructs the bladder outlet. Consequently, the bladder becomes distended and urine is retained. People with stool impaction experience urinary frequency and urge or overflow incontinence.

Pathologic mental changes create risks for incontinence in several ways. Dementing illnesses, such as Alzheimer's disease, directly affect the higher neurologic centers and can interfere with voluntary control over micturition. The manifestations of dementing illnesses, such as impaired memory and attention, also interfere with voluntary control over urination. In addition, older adults with dementia may lack the perceptual abilities that are necessary for finding and using appropriate facilities. One study of nursing home residents found that the development of urinary incontinence was strongly associated with dementia and the inability to walk and transfer independently (Ouslander et al., 1993).

Older adults and their caregivers may unintentionally exacerbate incontinence by limiting fluid intake in response to the fear or onset of incontinence. If bladder fullness is not adequately achieved, as in states of dehydration or limited fluid intake, the neurologic mechanism that controls bladder emptying will not function effectively, and incontinence will occur. Dehydration and inadequate hydration also cause increased bladder irritability, with subsequent uninhibited contractions.

Altered Thirst Perception

Although the exact causative mechanism is unclear, older adults may not experience thirst sensation in response to fluid deprivation. In a study of healthy, nonmedicated, men, aged 20 to 75 years, various aspects of thirst and dehydration were observed after the participants were deprived of fluid for 24 hours. The older men were found to be less thirsty than the younger men, and they reported feeling remarkably little thirst or dry mouth discomfort. Moreover, when the participants were given free access to water, the older men drank less water and, in contrast to the younger men, they did not drink enough water to rehydrate their body fluids to predeprivation levels (Phillips et al., 1984). In the presence of conditions that place additional demands on fluid and electrolyte balance, such as acute infection or elevated body temperature, reduced thirst sensation may interfere with the mechanisms that normally compensate for these physiologic stresses.

Medications

Medications influence micturition in a number of ways, and they are common risk factors in the development of urinary incontinence. For example, loop diuretics increase urinary output, placing additional demands on the urinary system and compounding the effects of an age-related decrease in bladder capacity. Anticholinergic medications, including over-the-counter antihistamines, can affect the muscles involved in urinary control. This adverse effect may be especially detrimental in the presence of prostatic hyperplasia or weakened pelvic floor muscles. Medications that can cause urinary incontinence and the associated mechanisms of action of these medications are listed in Table 9-1.

In addition to creating risk factors for incontinence, medications can compromise kidney function through the overstimulation of ADH secretion. This medication effect may compound age-related effects that predispose older adults to hyponatremia. Medications that stimulate ADH secretion include aspirin, narcotics, acetaminophen, amitriptyline, barbiturates, chlorpropamide, clofibrate, fluphenazine, and haloperidol.

Lifestyle Factors

Obesity (i.e., weight that exceeds average weights by more than 20%) increases the risk of incontinence, particularly for women. Smoking of cigarettes and other nicotine-containing products may increase the risk of urinary urgency, frequency, and urge incontinence. Also, smokers who develop chronic coughs may experience increased difficulty with stress incontinence (Penn et al., 1996).

TABLE 9-1
Medication Effects That Increase the Risk of Urinary Incontinence

Medication Type	Mechanism of Action
Loop diuretics (e.g., furosemide, bumetanide)	Increased diuresis can cause urgency, frequency, and polyuria.
Anticholinergic agents (e.g., antihistamines, antipsychotics, antidepressants, antispasmodics, belladonna alkaloids, anti-parkinsonian agents)	Decreased bladder contractility can cause urinary retention with frequency and overflow incontinence; anticholinergics may also impair cognition or mobility.
Adrenergics (e.g., decongestants)	Decreased bladder contractility and increased sphincter tone can cause urinary retention with frequency and overflow incontinence.
Alpha-adrenergic blockers (e.g., prazosin)	Decreased internal sphincter tone can cause urine leakage.
Calcium channel blockers (e.g., nifedipine, verapamil)	Decreased bladder contractility can cause urinary retention and overflow incontinence.
Hypnotics and anti-anxiety agents (e.g., benzodiazepines)	Sedation, delirium, and impaired cognition can contribute to incontinence.
Alcohol	Sedation, diuresis, delirium, and impaired cognition can contribute to incontinence.

Behaviors Based on Myths and Misunderstandings

Attitudes based on myths or lack of knowledge about urinary function can have a detrimental effect on the behavior of older adults and their caregivers. If older adults or their caregivers do not understand age-related changes, they may form hopeless attitudes about incontinence, or they may view incontinence as a normal consequence of aging. Studies indicate that 50% to 70% of incontinent people do not seek medical advice for the condition, and that as many as 82% do not view incontinence as abnormal (Holst and Wilson, 1988; Mitteness, 1990; Wyman et al., 1990; Goldstein et al., 1992). Health care professionals may reinforce these misperceptions and may even discourage patients from seeking treatment for incontinence. A study of older women revealed that less than 50% of the participants who reported incontinence to their primary care provider received a response indicating a need for further assessment (Simons, 1985).

Because of such attitudes of resignation, early signs and symptoms of urinary dysfunction may be ignored, and the problem may progress. For example, older adults often underestimate the interval between the perception of the urge to void and the actual need to empty the bladder. When incontinence occurs because of this, they may compensate by decreasing their fluid intake or urinating at more frequent intervals. However, these compensatory actions can lead to further urgency and incontinence, which, in turn, may reinforce the myth that incontinence is an inevitable problem of aging.

Incontinence may be precipitated by the attitudes and expectations of caregivers. When episodes of incontinence are noted soon after admission of an older adult to a long-term care facility, nursing staff members are likely to view the resident as having chronic incontinence, and their subsequent behaviors may reinforce the expectation of incontinence. For example, an older adult may initially experience episodes of incontinence because the toilet is too far away or cannot readily be located. However, if staff members assume that incontinence is the norm for that person, they might initiate use of absor-

bent pads by the resident, giving the older adult the message that voluntary control over urination is not expected.

In any setting, caregivers may believe that the use of pads or other incontinence products for the management of incontinence is easier and more convenient than preventing incontinence by assisting with toileting activities at the necessary intervals. In these situations, dependent older adults will behave according to the expectations of the caregivers, and incontinence will be the inevitable consequence. One study of a continence training program for nursing home residents found that nursing staff did not follow through with an individual toileting program designed to significantly reduce the number of incontinent episodes. Staff resistance was partially attributable to the longer amount of time required for toileting residents compared to the time required for changing wet incontinence products (Colling et al., 1992).

Functional Abilities

Despite the wide range of factors that may contribute to the development of incontinence in older adults, studies suggest that the most significant contributing condition is impaired cognitive or ambulatory ability. Studies of the relationship between various diagnoses and incontinence have failed to identify statistically significant differences between continent and incontinent older adults with the same diagnosis. When functional abilities have been examined in relation to urinary control, however, continent subjects have been found to be more independent in performing activities of daily living (ADL) than incontinent subjects.

A recent study of nursing home residents found that an impaired ability to perform ADL (particularly impairments in walking, dressing, toileting, and transferring) was the risk factor with the strongest association with urinary incontinence (Brandeis et al., 1997). Additional

DISPLAY 9-1
Environmental Risks That Can Contribute to Urinary Incontinence

- Houses with bathrooms on only one floor and with living and bedroom areas on two floors
- Any setting in which navigation of stairs is necessary to reach the bathroom
- Long-term care facilities or adult care homes with hallways separating bedrooms or living areas from bathrooms
- Any setting in which the distance between the toilet facilities and the older adult is more than 40 feet
- Adult care homes and other homes with a high proportion of residents per bathroom
- Small bathrooms and narrow doors and halls that do not accommodate walkers or wheelchairs

- Chair designs and bed heights that hinder mobility
- Poor color contrast, as between a white toilet and seat and light-colored floor or walls
- Restaurants, shopping malls, and other places with poorly visible or poorly color-contrasted signs designating gender-specific bathroom facilities
- Public places, such as restaurants, with dim lighting and out-of-the-way bathroom facilities
- Bright environments, where glare interferes with the perception of signs for bathrooms
- Mirrored walls, which reflect bright lights and create glare

risk factors identified by this study included delirium, restraints, and antipsychotic medications.

Environmental Influences

Environmental influences may impede or prevent older adults from reaching and using the toilet in home, public, and institutional settings. When these environmental obstacles are accompanied by mobility limitations and age-related changes that affect urinary function, incontinence may result. In a research study involving interviews with 559 caregivers of dependent older adults in their homes, caregivers of incontinent older adults reported more environmental barriers than did the caregivers of continent older adults. Environmental obstacles included the need to navigate stairs, an absence of grab bars and railings, and bathroom fixtures that were difficult to use (Noelker, 1987). Display 9-1 summarizes some environmental risk factors that may contribute to the incidence of incontinence in older adults.

Functional Consequences

Despite the many age-related changes in the urinary tract, the mechanisms involved in the elimination of wastes are not greatly affected in healthy, nonmedicated, older adults. However, in the presence of any unusual physiologic demands, such as may accompany the use of medications, the older adult is increasingly likely to experience functional consequences affecting homeostatic mechanisms and urinary control.

Although incontinence is the most obvious functional consequence of age-related changes and risk factors that affect urinary elimination, more subtle functional consequences may occur, many of which have serious effects. For example, age-related changes in kidney function may affect medication elimination, contributing to the increased incidence of adverse medication reactions among older adults. These adverse medication effects can significantly impair physical and mental abilities and have profound functional consequences. Other, more subtle, consequences may result from the age-related

TABLE 9-2
Age-Related Changes in Urinary Elimination

Change	Consequence
Kidneys	
• Decreased number of functioning nephrons	Decreased glomerular filtration rate
• Decreased blood flow	Delayed excretion of water-soluble medications
Renal Tubules	
• Fatty degeneration	
• Presence of diverticuli	Decreased efficiency of homeostatic mechanisms
• Loss of convoluted cells	
• Altered composition of basement membrane	Nocturia
Urinary Muscles	
• Hypertrophy of bladder muscle	
• Replacement of smooth muscle with connective tissue	Diminished bladder capacity
• Relaxation of pelvic floor muscles	
Neurologic Control	
• Degenerative changes in the cerebral cortex	Contractions during filling
	Incomplete bladder emptying
	Chronic residual urine
	Urinary urgency and frequency

changes that affect homeostasis and the elimination of the by-products of metabolism. Table 9-2 summarizes the age-related changes that affect urinary elimination.

Metabolism, Homeostasis, and Elimination of Metabolic Wastes

In healthy, nonmedicated, older adults, age-related changes have a quite limited effect on renal function. Such effects may include impaired absorption of calcium, a predisposition to hyponatremia, and a diminished ability to respond to physiologic stress. Relatively more serious functional consequences, however, are likely to occur in medicated older adults or in older adults with any condition affecting renal function, fluid and electrolyte balance, or plasma volume and osmolality. For instance, diuretics are more likely to cause hypovolemia and dehydration in older adults than in younger people.

Because the older body is less able to compensate for certain conditions, such as water deprivation or excessive fluid loss, the likelihood of serious dehydration is increased. For example, volume depletion may occur soon after the onset of fever-producing illnesses because of the inability to compensate for insensible fluid losses. Likewise, any condition or medication that stimulates ADH secretion, such as pneumonia or chlorpropamide, is likely to cause water intoxication and hyponatremia in older adults because of their diminished ability to compensate for excessive levels of ADH. Even with normal states of hydration, a decrease in GFR delays water excretion and may lead to hyponatremia. Because of declines in renal function, older adults require additional time to correct pH imbalances. Even normal daily activities can challenge the renal function of older adults because of diminished renal efficiency. For example, when older adults perspire during exercise, they may tire easily because of age-related delays in the mechanisms controlling water and sodium conservation.

Age-related changes in the kidney and in aldosterone secretion also impair the ability of the kidney to respond to alterations in sodium intake. Normally, increased sodium intake is accompanied by vasodilation, but this response is delayed in older adults. Similarly, when salt intake is restricted, older adults do not achieve low urinary sodium concentrations as readily as do their younger counterparts.

Medication Excretion

Perhaps the greatest functional consequence of age-related renal changes involves the excretion of water-soluble medications. The excretion of some medications, such as digoxin, cimetidine, and aminoglycoside antibiotics, is particularly dependent on the GFR. The excretion of other medications, such as penicillin and procainamide, is highly dependent on renal tubular function. Unless medication doses are adjusted to account for age-related changes in GFR and renal tubular function, excretion of inactive ingredients may be delayed, causing an accumulation of these toxic substances. As a rule, older adults require a 50% higher urine volume to excrete the same solute load as their younger counterparts.

Incontinence

As a result of age-related physiologic changes, the bladder of the older adult has a decreased capacity, empties incompletely, contracts during filling, and retains residual urine. Functionally, these age-related changes result in shorter intervals between voidings and less time between the perception of the urge to void and the actual need to empty the bladder. Consequently, urgency and frequency are often experienced during the day, and nocturia may occur several times nightly. In addition, chronic residual urine is likely to cause symptomatic or asymptomatic bacteriuria. Although these functional consequences do not necessarily cause incontinence, they are predisposing factors.

As defined by the International Continence Society, *incontinence* is a condition in which involuntary loss of urine is a social or hygienic problem and is objectively demonstrable. Incontinence is categorized as *transient* when it develops in response to acute conditions. It is considered to be *established* when it develops in response to a variety of chronic neural or genitourinary conditions. Incontinence can be further defined by specific characteristics and underlying mechanisms, as described in Table 9-3. In addition, incontinence may be classified as *mixed* when a person has a combination of the manifestations and underlying causes listed in Table 9-3.

Studies of older adults residing in nursing homes consistently cite at least a 50% prevalence rate for urinary incontinence. By contrast, estimates of the prevalence of incontinence in noninstitutionalized people older than 60 years of age range from 15% to 35%, with the prevalence in women being twice that in men (Urinary Incontinence Guideline Panel, 1996). One study of patterns of urinary incontinence in noninstitutionalized older adults revealed a self-reported prevalence of 18.9% in men and 37.7% in women. Women reported mixed incontinence and stress incontinence as primary conditions and urge incontinence as a secondary condition. Men reported urge incontinence as a primary condition, with stress incontinence developing as a secondary condition (Herzog et al., 1990)

Psychosocial Consequences for Older Adults

The psychosocial impact of age-related changes in urinary elimination patterns is influenced by a number of factors, such as self-esteem, attitudes, and usual activities outside the home. One research review has concluded that urinary incontinence is associated with many negative consequences affecting emotional and social well-being (Wyman et al., 1990). Wyman and colleagues cite studies that have found that as many as 75% of incontinent subjects report a negative impact on their mental health, and up to 52% report interference with their social activities. Studies have also found that urinary incontinence is frequently linked to interference with relationships, particularly sexual relationships (Wyman et al., 1990).

Even for older adults who are not inconti-

TABLE 9-3
Urinary Incontinence: Manifestations and Underlying Mechanisms

Type	Manifestations	Underlying Mechanisms
Transient	Acute onset, but may be ignored for a long time; associated with identifiable causes	Delirium, infections, pathologic conditions, fecal impaction, limited mobility, medications (see Table 9-1)
Stress	Sudden leakage of small amounts of urine as a result of an activity that increases abdominal pressure (e.g., coughing, lifting, laughing, sneezing, or exercise)	Medications, obesity, estrogen deficiency, weakness of the pelvic floor muscles, postradiation or postprostate surgery effects, urethral sphincter weakness
Urge	Inability to hold urine long enough to get to the toilet despite the perception of the urge to void (Cognitive impairments can impair this perception.)	Medications, stroke, dementia, parkinsonism, urinary tract infection, detrusor overactivity or instability
Overflow	Leakage of small amounts of urine, periodically or continually, without the urge to void or without being able to pass large amounts	Medications, fecal impaction, enlarged prostate, diabetic neuropathy, severe pelvic prolapse
Functional	Intermittent or consistent total incontinence in a person with an intact urinary tract but with other functional impairments	Medications, mobility limitations or cognitive impairments in combination with external factors (e.g., caregiver inattention, restraints, environmental barriers)

nent, the sensation of urinary urgency may lead to fears and feelings of powerlessness and insecurity. For instance, older adults with urinary urgency or frequency may be afraid to venture far from the bathroom. Also, older adults who do not understand age-related changes may have exaggerated fears of progressive incontinence, triggered by the mere onset of urgency or frequency. One erroneous strategy for preventing incontinence is to limit fluid intake. However, this compensatory action can have many detrimental effects, as it increases the risk of dehydration, bacteriuria, incontinence, constipation, adverse drug effects, and impaired homeostatic mechanisms.

Older adults who have experienced episodes of incontinence may become preoccupied with covering up any evidence of wetness. In one study of self-care strategies for urinary inconti-

nence, 80% of the subjects significantly reduced their social activities because of their fear of having their incontinence discovered by others (Mitteness, 1987). When incontinence occurs, fears and anxieties may arise from shame and embarrassment. In social settings, embarrassment and social rejection are possible outcomes if the older adult has a detectable odor of urine or experiences an episode of incontinence. In addition to being embarrassed about their incontinence, older adults may be embarrassed about having to use toilet facilities more frequently than might be considered socially appropriate.

An association between incontinence and infantile behaviors can foster ageist attitudes (i.e., "old people should be treated just like children"). Infantalizing attitudes and behaviors on the part of caregivers can have a devastating

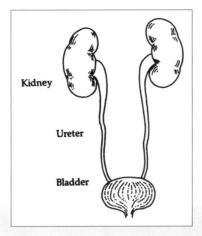

AGE-RELATED CHANGES

- Degenerative changes in cerebral cortex
- Decreased number of nephrons
- Decreased renal blood flow
- Decreased glomerular filtration rate
- Hypertrophy of muscles in the urinary tract
- Relaxation of pelvic floor muscles
- Contractions during bladder filling
- Decreased bladder capacity

NEGATIVE FUNCTIONAL CONSEQUENCES

- Decline in efficiency of homeostatic mechanisms
- Delayed excretion of water-soluble medications
- Diminished bladder capacity
- Nocturia
- Urinary urgency and frequency
- Chronic residual urine

RISK FACTORS

- Genitourinary disease (e.g., prostatic hyperplasia)
- Systemic disease (e.g., cerebrovascular accident, dementia, dehydration)
- Medications (e.g., diuretics, anticholinergics)
- Any factor that interferes with socially appropriate urinary elimination (e.g., impaired mobility)
- Environmental barriers
- Unfamiliar environments
- Indwelling catheters

FIGURE 9-1. Urinary function in older adults.

effect on the dignity and self-esteem of older adults, especially when absorbent briefs are used for the older adult and the caregiver uses words such as "diapers."

Psychosocial Consequences for Caregivers

For caregivers of dependent older adults in home settings, the onset of urinary incontinence may create additional stress, especially if urinary incontinence is compounded by environmental barriers or functional limitations. Caregivers report that tasks related to incontinence are some of the most difficult aspects of providing care, and they represent a major source of stress. Urinary incontinence has been identified as a major factor influencing the decision to seek institutional care.

Caregivers in home settings are likely to feel angry, guilty, frustrated, or inadequate when dealing with incontinence on a daily basis. In Noelker's study (1987) of 559 family caregivers of dependent older adults, caregivers of incontinent older adults reported the following: increased restrictions on their own social activities, increased doubts about their caregiving abilities, a greater perception of caregiving tasks having negative effects on family relationships, and a greater perception of caregiving tasks as being tiring, difficult, and emotionally upsetting. Lifelong attitudes about control over urination may contribute to feelings of disgust about the care demands, which may be further compounded by guilt feelings regarding this initial reaction to caregiving tasks. If the caregiver perceives intentionality on the part of the dependent person in his or her failure to control urination, these feelings will likely be intensified. In institutional settings, nursing staff and other caregivers may experience these same feelings to a lesser degree.

Figure 9-1 illustrates the age-related changes, risk factors, and negative functional consequences that can affect urinary elimination.

Nursing Assessment

Nursing assessment of urinary elimination is aimed at identifying: (1) risk factors that influence overall urinary function; (2) risk factors that increase the potential for incontinence; (3) signs and symptoms of any dysfunction involving urinary elimination; (4) fears and attitudes about urinary dysfunction; and (5) psychosocial consequences of incontinence. The nurse obtains most of this information by interviewing older adults and the caregivers of dependent older adults. In addition, the nurse obtains objective data from laboratory tests and by observing behaviors, behavioral cues, and environmental influences.

Interview Questions

Because urinary elimination is performed in the context of certain social expectations, discussion of this topic may be influenced by a person's attitudes and feelings. Although nurses usually learn to discuss urinary elimination with relative ease, older adults may feel uncomfortable with such a topic, especially if there are gender or age differences, or if a communication barrier, such as a hearing impairment, exists.

Terminology related to urinary elimination presents further difficulties in interviewing older adults. In social settings, euphemisms are commonly used to avoid directly discussing urination (e.g., "I'm going to the powder room," "I'm going to take a leak," "I have to use the john," and the like). Even the sounds associated with urinary elimination may be viewed as embarrassing, so people may run faucet water or flush the toilet to disguise the sound of urination when others are present.

Because of this social context, successful interviewing about urinary elimination depends on identifying the terms that are least embarrassing and most understandable to the older adult. "Pee," "urinate," "pass water," and "use the toilet" are phrases that might be used to refer to urinary elimination. If any hearing impairment is present, however, a term such as "urinate," which is not used in everyday social language, or a one-syllable word like "pee" may be difficult to understand. Although phrases like "use the toilet" and "go to the bathroom" are not specific to urinary elimination, they may prove to be acceptable, especially if additional questions are asked in order to distinguish between urinary and bowel elimination.

Similarly, the terminology related to incontinence is problematic for those who are not health care professionals because incontinence has a variety of meanings in different social contexts. For older adults, the term may be totally unfamiliar, or it may be associated with lack of control over sexual desires and activities. Hearing impairments, if present, may further interfere with comprehension of this word. Rather than using the term incontinence, it may be more acceptable to older adults to discuss "trouble holding their water." Older adults may tend to use phrases, such as "accidents," "leaking," "weak kidneys," or "bladder trouble," to describe incontinent episodes. The first task of the nurse in interviewing the older adult about incontinence is to discover and use the terms that are most acceptable and comprehensible to the person.

The nurse can set the stage for direct questions about urinary elimination by focusing initial questions on risk factors. Assessment of attitudes about urinary incontinence and its psychosocial consequences usually is accomplished indirectly by evaluating the responses to the interview questions. If incontinence has been acknowledged, questions about what the person has done about it may help to identify fears and attitudes that contribute to psychosocial consequences or interfere with interventions. If depression and social withdrawal were first noted at the time of onset of incontinence, this is a good clue that the person's self-esteem and usual activities have been affected by the condition. If older adults show a willingness to discuss their incontinence, direct questions can be asked about its impact on their daily activities and social life.

Display 9-2 summarizes interview questions related to urinary elimination. Some of the questions listed, such as medication patterns or medical history, may be asked in other parts of the interview. Although the questions should not be repeated, the information should be incorporated into the assessment of urinary elimination.

Behavioral Cues and Environmental Observations

Because of attitudes of resignation about urinary incontinence and the social stigma associated with it, older adults may deny any problems they may be experiencing. To obtain a comprehensive assessment of urinary elimination patterns, nurses must supplement the interview information with observations about behaviors related to urinary elimination. In institutional settings, particularly long-term care facilities, nurses have many opportunities to observe behavioral cues to incontinence. In home settings, caregivers of dependent older adults may observe behavioral cues and provide valuable information about urinary elimination patterns. Specific observations that may yield important information are listed in Display 9-3.

Home environments should be assessed for barriers that might interfere with the quick performance of urinary elimination (refer to Display 9-1). Stairways, long hallways, poor lighting, and cluttered surroundings may increase the time needed to get to the toilet, especially if the older adult has any functional impairment or uses assistive devices, such as a walker. Also, it is important to assess the environment for the presence of safety and assistive devices or their potential benefit to the individual. For instance, an elevated toilet seat, grab bars near the toilet, and grab bars on the walls leading to the toilet may improve the person's ability to urinate safely. Display

DISPLAY 9-2
Guidelines for Assessing Urinary Elimination

Interview Questions to Assess Risk Factors Influencing Urinary Elimination

- (Men) Have you had any surgery for prostate or bladder problems?
- (Men) Have you ever been told you had prostate problems? (Or Do you think you have prostate problems?)
- (Women) Have you had any children? (If yes, ask about the number of pregnancies and any problems with childbirth.)
- (Women) Have you had any surgery for pelvic, bladder, or uterine disorders?
- (Women) Have you had any infections in your vaginal area?
- Do you have any pain, burning, or discomfort when you urinate (pass water)?
- Have you had any urinary tract infections?
- Do you have any chronic illnesses?
- What medications do you take?
- Do you have any problems with your bowels?
- How much water and other liquids do you drink during the day? (Ask for details about timing and the amount of alcoholic, carbonated, and caffeinated beverages consumed.)

Interview Questions to Assess Risk Factors for Socially Appropriate Urinary Elimination

- Do you have any trouble walking or any difficulty with balance?
- Do you have any trouble reading signs or finding restrooms when you're in public places?

Interview Questions to Assess Signs and Symptoms of Urinary Dysfunction

- Do you ever leak urine?
- Do you ever wear pads or protective garments to protect your clothing from wetness?
- Do you ever have difficulty holding your urine (water) long enough to get to the toilet? (Or How long can you hold your urine after you first feel the need to go to the bathroom?)

- Do you have trouble holding your urine (water) when you cough, laugh, or make sudden movements?
- Do you wake up at night because you have to go to the bathroom to urinate (pass water)? (If the response is affirmative, try to differentiate between this symptom and the habit of going to the bathroom after waking up for some other reason.)
- Immediately after urinating (passing your water), does it feel like you haven't emptied your bladder completely?
- Do you have to exert pressure during urination to feel like your bladder is being completely emptied?
- (Men) When you urinate (pass water), do you have any difficulty starting the stream or keeping the stream going?

Interview Questions If Incontinence Has Been Acknowledged

- When did your incontinence begin?
- What have you done to manage the problem? (Have you cut down on the amount of liquids you drink? Do you empty your bladder at frequent intervals as a precautionary measure?)
- Are there certain things that make the problem worse or better?
- Does it happen all the time, or just at certain times?
- Do you have any pain when you urinate (pass water)?
- (Women) Do you feel any pressure in your pelvic area?

Interview Questions to Assess Fears, Attitudes, and Psychosocial Consequences of Incontinence

- Have you ever sought help or talked to a primary care provider or other health care professional about this problem?
- Have you changed any of your activities because you need to stay near a toilet?
- Do you avoid going to certain places because of difficulty holding your urine (water)?

DISPLAY 9-3
Guidelines for Assessing Behavioral Cues for and Environmental Influences on Incontinence

Behavioral Cues

- Does the older adult use disposable or washable pads or products?
- Is there an odor of urine on clothing or furniture (especially couches and stuffed chairs)?
- Has the older adult withdrawn from social activities, especially those held away from home?

Environmental Influences

- Where are the bathroom facilities located in relation to the older adult's usual daytime and nighttime activities?

- Does the person have to go up or down stairs to use the toilet at night or during the day?
- Are there any grab bars or other aids in, near, or on the way to the bathroom?
- Would the person benefit from using an elevated toilet seat?
- Does the person use a urinal or other aid to cut down on the number of trips to the bathroom?
- How many people share the same bathroom facilities?
- Is privacy ensured?

9-3 lists specific environmental factors that should be assessed for their influence on socially appropriate urinary elimination.

Laboratory Data

Data from urinalysis and blood chemistry tests contribute important information to the assessment of urinary elimination. Blood chemistry values that may be helpful in assessing renal function include the following: electrolyte level, creatinine level, creatinine clearance, nonprotein nitrogen level, and blood urea nitrogen level.

In older adults, the serum creatinine may not be an accurate indicator of the GFR. Rather, a 24-hour urine collection for creatinine clearance may have greater value as an indicator of renal functioning. Alternatively, the Crockcroft-Gault formula (described on page 262) can be used to estimate renal function in older adults. A urinalysis should also be performed on a midstream or second-void specimen. At the age of 80 years, the normal upper limit for specific gravity is 1.024, and slight proteinuria is normal in older adults. Other than these two variations, the urinalysis results should be within the normal range for healthy older adults.

Nursing Diagnosis

When the nursing assessment identifies any risk factors for incontinence or any complaints about or evidence of incontinence, an applicable nursing diagnosis would be Altered Patterns of Urinary Elimination. This is defined as "the state in which the individual experiences or is at risk for experiencing urinary elimination dysfunction" (Carpenito, 1997, p. 904). Major defining characteristics commonly found in older adults include urgency, frequency, dribbling, nocturia, hesitancy, and incontinence. Further assessment may provide enough additional information about the history and current manifestations of incontinence to enable the nurse to identify a specific pattern of urinary elimination: Urinary Retention, or Stress, Urge, Reflex, Total, or Functional Incontinence (Carpenito, 1997).

Nurses may identify one or more of the following factors as contributing to incontinence in an older adult: fecal impaction, estrogen deficiency, prostatic enlargement, environmental barriers, urinary tract infections, adverse medication effects, cognitive impairments, and functional impairments (especially impaired vision or mobility). When older adults have one or several of these factors, the nursing diagnosis of high risk for a particular type of urinary incontinence might be used. For example, an older man with prostatic enlargement who is taking an anticholinergic agent is at High Risk for Urinary Retention. Similarly, an 86-year-old woman who restricts her fluid intake to 500 mL/day because her arthritis interferes with her ability to get to the bathroom is at High Risk for Functional Incontinence.

Knowledge Deficit related to normal urinary function is a nursing diagnosis that might be used when older adults falsely attribute incontinence to normal aging, especially when this misperception interferes with further assessment and potential interventions. Additional nursing diagnoses should be addressed when negative consequences are identified in the older adult or their caregivers. Nursing diagnoses that address psychosocial consequences include Anxiety, Social Isolation, Altered Sexuality Patterns, Body Image Disturbance, and Caregiver Role Strain (or High Risk for such). Nursing diagnoses that might address the physical consequences of incontinence include Sleep Pattern Disturbance, High Risk for Infection, and High Risk for Impaired Skin Integrity.

Nursing Goals

Nursing care plans are directed toward preventing, minimizing, or compensating for the effects of age-related changes on urination, homeostasis, and medication excretion. One nursing goal related to urinary function is to alleviate the factors that increase the risk of urinary incontinence in older adults. This is achieved through direct nursing actions that address risk factors and through health education, as discussed in the following section. Another goal related to urinary function is to maintain homeostasis. This goal is addressed through health promotion activities that improve or maintain adequate renal function.

The initial nursing goal for incontinent older adults is to control and alleviate the incontinence. This is achieved through nursing and medical interventions that are based on a comprehensive evaluation to identify the underlying cause. If incontinence cannot be alleviated, nursing care is directed toward preventing negative consequences of the incontinence. For example, one goal might be for the older adult to manage the incontinence in such a way that his or her skin remains intact. Another goal would be for the older adult to maintain quality of life by managing the incontinence so he or she can participate in daily and desirable activities. This goal is achieved through environmental modifications and through the use of appropriate incontinence products and continence aids.

Nursing Interventions

Alleviating Risk Factors

Perhaps the risk factor most amenable to nursing interventions is the false perception of incontinence as an inevitable effect of aging for which nothing can be done. Because this attitude is based on myths or a lack of information, it can be changed through education. Nurses must teach older adults and their caregivers about normal age-related changes and risk factors that contribute to incontinence, and about the need for a comprehensive evaluation of any problems with urinary elimination. Education must also focus on health promotion activities aimed at preventing incontinence and other complications associated with age-related changes affecting urinary elimination. For example, pelvic muscle exercises (PME) can be performed by men and women who have any age-related changes or risk factors that increase their risk for experiencing urinary incontinence. Display 9-6 can be used to teach older adults about PME, as discussed later.

Teaching older adults the rationale for maintaining adequate fluid intake as a means of preventing incontinence is a simple but important intervention. Older adults are less likely to restrict their fluid intake if they understand that the signal to void from a full bladder is a requirement for voluntary control over urination. In addition, they should understand that concentrated urine as a result of fluid restriction may cause incontinence by stimulating bladder contractions. Finally, when nurses discuss the need to maintain adequate fluid intake, they should explain that older adults may not experience the sensation of thirst, even in the presence of dehydration. Thus, if older adults depend on their thirst sensation to indicate a need for fluids, their intake of liquids may be inadequate. Interventions to promote adequate fluid intake should include the identification of nonalco-

holic, noncaffeinated, and noncarbonated beverages that are most acceptable to the older adult and that will be consumed readily, even in the absence of thirst sensation.

When a risk factor interferes with normal urinary elimination, interventions should be directed toward optimal management of the precipitating factor. For example, if postmenopausal estrogen depletion leads to vaginitis and trigonitis, the older woman should be encouraged to seek medical treatment for the underlying condition. When fecal impaction or chronic constipation are risk factors for urinary incontinence, interventions should be aimed at attaining and maintaining good bowel function, as discussed in Chapter 8. Display 9-4 summarizes the teaching points that should be empha-

---

DISPLAY 9-4
Education Related to Urinary Elimination

Correction of Myths About Incontinence

- Incontinence is not an inevitable age-related change.
- The usual age-related changes affecting urination include a shortened interval between the perception of the urge to void and the actual need to empty the bladder, an increased frequency of voiding, and the need to get up to urinate several times during the night.
- Actions can be taken to minimize the consequences of age-related changes.
- Nocturia, urgency, and frequency do not necessarily lead to total incontinence.
- If actual incontinence occurs, a pathologic condition or other influencing factor can usually be identified through a comprehensive evaluation.
- One of the requirements for voluntary control over urination is the signal of the need to void because of a full bladder. Restricting fluid intake interferes with this signal.
- Highly concentrated urine, from inadequate fluid intake, will stimulate involuntary bladder contractions and may lead to incontinence.

- Consistently emptying the bladder at intervals of less than 1 or 2 hours will not resolve, but will rather contribute to, problems with incontinence.

Health Promotion Activities

- Seek medical advice from a knowledgeable practitioner about any difficulties with urinary continence.
- Drink 8 to 10 glasses of noncaffeinated liquid every day, with limited intake during the evening hours.
- Do not depend on thirst sensation as an accurate indicator for adequate fluid intake. Drink liquids even if you do not feel thirsty.
- Avoid excessive use of alcoholic, caffeinated, or carbonated beverages, especially before bedtime.
- Take steps to prevent constipation (refer to Display 8-4).
- Drink one or two glasses of fluid before, and every 15 minutes during, periods of sweat-producing exercise or activity.

ALTERNATIVE
AND
PREVENTIVE
HEALTH
CARE
PRACTICES

Preventing or Alleviating Prostate Problems

Herbs
- Pygeum, horsetail, pipsissewa, saw palmetto, pumpkin seeds, stinging nettle, uva ursi

Homeopathic Remedies
- Saw palmetto, baryta, barberry

Nutritional Considerations
- Zinc, vitamins C and E
- Avoidance of caffeine and alcohol

Preventive Measures and Additional Approaches
- No smoking
- Aromatherapy: geranium, clary sage
- Yoga, imagery, reflexology, acupuncture

sized to address risk factors that affect urinary function. In addition, there are certain alternative and preventive health care practices, summarized in the box at the end of this section, that may be used to address prostate problems.

Maintaining Homeostasis

In performing normal day-to-day activities, healthy, nonmedicated, older adults will not be greatly affected by age-related kidney changes. However, under any condition of physiologic stress, such as that associated with exercise, compensatory actions must be taken to prevent detrimental effects on homeostasis. Exercising in a cool environment and increasing one's fluid intake prior to exercise, for example, may compensate for the age-related inefficiency of sodium and water conservation. In conditions of extreme heat and humidity, older adults can take protective measures, such as increasing their fluid intake, avoiding alcoholic, carbonated, and caffeinated beverages; and staying in cool, nonhumid environments. Display 9-4 summarizes some of the health promotion activities that address overall urinary function, including maintenance of homeostasis.

Older adults taking normal doses of water-soluble medications are likely to experience adverse medication effects because of diminished renal function. Therefore, when water-soluble medications are prescribed for older adults, doses should be adjusted according to accurate measurements of kidney function and serum drug levels. Nurses should be aware of the increased potential for adverse medication effects, especially when the older adult is taking more than one medication. Further information about adverse medication effects and interventions for medication management are discussed in Chapter 18.

Controlling and Alleviating Incontinence

When incontinence occurs, initial interventions are directed toward controlling and alleviating, rather than simply managing, the symptoms. Before any interventions are considered, however, a comprehensive evaluation must be done to determine the underlying cause of the incontinence. Recent nursing articles provide guidelines for nursing assessment and interventions of incontinence in cognitively impaired adults (Thompson and Smith, 1998) and in acute care (Bradway et al., 1998) and long-term care facilities (Smith, 1998).

Nurses should be familiar with any specialty clinics in their geographic area that deal with incontinence. If a continence clinic is not available, a geriatric assessment program may be a good resource for an evaluation. In addition to considering the underlying mechanisms for incontinence, other factors that should be considered when planning interventions include: environmental conditions, resources and abilities of caregivers, functional and cognitive abilities of the older adult, and negative effects and social acceptability of the intervention.

The following interventions may be used singly or in combination for control of incontinence: surgery, medications, biofeedback, continence retraining, environmental modifications, PME, and a variety of minimally invasive procedures. Medication is not always the best intervention and should not be the first line of treatment. Medications for incontinence are often ineffective, particularly when prescribed without accurately determining the cause of incontinence. Older adults are particularly susceptible

to adverse medication effects. Therefore, nurses should encourage the use of nonpharmacologic interventions, such as PME or continence retraining, as an initial approach to dealing with urinary incontinence. If incontinence cannot be alleviated through these interventions, urinary elimination may be managed with an array of aids and equipment.

Environmental Modifications

When incontinence is primarily caused by the time interval between the perception of the urge to void and the ability to reach an appropriate receptacle, modifications of the environment may be the simplest and most effective intervention. If environmental adaptations cannot be made, as in public places, older adults should become familiar with the location and arrangement of the bathroom facilities before the need to urinate is imminent. In home and institutional settings, the provision of bedside commodes and privacy may be an effective intervention. If space is limited, however, or if privacy cannot be assured, bedside commodes may not be acceptable. Display 9-5 lists environmental modifications that should be considered for alleviating

---

DISPLAY 9-5
Environmental Modifications for Preventing Incontinence

Modifications to Enhance Visibility of Facilities

- Use contrasting colors for the toilet seat and surroundings.
- Provide adequate lighting in and near toilet areas, but avoid creating glare.
- Use night-lights in the pathway between the bedroom and bathroom.

Modifications to Improve the Ability to Use the Toilet in Time

- Encourage the use of chairs or beds that are designed to help the person arise unaided after sitting or lying.
- Install handrails in the hallway(s) leading to the bathroom.

- Make sure the pathway to the bathroom is safe and uncluttered.

Modifications to Improve the Ability to Use the Toilet

- Place grab bars at appropriate places to facilitate getting on and off the toilet and to assist men in maintaining their balance when standing at the toilet.
- Use elevated toilet seats or an over-the-toilet chair to compensate for any functional limitations of the lower extremities.
- If the person has functional limitations involving the upper extremities, clothing for the lower body should feature easy-open closures, such as Velcro or elastic waistbands.

incontinence when functional limitations, such as vision or mobility impairments, contribute to the incontinence.

Medications

Medications have been used, with varying degrees of success, in the control of incontinence. They also may be effective in the treatment of underlying conditions, such as vaginitis and urinary tract infections. In recent years, several types of medications have been used effectively to manage the irritative symptoms of benign prostatic hyperplasia, including urgency and urge incontinence (Beduschi et al., 1998). If medications are prescribed, nurses should be familiar with their expected positive effects, as well as their potentially negative side effects. Medications that act on the autonomic nervous system are the ones most often used for control of incontinence. Alpha-adrenergic agents are used to control stress incontinence by increasing bladder outlet resistance through stimulating receptors at the trigone and internal sphincter. Anticholinergic medications may be used to control the uninhibited or unstable bladder by blocking the transmission of nerve impulses. Cholinergic medications are used to prevent urinary retention and overflow incontinence by stimulating bladder contractions or increasing intravesical pressure. Alpha-adrenergic blocking agents may be used, either alone or in combination with cholinergic agents, to decrease bladder outlet resistance in the treatment of overflow incontinence. Table 9-4 summarizes the specific types and modes of actions for medications used in the treatment of incontinence.

Surgery

Various surgical procedures may be used to control incontinence when structural abnormalities, such as a cystocele, are identified as the underlying cause. For example, one of several bladder suspension procedures might be used in the treatment of stress incontinence. The goal of bladder suspension surgery is to reposition the urethra so that the pelvic floor muscles can squeeze it more effectively. When urinary incontinence is caused by loss of sphincter control, it may be treated successfully by surgical implantation of an artificial urinary sphincter. This is a device with an inflatable cuff that is placed around the urethra to hold it closed. To operate the artificial urinary sphincter, men squeeze a pump in the scrotum, whereas women press a valve in the labia to deflate the cuff, which automatically reinflates after voiding is completed. If incontinence is attributable to prostatic hyperplasia, surgical intervention to correct the underlying problem may alleviate the incontinence.

TABLE 9-4
Medications for Treating Urinary Incontinence

Medication	Action	Type of Incontinence
Phenylpropanolamine Pseudoephedrine Estrogen	Stimulation of alpha-adrenergic receptors to induce or strengthen muscle contraction	Stress (urethral sphincter insufficiency)
Oxybutynin Propantheline Dicyclomine	Anticholinergic or antispasmodic action to inhibit uncontrolled bladder contractions	Urge (detrusor hyperactivity)
Bethanecol	Cholinergic action to stimulate bladder contractions	Urinary retention with overflow
Phenoxybenzamine	Alpha-adrenergic blocking action to relax the internal sphincter	Overflow secondary to outlet obstruction

Self-Insertion Devices and Minimally Invasive Procedures

A variety of intravaginal or intraurethral devices are available for resolving stress incontinence. Pessaries have been used for many decades to treat cystocele in women. They come in many sizes and shapes and are individually fitted by a primary care practitioner. Pessaries need to be removed and reinserted at intervals ranging from nightly to once every few months, depending on the type of pessary that is used. Also, several types of disposable devices are available for self-insertion into the urethra. One type of device controls urination through the inflation and deflation of a small balloon that rests at the bladder neck. Another recent development is the use of a bladder neck prosthesis to control stress incontinence in women. Because the availability of nonsurgical devices for the control of urinary incontinence in men and women is rapidly evolving, people with urinary incontinence should be encouraged to obtain current information from a health care provider or from the National Association for Continence, listed in the Educational Resources at the end of this chapter.

In recent years, several minimally invasive procedures have been developed for the treatment of incontinence. For example, periurethral injections of collagen may be effective in treating stress incontinence in men and women; however, several injections may be required, especially in men. Minimally invasive surgical procedures, such as visual laser ablation and transurethral electrovaporization, are also being used to treat benign prostatic hyperplasia.

Pelvic Muscle Exercises

When weakening of the pelvic floor musculature causes incontinence, exercises to strengthen these muscles can cure or improve incontinence. PME were first advocated in the late 1940s by an American gynecologist, A. H. Kegel, for postpartum therapy. Since then, many variations of these exercises have been promoted, both for control of incontinence and for enhancement of sexual pleasure. A recent review of the literature on the use of PME to treat women with stress incontinence revealed cure rates as high as 73% and improvement rates as high as 96% (Wells, 1990). Studies have also documented the benefits of PME for patients with urge incontinence, for men following prostatic surgery, and for women who have undergone multiple surgical repairs (Urinary Incontinence Guideline Panel, 1996). PME are sometimes combined with other interventions, such as medications, biofeedback, or pelvic floor electrical stimulation. Recently, vaginal weight cones have become available to assist women in performing PME. Information about vaginal weight cones and other devices that might be helpful in performing pelvic muscle rehabilitation exercises is available from the identified references listed in the Educational Resources section of this chapter.

The goal of PME, also known as pelvic muscle rehabilitation, is improvement of urethral resistance through active exercise of the pubococcygeal muscle. There are no contraindications for or negative effects of these exercises, which can be initiated by any motivated person. They are recommended for women with stress incontinence and for men and women as adjuncts to bladder training for urge incontinence (Urinary Incontinence Guideline Panel, 1996). A very important aspect of teaching about PME is to help the person accurately identify the pubococcygeal muscle. Once the pubococcygeal muscle is identified, the person must practice contracting and relaxing this muscle, gradually increasing their ability to hold the contraction. It is important to emphasize that improvement is very gradual, and full effects are not noticed until 3 to 6 months of regular exercise have been completed. Even after full effects are achieved, daily maintenance exercises must be continued. Display 9-6 summarizes the points that should be covered when teaching adults to do these exercises.

DISPLAY 9-6
Instructions for Performing Pelvic Muscle Exercises

Purpose: To prevent the involuntary loss of urine by strengthening the pelvic floor muscles

Frequency: Minimum of 60 times daily for at least 6 weeks; ideally working up to 150 contractions daily in several sessions of at least 15 exercises per session (e.g., 3 to 10 sets of 15 exercises, or 4 to 6 sets of 20 exercises), continued indefinitely

Position: Lying, sitting, or standing

Identifying the Pubococcygeal Muscle

- Identify the pubococcygeal muscle by contracting the muscle that stops the flow of urine. Do NOT do this regularly when urinating.
- (*Women*) Lie down and insert a finger about three quarters of the way up your vagina. Squeeze the vaginal wall so you feel pressure on your finger and a sensation in your vagina.
- (*Men*) Stand in front of a mirror and try to make your penis move up and down without moving the rest of your body.
- Biofeedback, weighted vaginal cones, or a perineometer (a balloon-like device that is placed in the vagina) can be used to assist in identifying the pubococcygeal muscle and in measuring the strength of the contraction.

Method

- Tighten your pubococcygeal muscle and hold for a period of 3 seconds.
- Relax this muscle for an equal period.
- Repeat the contraction/relaxation cycle (one exercise) for your scheduled number of times.
- Breathe normally during these exercises and do NOT tighten other muscles at the same time. Be careful not to contract your legs, buttocks, or abdominal muscles while you are contracting your pubococcygeal muscle.
- Repeat this exercise daily in several sessions for a total of 60 to 150 exercises.
- For each of the daily sessions, vary your position (e.g., perform the exercise while lying down in the morning, standing in the afternoon, and sitting in the evening).
- Gradually increase the duration of each exercise up to a count of 10 for a contraction and 10 for a relaxation.

Additional Information: The National Association for Continence (800)252-3337 has audiotapes and written materials available about pelvic muscle exercises.

Continence Training

Continence training can variously be categorized as: (1) methods that are self-directed by motivated and cognitively intact people; or (2) methods that are directed by motivated caregivers of cognitively impaired people. A variety of terms and techniques are applied to continence training programs. Display 9-7 describes the various terms, and the next sections discuss the general principles of continence training programs.

The goal of continence training is to achieve a continent interval of 2 to 4 hours between voidings. These intervals will not necessarily be equal, and they will usually be longer during the night. In self-directed programs, the person hopes to regain voluntary urinary control, whereas in caregiver-directed programs the caregiver hopes to reduce the episodes of incontinence. Self-directed continence training, alone or in combination with biofeedback or medications, is most successful with urge incontinence. Continence training cannot be effective if the bladder capacity is less than 150 mL.

DISPLAY 9-7
Terms Used for Continence Training Programs

Self-Directed Program
Bladder drill
Bladder training
Bladder retraining
Bladder exercise
Bladder retention exercise

Caregiver-Directed Program
Scheduled toileting
Routine toileting
Prompted voiding
Timed voiding
Habit training

Caregiver-directed programs are most successful when they are based on a good assessment of individual voiding patterns. The nursing literature cites examples of successful incontinence programs instituted in nursing homes (e.g., Colling et al., 1992). Caregiver-directed programs may include the use of electronic devices or behavior modification techniques. One study documented the success of a combined regimen of prompted voiding and use of a bell-pad (an electronic alarm device) to improve daytime continence in cognitively impaired older adults (McCormick et al., 1992).

Essential elements of any continence training program include motivation, an assessment of continence and incontinence habits, a regulated fluid intake of 2000 to 3000 mL per day, timed voiding in the most appropriate place, and ongoing monitoring. During the initial assessment, symptom diaries are used to record times and circumstances of toileting, and times of and reasons for any episode of incontinence. After the usual voiding pattern has been identified, the older adult is encouraged to resist the sensation of urgency and to postpone voiding rather than responding immediately to an urge. With caregiver-directed methods, the caregiver determines the times of voiding. These methods are most successful when the timed intervals are flexible and are based on the person's needs. Caregivers often use some form of behavior modification to reward dryness and urination at appropriate intervals, and they may use negative reinforcement techniques when incontinence occurs. Display 9-8 summarizes the steps involved in a continence training program.

Biofeedback

Biofeedback is sometimes used as an intervention for urge or stress urinary incontinence, either alone or in conjunction with other treatment modalities. Biofeedback therapy involves using electronic or mechanical instruments to provide information to incontinent people about the physiologic activity involved in urination. This information is used to change the physiologic responses that control bladder function. Studies of the use of biofeedback in combination with behavioral therapies show continence improvement rates ranging from 54% to 95% (Urinary Incontinence Guideline Panel, 1996). Studies have found that biofeedback may be more effective than PME for some older women (Burns et al., 1993).

Managing Incontinence

When incontinence cannot be alleviated or controlled, it may be managed with the use of various aids and equipment, including disposable and washable incontinence products; indwelling, external, or intermittent catheters; and collecting devices, such as urinals and commodes. Because continence aids can be beneficial as well as detrimental, they should be used only after careful consideration of a number of factors.

DISPLAY 9-8
Continence Training

Purpose: To achieve voluntary control over urination at intervals of 2 to 4 hours

Method

Step 1: Identify the usual voiding pattern, noting the times of incontinence and information about fluid intake. During the first few days, keep a diary to record the following information at hourly intervals: dry or wet, amount voided, place of voiding, fluid intake, and sensation and awareness of need to void.

Step 2: Using information from the voiding diary, establish a schedule that allows for emptying of the bladder before incontinence is likely to occur.

Step 3: Provide the equipment and assistance necessary for optimal voiding at scheduled times.

Step 4: Provide 2000 to 3000 mL of noncaffeinated liquids per day for liquid intake. The largest amounts should be consumed during the early part of the day, and fluid intake should be limited about 2 to 4 hours before bedtime.

Step 5: Gradually increase the length of time between voidings until the interval is 2 to 4 hours long.

When used in conjunction with environmental modifications to increase accessibility of toilet facilities, such equipment usually has beneficial effects; however, when aids and equipment are used by caregivers of dependent older adults as substitutes for other methods of achieving continence, they are beneficial only to the caregiver and are detrimental to the older adult. For example, if protective products are used to manage incontinence, the positive effect for the caregiver may be that this method facilitates ease of care; however, the negative effects for the older adult include the likelihood of skin breakdown and decreased self-esteem. Except when used in conjunction with environmental modifications to control incontinence, aids and equipment should be considered only after other means of alleviating incontinence have been attempted, or when the needs of the caregiver take precedence over the needs of the older adult.

When an older adult depends on a caregiver for assistance with urinary elimination, the needs, limitations, and abilities of the caregiver must be considered in planning interventions.

In institutional settings, different demands may be placed on caregivers, who are expected and trained to care for incontinent patients/residents using the most appropriate interventions. In home settings, the total caregiving situation must be considered, and the needs of the caregiver may take precedence over the needs of the older adult, especially if the caregiver has functional limitations. Display 9-9 lists factors to be considered in selecting and using various types of aids and equipment for managing urinary incontinence. Nurses can keep up-to-date on new developments in incontinence products by visiting the Internet sites listed in the Educational Resources section of this chapter.

Maintaining Quality of Life

Urinary incontinence has many serious detrimental effects that can interfere with the quality of life, as discussed in the section on Functional Consequences. For example, urinary incontinence may lead to social isolation and withdrawal from desirable activities. Interventions

DISPLAY 9-9
Considerations Regarding Continence Aids and Equipment

Assessment Considerations

- What is the cost of various disposable and washable products, both initially and over a period of time?
- What are the needs and abilities of the caregivers of dependent older adults in home settings? (Can the caregiver manage the tasks involved in toileting?)
- What are the secondary benefits of various aids? (For example, in home settings, if the care of an individual with an indwelling catheter is covered by Medicare as skilled care, will additional services, such as home health aide assistance, also be covered?)
- What will the consequences be if the incontinence cannot be managed in the home setting? (For example, will the older adult be institutionalized?)

Teaching Related to Equipment

- Commodes are useful in diminishing the distance between the place of usual activities and toilet facilities.
- If commodes are viewed as socially unacceptable, measures can be taken to ensure privacy and increase their social acceptability.
- Commodes are now available that are attractively designed to resemble normal furniture items.
- Privacy can be ensured by placing an attractive screen around the commode.
- A bedpan can be placed on a regular chair, especially in the bedroom, and removed when not in use.

ALTERNATIVE
AND
PREVENTIVE
HEALTH
CARE
PRACTICES

Preventing or Alleviating Incontinence and Promoting Urinary Function

Herbs

- Buchu, yarrow, nettle, parsley, cranberry, bearberry, Echinachea, couch grass, uva ursi, celery seed, marsh mallow

Homeopathic Remedies

- Cantharis, staphysagria, Causticum, pulsatilla, couch grass, damiana, mullein, Gelsemium

Nutritional Considerations

- Fluid intake of at least 2000 mL daily; blueberries, cranberries, yogurt with live cultures
- Avoidance of sugar, coffee, alcohol, tomatoes, black tea, chocolate, excess salt, carbonated or caffeinated beverages, artificial sweeteners, and heavily spiced foods
- Thiamin

Preventive Measures and Additional Approaches

- Aerobic exercise 30 minutes 3 times weekly
- No smoking; maintenance of ideal body weight
- Yoga, acupuncture, biofeedback, relaxation, imagery, reflexology, PME (see Display 9-6)

that successfully control, alleviate, and manage urinary incontinence may also improve the person's quality of life. Alternative and preventive health care practices, as summarized in the box on page 287, may improve quality of life with regard to urinary function and incontinence.

Evaluating Nursing Care

Nursing care for older adults with urinary incontinence or other problems affecting urinary function is evaluated by measuring the extent to which identified goals have been achieved. The initial goal for any incontinent person is to achieve periods of continence that are as long as possible. When older adults attribute incontinence to aging processes, the effectiveness of nursing interventions may be evaluated by the person verbalizing accurate information about age-related changes and risk factors that affect urinary elimination. Another measure of the effectiveness of nursing interventions in such cases would be that the person seeks evaluation for his or her incontinence, rather than accepting this condition as inevitable. For older adults with stress urinary incontinence, a measure of the effectiveness of nursing interventions might be their performance of 60 PME daily.

If incontinence cannot be resolved, the goals of nursing care are directed toward managing urinary elimination in such a way as to maintain the dignity of the older adult and prevent negative consequences. In these situations, nursing care might be measured by the extent to which the person maintains their daily activities. For example, if older adults restrict their social activities because of incontinence, a measure of the success of nursing interventions might be that they begin using incontinence products to permit them to be away from their home for 4 hours at a time. For people with total incontinence, a measure of the effectiveness of nursing interventions would be the absence of skin irritation and breakdown.

Chapter Summary

Older adults are at risk of developing urinary incontinence because of the following consequences of age-related changes: diminished bladder capacity, bladder contractions during filling, incomplete bladder emptying, urinary urgency and frequency, and relaxation of the pelvic floor musculature. Additional consequences of age-related changes that affect urinary elimination include delayed excretion of water-soluble medications and decreased efficiency of homeostatic mechanisms.

Risk factors that increase the probability of the development of urinary incontinence include fecal impaction, adverse medication effects, diseases (e.g., dementia, prostatic hyperplasia), impaired physical function (e.g., limited mobility), and environmental barriers (e.g., long distance to the bathroom). Older adults, as well as professional and nonprofessional caregivers, commonly blame incontinence on age-related processes. These myths and misunderstandings may interfere with older adults' seeking and receiving help for their incontinence. When urinary incontinence is not addressed, older adults are likely to restrict their social activities and experience additional negative consequences.

Nursing assessment of urinary elimination focuses on the identification of any factors that influence overall urinary elimination or increase the risk of urinary incontinence. Nurses also assess signs and symptoms of urinary incontinence and identify any negative consequences. Applicable nursing diagnoses include Urinary Retention, Altered Urinary Elimination, and specific types of urinary incontinence (e.g., Stress, Urge, Total). Nursing care addresses the identified risk factors and is directed toward alleviating incontinence. When incontinence cannot be resolved or prevented, nursing goals address the actual and potential negative consequences (e.g., social isolation, impaired skin integrity). Evaluation of nursing care is measured by the extent to which the person achieves continence or, if continence cannot be achieved, by the success with which negative consequences are prevented.

Critical Thinking Exercises

1. Describe how each of the following age-related or risk factors might influence urinary function in older adults: medications, renal function, functional abilities, environmental conditions, altered thirst perception, changes in the urinary tract and nervous system, and myths and misunderstandings on the part of older adults, their caregivers, and health care professionals.
2. What are the psychosocial consequences of urinary incontinence for older adults and their caregivers?
3. Describe how you would address the following statement made by a 74-year-old woman: "Of course I have to wear pads all the time, just like when I was a teenager. I haven't talked to the doctor because I figured this was pretty normal at my age."
4. Describe the nursing assessment, with regard to urinary elimination, for a 75-year-old man and a 75-year-old woman.
5. You are asked to give a health education talk on "Problems with Urine Control" at a senior center. What information would you include about each of the following topics: normal changes of aging, why incontinence is common, and what treatment options are available for incontinence?

Case Example and Nursing Care Plan

Pertinent Case Information

Ms. U., who is 79 years old, is being transferred to a nursing home for rehabilitation after sustaining a hip fracture. A Foley catheter was inserted before her surgery 7 days ago, and it was removed yesterday. She is ambulating with a walker but needs one-person assistance. The discharge summary describes her as incontinent of urine. Ms. U. hopes to regain her independence in performing ADL so that she can return to her own home, which she shares with her friend.

Nursing Assessment

During your functional assessment, Ms. U. tells you she has had "trouble holding her water" since they removed the catheter yesterday. She is quite embarrassed about this and has not talked with any other health care practitioner about this. She says that she had too many other questions to discuss with her orthopedic surgeon, and she states that the nurses kept a large absorbent pad on her bed so she wouldn't have to walk to the bathroom. When she went to physical therapy, she used sanitary napkins, which her friend brought to her. She limited her fluid intake to a cup of coffee with each meal and a few sips of water with her pills.

Further assessment of Ms. U's incontinence reveals that, for many years, she has had difficulty with "leaking," particularly when she coughs, sneezes, or exercises. Also, she gets up to urinate about 4 to 5 times nightly. In fact, it was during one of these trips to the bathroom that she tripped and fractured her hip. She says she wakes up a lot during the night and goes to the bathroom because she's afraid of wetting the bed. She does not feel the need to urinate every time she wakes up, but she goes to the bathroom to prevent any leakage. She limits her fluid intake to 6 glasses per day and does not drink anything after 5 P.M. In the past few years, she has not left her house for longer than 2 hours at a time because she is afraid of "accidents." She tearfully confides that she thinks the orthopedic surgeon damaged a nerve in her bladder, which she believes is the reason she has such little "control over my water" since the surgery. She thinks they inserted the catheter because she has "weak kidneys." She states, "Before I had this fractured hip, I just had the usual problems that any older woman would have. Now I'll never be able to hold my water. I wish you'd just put that tube back in me so I can go home again."

Nursing Diagnosis

In addition to the nursing diagnoses that are related to Ms. U.'s impaired mobility, you address her problem with urinary incontinence. In deciding which type of urinary incontinence to include in your nursing diagnosis, you conclude that both Stress Incontinence and Functional Incontinence are appropriate because of the combination of long-term and recent factors that contribute to her incontinence. Your nursing diagnosis is Stress/Functional Incontinence related to limited mobility, recent indwelling catheter, and insufficient knowledge of normal urinary function and pelvic muscle exercises. Evidence for this diagnosis can be found in Ms. U.'s statements reflecting misconceptions and lack of information and in her description of current and past problems with incontinence. Evidence also is derived from your observations that she needs one-person assistance for walking and that she uses sanitary napkins and bedpads for urinary incontinence.

Goals	Nursing Interventions	Evaluation Criteria
To increase Ms. U.'s knowledge of normal urinary function	Discuss and describe normal urinary function, using a balloon partially filled with water and a simple illustration of the female urinary tract. Emphasize the relationship between adequate fluid intake and the maintenance of continence.	Ms. U. will be able to describe normal urinary function and the mechanisms involved in maintaining continence.
To increase Ms. U.'s knowledge about causative factors for incontinence	Describe age-related changes that contribute to incontinence, using the information contained in Display 9-4. Discuss the effects of frequent bladder emptying and limited fluid intake on the maintenance of continence. Discuss the relationship between limited mobility and urinary incontinence.	Ms. U. will describe age-related changes that influence urinary elimination. Ms. U. will identify risk factors that contribute to her incontinence.

To correct Ms. U's misconceptions about her urinary incontinence	Emphasize that as Ms. U. regains her mobility, she will regain her ability to maintain continence.	Ms. U. will state correct information about the relationship between her hip surgery and her incontinence.
	Emphasize that urinary incontinence is not an inevitable consequence of aging.	Ms. U. will express confidence in regaining urinary control.
	Explain that the orthopedic surgeon was not operating on or near her bladder or urinary tract.	
	Explain that the Foley catheter probably contributed to her current incontinence, but that this is a temporary situation that will resolve with proper interventions.	
	Emphasize that the nursing home staff will work with her to improve or alleviate her incontinence.	
To eliminate factors that contribute to functional incontinence	Provide a bedside commode for Ms. U.'s use until she regains her ability to walk to the bathroom without assistance.	Ms. U. will be continent of urine, except for stress incontinence.
	Work with the physical therapy staff to teach Ms. U. a proper technique for independent transfer to the commode.	
	The nursing and dietary staff will provide 2500 mL of fluids/day, taking into consideration her preferences.	
	The nursing and dietary staff will work with Ms. U. to schedule her fluid intake at acceptable times of the day, with minimal intake in the evening.	
	Talk with Ms. U. about eliminating the bedpads as soon as she feels confident about maintaining continence.	
Ms. U. will regain full control over urination.	Suggest that Ms. U. seek a comprehensive assessment of her urinary incontinence.	Ms. U. will report a reduction in or elimination of her stress incontinence.
	Teach Ms. U. to perform PME.	
	Give Ms. U. a copy of Display 9-6 for use as a guide for performing PME.	
	Emphasize the need to perform PME on an ongoing basis for alleviation of stress incontinence.	
	Give Ms. U. information about educational resources that might be helpful for her.	

Educational Resources

American Foundation for Urologic Disease
300 West Pratt Street, Suite 401
Baltimore, MD 21201
(800) 242-2383
• Educational brochures about urinary
incontinence, prostate disease, erectile
dysfunction, and other aspects of urinary function
(some available in Spanish)

Kimberly-Clark Corporation
P.O. Box 349, Department M, Neenah, WI 54957-9973
(800) 524–3577
• Community education kit and an ANA-approved
continuing education program

National Association for Continence (NAFC)
(formerly called Help for Incontinent People)
P.O. Box 8310, Spartanburg, SC 29305-8310
(800) 252-3337
www.nafc.org
• Resource guide, continence referral service,
audiovisuals, newsletters, and other publications
about incontinence

Procter & Gamble
1 Procter & Gamble Plaza, Attention: ATTENDS
Brand Manager, Cincinnati, OH 45202
(800) 428-8363
• Newsletter for nursing assistants in facilities that
use ATTENDS products
• Videotape for anyone who uses incontinence
products

The Simon Foundation for Continence
P.O. Box 835, Wilmette, IL 60091
(800) 237-4666
• Audiovisuals and publications about incontinence
• I Will Manage, education/support group for
people with incontinence

*U.S. Department of Health and Human Services
Agency for Health Care Policy and Research*
AHCPR Publications Clearinghouse, P.O. Box
8547, Silver Spring, MD 20907
(800) 358–9295
www.ahcpr.gov
• Patient's guide, caregiver's guide, clinician's
reference guide, and Spanish-language patient's
guide on incontinence
• Guide to establishing, implementing, and
continuing an effective continence program in a
long-term care facility

References

Beduschi, R., Beduschi, M. C., & Oesterling, J. E. (1998). Benign prostatic hyperplasia: Use of drug therapy in primary care. *Geriatrics, 53*(3), 24–40.

Bradway, C., Hernly, S., & the NICHE faculty. (1998). Urinary incontinence in older adults admitted to acute care. *Geriatric Nursing, 19*, 98–101.

Brandeis, G. H., Baumann, M. M., Hossain, M., Morris, J. N., & Resnick, N. M. (1997). The prevalence of potentially remediable urinary incontinence in frail older people: A study using the minimum data set. *Journal of the American Geriatrics Society, 45*, 179–184.

Burns, P. A., Pranikoff, K., Nochajski, T. H., Hadley, E. C., Levy, K. J., & Ory, M. G. (1993). A comparison of effectiveness of biofeedback and pelvic muscle exercise treatment of stress incontinence in older community-dwelling women. *Journal of Gerontology: Medical Sciences, 48*(4), M167-M174.

Carpenito, L. J. (1997). *Nursing diagnosis: Application to clinical practice* (7th ed.). Philadelphia: J. B. Lippincott.

Colling, J., Ouslander, J., Hadley, B. J., Eisch, J., & Campbell, E. (1992). The effects of patterned-urge-response toileting (PURT) on urinary incontinence among nursing home residents. *Journal of the American Geriatrics Society, 40*, 135–141.

Creason, N. S., Burgener, S. C., & Farrand, L. (1992). Guidelines for assessment of incontinence in elderly institutionalized women. *Geriatric Nursing, 13*(2), 76–79.

Freundl, M., & Dugan, J. (1992). Urinary incontinence in the elderly: Knowledge and attitude of long-term care staff. *Geriatric Nursing, 13*(2), 70–75.

Goldstein, M., Hawthorne, M. E., Engeberg, S., McDowell, B. J., & Burgio, K. L. (1992). Urinary incontinence: Why people do not seek help. *Journal of Gerontological Nursing, 18*(4), 15–20.

Herzog, A. R., Diokno, A. C., Brown, M. B., Normolle, D. P., & Brock, B. M. (1990). Two-year incidence, remission, and change patterns of urinary incontinence in noninstitutionalized older adults. *Journal of Gerontology: Medical Sciences, 45*, M67–M74.

Holst, K., & Wilson, P. D. (1988). The prevalence of female urinary incontinence and reasons for not seeking treatment. *New Zealand Medical Journal, 101*, 756–758.

Lindeman, R. D. (1992). Renal and electrolyte abnormalities. In E. Calkins, A. B. Ford, & P. R. Katz (Eds.), *Practice of geriatrics* (pp. 436–453). Philadelphia: W. B. Saunders.

Lindeman, R. D. (1996). Renal and urinary tract function. In J. E. Birren (Ed.), *Encyclopedia of gerontology: Age, aging, and the aged* (Vol. 2, pp. 407–417). New York: Academic Press.

Luft, J., & Vriheas-Nichols, A. A. (1998). Identifying the risk factors for developing incontinence: Can we modify individual risk? *Geriatric Nursing, 19*, 66–70.

McCormick, K. A., Burgio, L. D., Engel, B. T., Scheve, A., & Leahy, E. (1992). Urinary incontinence: An augmented prompted void approach. *Journal of Gerontological Nursing, 18*(3), 3–10.

Mitteness, L. S. (1987). The management of urinary incontinence by community-living elderly. *Gerontologist, 27,* 185–192.

Mitteness, L. S. (1990). Knowledge and beliefs about urinary incontinence in adulthood and old age. *Journal of the American Geriatrics Society, 38,* 374–378.

Noelker, L. S. (1987). Incontinence in elderly cared for by family. *The Gerontologist, 27,* 194–200.

Ouslander, J. G., Palmer, M H., Rovner, B. W., & German, P. S. (1993). Urinary incontinence in nursing homes: Incidence, remission and associated factors. *Journal of the American Geriatrics Society, 41,* 1083–1089.

Penn, C., Lekan-Rutledge, D., Joers, A. M., Stolley, J. M., & Amhof, N. V. (1996). Assessment of urinary incontinence. *Journal of Gerontological Nursing, 22*(1), 8–19.

Phillips, P. A., Phil, D., Rolls, B. J., Ledingham, J. G. G., Forsling, M. L., Morton, J. J., Crowe, M. J., & Wollner, L. (1984). Reduced thirst after water deprivation in healthy elderly men. *The New England Journal of Medicine, 311,* 753–759.

Rowe, J. W., Andres, R., Tobin, J. D., Norris, A. H., & Shock, N. W. (1976). The effect of age on creatinine clearance in men: A cross-sectional and longitudinal study. *Journal of Gerontology, 31,* 155–163.

Simons, J. (1985). Does incontinence affect your client's self-concept? *Journal of Gerontological Nursing, 11*(6), 37–41.

Smith, D. B. (1998). A continence care approach for long-term care facilities. *Geriatric Nursing, 19,* 81–86.

Thompson, D. L. & Smith, D. A. (1998). Continence restoration in the cognitively impaired adult. *Geriatric Nursing, 19,* 87–90.

Urinary Incontinence Guideline Panel. (1996 Update). *Managing acute and chronic urinary incontinence: Clinical practice guideline update.* (AHCPR Pub. No. 96-0686). Rockville, MD: Agency for Health Care Policy and Research, Public Health Service, U.S. Department of Health and Human Services.

Wells, T. J. (1990). Pelvic (floor) muscle exercise. *Journal of the American Geriatrics Society, 38,* 333–337.

Wyman, J. F., Harkins, S. W., & Fantl, J. A. (1990). Psychosocial impact of urinary incontinence in the community-dwelling population. *Journal of the American Geriatrics Society, 38,* 282–288.

Cardiovascular Function

Chapter

10

Learning Objectives	
	1. *Delineate age-related changes that affect cardiovascular function.*
	2. *Delineate risk factors for atherosclerosis, postural hypotension, and overall cardiovascular function.*
	3. *Discuss the functional consequences of age-related changes and risk factors that affect cardiovascular function.*
	4. *Describe the assessment of cardiovascular function and risks for cardiovascular disease in older adults.*
	5. *Identify interventions directed toward achieving optimal cardiovascular performance, reducing risk factors for cardiovascular disease, and preventing postural hypotension in older adults.*

*C*ardiovascular function is responsible for the life-sustaining activities of maintaining homeostasis, circulating blood cells, removing carbon dioxide and other waste products, and delivering oxygen, nutrients, and other substances to all the body organs and tissues. Along with respiratory function, cardiovascular function is essential for human life. Like many other physiologic systems, the cardiovascular system has a tremendous adaptive capacity to compensate for age-related changes. For example, moderate myocardial hypertrophy successfully compensates for increases in arterial pressure and serves to maintain heart volume and normal pumping action despite age-related changes (Lakatta, 1988). Healthy older adults, therefore, will not notice any significant change in cardiovascular performance because of age-related changes. In the presence of risk factors, however, the cardiovascular system is less efficient in performing life-sustaining activities, and serious negative functional consequences can occur.

Age-Related Changes

As with many other aspects of physiologic function, it is difficult to determine whether the changes in cardiovascular function that commonly affect older adults are attributable to age or disease. Knowledge about distinct age- or disease-related changes in cardiovascular function is confounded by the fact that only in recent years has medical technology enabled researchers to identify older subjects who are free of disease. Before these technological advances, subjects were likely to be excluded from studies on the basis of symptoms of cardiac disease, but not on the basis of asymptomatic pathologic processes. For example, studies based on autopsy findings and stress-test technology indicate that the prevalence of coronary atherosclerosis in older adults is about twice as high as estimates based on clinical history and resting electrocardiograms suggest (Rodeheffer and Gerstenblith, 1985). It is now estimated that about half of the population aged 65 years or older has at least a 50% occlusion of at least one major coronary artery (Lakatta, 1988). Therefore, at least some of the conclusions drawn from early research are now being challenged by newer studies of older subjects who have been carefully screened for asymptomatic heart disease. These recent studies suggest that some of the earlier findings regarding cardiovascular changes were based on studies that included older subjects with underlying diseases. Although these studies might offer accurate information about common cardiovascular changes that affect older people, they do not provide information about age-related changes.

In addition to differentiating between age- and disease-related changes in cardiovascular function, researchers are trying to distinguish between changes that are age-related and those that can be linked to risk factors. Perhaps more than any other aspect of physiologic function, lifestyle factors significantly influence cardiovascular performance. It is now known, for example, that stress, smoking, dietary habits, and physical exercise have long-term effects on cardiovascular function. Less is known about how these long-term effects can be differentiated from age-related processes, particularly when whole societies are affected by these factors. Blood pressure (BP), for example, has been found to increase gradually in adulthood in people who live in Western societies. This change is not found, however, in those from less industrialized societies. Therefore, changes that are thought to be age-related because they occur consistently in large population samples may be found to be related to lifestyle when cross-cultural studies are done. Lifestyle and environmental influences are important factors in explaining the wide range of variability in cardiovascular function among older adults, even for changes that are not disease-related. Finally, even when changes in the cardiovascular system are identified, their functional consequences are not always clear. With these limitations in mind, the following sections describe the age-related changes that may affect cardiovascular performance.

Myocardium

Although anatomic changes of the myocardium have been identified in older hearts, many questions have been raised about whether the changes are attributable to aging, disease, or risk factors. Furthermore, the functional significance of these changes, if any, has not been determined. In brief, some of the identified changes, which may be age-related or disease-related, are amyloid deposits, lipofuscin accumulation, basophilic degeneration, valvular thickening and stiffening, and increased amounts of connective tissue. Studies of changes in heart size in older adults have variously shown atrophy as well as hypertrophy, but these changes are not necessarily age-related. It is now thought that these findings are predominantly disease-related, and there is some agreement that the primary age-related change in heart size is a slight left ventricular hypertrophy that develops gradually between the ages of 30 and 70 years. This left ventricular hypertrophy is attributed to dilation of the aorta and elevation of the systolic BP (SBP). Changes in the left ventricle are important in terms of the functional impact on circulatory efficiency.

Cardiac Physiology

Age-related changes in cardiac physiology are minimal, and the changes that occur affect cardiac performance only under conditions of physiologic stress. Even under stressful conditions, the heart in healthy older adults is able to adapt, although the adaptive mechanisms may differ from those of younger adults or be slightly less efficient. The age-related changes that cause functional consequences primarily involve the electrophysiology of the heart, or the conduction system. Age-related changes in the neuro-conductive system include a decrease in the number of pacemaker cells, increased irregularity in the shape of pacemaker cells, and a thickening of the shell around the sinus node. In addition, increased amounts of myocardial fat, collagen, and elastic fibers affect the sinus node.

Other changes that are thought to be age-related include thickening of the atrial endocardium, thickening of the atrioventricular valves, and calcification of at least part of the mitral annulus of the aortic valve. The end result of these changes is interference with the ability of the heart to contract completely. With less effective contractility, more time is required to complete the cycle of diastolic filling and systolic emptying. In addition, the myocardium becomes increasingly irritable and less responsive to the impulses from the sympathetic nervous system. One consequence of this is the increased likelihood of cardiac arrhythmias.

Vasculature

Age-related changes affect two of the three vascular layers, and functional consequences vary, depending on the layer that is affected. Changes in the tunica intima, for example, have the most serious functional consequences in the development of atherosclerosis. The outermost layer, called the tunica adventitia, is the one layer that does not seem to be affected by age-related changes. This layer is composed of loosely meshed adipose and connective tissue. It supports nerve fibers and the vasa vasorum, the blood supply for the tunica media.

The tunica media, the second layer, is composed of single or multiple layers of smooth muscle cells surrounded by elastin and collagen. The smooth muscle cells participate in the tissue-forming functions of producing collagen, proteoglycans, and elastic fibers. The tunica media also provides structural support for the artery and functions in expansion and contraction. Thus, it is the layer that is affected by increased BP.

Age-related changes that affect the tunica media include an increase in collagen and a thinning and calcification of elastin fibers, with the end result being stiffened blood vessels. Consequences of these changes include increased peripheral resistance, impaired baroreceptor function, and diminished ability to increase organ blood flow. These changes are particularly pronounced in the aorta, where the diameter of the lumen increases to compensate for the age-related arterial stiffening. Although these changes are currently viewed as age-related, longitudinal and cross-cultural studies are beginning to raise questions about the impact of lifestyle variables on arterial stiffness. In contrast to the disease-related changes of atherosclerosis, these changes do not cause serious vascular narrowing or actual diseases. They do, however, interfere with cardiac function by altering the resistance to blood flow from the heart. As a result of age-related vascular changes, the pulsatile flow of blood is impaired, and pulse wave velocity increases. The left ventricle is forced to work harder, and the baroreceptors in the large arteries lose their effectiveness in controlling BP, especially during postural changes. An end result is a slightly increased SBP.

The innermost layer, called the tunica intima, consists of a single layer of endothelial cells on a thin layer of connective tissue. The tunica intima controls the entry of lipids and other substances from the blood into the artery wall. Intact endothelial cells allow blood to flow freely without clotting; however, when the endothelial cells are damaged, they function in the clotting process. The tunica intima is the layer most directly affected by age-related changes and most involved with atherosclerotic processes. With increasing age, the tunica intima thickens as a result of fibrosis, cellular proliferation, and lipid and calcium accumulation. In addition, the endothelial cells become irregular in size and shape. These changes make the arterial walls more vulnerable to atherosclerosis, as discussed in the section on Functional Consequences.

Veins undergo changes similar to those affecting the arteries, but to a lesser degree. Veins become thicker, more dilated, and less elastic with increasing age. Valves of the large leg veins become less efficient in the return of blood to the heart. Peripheral circulation is further influenced by an age-related reduction in muscle mass and a concurrent reduction in the demand for oxygen.

Baroreflex Mechanisms

Control of BP and other aspects of cardiovascular performance depend on the baroreflex mechanisms and are therefore affected by age-related baroreflex changes. In part, BP is regulated by baroreflex mechanisms that increase heart rate and peripheral vascular resistance to compensate for transient decreases in arterial pressure. Similarly, to compensate for transient increases in arterial pressure, baroreflex mechanisms decrease the heart rate and vascular tone. In older adults, the compensatory response to both hypertensive and hypotensive stimuli is blunted; the heart rate does not increase or decrease as efficiently as in younger adults. The age-related changes that are thought to alter baroreflex mechanisms include arterial stiffening and reduced cardiovascular responsiveness to adrenergic stimulation.

Risk Factors

The most significant risk factors that affect cardiovascular function are those that lead to atherosclerosis, and these risks are the same for both younger and older adults. Other risks are of minimal importance in comparison to the major consequences of atherosclerosis. The only risk factors that affect the cardiovascular function of older adults more than that of younger adults are those that contribute to postural (orthostatic) hypotension. Even healthy older adults, however, will be affected by age-related cardiovascular changes under conditions of physical stress. Therefore, physical deconditioning is a risk factor for diminished cardiovascular function in older adults.

Risks for Atherosclerosis and Cardiovascular Disease

Atherosclerosis is a disease process associated with the following risk factors: obesity, diabetes, heredity, hypertension, male gender, increased age, physical inactivity, cigarette smoking, personality factors, and dietary habits that contribute to hyperlipidemia. A recent study found that

people who spend 1 hour or more per week in close contact with one or more smokers had a significantly increased risk of developing atherosclerosis (Howard et al., 1998). With increased age, gender differences diminish, so that the risks for coronary heart disease are about the same for men and women older than 70 years of age.

Longitudinal data from the Framingham Study indicate that increased age is the most important risk factor for cardiovascular disease. Of the remedial factors, however, hypertension, including isolated systolic hypertension, is the most important risk factor in older people (Kannel and Vokonas, 1985). Additional conclusions about significant risk factors for cardiovascular disease in older people include the following (Kannel and Vokonas, 1985; Aronow, 1990; Finucane et al., 1993):

1. Exercise may exert a protective benefit.
2. High levels of low-density lipoprotein (LDL) and low levels of high-density lipoprotein (HDL) are risk factors for coronary artery disease.
3. Cigarette smoking increases the risk for cardiovascular mortality, but this excess risk is reversed within 1 to 5 years after smoking cessation.
4. Postmenopausal use of hormones is associated with decreased risks of cardiovascular disease, coronary heart disease, and stroke incidence and mortality in older women.

Risks for Postural Hypotension

Postural hypotension can occur in healthy older adults as a result of age-related changes, but it is more likely to occur in older adults who have additional risk factors. Although postural hypotension might seem to be a relatively harmless phenomenon, it can affect the safety and quality of life of older adults and can lead to serious negative functional consequences. It can contribute to falls and fractures, particularly in the

DISPLAY 10-1
Risk Factors for Postural Hypotension

Disease-Related Conditions

Hypertension, including isolated systolic hypertension

Volume depletion (e.g., dehydration)

Parkinson's disease

Cerebral infarct

Diabetes

Anemia

Peripheral neuropathy

Arrhythmias

Electrolyte imbalances (e.g., hyponatremia, hypokalemia)

Miscellaneous

Age of 75 years or older

Prolonged bed rest

Surgical sympathectomy

Valsalva maneuver during voiding

Medications

Antihypertensives

Anticholinergics

Phenothiazines

Antidepressants

Levodopa

Vasodilators

Nitrates

Barbiturates

Alcohol

---

presence of additional risk factors, such as impaired vision and environmental barriers. Even older adults without any risk factors may experience postural hypotension, as discussed in the section on Functional Consequences. Any of the risk factors listed in Display 10-1 may increase the possibility of postural hypotension.

Physical Deconditioning

Physical deconditioning, or lack of exercise, significantly influences many aspects of cardiovascular function, including BP, heart rate, and oxygen consumption. Deconditioning can accentuate the functional consequences of age-related changes, particularly in the presence of physiologic stress. For example, one study found that the decline in maximum oxygen uptake that usually occurs between the ages of 25 and 65 years was 40% slower in physically fit men than in sedentary men (Ogawa et al., 1992). Therefore, any factors that contribute to deconditioning are risk factors for poor cardiovascular function. These factors include acute illness, a sedentary lifestyle, mobility limitations, cardiac disease or other diseases that interfere with physical activity, and psychosocial influences, such as depression or lack of motivation.

Functional Consequences

Healthy older adults experience no significant cardiovascular effects in the resting state, although their cardiovascular performance is less efficient during exercise. Older adults do, however, have a high prevalence of atherosclerosis and other disease-related cardiovascular conditions, and these conditions account for many of the negative functional consequences that affect this population. In the following sections, the functional consequences of specific aspects of cardiovascular performance are discussed. In addition, atherosclerosis is discussed as a negative functional consequence because it is so prevalent with increasing age.

Rate and Rhythm

The resting and average heart rates of healthy older people do not change, but the maximum heart rate achieved during strenuous exercise is diminished. Whereas a younger adult's heart rate speeds up to 180 to 200 beats per minute under stress, the heart rate of a 70- to 75-year-old person accelerates to only 140 to 160 beats per minute (Svanborg, 1996).

In healthy older people, the prevalence of cardiac arrhythmias is thought to increase as a result of the age-related changes that affect the conduction mechanism. The results of the Baltimore Longitudinal Study of Aging indicate that 88% of the healthy older subjects tested had supraventricular ectopic beats, and 80% had ventricular ectopic beats (Fleg and Kennedy, 1982). Another study found that 17.2% of healthy older subjects had premature ventricular beats in excess of the normal upper limit of 200 per 24 hours (Tammaro et al., 1986).

Cardiac Output

Cardiac output is considered to be the most important overall measure of cardiac performance because it represents the heart's ability to meet the oxygen requirements of the body. It is influenced by the heart rate and stroke volume and is defined as the amount of blood pumped by the heart per minute. Although many gerontological references state that resting cardiac output decreases with advanced age, this so-called age-related change is now being attributed to disease-related processes. It is now thought that healthy older adults do not have any age-related change in resting cardiac output. One gerontologist, however, qualifies this conclusion by stating that, although there is no age-related change noted in the upright resting cardiac output of older adults, there is an age-related decrease in the supine resting cardiac output and stroke vol-

ume (Wei, 1988). This diminished ability to increase cardiac output when recumbent may be attributable to decreased myocardial compliance and increased diastolic stiffness (Wei, 1988). Despite this disagreement about age-related alterations in resting cardiac output, there is consistent agreement about an age-related decline in cardiac output under conditions of physiologic stress.

Response to Exercise

A negative functional consequence that affects cardiovascular performance in healthy older adults is a blunted adaptive response to physical exercise. Physiologic stress, such as that associated with exercise, increases the demands on the cardiovascular system by 4 to 5 times the basal level. The adaptive response involves many aspects of physiologic function, including the respiratory, cardiovascular, musculoskeletal, and autonomic nervous systems. With increasing age, there is a steady decline in the maximal attainable heart rate during intense physical exercise, but there is little or no effect at submaximal exercise levels in the absence of heart disease or other risk factors.

Before the late 1980s, it was widely believed that this consequence was primarily the result of decreased cardiac output. However, this conclusion has been questioned recently because the studies on which it is based included subjects with asymptomatic coronary artery disease. Furthermore, studies that have drawn this conclusion have not controlled for the impact of lifestyle and physical conditioning (Lakatta, 1988). Research indicates that age-related cardiac output changes are not necessarily the primary cause of the older person's diminished ability to adapt to stress. Data from the Baltimore Longitudinal Study of Aging suggest that the underlying mechanism is an age-related decrease in the cardiovascular response to beta-adrenergic stimulation (Rodeheffer et al., 1984; Lakatta, 1988).

Research does not question the conclusion that, in older adults, the adaptive response to intense exercise is diminished. What is questioned is the underlying mechanism, particularly the theory that diminished cardiac output is the responsible mechanism. This is an important concept for nurses and other health care providers to consider when addressing risk factors that interfere with functional abilities, particularly lifestyle factors. For example, if lack of physical activity, rather than inevitable age-related changes, is responsible for the diminished response to stress exercise, the cardiovascular function of older adults might be improved through increased physical activity.

Blood Pressure

A major longitudinal and cross-sectional study of adults screened for disease and medication has identified the following age-related changes affecting BP in healthy adults in Western societies (Pearson et al., 1997):

1. In men, diastolic BP (DBP) increases steadily at a rate of 1 mm Hg per decade without any plateau or decline.
2. In women, DBP is relatively stable until it increases significantly between the ages of 40 and 60 years, after which it stabilizes and may even decline slightly after the age of 70 years.
3. SBP is relatively stable until about the age of 50 years in men and 40 years in women; thereafter, it increases by 5 to 8 mm Hg per decade.
4. Between the ages of 30 and 70 years, SBP increases to a greater degree than DBP, with an average increase in SBP of 15 mm Hg in men and 21 mm Hg in women and an average DBP increase of 3.5 mm Hg in men and 5 mm Hg in women.
5. After the age of 70 years, SBP may plateau or decline in women but not in men.

Another recent study found that women older than 62 years of age who were not taking estrogen replacement medication had a greater increase in SBP, mean BP, and pulse pressure than did men of any age or women younger than age 62 included in the study. This study concluded that increased age was an independent risk factor for increased BP in women, but not in men (Gardner and Poehlman, 1995). These trends do not occur in non-Western societies, so they cannot be viewed solely as age-related changes. Cross-cultural studies suggest that BP levels increase with increased weight and are influenced by lifestyle factors, such as cigarette smoking and physical activity.

Postural and Postprandial Hypotension

Postural hypotension is most commonly defined as a reduction in SBP of 20 mm Hg or more after at least 1 minute of standing. Sometimes, distinctions are made between symptomatic and asymptomatic hypotension, and between postural systolic hypotension and postural hypotension, as discussed in the Nursing Assessment section (see Table 10-2). Common complaints accompanying symptomatic postural hypotension include dizziness, faintness, and lightheadedness. Less commonly, symptomatic postural hypotension may be accompanied by impotence, constipation, blurred vision, urinary incontinence, abnormal sweating, and other evidence of autonomic insufficiency. When this occurs, the postural hypotension is the result of diseases that affect the autonomic and sympathetic nervous systems, such as Parkinson's disease or dementia of the vascular or Alzheimer's type.

Studies indicate that 10% to 33% of all older adults are affected by postural hypotension, but that less than 7% of healthy, nonmedicated, older adults are so affected (Harris et al., 1991; Patel et al., 1993). Because the prevalence of postural hypotension increases with advanced age, an age of 75 years and older is often considered to be a risk factor. Consequences of postural hypotension include syncope, frequent falling, and difficulty with walking (Rutan et al., 1992).

Postural hypotension is a complex functional consequence that is at least partially attributable to age-related changes in the baroreflex mechanisms. Studies have consistently shown an age-related blunting of the baroreflex-mediated heart rate response to both hypotensive and hypertensive stimuli. Blood pressure regulation is also affected by age-related and disease-related cardiovascular changes (e.g., atherosclerosis). In addition, the age-related increase in SBP that is common in Western societies further interferes with BP homeostasis (Lipsitz, 1989). Consequently, older adults are increasingly susceptible to postural hypotension, and their BP is more labile.

Studies have shown that postprandial hypotension, or a BP reduction of 20 mm Hg within 1 hour of eating a meal, occurs in about one third of healthy older adults (Lipsitz and Fullerton, 1986). Postprandial reductions in BP have not been demonstrated in younger subjects. Postprandial hypotension is thought to result from a combination of factors, including impaired baroreflex mechanisms and the release of vasoactive gastrointestinal hormones. Postprandial hypotension is associated with the consumption of carbohydrates, particularly glucose, which causes insulin release (Jansen and Hoefnagels, 1991). In addition to increased age, the risk factors for postprandial hypotension include hypertension, hypotensive medications ingested before meals, and conditions that cause autonomic dysfunction. One study found that postprandial hypotension was accompanied by a small increase in cerebrovascular resistance (Krajewski et al., 1993). This study suggested that people with already compromised cerebral blood supply may be at greatest risk of postprandial cerebral ischemia. A high carbohydrate meal may increase the risk of postprandial hypotension, but caffeinated beverages ingested immediately after a high-carbohydrate meal may prevent postprandial hypotension (Heseltine et al., 1991). Postprandial hypotension in nursing home residents has been associated with a higher incidence of falls, syncope, new stroke, and new coronary events (Aronov and Ahn, 1997).

Additional Functional Consequences

Several additional functional consequences occur because of age-related changes, but little is known about the underlying mechanisms. For example, in older adults, the increase in SBP that occurs in response to aerobic exercise is sustained for a longer period of time after exercise ceases than in younger populations. Another consequence of age-related changes is an attenuation of the cardiovascular reflex responses to common activities, such as coughing, digestion, and the Valsalva maneuver. This consequence may be associated with altered baroreflex function. Age-related changes in cardiovascular and baroreflex mechanisms can reduce cerebral blood flow, particularly in the presence of risk factors. Studies have shown a reduction in cerebral blood flow in healthy older adults and a further reduction in those with risk factors for cerebrovascular disease, such as diabetes, hypertension, hyperlipidemia, and heart disease. Finally, increased tortuosity and dilation of the veins, along with decreased efficiency of the valves, lead to impaired venous return from the lower extremities. Consequently, the older adult may have stasis edema of the feet and ankles and an increased susceptibility to certain diseases or conditions, such as venous stasis ulcers. Table 10-1 summarizes the age-related changes and functional consequences that are thought to occur in healthy older adults.

Atherosclerosis

Atherosclerosis is viewed as a negative functional consequence resulting from a combination of age-related vascular changes and risk factors. It differs from other functional consequences discussed in this text, however, in that it is a disease process. It is discussed here because it occurs so commonly in older adults and be-

TABLE 10-1
Age-Related Changes Affecting
Cardiovascular Performance

Change	Consequence
Stiffening of vasculature, especially in aorta	Thickening of left ventricular wall; progressive increase in blood pressure
Altered response to adrenergic stimulation plus additional age-related changes	Diminished adaptive response to intense physical exercise
Age-related changes in conduction tissue	Increased frequency of and susceptibility to arrhythmias
Altered baroreflex mechanisms	Increased susceptibility to postural and postprandial hypotension
Cardiovascular changes plus altered baroreflex mechanisms	Reduction in cerebral blood flow
Thicker, less elastic, and more dilated veins	Increased susceptibility to varicosities and venous stasis

cause it is caused by risk factors that can be addressed through health education. In addition, it is included in this text because it is so closely linked to aging that it has been identified as "almost a universal age-related phenomenon in human populations" (Bierman, 1985, p. 842). Although the physiologic changes of atherosclerosis begin in early adulthood, the morbidity and mortality associated with this process are most detrimental in older adulthood, as is evident from the following statistics: atherosclerosis accounts for 25% of the deaths in people younger than 65 years of age, and it is the leading cause of death in people older than 65 years of age (Crow et al., 1996).

Atherosclerosis is the most common form of arteriosclerosis, which is the broad category of disorders that cause hardening and thickening of the arterial walls. The term comes from the Greek word *athera*, meaning "gruel." This term accurately describes the gruel-like material

found in the central portion of atherosclerotic plaques (Adelman, 1988).

The "reaction to injury" theory, first described by Ross and Glomset (1976), is a widely accepted explanation for the development of atherosclerosis. According to this theory, atherogenesis is a cyclical process that proceeds as follows:

1. The integrity of the intimal endothelium is injured as a result of repeated or continuing insults.
2. Circulating blood platelets arrive and aggregate at the site.
3. Compensatory processes eventually lead to migration of medial smooth muscle cells into the intima and the proliferation of these cells at the site of injury.
4. Lipids and connective tissue accumulate.

The initial injury may be caused by chemicals (as in hypercholesterolemia), mechanical stress (as with hypertension), or immunologic factors (as with renal transplantation). With repeated or chronic injury, this process continues; the intima becomes thicker, and blood flow over the injured sites is altered, thereby increasing the risk of further injury. The sequence of events is a vicious cycle that eventually leads to serious pathologic conditions, such as myocardial infarction or cerebrovascular accidents.

Two important factors that determine the ultimate outcome of this process are: (1) whether the injury is acute or chronic; and (2) whether the presence of LDL contributes to the progression of steps 3 and 4. This process can be halted, therefore, by eliminating the cause of injury and by decreasing the amount of LDL. This theory has been used to explain: (1) how age-related changes in the intima might contribute to atherosclerosis; (2) how risk factors might enhance lesion formation; (3) how inhibitors of platelet aggregation could interfere with lesion formation; and (4) how the process might be interrupted or retarded (Bierman, 1985).

Figure 10-1 summarizes the age-related changes, risk factors, and negative functional

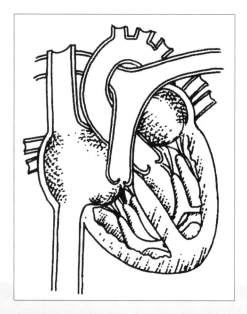

AGE-RELATED CHANGES

- Stiffening of vasculature
- Hypertrophy of left ventricular wall
- Thicker, less elastic, more dilated veins
- Altered baroreflex mechanisms
- Changes in conduction mechanism
- Increased peripheral resistance

NEGATIVE FUNCTIONAL CONSEQUENCES

- Increased blood pressure
- Diminished adaptive response to intense exercise
- Decreased cerebral blood flow
- Increased susceptibility to arrhythmias
- Increased susceptibility to postural and postprandial hypotension
- Atherosclerosis
- Varicosities

RISK FACTORS

- Hypertension
- Obesity
- Tobacco smoking
- Dietary habits that contribute to hyperlipidemia
- Inactivity

FIGURE 10-1. Cardiovascular function of older adults.

consequences that affect cardiovascular performance.

Nursing Assessment

Nursing assessment of cardiovascular function does not differ significantly in older and younger adults. In adults of any age, what is most important is to identify risks for cardiovascular disease. The primary differences between younger and older adults are the relative degree of risk associated with different factors and the manifestations of some cardiac diseases. The following sections discuss the facets of assessment specific to older adults; these can be used in conjunction with the usual methods of assessing cardiovascular function. Display 10-2 provides guidelines for assessing cardiovascular function in older adults.

Rate and Rhythm

The normal range for heart rate in older adults is the same as that for all adults, but auscultation of heart sounds differs slightly in older and younger adults. The following changes may be observed in healthy older adults, but they are insignificant in the absence of symptoms or other abnormal findings: (1) a fourth heart sound may be heard; (2) short systolic ejection murmurs are commonly heard; (3) heart borders may be difficult to percuss; and (4) heart sounds may be diminished or distant. Electrocardiographic changes observed in healthy older adults include arrhythmias, left axis deviation, bundle branch blocks, ST-T wave changes, and prolongation of the P-R interval. Other than these variations, physical assessment criteria are the same for younger and older adults. Similarly, peripheral pulses do not differ significantly between healthy older and younger adults, but disease-related conditions, such as venous stasis, are known to occur more commonly in older adults.

If a murmur, arrhythmia, or any other unusual finding is detected, it is important to determine whether it reflects a new development, a pre-existing condition that had not been identified previously, or a pre-existing condition that has already been evaluated. The nurse should ask questions to determine the person's awareness of such abnormal findings. Any of the following terms might be used by older adults to describe arrhythmias: fluttering, palpitations, skipped beats, extra beats, or flip-flops. It is advisable to ask the older person about a history of arrhythmias before auscultation, as such an inquiry immediately after auscultation could cause undue concern. Arrhythmias may be caused by cardiac diseases, electrolyte imbalances, physiologic disturbances, or adverse medication effects; alternatively, they may be harmless manifestations of age-related changes. Likewise, murmurs may be caused by age- or disease-related conditions. Therefore, when murmurs or arrhythmias are detected, their meaning should be assessed in relation to the person's history, as well as in relation to the potential underlying causes. It is also important to find out the date of the person's last electrocardiogram, because this may provide baseline information regarding the duration of asymptomatic changes.

Blood Pressure

Assessment of BP in older adults is aimed at detecting hypertension, as well as postural hypotension. The approach to treating hypertension varies according to whether one views increased BP as a harmless age-related change, a risk factor for a disease process, or an indicator of a disease process. Although only a few nurses have primary responsibility for decisions regarding medical treatment of BP, all nurses are responsible for accurate assessment of BP and for decisions regarding the implications of these findings.

Assessment of BP in older adults is complicated by the fact that their BP has an increased

DISPLAY 10-2
Guidelines for Assessing Cardiovascular Function

Interview Questions to Assess for Risk Factors

- Have any of your blood relatives had heart problems or died of heart disease (e.g., stroke, hypertension, myocardial infarctions, or peripheral vascular disease)?
- Do you have diabetes? When was the last time you had your blood sugar (glucose) level checked?
- Do you smoke, or have you ever smoked? (If yes, ask additional questions, such as those appropriate for assessing respiratory function, Chapter 11.)
- Have you ever been told you have high blood pressure, or "borderline" high blood pressure? (If yes, ask the usual questions about duration of therapy, treatment, medical care, and the like.)
- Have you ever taken any medications for blood pressure or any heart problem? (If yes, ask the usual questions about type, dose, duration of therapy, and so on.)
- What is your usual pattern of exercise?

Additional Considerations Regarding Risk Factors

- Compare the person's ideal weight to his or her present weight.
- Determine usual dietary habits, paying particular attention to the person's intake of sodium, fiber, and types of fat. This information is usually obtained during the nutritional assessment.

Interview Questions to Assess for Cardiovascular Disease

- Have you ever had a heart attack, or any problems with your heart? (If yes, ask the usual additional questions.)
- When was the last time you had an electrocardiogram done?
- Do you ever have chest pain or tightness in your chest? (If yes, ask the usual questions to explore the type, onset, duration, and other characteristics.)

- Do you ever have difficulty breathing? (If yes, ask the usual questions regarding onset and other characteristics.)
- Do you ever feel lightheaded or dizzy? (If yes, ask about specific circumstances, medical evaluation, and methods of dealing with symptoms and ensuring safety.)
- Do you ever feel like your heart is racing, is irregular, or has extra or skipped beats? (If yes, ask about any prior medical evaluation.)
- Have you ever been told you had a heart murmur? (If yes, ask about any prior medical evaluation.)

Interview Questions to Assess for Postural Hypotension

- Do you ever feel lightheaded or dizzy, especially when you get up in the morning or after you've been lying down?
- (If yes) Is this feeling accompanied by any additional symptoms, such as sweating, nausea, or confusion?
- (If yes) Do any of the risks listed in Display 10-1 apply to you? (If yes, ask about any prior medical evaluation.)

Interview Questions That May Be Asked During Other Portions of an Assessment but That Are Useful in Assessing Cardiovascular Function

- Do you tire easily or feel you need more rest than is ordinarily required?
- Do you have any problems with indigestion?
- Do your feet or ankles ever get swollen?
- Do you wake up at night because of difficulty breathing or because of any other discomfort?
- Have you made any adjustments in your sleeping habits because of difficulty breathing (e.g., do you use more than one pillow or sleep in a chair)?
- Do you have any pain in your upper back or shoulders?

tendency to fluctuate in response to postural changes and other factors. In addition, a confusing array of terminology is used with regard to BP in older adults. The term "pseudohypertension" describes the phenomenon of elevated SBP readings that result from the inability of the external cuff to compress the arteries in older people with arteriosclerosis. This phenomenon explains the finding of extremely elevated SBP readings in persons without any evidence of end-organ damage and with normal DBP readings. Finally, assessment is complicated by the evolving viewpoints about which BP parameters, particularly for SBP, are normal or harmless in older adults.

The Joint National Committee on Detection, Evaluation, and Treatment of High Blood Pressure (JNC) has published six reports, the latest of which was issued in 1997. Several of these reports have revised the classification of high BP, so a BP measurement that was considered to be "normal" in 1980 could be deemed "pathologic" in the 1990s. The JNC now rec-

ommends a classification of hypertension by stages to emphasize the risk of any degree of high BP as a factor in cardiovascular disease (JNC, 1997).

To clarify various terms, Table 10-2 defines some of the criteria used with regard to BP in older adults. Information in this table is based on a consensus of medical information from recent publications, including the 1997 guidelines published by the JNC. Display 10-3 summarizes the correct method for measuring BP, which is reviewed here to emphasize the importance of accurately assessing BP and checking for postural hypotension in older adults.

Risks for Cardiovascular Disease

The assessment of risks for cardiovascular disease provides a basis for educational interventions directed toward preventing negative functional consequences. Hypertension, including isolated systolic hypertension, has been identified as the most important remediable risk for

TABLE 10-2
Blood Pressure (BP) Terms and Definitions

Adult BP	Systolic (mm Hg)		Diastolic (mm Hg)
Optimal	<120	and	<80
Normal	<130	and	<85
High normal	130–139	or	85–89
Hypertension, Stage 1	140–159	or	90–99
Hypertension, Stage 2	160–179	or	100–109
Hypertension, Stage 3	≥180		≥110
Isolated Systolic Hypertension	≥160		<90

Definitions

Pseudohypertension: Inaccurately high readings because of arteriosclerosis

Postural systolic hypotension: A drop in systolic blood pressure of 20 mm Hg upon standing for at least 1 minute after sitting or lying for at least 5 minutes

Postural hypotension: A drop in systolic blood pressure of 20 mm Hg and a concomitant reduction in diastolic blood pressure of 10 mm Hg upon standing for at least 1 minute after sitting or lying for at least 5 minutes

Source: JNC, (1997), The sixth report of the Joint National Committee on Prevention, Detection, Evaluation, and Treatment of High Blood Pressure, *Archives of Internal Medicine, 157,* 2413–2446.

DISPLAY 10-3
Guidelines for Assessing Blood Pressure (BP)

Factors That Influence BP Measurement in Older Adults

- BP readings are more variable and more sensitive to external factors, such as food digestion or postural changes.
- The person should not have eaten a meal within 1 hour prior to having his or her BP checked.
- The person should not have ingested caffeine or smoked a cigarette within $\frac{1}{2}$ hour prior to having his or her BP checked.
- The person should be seated and resting for 5 minutes before having his or her BP checked.
- Obtain BP readings with the person in a sitting or lying position, and then again after he or she has been standing for 1 to 3 minutes (to assess for postural hypotension).
- BP measurements may be lower in hot weather or at very warm indoor temperatures.

Method of Assessing BP

- The person should be seated with arm bared and feet flat on the floor.
- Support the person's arm as near to the heart level as possible.
- Ask the person to refrain from talking while you check his or her BP.
- Use a sphygmomanometer that has been checked for accuracy.
- Use an appropriate-sized cuff (i.e., the length of the cuff bladder should be at least 80% of the circumference of the arm, and the width should be 20% wider than the diameter of the arm).
- Record the cuff size that is used. (Cuffs that are too small will yield falsely high readings, whereas cuffs that are too large will yield falsely low readings.)
- Fit the deflated cuff firmly around the upper arm, with the center of the cuff bladder over the brachial artery and the bottom of the cuff about 1 inch to 1-1/2 inches above the bend of the arm.

- Inflate the cuff to 20 or 30 mm Hg above the palpated SBP.
- Deflate the cuff at a rate of 2 to 3 mm Hg per second.
- Measure SBP at the first sound and DBP at the onset of silence.
- If auscultatory gaps are heard, estimate the SBP by applying the cuff, palpating the radial pulse, and inflating the cuff until the pulse is no longer felt. Record the magnitude and range of the gap (e.g., 184/82, auscultatory gap 176–148).
- If a very low DBP is heard, record the onset of Korotkoff phases IV and V (e.g., 138/72/10). Also, be sure not to press too hard on the stethoscope.
- Measure BP in both arms the first time. On subsequent determinations, measure BP in the arm with the higher reading.
- If sounds are difficult to auscultate, support the person's arm above his or her head for 30 seconds. Then inflate the cuff, have the person lower the arm, and measure the BP.
- If it is necessary to recheck the BP in the same arm, deflate the cuff fully before reinflating it and wait at least 2 minutes before taking another measurement.

Normal Findings

- Normal BP is less than 130 mm Hg SBP, and less than 85 mm Hg DBP.
- The normal difference between lying/sitting and standing SBPs is 20 mm Hg or less after standing for 1 minute.
- The normal difference between lying/sitting and standing DBPs is 10 mm Hg or less after standing for 1 minute.

older adults. The degree of risk from hypertension remains high at any age, but the degree of risk from other factors changes with age. Within the broad category of "older adult," the relative risks for young-old and very old people may differ. For example, gender differences and total serum cholesterol levels become less important with advanced age. It would be more important, therefore, to identify these specific risks in a 60-year-old man than in an 85-year-old man or woman.

During the 1980s, saturated and polyunsaturated fats became household words, and much public attention was focused on the role of cholesterol as a risk factor for cardiovascular disease. By the late 1980s, mass screening programs for serum cholesterol levels were as popular as the mass BP screenings of the 1970s. Although these are especially important detection programs for younger, middle-aged, and young-old adults, their value for people aged 75 years and older is now being questioned. Based on longitudinal and cross-sectional studies, gerontologists have concluded that serum cholesterol levels in men increase until the age of about 55 years, plateau around the age of 65 years, and then decline. In women, serum cholesterol levels increase until the age of 60 to 70 years, then decline (Bowlin et al., 1997). Although there is agreement about the diminishing importance of serum cholesterol levels as a risk for older adults, there is no consensus on the exact age at which this risk factor diminishes in importance.

Recent lipid research supports the increased importance of LDL and HDL levels as predictors of cardiovascular risk in older adults. High levels of HDL are considered to be protective against atherosclerosis, and they are associated with a lower risk for cardiovascular disease. In contrast, high levels of LDL are considered to be risk factors for cardiovascular disease and are potent predictors of atherosclerosis. Therefore, rather than assessing total serum cholesterol in older adults, an LDL/HDL ratio of 3.0 or

greater is recommended as the parameter for concern in this population.

Obesity, cigarette smoking, physical inactivity, glucose intolerance, and left ventricular hypertrophy are additional factors that can pose risks for cardiovascular disease in both older and younger adults. Although assessment of these factors does not vary according to age, the implications are different for older adults. Display 10-4 summarizes the risks for cardiovascular disease, with emphasis on age-specific factors. It is important to keep in mind that knowledge about risk factors for adults of any age is still evolving, and that knowledge of age-specific aspects of cardiovascular risks is one step behind in this evolution.

Manifestations of Cardiac Disease

Some cardiac diseases can easily be overlooked in older adults because the primary symptom often differs from the expected manifestations. Congestive heart failure, for example, often begins very subtly, and the early manifestations may be mental changes secondary to the physiologic stress. Consequently, older adults are likely to be in more advanced stages of heart failure before an accurate diagnosis is made (Tresch, 1997). Likewise, it has long been recognized that older people with angina and acute myocardial infarctions are likely to have subtle and unusual manifestations, rather than the classic symptom of chest pain. Studies indicate that up to 75% of all episodes of myocardial ischemia may not be accompanied by symptoms; when symptoms do occur, they often are attributed to other problems (Gottlieb and Gerstenblith, 1988). One review concluded that 40% of older patients and 25% of younger patients will present with so-called nonclassic manifestations (MacDonald, 1984).

In the Framingham Study, electrocardiograms demonstrated that 25% of acute myocardial infarctions were either silent or unrecognized; interviews of these subjects indicated that fewer than 50% were silent and that slightly more than 50% were unrecognized by the patient or the primary care provider (Kannel and Abbott, 1984). Rather than complaining of chest pain, older adults are likely to have vague symptoms, such as fatigue, dyspnea, syncope, indigestion, and mental or behavioral changes. In addition, older adults who have mobility impairments or other functional limitations may not be active enough to experience exertion-related symptoms. Therefore, the absence of chest pain in older adults is not a good indicator of the absence of coronary artery disease.

When manifestations of myocardial ischemia or other cardiac disturbances differ from what is expected, they may be attributed to a noncardiac

cause. Therefore, any complaints about digestion, respiration, or the upper trunk must be considered to be potential indicators of cardiac disease. Assessment of these complaints is complicated by the fact that older adults often have more than one underlying condition that could be responsible for the symptoms. It is not unusual, for example, for an older person to have an esophageal reflux disorder as well as a history of ischemic heart disease. In addition to asking questions specifically related to cardiovascular function, the nurse must consider assessment information regarding other functional areas. Also, a baseline electrocardiogram is helpful in establishing the possibility of silent or atypical myocardial ischemia. Display 10-2 summarizes the guidelines for assessing cardiovascular func-

---

DISPLAY 10-4
Guidelines for Assessing Risks for Cardiovascular Disease

Increased Blood Pressure as a Risk Factor

- At any age, high BP is associated with an increased risk of morbidity and mortality from stroke, heart disease, and peripheral vascular disease.
- For older adults, hypertension is the most important remediable risk factor for cardiovascular disease.
- Increased DBP and SBP, and an elevated pulse pressure, are important risk factors for stroke, cardiovascular disease, and coronary heart disease.
- Studies have shown that successful treatment of hypertension reduces the risks of cardiovascular morbidity and mortality.
- In 1992, the Joint National Committee on Detection, Evaluation, and Treatment of High Blood Pressure concluded that the value of treating hypertension in older patients had been well established.

Blood Lipids

- After the age of 60 years in men and 70 years in women, the level of total serum cholesterol becomes less important as a risk factor.

- With increasing age, low serum levels of HDL and high levels of LDL become increasingly important as risk factors for cardiovascular disease.

Additional Risk Factors and Considerations

- With increased age, cigarette smoking remains a significant risk factor for respiratory diseases, cardiovascular mortality, and specific cardiovascular diseases, such as stroke and intermittent claudication.
- Diabetes mellitus is an important risk factor for cardiovascular morbidity and mortality, particularly in older women.
- Obesity is less significant as a risk factor in older women than in younger women, but it remains a risk factor, particularly for older men.
- Low vital capacity is highly associated with increased risk for cardiovascular mortality, particularly in older women.
- Vigorous exercise may be beneficial in reducing the risks of cardiovascular disease.

tion in older adults. This guide emphasizes the assessment components that are unique to older adults and refers to additional assessment components that apply to adults in general.

Nursing Diagnosis

If the nursing assessment identifies risks for impaired cardiovascular function in a healthy older adult, a nursing diagnosis of Altered Health Maintenance may be applicable. This is defined as "the state in which an individual or group experiences or is at risk of experiencing a disruption in health because of an unhealthy life-style or lack of knowledge to manage a condition" (Carpenito, 1997, p. 427). Related factors common in older adults include lack of regular aerobic exercise, cultural influences on patterns of food intake and preparation, and insufficient knowledge about low-sodium diets, dietary measures to control cholesterol levels, and the effects of tobacco use. The case example at the end of this chapter addresses this type of nursing diagnosis.

For older adults with impaired cardiovascular function, applicable nursing diagnoses may include Activity Intolerance, Decreased Cardiac Output, Altered Cardiopulmonary Tissue Perfusion, and Potential Complication: Cardiac/Vascular. The nursing diagnosis of High Risk for Injury may be appropriate for older adults with postural or postprandial hypotension, particularly in the presence of additional risk factors for falls and fractures (e.g., osteoporosis, neurologic disorders, and medication side effects).

Nursing Goals

One nursing goal for improved cardiovascular function in older adults is to alleviate the risk factors that cause or contribute to cardiovascular disease. This is achieved primarily through interventions that address hypertension and

through dietary modifications to reduce cholesterol levels. Lifestyle interventions, such as exercise, are important preventive measures in reducing the risk of cardiovascular disease. Preventive measures are particularly important in young-old adults, but should not be overlooked even in nonagenarians.

Another goal for improved cardiovascular function is to prevent postural hypotension or to minimize its negative consequences if it cannot be prevented. This is achieved through health education regarding the prevention of postural hypotension and through interventions that address the effects of postural hypotension. These interventions are important because postural hypotension can lead to serious consequences, such as falls and fractures.

A third goal is maintaining quality of life by enhancing the older adult's adaptive response to physiologic stress. Physical exercise is the primary intervention for enhancing one's adaptive response to physical stress. This preventive measure also reduces the risks of cardiovascular disease and postural hypotension.

Nursing Interventions

Eliminating Hypertension as a Risk Factor for Cardiovascular Disease

As emphasized earlier, the single most important and remediable risk factor for cardiovascular disease in older adults is hypertension. Although this is the most important area of intervention, geriatric practitioners may differ significantly in their approaches to medical interventions. The evolving recommendations about hypertension can be particularly problematic for nurses, even though decisions about medication are generally made by primary care providers. Nurses assess BP much more frequently than do primary care providers, and they are responsible for making decisions about the appropriate steps to take based on BP findings. In institutional settings, nurses administer prescribed antihypertensive medications and make decisions about the effects of medical interventions. In home and community settings, nurses educate older adults and their caregivers regarding the significance of BP readings. In all settings, nurses decide whether a primary care provider should be contacted regarding BP findings. Additionally, they are responsible for evaluating the response of an older person to prescribed medications and for educating older adults and their caregivers about medication interventions. Nurses, therefore, have a great deal of decision-making responsibility regarding the management of hypertension, and they must base their decisions on up-to-date and reliable information.

Because nurses work in conjunction with many primary care providers in planning and carrying out medical interventions for hypertension, it is helpful to understand the different medical approaches to the evaluation and treatment of hypertension. The approach of primary care providers who formed their opinions before 1980 and have not changed their approach since then may differ from the approach of primary care providers who base their practice on the most recent recommendations of the JNC. These are important considerations because, since the mid-1980s, two of the commonly accepted beliefs about hypertension in older adults have been challenged.

First, the premise that an SBP of "100 plus your age" is both normal and harmless has been challenged by studies showing that the oldest age groups have the greatest relative risk for any given SBP. Indeed, based on the recommendations of the JNC, this adage is applicable only up until the age of 40 years! The 1997 JNC report recommended a classification of high BP applicable to all adults (see Table 10-2). The report emphasized the importance of treating hypertension in older people, basing this recommendation on studies demonstrating the benefits of treatment regardless of age, race, sex, and BP subclassifications. One precautionary statement

issued by the JNC emphasizes that antihypertensive drug therapy should be initiated and monitored with increasing caution in older adults. Specifically, the JNC suggests that the starting dose of a medication should be about half of that used in younger patients, and that drugs that can cause hypotension or cognitive dysfunction be avoided (JNC, 1997). In addition, the JNC emphasizes the importance of lifestyle modifications in the treatment and prevention of hypertension. Specific recommendations regarding lifestyle modifications and pharmacologic interventions for hypertension in older adults are presented in Display 10-5.

Second, the premise that the risks of antihypertensive medication are greater than the risks of nontreatment has been refuted by numerous studies. Clinical trials of diuretics, for example, show that these are safe agents for controlling hypertension and reducing the risk of cardiovascular events. Although adverse effects of antihypertensive medications commonly occur, they are no more common in older than in younger adults.

Consideration also must be given to the cost of medications, their potential side effects, and drug-drug interactions, including interactions with over-the-counter preparations. For example, oral decongestants can interact with many types of antihypertensive agents. No matter what pharmacologic approach is taken, adverse effects must be considered on an individualized basis. With the great variety of antihypertensive agents available, the choice of medication is based on both its therapeutic effectiveness and its potential for adverse effects. This is an important consideration for older adults with functional impairments, as the degree of risk from adverse effects is at least partially related to the type of functional impairment that exists. For example, if postural hypotension is an adverse effect of a medication, this is potentially more detrimental to a frail but ambulatory 85-year-old woman than to a nonambulatory older

DISPLAY 10-5
Guidelines for Nursing Management of Hypertension

Considerations Regarding the Treatment of Hypertension

- Risks from and definitions of hypertension apply to all age categories (refer to Table 10-2 for criteria).
- A person's BP should be measured at least 3 times before making any decisions about treatment.
- When hypertension is diagnosed, its probable duration should be considered when deciding on the initial treatment step. (For example, if a 90-year-old person has a BP reading of 180/95 but has not had a BP check in 5 years, this condition has probably developed gradually and so should be treated conservatively.)
- Studies have demonstrated the safety and effectiveness of medications for treating hypertension in older adults.
- The safety of antihypertensive agents is improved by carefully selecting the medication, starting with low doses, and changing the medication regimen gradually, in small increments, if necessary.

Treatment Goals

- The goals of hypertensive treatment are to control BP by the least intrusive means and to prevent cardiovascular morbidity and mortality.
- Treatment is directed toward achieving and maintaining an SBP of less than 140 mm Hg and a DBP of less than 90 mm Hg.
- BP reduction to 130/85 mm Hg is recommended if this can be achieved without compromising cardiovascular function.

- For older adults with isolated systolic hypertension or SBP levels of 140 to 160 mm Hg, lifestyle modifications should be the first treatment step.
- The initial goal of therapy for those with a SBP of greater than 180 mm Hg is to reduce the SBP to less than 160 mm Hg.
- For older adults with SBP measurements of between 160 and 179 mm Hg, the initial goal is to reduce the SBP by 20 mm Hg.
- If initial treatment is well tolerated, further reduction of the SBP should be considered.

Treatment Approaches

- Lifestyle modifications can be used as an initial step for a 3- to 6-month trial.
- Lifestyle modifications that are recommended for preventing and treating high BP include: (1) avoidance of tobacco; (2) a no-added-salt or 2-g sodium diet; (3) weight reduction when appropriate (i.e., when the person weighs more than 110% of his or her ideal weight); (4) regular physical exercise (i.e., 30 to 45 minutes of brisk walking 3 to 5 times weekly); and (5) limitation of alcohol intake to 1 oz per day (e.g., 2 oz of 100-proof whiskey, 8 oz of wine, or 24 oz of beer).
- Lifestyle modifications that can reduce the risk of cardiovascular disease should also be incorporated into the treatment plan (see Display 10-6).

adult. When antihypertensive medications are used judiciously, their benefits far outweigh their risks.

The stepped-care approach to hypertension, initially recommended in the first JNC report published in the 1970s, has become widely accepted since then. In the subsequent five reports,

the stepped-care approach was consistently recommended, but the specific types of medications used in each step have changed as newer agents have been developed. Using the stepped-care approach, lifestyle modifications might be tried initially, followed by drug therapy with diuretics or beta-blockers. Although many newer and equally effective antihypertensive medications are now available, the JNC does not recommend these for initial drug therapy because of the lack of long-term, controlled trials to demonstrate their efficacy in reducing morbidity and mortality. Also, the newer drugs are generally more expensive than the older drugs, so the cost of the medication must be considered, particularly in the case of older adults for whom medication costs are usually out-of-pocket expenses. Another consideration governing the selection of antihypertensive drugs is that, in general, Blacks are more responsive to diuretics and calcium antagonists than to beta-blockers or angiotensin-converting enzyme (ACE) inhibitors. Additional cultural aspects of hypertension prevalence and treatment are summarized in the Culture Box. Age and gender have not been found to affect drug responsiveness (JNC, 1997).

Display 10-5 presents guidelines for nursing decisions regarding interventions for hypertension. This information is based primarily on the 1997 recommendations of the JNC. These guidelines can be used for nursing decisions regarding all of the following interventions: administering prescribed medications, communicating with primary care providers about BP findings, and educating older adults and their caregivers about hypertension.

Addressing Lifestyle Factors and Other Risks for Cardiovascular Disease

Physical exercise provides significant benefits to older adults in terms of improving cardiovascular performance and reducing risks for impaired cardiovascular function. Studies of age-matched sedentary and physically active older people have identified the following positive consequences of physical conditioning: lower body fat ratios, lower BP measurements, lower resting heart rates, improved physical working capacity, and lower rates of myocardial infarction. Numerous studies suggest that the positive effects of three $\frac{1}{2}$-hour periods of aerobic exercise per week include a significant improvement in cardiovascular function. One recent study of older and younger male runners concluded that the men who were age 60 years and older had reduced heart disease risk in proportion to their vigorous activity (Williams, 1998). Additional positive effects of exercise in other functional areas are noted throughout this text, and this information can be used in educating older

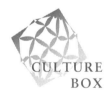

CULTURE
BOX

Cultural Aspects of Hypertension Prevalence and Treatment

- The prevalence of hypertension is higher in Blacks than in Whites.
- Hypertension tends to appear at an earlier age, to be more severe, and to be associated with higher rates of morbidity and mortality in Blacks than in Whites.
- Hypertension has increased among American Indians since the 1950s, but it is still lower than in other ethnic groups in the United States.
- Response to hypertension medications may vary by race (e.g., Blacks tend to respond better to diuretics or calcium channel blockers, Whites may respond better to beta blockers and ACE inhibitors).
- Chinese Americans and some other cultural groups are likely to use herbal medicines for hypertension.

adults about the many positive functional consequences of regular physical exercise.

Additional preventive measures are directed toward early detection of risks from hypertension and hyperlipidemia. Health measures are also directed toward eliminating risks associated with lifestyle. Dietary measures aimed at lowering blood cholesterol levels, which are no less important in older adults than in younger adults, are summarized in Display 10-6 and reviewed in the article by Yen (1998) listed in the References at the end of this chapter. Interventions that address the risks for cardiovascular disease are summarized in Display 10-6, which is written in nontechnical terms so that it can be used in educating older adults.

In recent years, there has been a growing consensus that hormonal replacement therapy in menopausal women confers a protective effect against stroke, myocardial infarction, ischemic heart disease, and coronary artery disease. However, controversy persists about the risks associated with hormonal replacement therapy, and menopausal women are advised to discuss both the risks and benefits with their primary care provider. Details concerning the risks and benefits of hormonal replacement therapy are discussed in Chapter 16 and summarized in Display 16-6. In the past few years, there has also been increasing consensus regarding the role of low-dose aspirin therapy in preventing and treating cardiovascular disease. Because aspirin therapy, even when administered in low doses, is accompanied by the risks of gastrointestinal distress and bleeding, people should consult their health care provider before initiating this measure. Certain alternative and preventive health care practices, as summarized in the box below, also may be effective in addressing the risks that affect cardiovascular function.

ALTERNATIVE AND PREVENTIVE HEALTH CARE PRACTICES

Promoting Cardiovascular Function

Herbs
- For atherosclerosis: garlic, hawthorn, alfalfa
- For reducing cholesterol: garlic, hawthorn, bilberry, fenugreek, capsaicin, gogulipid, oat bran
- For circulatory problems: ginger, ginkgo, hawthorn
- For high blood pressure: garlic, hawthorn

Homeopathic Remedies
- Hawthorn

Nutritional Considerations
- Zinc, calcium, magnesium, potassium, coenzyme Q_{10}, and vitamins A, B-complex, C, and E
- A diet high in fiber, garlic, and potassium, and low in salt, sugar, caffeine, and saturated fats

Preventive Measures and Additional Approaches
- Aerobic exercise for 30 minutes 3 times weekly
- No smoking; maintenance of ideal body weight
- Yoga, music, relaxation, meditation, imagery, acupuncture, reflexology, biofeedback, t'ai chi, autogenic training
- Aromatherapy: rose, lavender, peppermint, marjoram

DISPLAY 10-6
Education Regarding Risks for Cardiovascular Disease

Detection of Risks in Healthy Older Adults

- Have blood pressure checked annually.
- If the total serum cholesterol level is less than 200 mg/dL, have it rechecked every 5 years.
- If the total serum cholesterol level is between 200 and 239 mg/dL, follow dietary measures to reduce it and have it rechecked annually.
- If the total serum cholesterol level is 240 mg/dL or more, obtain a further medical evaluation.

Reduction of Risks

- Maintain weight at a level less than 110% of ideal weight.
- Exercise daily, and engage in aerobic exercise (i.e., exercise that increases the pulse rate) several times weekly for 30 to 45 minutes each time.
- If you smoke, quit.
- Avoid "passive smoking" (i.e., inhaling smoke from other people's cigarettes).
- Avoid foods that are high in sodium, and follow dietary measures to reduce serum cholesterol levels.
- Discuss with your primary care provider the use of low-dose aspirin therapy as a preventive measure, particularly if there is any history of coronary artery disease or cerebrovascular events.
- Menopausal and postmenopausal women should discuss with their primary care provider the risks and benefits of hormonal replacement therapy.

Dietary Measures to Reduce Cholesterol Levels

- Limit total fat intake to less than 30% of your total daily calorie intake.
- Limit saturated fat intake to less than 10% of your total daily calorie intake.
- Limit total daily cholesterol intake to between 250 and 350 mg.

- Polyunsaturated and monounsaturated fatty acids are better for you than saturated fatty acids and hard fats.
- Vegetable oils (e.g., corn, olive, peanut, and safflower oils) generally are high in unsaturated fatty acids.
- The most common polyunsaturated fatty acid is linoleic acid, which can lower serum LDL cholesterol levels when it is substituted for saturated fatty acids in the diet.
- The most common monounsaturated fatty acid is oleic acid, which generally has a neutral or beneficial effect on cholesterol levels.
- Avoid the following saturated fatty acids, as they usually raise serum cholesterol levels: lauric, myristic, and palmitic.
- Stearic acid is one saturated fatty acid that is thought to lower serum cholesterol levels.
- Hard fats, which are derived from animal sources (e.g., dairy products) and certain plants (e.g., palm and coconut oils), tend to contain increased amounts of saturated fatty acids.
- Use skim or 1% milk rather than whole milk.
- Use nonfat or low-fat yogurt, sour cream, cream cheese, and cottage cheese.
- Use nonfat or low-fat dairy desserts (e.g., nonfat frozen yogurt).
- Limit consumption of butter or margarine.
- Limit consumption of egg yolks, including those in food, to two or three per week.
- Use egg whites or egg substitutes instead of whole eggs.
- Limit consumption of lean meats to five or fewer 3- to 5-ounce servings per week.
- Trim fat off meats and the skin off poultry.
- Avoid eating processed meats (e.g., bacon, bologna, sausage, hot dogs).
- Avoid gravies, fried foods, and organ meats.
- Include foods that are high in fiber content in your daily diet.

Preventing and Managing Postural Hypotension

Interventions aimed at preventing postural and postprandial hypotension can be initiated as overall health measures for older adults who have the risk factors listed in Display 10-1. It should be noted that this includes all people aged 75 years and older. For older adults with symptomatic postural hypotension, interven-tions to alleviate the problem are important in terms of maintaining quality of life and pre-venting serious consequences. When symptom-atic postural hypotension cannot be alleviated, interventions must be directed toward ensuring the individual's safety, particularly in terms of preventing falls and fractures. These three levels of interventions are summarized in Display 10-7.

DISPLAY 10-7
Education Regarding Postural Hypotension

Prevention of Postural and Postprandial Hypotension

- Maintain adequate fluid intake.
- Avoid excessive alcohol consumption.
- Avoid medications that increase the risk for postural hypotension, particularly if addi-tional risk factors are present. (Refer to Dis-play 10-1.)
- Maintain good physical fitness, especially good muscle tone.
- Avoid sitting for prolonged periods or stand-ing still after meals.
- Avoid sources of intense heat (e.g., direct sun, electric blankets, and hot baths and showers), as these cause peripheral vasodi-lation.
- Minimize the risk of postprandial hypoten-sion by taking antihypertensive medications 1 hour after meals rather than before meals.
- Eat small, frequent meals to reduce the risk of postprandial hypotension.
- If taking nitroglycerin, do not take it while standing.

Management of Postural Hypotension

- Change your position slowly, especially when moving from a sitting or lying position to a standing position.
- Before standing up, sit at the side of the bed for several minutes after rising from a lying position.
- Avoid prolonged standing; try to sit while performing activities that can be done in a sit-ting rather than standing position.
- Maintain adequate fluid intake, but avoid di-uretic beverages (e.g., caffeinated beverages).

- Engage in regular, but not excessive, exercise. (Swimming is an excellent form of exercise because the hydrostatic pressure prevents blood from pooling in the legs.)
- Wear a waist-high elastic support garment or thigh-high elastic stockings during the day, and put them on before getting out of bed in the morning.
- Sleep with the head of the bed elevated on blocks.
- Avoid alcohol consumption.
- Avoid large meals.
- Avoid strenuous exercise, especially for 2 hours after meals.
- During the day, rest in a recliner chair with your legs elevated.
- Take measures to prevent constipation and avoid straining during bowel movements.
- Observe safety precautions (see below).

Prevention of Negative Functional Consequences If Hypotension Cannot Be Prevented

- Reduce the potential for falls and other nega-tive functional consequences of postprandial hypotension by remaining seated (or by lying down) after meals.
- Use a call system if help is needed with walking.
- Adapt the environment to minimize the risk and consequences of falling (e.g., ensure good lighting, install grab bars, keep pathways clear).

Evaluating Nursing Care

Nursing care is evaluated according to the degree to which nursing goals have been achieved. Short-term goals that address the risk factors for impaired cardiovascular function would be evaluated by the extent to which the older adult verbalizes correct information about the risks. Also, the older adult may verbalize an intent to change or eliminate the lifestyle factors that increase the risk of impaired cardiovascular function. For example, the older adult may agree to join an exercise program for seniors and to follow dietary measures to reduce serum cholesterol levels. Long-term goals would be measured by determining the actual reduction in risk factors. For example, the person's serum cholesterol level may decrease from 238 to 198 mg/dL after 6 months of regular exercise and dietary modifications. For older adults with impaired cardiovascular function, the nurse would evaluate the extent to which the person's signs and symptoms are alleviated. Evaluation would also address the extent to which the older adult verbalizes correct information about their impaired cardiovascular status.

Chapter Summary

Age-related changes in cardiovascular function increase the susceptibility of older adults to atherosclerosis, cardiac arrhythmias, and postural and postprandial hypotension. Age-related changes also interfere with their adaptive response to intense exercise. Factors that increase the risk of impaired cardiovascular function include obesity, hypertension, tobacco use, physical inactivity, and dietary habits that contribute to hyperlipidemia. Risk factors that contribute to postural hypotension include systemic diseases and adverse medication effects. Functional consequences include atherosclerosis and an increased susceptibility to cardiac arrhythmias.

Nursing assessment focuses on identifying remediable factors that increase the risk of cardiovascular disease. Cardiovascular assessment of older and younger adults does not differ significantly, but the manifestations of heart disease may be more subtle and less predictable in older adults. Relevant nursing diagnoses include Altered Health Maintenance, Decreased Cardiac Output, and Altered Cardiopulmonary Tissue Perfusion. Nursing interventions focus on the risk factors that actually or potentially interfere with cardiovascular function. For healthy older adults, nursing care is evaluated according to their increased knowledge of factors that influence cardiovascular function and their expressed intent to address the identified risk factors. For older adults with impaired cardiovascular function, nursing care is evaluated according to their improved comfort and level of function.

Critical Thinking Exercises

1. Discuss how each of the following factors influence cardiovascular function, including postural hypotension: lifestyle, medications, age-related changes, and pathologic conditions.
2. Demonstrate how you would teach a home health aide to assess blood pressure and postural hypotension correctly.
3. Describe the questions and considerations you would include in an assessment of cardiovascular function in an older adult who has no complaints of heart problems, but who has a history of falling twice in the past month and who has not been evaluated by a primary care provider in the past year.
4. You are asked to give a health education talk entitled "Keeping Your Heart Healthy" at a senior center. What information would you include in the presentation? What local resources (i.e., specific addresses and phone numbers of agencies or organizations in your area) would you suggest your audience contact for further information? What audiovi-

sual aids would you use? How would you involve the participants in the discussion?

5. You are working in an assisted-living facility and several of the residents have postural hy-potension. What would you include in your health education with regard to management of postural hypotension?

Case Example and Nursing Care Plan

Pertinent Case Information

Mr. C. is a 68-year-old African American who frequently comes to your Senior Wellness Clinic for a blood pressure check. He has been taking hydrochlorothia-zide, 25 mg, and verapamil, 120 mg, every morning, and his blood pressure measurements range between 130/84 and 126/80. Mr. C. sees his primary care provider once a year and obtains additional health care through community resources, such as health fairs. During his monthly appointment with you, he brings a paper with the results of a screening test indicating that his total cholesterol level is 220 mg/dL. Mr. C. states that, 6 months ago, his primary care provider told him he didn't have to worry about his cholesterol level. However, he doesn't know whether his cholesterol level was checked at that time. He does not want to return to his primary care provider until his annual appointment, but he is worried about his cholesterol level because his screening test results are "on the high side."

Nursing Assessment

You assess Mr. C.'s knowledge about the risks for impaired cardiovascular function, and you try to identify relevant risk factors. Mr. C. reports that his mother died in her early fifties from a heart attack, and that his father died in an accident at the age of 25 years. Mr. C. has had hypertension since the age of 24 years, and his daughter has been told she has "borderline high blood pressure." Mr. C. does not smoke tobacco, nor does anyone in the household. He gets very little exercise and weighs 210 pounds, which is about 30 pounds over his ideal weight. He knows that exercise is associated with weight control but is unaware of the relationship between exercise and cardiovascular function.

You find out that Mr. C. has no knowledge about dietary sources of choles-terol and that he consumes a diet high in what he terms "soul food." Although he says he has heard a lot about "good and bad cholesterol" in the news, he does not know which foods are good or bad. He tries to buy foods that say "no cholesterol" on the label, but he says the labels are too confusing about the different kinds of fats. Mr. C. and his wife live with their daughter and her teenage children. Mr. and Mrs. C. usually do the family grocery shopping, and his wife and daughter prepare the family meals.

A diet history reveals that the family usually eats fried fish or chicken about 4 times a week and pig's feet or ham hocks for the other main meals. Common side dishes are corn, okra, grits, cornbread, sweet potatoes, black-eyed peas, and fried greens. For cooking, they use lard, saltpork, or bacon drippings. Their usual beverage is decaffeinated coffee with sugar and cream. The family generally has cereal and toast for breakfast, but they have bacon and eggs on Saturdays and Sundays. Mr. and Mrs. C. eat their noon meal at the senior center 5 days a week.

Nursing Diagnosis

Your nursing diagnosis is Altered Health Maintenance related to lack of regular exercise, dietary habits that contribute to hyperlipidemia, and insufficient information about lifestyle factors that increase the risk of cardiovascular disease. Evidence of these risk factors comes from Mr. C.'s inactivity, eating patterns, history of hypertension, and family history of cardiovascular disease. Also, Mr. C. has verbalized insufficient information about the relationship between exercise and cardiovascular function and about dietary measures to control cholesterol.

Goals	Nursing Interventions	Evaluation Criteria
To increase Mr. C.'s knowledge of risk factors for cardiovascular impairment	Discuss the risk factors for impaired cardiovascular function, using information from Display 10-4. Emphasize the risk factors that can be addressed through lifestyle modifications (e.g., exercise, weight loss, and dietary measures to control cholesterol levels).	Mr. C. will be able to describe his risk factors for cardiovascular disease. Mr. C. will identify those risk factors that he can address through lifestyle changes.
To increase Mr. C.'s knowledge of the relationship between diet and serum cholesterol levels	Use teaching materials obtained from the American Heart Association to illustrate the relationship between diet and serum cholesterol levels. Provide a copy of these pamphlets for Mr. C. to take home. Suggest that Mr. C. discuss the information in the pamphlets with his wife and daughter. Ask Mr. C. to bring his wife to the nursing clinic next month so you can talk with both of them about dietary measures to control cholesterol.	Mr. C. will accurately describe the relationship between food intake and cholesterol levels. Mr. C. will identify family eating habits that contribute to his elevated serum cholesterol level.
Mr. C. will modify one dietary habit that contributes to his high cholesterol level.	Work with Mr. C. to make a list of the foods associated with high cholesterol levels (e.g., fried foods, ham hocks, lard, bacon and eggs).	Mr. C. will state that he is willing to change one eating habit that contributes to his high cholesterol level. Next month, Mr. C. will report

Give Mr. C. a copy of Display 10-6 and use this to discuss dietary measures to reduce cholesterol.

Ask Mr. C. to select one change in dietary habits that will have a positive effect on his cholesterol level (e.g., switching from lard to vegetable oil for frying foods).

that he has changed one eating pattern that contributes to high cholesterol levels.

Mr. C. will increase his knowledge about the relationship between exercise and cardiovascular function.

Use pamphlets from the American Heart Association to teach about the effects of aerobic exercise on cardiovascular function.

Review information about the relationship between exercise and weight.

Mr. C. will describe the beneficial effects of regular aerobic exercise.

Mr. C. will begin exercising on a regular basis.

Discuss ways in which Mr. C. can incorporate regular exercise into his daily activities.

Invite Mr. C. and his wife to participate in the daily "Eldercise" program that is offered following the noon meal at the senior center.

Mr. C. will verbalize a commitment to perform 30 minutes of exercise 3 days a week.

To eliminate lifestyle factors that increase the risk for cardiovascular disease

Ask Mr. C. to invite his wife to your monthly appointments so that she can also receive important health education.

Identify a plan that will enable Mr. and Mrs. C. to gradually incorporate additional dietary measures aimed at reducing cholesterol into the family meal plans.

Identify a plan that will enable Mr. and Mrs. C. to include 30 minutes of exercise 3 times a week.

Discuss weight reduction with Mr. C. and emphasize that dietary modifications and regular exercise are interventions that should facilitate weight loss.

Mr. C.'s total cholesterol level will be ≤200 mg/dL at the end of 6 months.

Mr. C.'s serum cholesterol level will remain below 200 mg/dL.

Mr. C. will report that he engages in 30 minutes of exercise 3 times weekly.

Mr. C. will report that he follows the dietary measures presented in Display 10-6.

Mr. C.'s weight will be reduced to between 180 and 198 pounds and he will maintain that weight.

Educational Resources

American Heart Association
7272 Greenville Avenue
Dallas, TX 75231-4596
(214) 373-6300; (800) 242-8721
www.americanheart.org

National Heart, Lung, and Blood Institute
Information Center
National High Blood Pressure Education Program
Latino Cardiovascular Health Resources
P.O. Box 30105
Bethesda, MD 20824-0105
(301) 251-1222
www.nhlbi.nih.gov/nhlbi/nhlbi.htm

National Stroke Association
96 Inverness Drive East, Suite I
Englewood, CO 80112-5112
(800) 787-6537
www.stroke.org

References

Adelman, B. (1988). Peripheral vascular disease. In J. W. Rowe & R. W. Besdine (Eds.), *Geriatric medicine* (pp. 219–230). Boston: Little, Brown.

Aronow, W. S. (1990). Cardiac risk factors: Still important in the elderly. *Geriatrics, 45*(1), 71–80.

Aronow, W. S., & Ahn, C. (1997). Association of postprandial hypotension with incidence of falls, syncope, coronary events, stroke, and total mortality at 29-month follow-up in 499 older nursing home residents. *Journal of the American Geriatrics Society, 45,* 1051–1053.

Bierman, E. L. (1985). Arteriosclerosis and aging. In C. E. Finch & E. L. Schneider (Eds.), *Handbook of the biology of aging* (pp. 842–868). New York: Van Nostrand Reinhold.

Bowlin, S. J., Medalie, J. H., & Pearson, T. A. (1997). Cholesterol and vascular disease in the elderly. *Nutrition, Health & Aging, 1*(1), 51–61.

Carpenito, L. J. (1997). *Nursing diagnosis: Application to clinical practice* (7th ed.). Philadelphia: J. B. Lippincott.

Crow, M. T., Bilato, C., & Lakatta, E. G. (1996). Atherosclerosis. In J. E. Birren (Ed.), *Encyclopedia of gerontology: Age, aging, and the aged* (Vol. 1, pp. 123–129). New York: Academic Press.

Finucane, F. F., Madans, J. H., Bush, T. L., Wolf, P. H., & Kleinman, J. C. (1993). Decreased risk of stroke among postmenopausal hormone users: Results from a national cohort. *Archives of Internal Medicine, 153,* 73–79.

Fleg, J. L., & Kennedy, H. L. (1982). Cardiac arrhythmias in a healthy elderly population. *Chest, 81,* 302–307.

Gardner, A. W., & Poehlman, E. T. (1995). Predictors of the age-related increase in blood pressure in men and women. *Journal of Gerontology: Medical Sciences 50A*(1), M1–M6.

Gottlieb, S. O., & Gerstenblith, G. (1988). Silent myocardial ischemia in the elderly: Current concepts. *Geriatrics, 43*(4), 29–33.

Harris, T., Lipsitz, L. A., Kleinman, J. C., & Cornoni-Huntley, J. (1991). Postural change in blood pressure associated with age and systolic blood pressure: The National Health and Nutrition Examination Survey II. *Journal of Gerontology: Medical Sciences, 46,* M159–M163.

Heseltine, D., Dakkak, M., Woodhouse, K., Macdonald, I. A., & Potter, J. F. (1991). The effect of caffeine on postprandial hypotension in the elderly. *Journal of the American Geriatrics Society, 39,* 160–164.

Howard, G., Wagenknecht, L. E., Burke, G. L., Diez-Roux, A., Evans, G. W., McGovern, P., et al. (1998). Cigarette smoking and progression of atherosclerosis. *Journal of the American Medical Association, 279,* 119–124.

Jansen, R. W. M. M., & Hoefnagels, W. H. L. (1991). Hormonal mechanisms of postprandial hypotension. *Journal of the American Geriatrics Society, 39,* 1201–1207.

Joint National Committee on Prevention, Detection, Evaluation, and Treatment of High Blood Pressure (JNC). (1997). The sixth report of the Joint National Committee on Prevention, Detection, Evaluation, and Treatment of High Blood Pressure (JNC VI). *Archives of Internal Medicine, 157,* 2413–2446.

Kannel, W. B., & Abbott, R. D. (1984). Incidence and progress of unrecognized myocardial infarction: Based on 26 years' follow-up in Framingham study. In W. Rutishouser & H. Roskamm (Eds.), *Silent myocardial ischemia* (pp. 131–137). Berlin: Springer-Verlag.

Kannel, W. B., & Vokonas, P. S. (1985). Cardiovascular risk factors in the elderly: The Framingham study. In G. L. Maddox & E. W. Busse (Eds.), *Aging: The universal human experience* (pp. 134–152). New York: Springer.

Krajewski, A., Freeman, R., Ruthazer, R., Kelley, M., & Lipsitz, L. A. (1993). Transcranial Doppler assessment of the cerebral circulation during postprandial hypotension in the elderly. *Journal of the American Geriatrics Society, 41,* 19–24.

Lakatta, E. G. (1988). Cardiovascular system aging. In B. Kent & R. N. Butler (Eds.), *Human aging research: Concepts and techniques* (pp. 199–219). New York: Raven Press.

Lipsitz, L. A. (1989). Altered blood pressure homeostasis in advanced age: Clinical and research implications. *Journal of Gerontology: Medical Sciences, 44,* M179–M183.

Lipsitz, L. A., & Fullerton, K. J. (1986). Postprandial blood pressure reductions in healthy elderly. *Journal of the American Geriatrics Society, 34,* 267–270.

MacDonald, J. B. (1984). Presentation of acute myocardial infarction in the elderly: A review. *Age and Ageing, 13,* 196–200.

Ogawa, T., Spina, R. J., Martin, W. H., Kohrt, W. M.,

Schechtman, K. B., Holloszy, J. O., & Ehsani, A. A. (1992). Effects of aging, sex, and physical training on cardiovascular responses to exercise. *Circulation, 86,* 494–503.

Patel, A., Maloney, A., & Damato, A. N. (1993). On the frequency and reproducibility of orthostatic blood pressure changes in healthy community-dwelling elderly during 60-degree head-up tilt. *American Heart Journal, 126,* 184–188.

Pearson, J. D., Morrell, C. H., Brant, L. J., Landis, P. K., & Fleg, J. L. (1997). Age-associated changes in blood pressure in a longitudinal study of healthy men and women. *Journal of Gerontology: Medical Sciences, 52A*(3), M177–M183.

Rodeheffer, R. J., & Gerstenblith, G. (1985). Effect of age on cardiovascular function. In H. A. Johnson (Ed.), *Relations between normal aging and disease* (pp. 85–99). New York: Raven Press.

Rodeheffer, R. J., Gerstenblith, G., Becker, L. C., Fleg, J. L., Weisfeldt, M. L., & Lakatta, E. G. (1984). Exercise cardiac output is maintained with advancing age in healthy human subjects: Cardiac dilatation and increased stroke volume compensate for a diminished heart rate. *Circulation, 69,* 203–213.

Ross, R., & Glomset, J. (1976). The pathogenesis of atherosclerosis. *New England Journal of Medicine, 295,* 369, 420.

Rutan, G. H., Hermanson, B., Bild, D. E., Kittner, S. J., LaBaw, F., & Tell, G. S. (1992). Orthostatic hypotension in older adults: The Cardiovascular Health Study. *Hypertension, 19,* 508–519.

Svanborg, A. (1996). Cardiovascular system. In J. E. Birren (Ed.), *Encyclopedia of gerontology: Age, aging, and the aged* (Vol. 1, pp. 245–251). New York: Academic Press.

Tammaro, A. E., Casale, G., & deNicola, P. (1986). Circadian rhythms of heart rate and premature ventricular beats in the aged. *Age and Ageing, 15,* 93–98.

Tresch, D. D. (1997). The clinical diagnosis of heart failure in older patients. *Journal of the American Geriatrics Society, 45,* 1128–1133.

Wei, J. Y. (1988). Cardiovascular system. In J. W. Rowe & R. W. Besdine (Eds.), *Geriatric medicine* (pp. 167–192). Boston: Little, Brown.

Williams, P. T. (1998). Coronary heart disease risk factors of vigorously active sexagenarians and septuagenarians. *Journal of the American Geriatrics Society, 46,* 134–142.

Yen, P. K. (1998). Stopping heart disease with diet. *Geriatric Nursing, 19,* 50–51.

Respiratory Function

Chapter

11

*T*he primary functions of respiration are to supply oxygen to the blood and remove carbon dioxide. Adequate respiratory performance is essential to life because all body organs and tissues need oxygen. For these reasons, it is noteworthy that respiratory function shows very little age-related decline in healthy, nonsmoking, older adults. The age-related changes that do affect respiratory performance are so subtle and gradual that older adults compensate well for these changes. When a complicating factor, such as illness, places extraordinary demands for oxygen on the body, age-related respiratory changes may influence the overall function of the older adult. Of all aspects of physiologic function in older adults, respiratory performance seems to be least affected by age-related changes and most able to compensate for those changes that do occur.

Age-Related Changes

As with other body functions, it is difficult to separate the effects of age-related changes from those caused by disease processes and external influences, such as tobacco smoking. These influences occur throughout the life span, but because their effects are cumulative, their impact is more pronounced in older adults. In addition,

their cumulative effect may cause negative functional consequences only when they interact with age-related changes, such as diminished immune response, or with risk factors, such as diminished mobility.

Upper Respiratory Structures

Although the nose is often overlooked in discussions of respiratory function, age-related changes of the upper respiratory structures can influence both comfort and function. Age-related connective tissue changes cause the nose in older persons to have a retracted columella (the lower edge of the septum) and a poorly supported, downwardly rotated tip. Although these consequences may be viewed as more cosmetic than functional, they can impair the flow of air through the nasal cavity. These minor changes may cause mouth breathing during sleep, which causes snoring. Because of a combination of mouth breathing during sleep and diminished saliva production, an older adult might awaken with a dry mouth and sore throat.

The epiglottis and upper airway structures expel mucus and unwanted material from the lungs, and they protect the lower airway from harmful substances, ranging in size from microorganisms to large pieces of food. One of the age-related changes that affects these structures is calcification of the cartilage, which causes the trachea to stiffen. Another is blunting of the cough and laryngeal reflexes, with a concomitant decrease in coughing in older adults. Age-related reductions in the number of laryngeal nerve endings have also been noted and these may contribute to diminished efficiency of the gag reflex.

Chest Wall and Musculoskeletal Structures

Together, the chest wall and lungs function like a bellows, with the chest expanding outward in relation to lung expansion. The rib cage and the vertebral musculoskeletal structures are affected by the same kind of age-related changes that affect other musculoskeletal tissue. That is, the ribs and vertebrae become osteoporotic, the costal cartilage becomes calcified, and the respiratory muscles become weaker. As a result of these age-related processes, the following structural changes occur, which can affect respiratory performance: kyphosis, shortened thorax, chest wall stiffness, and increased anteroposterior diameter of the chest. The overall impact on respiratory performance includes diminished respiratory efficiency and reduced maximal inspiratory and expiratory force. To compensate for these and other age-related changes (discussed later), older adults depend increasingly on accessory muscles, particularly the diaphragm, and are, therefore, increasingly sensitive to any changes in intra-abdominal pressure. In summary, older adults expend more energy to achieve the same respiratory efficiency as younger adults, but the overall functional consequences for healthy older people are minimal.

Lungs

Even in healthy older adults, lungs become smaller and flabbier, and their weight diminishes by approximately 20%. The age-related changes that have the most significant functional consequences are those that occur in the lung parenchyma, or the part of the respiratory system where gas exchange takes place. The affected structures include the terminal bronchioles, alveolar ducts, alveoli, and capillaries. Beginning at around the age of 30 years, the alveoli progressively enlarge and their walls become thinner. This process of duct ectasia continues throughout adulthood, causing approximately a 4% loss of alveolar surface area per decade. Age-related changes also affect the pulmonary vasculature. The trunk of the pulmonary artery becomes thickened and less extensible, and its diameter widens. The number of capillaries also diminishes, and there is a decrease in pulmonary capillary blood volume. Finally, the mucosal bed, where diffusion takes place, thickens.

Elastic recoil is the characteristic that enables lung tissue to resist expansion as it fills with air. Elastic recoil assists in maintaining a positive pressure across the lung surface during inspiration, so as to hold the small airways open. During expiration, elastic recoil is responsible for keeping the airways open until the pressure placed on them by the respiratory muscles forces them to collapse. If the airways close prematurely, air is trapped and the lungs cannot expire to their maximum capacity. In healthy older adults, elastic recoil diminishes by a small degree, owing to a combination of age-related changes in the parenchyma and alterations in the elastic fibers. The end result is early airway closure, the mechanism that is primarily responsible for age-related changes in lung volumes and air flow rates.

Lung Volumes and Airflow Rates

Specific aspects of lung function, such as air volumes and flow rates, are measured by pulmonary function tests. In older adults, air volumes are altered because of the age-related changes in the chest wall and in lung elastic recoil. Because various lung volumes are interrelated, however,

TABLE 11-1
Age-Related Changes in Some Indicators of Lung Function

Indicator	Definition	Age-Related Change
Tidal volume	Amount of air moved in and out during a normal breath	None
Residual volume	Amount of air left in the lungs after a forced expiration	Increased by 50%
Vital capacity	Maximum volume of air that can be expelled following a maximum inspiration	Decreased by 25%
Total lung capacity	Amount of air that can be held in the lungs after a maximum inspiratory effort	Unchanged, as a result of compensatory mechanisms
Forced expiratory volume	Amount of air expelled within 1 second after a maximum inspiration	Decreased

the total lung capacity remains essentially the same owing to compensatory mechanisms. Airflow rates are affected to a small degree by age-related changes and to a greater degree by additional variables, such as height, gender, and lung volumes. Overall, there is an age-related decline in all airflow rates, but because of the many influencing factors, there is a wide range of normal levels. Table 11-1 summarizes the age-related changes that affect some parameters of lung function.

Gas Exchange

Because gas exchange is the primary function of the respiratory system, this is the most important functional aspect to consider. Oxygen–carbon dioxide exchange depends on a close match between ventilation, or the amount of air in the lungs, and perfusion, or the amount of blood flowing into the lungs. Because of age-related changes, particularly early airway closure, gas exchange is more likely to be compromised in the lower than the upper lung regions. As a consequence, inspired air is preferentially distributed in the upper regions, and a ventilation-to-perfusion mismatch results. The end result of this mismatch is a gradual decrease in

arterial PO_2 (oxygen pressure) of approximately 4 mm Hg per decade.

Response to Hypoxia and Hypercapnia

Compensatory changes in respiratory rate are made under conditions of hypercapnia (too much carbon dioxide) or hypoxia (too little oxygen). The response mechanism varies, depending on the stimulus. The response to hypercapnia is initiated by the central chemoreceptor, located in the medulla, whereas the response to hypoxia is initiated by peripheral chemoreceptors, located in the carotid and aortic bodies. When these mechanisms operate efficiently, the respiratory rate and depth increase in response to either low levels of oxygen or high levels of carbon dioxide. Although many researchers maintain that both responses are diminished by age-related changes, research-based conclusions about the effects of aging on responses to hypoxia and hypercapnia vary. One recent summary of research concluded that older adults generally have a blunted response to hypercapnia but that there is no statistically significant group difference for older adults because of the high degree of individual variation. The probable underlying mechanism for any age-related changes that occur is diminished neural output from the central nervous system to the respiratory muscles (Cherniach and Altose, 1996).

Risk Factors

For people at any age, tobacco smoking, particularly cigarette smoking, is the single most important risk factor for lung disease and impaired respiratory function. For smokers who have not succumbed to the detrimental effects before later adulthood, the risks of smoking are both immediate and cumulative. In comparison to smoking, all other risk factors pale in significance, but other risks are mentioned because, particularly for nonsmokers, these may be the factors that can be addressed through interventions to improve respiratory function. For smokers, however, these other risks are of minimal importance, and attention must be focused on the serious negative consequences of smoking.

Smoking and Other Lifestyle and Environmental Risk Factors

Tobacco smoking causes detrimental effects through heat and chemical actions on the respiratory system. Toxic gases released from burning cigarettes include carbon monoxide, hydrogen cyanide, and nitrogen dioxide. In addition, burning cigarettes release tobacco tar, which contains nicotine and many other harmful chemicals. Harmful physiologic effects on the respiratory system include, but are not limited to: (1) bronchoconstriction; (2) inflammation of the mucosa throughout the respiratory tract; (3) early airway closure (which is also an age-related change); and (4) inhibited ciliary action, leading to increased coughing and mucous secretions and diminished protection from harmful organisms. Risks for older adults are compounded by age-related changes and the cumulative effects of cigarette smoking. Even in otherwise healthy people, smokers have a doubled or

tripled rate of decline, compared with nonsmokers, in the forced expiratory volume at 1 second. This is an accelerated and exacerbated age-related change that increases the risk for diseases.

The negative effects of "passive smoking" (i.e., the inhalation of tobacco smoke in enclosed environments) were first reported to the public in the 1972 Surgeon General's Report. Although this report was initially viewed with some skepticism, there is mounting evidence that nonsmokers exposed to cigarette smoke may be affected by the cumulative and negative consequences of this risk factor. In fact, reports have indicated that "sidestream" smoke, or the smoke that is released from burning cigarettes, may contain up to 50 times as many carcinogens as the smoke inhaled by the smoker (Berger, 1987). Studies have found an association between passive smoking and increased risk of atherosclerosis, lung cancer, brain tumors, breast cancer, nasal carcinoma, and coronary artery disease (Lee and D'Alonzo, 1993; Howard et al., 1998). Although public awareness about the health risks of passive smoking has increased significantly in the past 2 decades, older adults are less knowledgeable than younger populations about the health hazards of active and passive smoking. Women, less educated people, and current smokers are other groups of people that are less knowledgeable about the health risks of passive smoking (Brownson et al., 1992).

An environmental risk factor that can lead to negative functional consequences is the inhalation of air pollutants. Along with the skin, the respiratory system is the area of physiologic function most directly influenced by environmental factors, such as air quality. Like the effects of cigarette smoking, the effects of air pollution are cumulative over many years and, therefore, have an increased impact on older adults who have been exposed to these risks over much of their lifetime. For example, older adults who have lived their entire lives in urban environments may have been exposed to air pollutants for as many as 7 or 8 decades.

Older adults who previously worked in certain occupations may have been exposed to toxic substances with long-term effects. Because hazards in the workplace were largely unregulated before the 1970s, many older people never benefited from the protections enforced under the Occupational Safety and Health Act. In addition, much of the information now available on the harmful effects of certain chemicals was not understood when these older adults were part of the work force. Therefore, older adults are more likely than younger adults to experience the long-term effects of occupational exposure to harmful substances. Some of the job categories that may be associated with an increased risk of respiratory disease are summarized in Display 11-1.

Additional Risk Factors

In addition to the age-related changes that involve the respiratory system, age-related changes affecting other aspects of function can also affect respiratory performance. For example, kyphosis, which is caused by age-related skeletal changes, interferes with maximum respiratory performance. A decline in immune response and host defense mechanisms is an age-related change that is thought to contribute to the increased morbidity and mortality noted in older adults with pneumonia and other lower respiratory infections.

Any chronic illness that interferes with mobility or activity increases the risk for impaired respiratory function. Restricted activity levels and a recumbent position exacerbate the effects of age-related changes and result in compromised respiratory performance in older adults. The function of the respiratory muscles, for example, is compromised by assuming a recumbent position or by any condition that contributes to shallow breathing. Therefore, any older adult who is on bed rest, even for short periods of time, is at increased risk for impaired respiratory function. The negative functional consequences of bed rest are attributable, at least in part, to the fact that the recumbent position interferes with chest wall expansion, which is already compromised by age-related changes. Obesity also can interfere with respiratory function, through its impact on an individual's overall activity level.

Reduced Maximum Pulmonary Function

A unique characteristic of respiratory performance is that the maximum level of function

---

DISPLAY 11-1
Occupations Associated with an Increased Risk
of Harmful Respiratory Effects

Firefighters	Asbestos workers
Traffic controllers	Quarry workers
Shipyard workers	Miners
Rubber workers	Grain workers
Aluminum workers	Construction workers
Iron and steel foundry workers	Workers exposed to the following: nickel,
Tunnel and street repair workers	arsenic, beryllium, chromium, or radiation

From T. Ferguson, (1987), *The smoker's book of health* (pp. 51–52) (New York: G. P. Putnam & Sons).

in middle and later adulthood is significantly influenced by the maximum level of function reached during the 3rd decade of life. In turn, the maximum level of function attained in the early twenties depends significantly on factors that affected respiratory development in early life, such as inhalation of household cigarette smoke. Although these effects cannot be reversed, it is important to consider their consequences, as respiratory complaints develop when pulmonary function is reduced to half of the maximally attained level. Therefore, if the maximum level of pulmonary function attained in early adulthood was high, the older person should be able to tolerate a relatively greater degree of age-related changes and exposure to risk factors before experiencing respiratory dysfunction. Conversely, if the maximum level attained was low, respiratory symptoms are likely to develop at an earlier point, when the impact of age-related changes or risk factors is still minimal.

Functional Consequences

In the absence of smoking and other risk factors, healthy older adults will not experience any negative functional consequences related to their respiratory performance during day-to-day activities. Under conditions of physical stress, however, older adults may become dyspneic and fatigued because their respiratory system is less efficient in gas exchange. However, even this effect may be at least partially compensated for through physical conditioning. Thus, healthy and physically conditioned older adults do not experience negative functional consequences from age-related changes alone.

The overall functional consequences of age-related changes are summarized in Table 11-2. Even in the presence of risk factors, the negative functional consequences for older adults do not differ from those that affect the respiratory function of adults of any age. That is, in the presence of risk factors, such as cigarette smoking and air pollutants, people of any age are more likely to have cancer and chronic lung diseases than those without those risk factors. In fact, people who smoke cigarettes during their early adult years are less likely to live long enough to experience any age-related changes because they tend to die at a younger age than do nonsmokers.

The only negative functional consequence of age-related changes and risk factors that is unique to older adults is an increased susceptibility to lower respiratory infections. In addition, respiratory infections have more serious

TABLE 11-2
Age-Related Changes Affecting Respiratory Function

Change	Consequences
Upper airway changes: calcification of cartilage; altered neuromuscular function and reflexes	Mouth breathing, snoring, diminished coughing, decreased efficiency of gag reflex
Increased anteroposterior diameter, chest wall stiffness, and weakened muscles	Increased use of accessory muscles; increased energy expended for respiratory efficiency
Enlargement of alveoli, thinning of alveolar walls, and diminished number of capillaries	Diminished efficiency of gas exchange; decreased arterial PO_2 value
Decreased elastic recoil and early airway closure	Changes in lung volumes; slight decrease in overall efficiency
Tidal volume unchanged; increased residual volume; decreased vital capacity	Total lung capacity unchanged

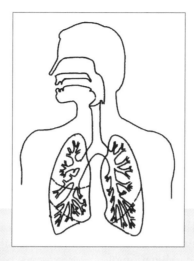

AGE-RELATED CHANGES

- Upper airway changes
- Increased anteroposterior diameter of chest wall
- Chest wall stiffness
- Weakened respiratory muscles
- Diminished vital capacity
- Enlargement of alveoli
- Decreased elastic recoil
- Early airway closure

NEGATIVE FUNCTIONAL CONSEQUENCES

- Increased use of accessory muscles
- Increased energy expended for respirations
- Decreased efficiency of gas exchange
- Diminished cough reflex
- Decreased efficiency of gag reflex
- Increased susceptibility to lower respiratory infections

RISK FACTORS

- Tobacco smoking
- Exposure to air pollutants
- Occupational exposure to toxic substances
  (e.g., asbestos)

FIGURE 11-1. Respiratory function in older adults.

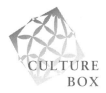

Cultural Aspects of Respiratory Function

- Cigar and cigarette smoking is an important social activity in many cultural groups; educational efforts directed toward smoking cessation need to address these issues.
- Whites have higher pulmonary function values than Blacks or Asians.
- Tuberculosis is more prevalent in African Americans, American Indians, Asian Americans, and Hispanics than in Whites.

consequences in older adults and are more likely to lead to death or cause a decline in functional status (Barker et al., 1998). The combination of age-related changes in respiratory function and age-related changes in immunity contributes to the increased risk of acquiring pneumonia and influenza in older adulthood. Mortality rates from pneumonia show an age-related increase from a rate of 24 per 100,000 for people aged 60 to 64 years to 1032 per 100,000 for people aged 85 years and older (Callahan and Wolinsky, 1996).

In addition to being increasingly susceptible to pneumonia and influenza, older adults are also more susceptible to tuberculosis than their younger counterparts. The most common reason for this is the reactivation of dormant tuberculosis, particularly in the presence of risk factors, such as smoking, diabetes, malnutrition, a debilitating illness, or long-term use of corticosteroids. The incidence of tuberculosis in community-living older adults is twice that of the general population; for older adults in nursing homes, the incidence is 4 times higher than that in the general population. Some of the cases of tuberculosis that affect nursing home residents are attributable to the ease with which this disease can spread among residents. Moreover, identification and treatment of tuberculosis may be delayed in older adults because disease manifestations are altered and usually more subtle in this population (as discussed in the Nursing

Assessment section). Mortality rates for older adults with tuberculosis are higher than those for younger populations.

Figure 11-1 summarizes the age-related changes, risk factors, and negative functional consequences that affect respiratory function. The Culture Box identifies some cultural aspects of respiratory function.

Nursing Assessment

Nursing assessment of respiratory function in younger and older adults differs in only two respects. The first difference involves some minor variations in the physical assessment of the respiratory system, even in healthy, nonsmoking, older adults. The second difference involves the manifestations and effects of lower respiratory infections in older adults. In keeping with the format of this text, only these two assessment components are discussed at length because these are the aspects unique to older people. Display 11-2 summarizes an interview format that may be used to assess the age-related changes, risk factors, and negative functional consequences that affect respiratory function in older adults.

Physical Assessment

The usual methods of inspection, palpation, percussion, and auscultation are used to

---

DISPLAY 11-2
Guidelines for Assessing Respiratory Function

Interview Questions to Assess Overall Respiratory Function

- Have you had any respiratory problems, such as asthma, chronic lung disease, pneumonia, or other infections?
- Have you ever had tuberculosis?
- Do you have any problems with breathing?
- Do you have any wheezing?
- Do you have spells of coughing? (If yes) When do they occur? How do they last? What brings them on? Are they dry or productive? Does the phlegm come from your throat or lungs? What does the phlegm look like?
- Do you ever have trouble getting enough air during any particular activities or when you lie down at night?
- Have you stopped doing any particular activities because of problems breathing? For example, have you stopped going up or down stairs, or have you limited the amount of walking you do? (For people with mobility limitations, this question might not be relevant.)
- Do you ever have any chest pain, or feelings of heaviness or tightness in your chest?
- Do you use more than one pillow at night, or make any other adjustments, because of trouble with breathing?
- Do you wake up at night because of coughing or difficulty with breathing?
- Do you ever feel as though you can't catch your breath?
- Do you have trouble breathing when the weather is hot, cold, or humid?
- Have you ever worked in a job where you were exposed to dust, fumes, smoke, or other air pollutants (e.g., in mining, farming, or any of the occupations listed in Display 11-1)?

- Have you lived in neighborhoods where there was a lot of pollution from traffic or factories?
- Do you tire easily?
- Do you smoke now, or have you ever smoked? (If yes, continue with the following sections; if no, ask whether the person is or has been exposed to passive smoke in home, work, or social environments.)

Interview Questions to Assess Smoking Behaviors

- How long have you smoked?
- How much do you smoke?
- What do you smoke?
- Have you smoked other types of tobacco in the past?

Interview Questions to Assess Knowledge of the Risk of Smoking

- Do you think there are any harmful effects of smoking for people in general?
- Do you think you're at risk for any harmful effects from smoking?
- Do you think there are any benefits to quitting smoking?

Interview Questions to Assess Attitudes Toward Smoking

- Have you ever thought about quitting smoking?
- Has your primary care provider or any other health professional ever talked to you about quitting smoking?
- What do you think about the idea of quitting smoking?
- Have you ever tried to quit? (If yes): What was your experience with the attempt?

---

evaluate respiratory performance in both younger and older adults. Some minor differences in assessment findings that may be observed in healthy older adults include: (1) increased resonance on percussion; (2) increased anteroposterior diameter; (3) diminished intensity of lung sounds; (4) altered appearance (i.e., leaning forward) secondary to kyphosis; and (5) an increased tendency for adventitious sounds to be auscultated in the lower lungs.

Asking the older person to cough before

auscultation of the lungs, and having the person breathe as deeply as possible with their mouth open, will facilitate auscultation of lung sounds. When nurses have an opportunity to observe respirations in a sleeping older adult, they may see frequent but brief periods of apnea. Because this phenomenon is common in older adults, it is discussed in greater detail in Chapter 14. With regard to assessment of respiratory illnesses, the manifestations of most respiratory diseases, such as influenza and chronic lung disease, do not differ in older and younger adults. Two exceptions to this are the manifestations of pneumonia and tuberculosis in older adults, as discussed in the next section.

Detection of Lower Respiratory Infections

The term detection has been used with regard to lower respiratory infections, rather than assessment, because when older adults have pneumonia, they do not always meet the typical assessment criteria. Rather than presenting with a productive cough, elevated temperature, and elevated white blood count, older adults are more likely to have subtler and less specific disease manifestations that the nurse must detect.

Lethargy, anorexia, tachypnea, dehydration, changes in mental status, and a decline in overall function are the manifestations of pneumonia most commonly seen in older adults, particularly in the early stages of the disease. In addition, the changes in lung sounds that typically occur with pneumonia may not be present; in fact, the only respiratory sign may be tachypnea. In older adults with pneumonia, the most significant finding on physical assessment of the lungs may be a diminished intensity of lung sounds or the presence of rales and rhonchi, which are very nonspecific findings. Even an initial chest radiograph may not provide accurate diagnostic information. Nurses must keep in mind that, although older adults may exhibit the typical manifestations of pneumonia, the absence of these manifestations is not as significant

in older adults as it is in younger adults. In older adults, a change in mental status or another alteration in functional status may be the major clue to a diagnosis of pneumonia. A recent study comparing the presentation of pneumonia in younger and older adults revealed that older adults had relatively fewer symptoms, particularly those associated with pain and fever, and were symptomatic for a longer period before a diagnosis of pneumonia was established (Metlay et al., 1997).

In addition to being aware of the different manifestations of pneumonia in older adults, nurses must also be aware of the increased rates and varied manifestations of tuberculosis in this population. As with pneumonia, manifestations of tuberculosis in this age group are likely to be subtle and nonspecific. In contrast to younger adults, older adults with tuberculosis are less likely to have hemoptysis, night sweats, and chest pain, and they are more likely to have cough, dyspnea, and vague manifestations, such as anorexia and weight loss. Some older adults may not have any respiratory manifestations, or they may have no symptoms at all (Van den Brande et al., 1991).

Another factor that makes it more difficult to detect tuberculosis in older adults is the high incidence of false-negative tuberculin skin test reactions in this population. One study found that 92% of younger subjects with tuberculosis, but only 55% of older subjects with tuberculosis, tested positive to tuberculin skin tests (Van den Brande et al., 1991). Other studies have indicated that 20% of younger adults and 30% of older adults with tuberculosis do not react to tuberculin skin tests (Creditor et al., 1988). Because tuberculosis often occurs as a reactivation of dormant disease, nurses must be particularly alert for manifestations of this disease in older adults who have a history of tuberculosis.

Smoking

Although smoking affects all people, regardless of age, some aspects of smoking behaviors differ according to age cohorts. Therefore, an assessment of smoking as a risk factor must address the age-related factors that affect these behaviors. It is important to realize, for example, that the cohort of people born in the early 1900s is the first age group to be exposed to the social pressures that encouraged smoking without knowing about the detrimental effects of smoking. As a consequence, people who began smoking in the early 1920s, when this became a popular habit for men in the United States, may have engaged in this habit for 4 or 5 decades before finding out that it was harmful. It was not until 1964 that the first report on the detrimental effects of cigarette smoking, entitled *Smoking and Health*, was issued by the U.S. Surgeon General. By this time, men had been smoking for 4 decades and women had been smoking for 2 decades. Thus, people in their seventies or eighties may be likely to adopt the attitude, "If I've smoked this long and am still alive, why should I quit now?"

For women in the United States, smoking was not socially acceptable until the mid-1940s. Thus, the cohort of smoking women who are now in their sixties is the first group of women who have smoked throughout their adulthood. The long-term consequences of smoking for older women are just now beginning to be recognized, as evidenced by the recent increase in lung cancer rates among older women.

In addition to assessing attitudes about smoking, nurses should assess past and present smoking patterns. Frequency of smoking and type of tobacco smoked are important determinants of the relative risk of smoking. Pipe and cigar smoking, for example, are not as detrimental to respiratory and cardiovascular function as cigarette smoking, but they do increase the risk of oral cancer. Moreover, cigarettes vary in the amount of nicotine they contain, and this variable influences the degree of risk associated with a particular type of cigarette. In contrast to younger adults, who began smoking when cigarettes had filters and were lower in nicotine, older adults began smoking when cigarettes had

no filters and contained greater amounts of tar and nicotine. Older adults, therefore, are more likely than younger adults to smoke cigarettes that have higher nicotine levels and thus are more harmful. Older adults, in fact, may still roll their own cigarettes using loose tobacco. Assessment questions designed to help the nurse determine smoking habits and attitudes about smoking are included in Display 11-2.

Additional Risk Factors

Risk factors that have less important effects on respiratory function than smoking should also be assessed. Information about factors that may have influenced respiratory development in early life, such as nutrition, respiratory infections, and chronic exposure to cigarette smoke, may be helpful in assessing the older adult's maximum respiratory function. Although the maximum respiratory function is attained by early adulthood, an understanding of the factors that influenced this level will provide information about the person's vulnerability to the effects of age-related changes and risk factors.

For this reason, questions about exposure to sidestream smoke and harmful air pollutants should be incorporated in the assessment. Occupational exposure to certain harmful substances is particularly important for smokers, because the risk of either one of these factors is compounded when the other factor is present. Information about the person's level of activity and about any factors that may interfere with mobility or routine activities will be helpful in assessing the degree to which additional exercise can be encouraged. If, for example, the person has severe mobility impairments as a result of arthritis, the potential for vigorous physical exercise may be quite limited. However, these individuals may benefit greatly from water exercises. Finally, information about the older adult's understanding of influenza and pneumonia vaccinations will provide a basis for education about these preventive measures. Display 11-2 summarizes information that must be included in a nursing assessment of respiratory function in older adults.

Nursing Diagnosis

The nursing diagnosis of Risk for Altered Respiratory Function is applicable when the nursing assessment identifies factors that may impair the older adult's respiratory function. This diagnosis is defined as "the state in which the individual is at risk of experiencing a threat to the passage of air through the respiratory tract and to the exchange of gases (O_2–CO_2) between the lungs and the vascular system" (Carpenito, 1997, p. 705). Related factors common in older adults include smoking, kyphosis, influenza, infection, chronic illnesses, and limited mobility. The case example at the end of this chapter addresses this nursing diagnosis. If only one aspect of respiratory function is impaired or is at risk for impaired function, then a nursing diagnosis, such as Ineffective Airway Clearance, might be appropriate. If impaired respiratory function interferes with activities of daily living, a nursing diagnosis of Activity Intolerance might be appropriate.

Debilitated or chronically ill older adults who live in group settings may be at high risk for infections, particularly influenza and tuberculosis. For example, if a nursing home resident has active tuberculosis, the nursing staff might address the nursing diagnosis of High Risk for Infection Transmission for the affected resident and the nursing diagnosis of High Risk for Infection for all other residents. Likewise, when influenza affects one or more residents or staff of a nursing home or group living facility, these nursing diagnoses may be applicable. Altered Health Maintenance is a nursing diagnosis that may be used for older adults who have insufficient knowledge about the detrimental effects of active or passive smoking. When nurses provide pneumonia or influenza immunizations for older adults, a nursing diagnosis of Health-Seeking Behaviors may be appropriate.

Nursing Goals

As emphasized throughout this chapter, negative functional consequences affect the respiratory performance of older adults primarily because of the risks of cigarette smoking or exposure to air pollutants. In the absence of these risks, the only negative functional consequence of concern to older adults is their increased vulnerability to lower respiratory infections. Two nursing goals that address these negative functional consequences are to prevent lower respiratory infections and to eliminate the risk factors for impaired respiratory function. Both of these goals are achieved through health education, as discussed in the following sections. One outcome of successful health education might be that older adult smokers quit smoking. Another outcome might be that older adults obtain immunizations against pneumonia and influenza and that they take other protective measures against respiratory infections. The goal of maintaining optimal respiratory function also may be achieved through physical exercise and other health promotion measures. Older adults with limited mobility should be taught to perform deep breathing exercises and should be instructed to do these several times daily.

Nursing Interventions

Preventing Lower Respiratory Infections

Interventions to prevent pneumonia and influenza are particularly important, as collectively, these two conditions constitute the fourth leading cause of death in people older than 65 years of age. Moreover, of all the leading causes of death in older adults, pneumonia and influenza are the only ones that can be prevented with investment of very little time, money, or motivation. Therefore, education about pneumonia and influenza vaccinations is an essential nursing intervention in caring for older adults. Although annual influenza immunizations are well accepted and well publicized, pneumonia vaccinations have received less attention. The Centers for Disease Control and Prevention (CDC) recommends pneumonia vaccinations for all people aged 65 years and older. Since 1997, the CDC has recommended a one-time booster dose for all people aged 65 years or older whose initial pneumonia vaccination was received 5 (or more) years earlier. Pneumonia vaccinations are also recommended for older adults who are uncertain about their vaccination status. Current information about influenza and pneumonia immunizations is summarized in Display 11-3, along with information about risk factors for these illnesses. This information is given in nontechnical language so that it can be used for educating older adults.

Nurses working in long-term care or other group living facilities are assuming responsibility for implementing programs to detect and address tuberculosis. Nursing models of prevention and intervention programs in long-term care facilities can be found in the gerontological literature (e.g., Hopkins and Schoener, 1996; Gubser, 1998). These programs include protocols for skin testing and other screening and diagnostic methods, as well as interventions for residents with tuberculosis and for prevention of the spread of the infection among staff and residents. Any nurse or direct-care staff member working with older adults should undergo periodic skin testing to screen for exposure to tuberculosis.

Eliminating the Risk of Cigarette Smoking

An assessment of attitudes about smoking provides a basis for planning educational interventions that will help older smokers eliminate this risk factor. If the assessment reveals an "I'm-too-old-to-change" attitude, the initial intervention might be to explore the older adult's understanding of his or her ability to change behavioral patterns. Using information about psychosocial development in older adulthood, the nurse might challenge such an attitude and encourage the older person to consider the possibility of a behavioral change.

Closely related to the "I'm-too-old-to-change" attitude is the "It's-too-late-to-do-any-good" attitude. Whenever older adults express such an attitude, nurses must challenge the underlying assumptions. This attitude might be prevalent among older adults because smokers older than 50 years of age are less likely than other smokers to think that smoking affects their health now, and to believe that there is a strong likelihood of serious health problems from smoking (Clark et al., 1997). Nurses can inform older adults that substantial health benefits are derived from quitting smoking, not only in terms of improved respiratory function, but also in terms of the reduced risk for heart disease. Studies indicate that many of the risks from smoking are negligible or significantly reduced within 2 years after the habit is discontinued. Within 10 to 15 years of quitting smoking, most or all of the negative effects are eliminated (Lee and D'Alonzo, 1993). Health education about the many beneficial effects of quitting smoking may enhance the older adult's motivation to quit smoking.

Older adults are most likely to quit smoking after a smoking-related illness develops, as evidenced by a 50% quit rate among smokers who survive heart attacks (Timmreck and Randolph, 1993). Recent clinical practice guidelines emphasize the importance of health care providers initiating the topic of smoking cessation and routinely identifying and intervening with all tobacco users at every opportunity (Fiore et al., 1996). Guidelines for nursing interventions for smoking cessation can be found in nursing literature (e.g., Wynd, 1997). Health education should include information about the variety of approaches to smoking cessation. Smokers may want to discuss with their primary care provider

---

DISPLAY 11-3
Education About Pneumonia and Influenza

Factors That Increase the Risk for Pneumonia and Influenza

- Diabetes or any chronic lung, heart, or kidney disease
- Hospitalization within the past year for heart or lung diseases
- Severe anemia or a debilitating condition
- Confinement to bed or very limited mobility
- Residence in a nursing home or other group living setting
- Immunosuppressive medications

Protection Against Influenza

- New vaccinations are developed every year, based on information about the strains of viruses that are most likely to affect people during the influenza season.
- Vaccines are made from inactivated viruses and, therefore, should have few or no side effects.
- People who are allergic to eggs and egg products should NOT receive influenza immunizations.
- Immunizations do not offer immediate protection, as there is a 2- to 3-week delay in developing an antibody response.
- Every year, the manufacturers of the influenza vaccination provide recommendations as to the best time for administering the immunizations for optimal effectiveness. The best time is during the late fall, but the exact time period will vary slightly from year to year.

- Vaccines are not 100% effective, but they are helpful for most older people.
- Influenza immunizations provide protection against the most serious viruses, but not against all types of respiratory infections.
- The duration of effectiveness of vaccinations may be shorter than 6 months in some older people; therefore, one vaccination might not protect the person through the entire season.
- In 1993, Medicare began paying for flu shots.
- People can protect themselves from respiratory infections by washing their hands frequently, by avoiding hand-to-mouth or hand-to-eye contact, and by not inhaling air that has been contaminated by particles from the cough or sneeze of someone with an infection.

Pneumonia Vaccinations

- Pneumonia vaccinations are recommended for people older than 65 years of age.
- Pneumonia vaccinations were considered one-time-only immunizations, but boosters are now being recommended for older adults who received their initial immunization 5 or more years ago.
- Common side effects include a slight fever accompanied by pain, redness, or tenderness at the injection site.
- Side effects, if they occur, are not serious and will subside within a few days.
- Pneumonia vaccinations are covered by Medicare.

---

various prescription or over-the-counter pharmacologic therapies that can help treat their nicotine addiction. In the past few years, several new prescription and over-the-counter smoking cessation products have been approved for use in the United States. Available methods for delivering nicotine substitutes include gum, patches, inhalants, and nasal sprays. In addition

to nicotine substitution products, a sustained-release form of buproprion has been available since 1997 as a non-nicotine aid to smoking cessation. A citric acid aerosol product also has been found to be effective as a smoking cessation product (Westman, et al., 1995). Combinations of products and methods are often used to improve the effectiveness of a smoking cessation

---

DISPLAY 11-4
Education About Cigarette Smoking

Attitudes About Smoking

- Stopping smoking at any age is more beneficial than continuing to smoke.
- Many of the harmful effects of smoking are reversed once the smoker quits.
- Although some of the effects of past smoking are irreversible, all of the harmful effects of future smoking can be avoided by quitting now.
- Smoking is a major risk factor for lung disease and heart diseases, including high blood pressure and heart attacks.
- Passive smoking (inhaling smoke from the air) is associated with an increased risk for many diseases.

Type of Tobacco

- The lower the tar and nicotine content of cigarettes, the less harmful the effects. Many cigarettes with lower tar and nicotine levels, however, have additional chemical additives that can be harmful.
- Pipe and cigar smokers are at a higher risk for chronic lung disease than nonsmokers, just as cigarette smokers are.
- The harmful effects of tobacco use on the mouth and upper respiratory tract are equal for all types of tobacco, including "smokeless tobacco." All smokers have the same risk for developing cancer of the mouth and upper respiratory tract.

- Snuff, chewing tobacco, and smokeless tobacco contain nicotine and many other harmful chemicals. The only advantage of smokeless tobacco is that it does not affect other people nearby.

Approaches to Quitting

- Any reduction in present tobacco use is better than maintaining the current level. The negative effects of smoking are directly proportional to the number of cigarettes inhaled.
- Various forms of prescription and over-the-counter nicotine substitutes (e.g., gum, skin patches, and nasal sprays) are available and may be helpful, especially when used in conjunction with counseling and self-help techniques.
- Besides nicotine substitutes, some non-nicotine prescription medications and over-the-counter products may be effective as a component of a smoking cessation program.
- People who are trying to quit smoking should discuss this with a health care professional to identify the methods that might be most effective.
- Many self-help programs are available for support and education regarding quitting smoking.
- Information about group programs can be obtained through the Internet or by calling the local office of any of the following organizations: American Lung Association, American Heart Association, or the American Cancer Society.

---

program. Regardless of the methods that are used, it is widely agreed that counseling from a health professional is an important component of any smoking cessation efforts. Educational materials about group and individual self-help programs are available through the organizations listed in the Educational Resources section.

Display 11-4 summarizes educational interventions that may be effective in helping older adults quit smoking. As in Display 11-3, this information is presented in nontechnical terms so that nurses can use it as a guide to teaching older adults. Alternative and preventive health care practices also may be effective in promoting

ALTERNATIVE
AND
PREVENTIVE
HEALTH
CARE
PRACTICES

Quitting Smoking and Maintaining Respiratory Health

Herbs
- For colds or coughs: thyme, yarrow, garlic, coltsfoot, peppermint, lobelia,* Echinacea, elecampane, marsh mallow, slippery elm, hyssop, licorice, red sage, Astragalus root
- For smoking cessation: lobelia* (Indian tobacco), combination of coltsfoot and plantain

Homeopathic Remedies
- For colds or coughs: aconite, bryonia, drosera, pulsatilla, nux vomica, antimonium tartaricum
- For smoking cessation: plantain, nux vomica

Nutritional Considerations
- Zinc; vitamins A, B-complex, C, and E

Preventive Measurements and Additional Approaches
- Humidifier, vaporizer, mustard poultice, steam therapy
- Aromatherapy: thyme, lemon, menthol, camphor, eucalyptus, lavender, tea tree
- For smoking cessation: exercise, music, imagery, massage, meditation, affirmations, hypnotherapy, deep breathing, stress reduction, individual or group counseling
- Acupuncture may be used for coughs, influenza, upper respiratory infections, nasal allergic conditions, and chronic respiratory conditions.

Special Precautions
- The side effects of lobelia include weakness, mental changes, gastrointestinal symptoms, and hearing and vision problems.

respiratory function and smoking cessation (see box above).

Evaluating Nursing Care

Evaluation of the effectiveness of nursing care is based on the nursing goals. A short-term goal for older adults with altered respiratory function might be that they can accurately identify factors that can be addressed to improve their respiratory function. For example, the person might verbalize knowledge about the detrimental effects of smoking. A long-term goal for older adults who smoke might be to quit smoking. Evaluation criteria for this goal are described in the case example that follows. If nursing care is directed toward preventing the spread of respiratory infections in long-term care settings, a goal would be to have all residents receive immunizations for pneumonia and influenza. Evaluation of this goal would be based on the number of residents who were immunized.

Chapter Summary

Under normal circumstances, healthy, non-smoking, older adults compensate well for any age-related changes that affect respiratory function. Respiratory performance may be compromised by risk factors, such as illness, tobacco use, or exposure to environmental pollutants. Older adults are more likely than younger adults to have lower respiratory infections, such as pneumonia, influenza, and tuberculosis. When lower respiratory infections occur in older adults, the manifestations are more subtle and the consequences are likely to be serious or life-threatening.

Nursing assessment of respiratory function in older adults focuses on identifying risk factors, such as cigarette smoking and inadequate immunizations against pneumonia and influenza. Nursing assessment of smokers concentrates on their knowledge about the harmful effects of active and passive smoking and on their attitudes about quitting smoking. For older adults who are at risk for lower respiratory infections, nursing assessment focuses on detecting the subtle manifestations of pneumonia or tuberculosis. Relevant nursing diagnoses include Altered Health Maintenance and High Risk for Altered Respiratory Function.

Nursing care is directed toward alleviating risk factors that interfere with optimal respiratory function. Health education includes information about quitting smoking and obtaining pneumonia and influenza vaccinations. Nursing care may be directed toward the prevention and early detection of respiratory infections, especially in nursing homes and other group settings. Nursing care is evaluated by documented improvement in respiratory function, elimination of risk factors (e.g., cigarette smoking), and prevention of respiratory infections.

Critical Thinking Exercises

1. What will a healthy, nonsmoking, 83-year-old person experience in his or her daily life with regard to respiratory function?
2. What would you include in a health education program, designed for older adults, on the prevention of pneumonia and influenza?
3. How would you address the following statement made by a 71-year-old person: "I've lived this long and don't have lung cancer, why should I start worrying now?"?
4. Find the names, addresses, and phone numbers of local agencies that would be appropriate resources for someone interested in quitting smoking. Contact at least one of these organizations to find out specific information about support groups, written materials, and other resources.

Case Example and Nursing Care Plan

Pertinent Case Information

Mr. R., a 74-year-old, recently moved into an assisted living complex where you are employed as the nurse at the Senior Wellness Clinic. When he comes in for his flu shot, he asks you how he can get some nicotine gum, because he has heard that this is a good way to cut down on cigarettes. Now that he lives in the assisted living complex, he can't smoke in the dining room, and he'd like to chew nicotine gum before and after he eats. He admits that he smokes a pack of cigarettes a day, but he denies having experienced any bad effects from smoking. Mr. R. sees his doctor annually for routine care, and he takes hydrochlorothiazide, 25 mg, daily for his blood pressure.

Nursing Assessment

You begin your nursing assessment by exploring Mr. R.'s attitudes about smoking and ascertaining his knowledge about the harmful effects of cigarette smoking. Mr. R. says he never tried to quit smoking because his wife smoked until she died a few months ago, and he felt it would be too hard to quit as long as she was smoking two packs per day. He states that he's been smoking for 40 years, and if he hasn't gotten lung cancer by now, he's not going to get it at his age. He also states that he's heard a lot about passive smoking. Again, though, he figured it wasn't worth quitting as long as his wife smoked. To comply with the rules in the assisted living facility, Mr. R. says he plans to chew nicotine gum when he can't smoke cigarettes, but he sees no reason to quit smoking.

In assessing Mr. R.'s knowledge about the effects of cigarette smoking, you determine that he is aware of some of the harmful effects of passive smoking but has very little information about the detrimental effects of cigarette smoking. He relates that his wife died of lung cancer, but he attributes her death to a history of breast cancer, which she had 10 years before the lung cancer. Mr. R. has no knowledge about cigarette smoking as a risk factor for cardiovascular disease, nor does he realize that his hypertension poses an additional risk. Mr. R. reports that he has experienced no ill effects from cigarette smoking, but when you ask about his history of respiratory infections, he admits he had pneumonia 3 years ago. He says he received a pneumonia shot 2 years ago, so he doesn't have to worry about getting pneumonia again. He says he's had bronchitis several times, but now that he won't be out shoveling snow, he doesn't worry about getting any lung infections.

Nursing Diagnosis

You use the nursing diagnosis of Altered Health Maintenance, related to insufficient knowledge about the effects of tobacco use and self-help resources. Some of Mr. R.'s statements reflect a lack of accurate information about the harmful effects of cigarette smoking, particularly regarding risks for respiratory infections and impaired cardiovascular function. Other statements probably reflect an intellectualization of his continued smoking. You intuit that, with some education and support, he may be willing to quit smoking.

Goals	Nursing Interventions	Evaluation Criteria
To increase Mr. R.'s knowledge about the harmful effects of cigarette smoking	Give Mr. R. brochures and illustrations provided by the Office on Smoking and Health and use these to discuss the effects of cigarette smoking.	Mr. R. will verbalize correct information about the risks of cigarette smoking. Mr. R. will describe the benefits derived from quitting smoking.

	Use brochures from the American Heart Association to discuss the risk factors for cardiovascular disease.	
	Discuss cigarette smoking as a risk factor for respiratory infections.	
	Give Mr. R. a copy of Display 11-4 and discuss the immediate and long-term benefits of quitting smoking.	
To increase Mr. R.'s knowledge about techniques to quit smoking	Using information from the American Lung Association, discuss some of the strategies for quitting smoking (e.g., quitting "cold turkey," using nicotine substitutes, participating in self-help groups).	Mr. R. will describe the advantages and disadvantages of the various methods of quitting smoking.
Mr. R. will quit smoking.	Identify the method Mr. R. prefers for quitting smoking.	Mr. R. reports that he has stopped or significantly reduced his smoking.
	Emphasize the importance of nutrition, exercise, and adequate fluid intake.	
	Agree on realistic goals for smoking cessation.	
	Discuss supportive resources. Set up weekly appointments at the Senior Wellness Clinic for support and further discussions.	

Educational Resources

Agency for Health Care Policy and Research
U.S. Department of Health and Human Services
AHCPR Publications Clearinghouse
P.O. Box 8547
Silver Spring, MD 20907
(800) 358–9295
www.ahcpr.gov
• Consumer guide, guide for primary care clinicians, and Spanish-language guide on quitting smoking

American Cancer Society
1599 Clifton Road, NE
Atlanta, GA 30329
(800) 227–2345
www.cancer.org

American Heart Association
7272 Greenville Avenue
Dallas, TX 75231–4596
(214) 373–6300; (800) 242–8721
www.americanheart.org

American Lung Association
1740 Broadway
New York, NY 10019–4374
(212) 315–8700
www.lungusa.org

National Heart, Lung, and Blood Institute Information Center
P.O. Box 30105
Bethesda, MD 20824–0105
(301) 251–1222
www.nhlbi.nih.gov/nhlbi/nhlbi.htm

Office on Smoking and Health
Centers for Disease Control and Prevention
Publications Catalog, Mail Stop K-50
4770 Buford Highway, NE
Atlanta, GA 30341–5705
(800) 232–1311
www.cdc.gov/tobacco

References

Barker, W. H., Borisute, H., & Cox, C. (1998). A study of the impact of influenza on the functional status of frail older people. *Archives of Internal Medicine, 158,* 645–650.

Berger, G. (1987). *Smoking not allowed: The debate* (p. 87). New York: Franklin Watts.

Brownson, R. C., Jackson-Thompson, J., Wilkerson, J. C. Davis, J. R., Owens, N. W., & Fisher, E. B. (1992). Demographic and socioeconomic differences in beliefs about the health effects of smoking. *American Journal of Public Health, 82,* 99–103.

Callahan, C. M., & Wolinsky, F. D. (1996). Hospitalization for pneumonia among older adults. *Journal of Gerontology: Medical Sciences, 51A*(6), M276–M282.

Carpenito, L. J. (1997). *Nursing diagnosis: Application to clinical practice* (7th ed.). Philadelphia: J. B. Lippincott.

Cherniach, N. S., & Altose, M. D. (1996). Respiratory system. In J. E. Birren (Ed.), *Encyclopedia of gerontology: Age, aging, and the aged* (Vol. 2, pp. 431–436). San Diego: Academic Press.

Clark, M. A., Rakowski, W., Kviz, F. J., & Hogan, J. W. (1997). Age and stage of readiness for smoking cessation. *Journal of Gerontology: Social Sciences, 52B*(4), S212–S221.

Creditor, M. C., Smith, E. C., Gallai, J. B., Baumann, M., & Nelson, K. E. (1988). Tuberculosis, tuberculin reactivity, and delayed cutaneous hypersensitivity in nursing home residents. *Journal of Gerontology: Medical Sciences, 43,* M97–M100.

Fiore, M. C., Bailey, W. C., Cohen, S. J., et al. (1996). *Smoking cessation. Clinical practice guideline No. 18.* AHCPR Publ. No. 96-0692. Rockville, MD: Agency for Health Care Policy and Research, Public Health Service, U.S. Department of Health and Human Services.

Gubser, V. L. (1998). Tuberculosis and the elderly: A community health perspective. *Journal of Gerontological Nursing, 24*(5), 36–41.

Hopkins, M. L., & Schoener, L. (1996). Tuberculosis and the elderly living in long-term care facilities. *Geriatric Nursing, 17,* 27–32.

Howard, G., Wagenknecht, L. E., Burke, G. L., Diez-Roux, A., Evans, G. W., McGovern, P., et al. (1998). Cigarette smoking and progression of atherosclerosis. *Journal of the American Medical Association, 279,* 119–124.

Lee, E. W., & D'Alonzo, G. E. (1993). Cigarette smoking, nicotine addiction, and its pharmacologic treatment. *Archives of Internal Medicine, 153,* 34–48.

Metlay, J. P., Schulz, R., Li, Y-H., Singer, D. E., Marrie, T. J., Coley, C. M., Hough, L. J., Obrosky, D. S., Kapoor, W. N., & Fine, M. J. (1997). Influence of age on symptoms at presentation in patients with community-acquired pneumonia. *Archives of Internal Medicine, 157,* 1453–1459.

Timmreck, T. C., & Randolph, J. F. (1993). Smoking cessation: Clinical steps to improve compliance. *Geriatrics, 48*(4), 63–70.

Van den Brande, P., Vijgen, J., & Demedts, M. (1991). Clinical spectrum of pulmonary tuberculosis in older patients: Comparison with younger patients. *Journal of Geronotology: Medical Sciences, 46,* M204–M209.

Westman, E. C., Behm, F. M., & Rose, J. E. (1995). Airway sensory replacement combined with nicotine replacement for smoking cessation. *Chest, 107,* 1358–1364.

Wynd, C. A. (1997). Smoking cessation. In B. M. Dossey (Ed.), *Core Curriculum for Holistic Nursing* (pp. 220–225). Gaithersburg, MD: Aspen.

Mobility and Safety

Chapter

12

1. *Delineate age-related changes that affect mobility.*
2. *Examine risk factors that increase the risk of osteoporosis and influence the safety and mobility of older adults.*
3. *Discuss the following functional consequences: musculoskeletal function, increased susceptibility to fractures, and increased susceptibility to falls.*
4. *Discuss the psychosocial and economic consequences of falls, fractures, and osteoporosis.*
5. *Describe methods of assessing overall musculoskeletal performance and risks for falls and osteoporosis.*
6. *Identify interventions directed toward safe mobility and the elimination of risks for falls and osteoporosis.*

Mobility is one of the most important aspects of physiologic function because it is essential for maintaining independence, and because serious consequences occur when independence is lost. For older adults, mobility is influenced to a small degree by age-related changes and to a large extent by risk factors. Because of the many risks that threaten mobility, falls are an unfortunately common occurrence in old age. Older adults, then, have the dual challenge of maintaining mobility skills and maintaining an upright position when they are walking. For these reasons, safety is considered to be an integral aspect of mobility.

Age-Related Changes

The bones, joints, and muscles are the body structures most closely associated with mobility, but many additional functional aspects are involved in safe mobility. Neurologic function, for example, influences all facets of musculoskeletal performance, and visual function influences the ability to interact safely with the environment.

Within the musculoskeletal system, osteoporosis is the age-related change that has the most significant overall impact, has been studied the most, and is most amenable to interventions aimed at prevention and management. For these reasons, a separate section of this chapter is devoted to osteoporosis, and this section is limited to all other age-related changes that affect mobility.

Bones

Bones provide the framework for the entire musculoskeletal system and work in conjunction with the muscular system to facilitate movement. Additional functions of bone in the human body include storage of calcium, production of blood cells, and support and protection of body organs and tissues. Bone is composed of a hard outer layer, called cortical or compact bone, and an inner, spongy meshwork, called trabecular or cancellous bone. The proportion of cortical to trabecular components varies according to bone type. Long bones, such as the radius and femur, may be as much as 90% cortical, whereas flat and vertebral bones are composed primarily of trabecular cells. Cortical and trabecular bone components are affected by age-related changes, but the rate and impact of age-related changes differ in the two types of bone. These changes are discussed in the separate section on osteoporosis and are summarized in Display 12-1 (p. 350).

Bone growth reaches maturity in early adulthood, but bone remodeling continues throughout one's lifetime. Age-related changes that affect this remodeling process include increased bone resorption, diminished calcium absorption, increased serum parathyroid hormone, impaired regulation of osteoblast activity, impaired bone formation secondary to reduced osteoblastic production of bone matrix, and a decreased number of functional marrow cells owing to replacement of marrow with fat cells. These age-related changes affect both men and women and account for the age-dependent type of osteoporosis. In addition, women are affected by menopausal changes that accelerate the rate of bone loss. These factors are discussed in greater detail in the section entitled Types of Osteoporosis. The following factors also can affect bone remodeling and are common in older adults: hyperthyroidism, decreased activity levels, chronic obstructive lung disease, deficiencies of calcium and vitamin D, and consumption of certain medications, such as glucocorticoids and anticonvulsants.

Muscles

All activities of daily living (ADL) are directly influenced by the function of the skeletal muscles, which are controlled by motor neurons. The age-related changes that have the greatest impact on muscle function are: (1) a loss of muscle mass as a result of decreases in the size and number of muscle fibers; (2) deterioration of muscle fibrils with subsequent replacement by connective tissue and, eventually, by fat tissue; and (3) deterioration of muscle cell membranes and a subsequent escape of fluid and potassium. By the age of 80 years, approximately 30% of the muscle mass is lost. In addition, there is an age-related loss of motor neurons, and this, too, affects muscular function. The end result of these age-related changes is a decline in motor function and a loss of muscle strength and endurance. Although these are considered to be age-related changes, exercise programs to increase strength and endurance may help to prevent negative functional consequences.

Joints and Connective Tissue

Numerous age-related changes affect the tissues responsible for the function of all musculoskeletal joints, including non-weight-bearing joints. Despite the fact that overall musculoskeletal function depends on the bones, muscles, and joints, it is the joints that are harmed, rather than helped, by continued use. In contrast to the bones or muscles, which benefit from exercise, the joints show the effects of wear and tear, even in early adulthood. In fact, degenerative processes that affect the functional efficiency of the joints begin to occur before skeletal maturity is reached. These changes begin in the 3rd decade and affect the tendons, ligaments, and synovial fluid.

Some of the most significant age-related joint changes include the following:

1. Diminished viscosity of synovial fluid;
2. Degeneration of collagen and elastin cells;
3. Fragmentation of fibrous structures in connective tissue;
4. Outgrowths of cartilaginous clusters in response to continuous wear and tear;
5. Formation of scar tissue and areas of calcification in the joint capsules and connective tissue; and
6. Degenerative changes in the arterial cartilage resulting in extensive fraying, cracking, and shredding, in addition to a pitted and thinned surface.

Some of the consequences of these changes include impaired flexion and extension movements, decreased flexibility of the fibrous structures, diminished protection from forces of movement, erosion of the bones underlying the outgrowths of cartilage, and diminished ability of the connective tissue to transmit the tensile forces that act on it.

Osteoarthritis has often been viewed as an extreme progression of age-related degenerative changes. Questions have been raised about this association, however, and attempts are being made to distinguish between age-related changes and disease-related changes (Hamerman, 1993). Gardner, for example, states that "load bearing cartilage surfaces, such as those of the femoral head, undergo at least two patterns of gross degenerative change, and these changes may be unrelated" (1983, p. 419). Similarly, another geriatrician maintains that osteoarthritis is not attributable to aging or wear and tear, and that striking differences exist between aged cartilage and osteoarthritis (Quinet, 1986). Because these changes are degenerative, not inflammatory, "osteoarthrosis" has been suggested as a term that would describe these changes more accurately (Gardner, 1983). Although this rationale is sound, the term osteoarthritis is the term that is commonly used to describe the degenerative joint diseases that commonly affect older adults.

Additional Changes That Affect Mobility and Safety

Mobility is most directly related to the function of the musculoskeletal system, but it is influenced by many other aspects of function. For example, safe mobility is influenced at least as much by changes in sensory ability and other areas of function as by changes in musculoskeletal performance. Vision and hearing influence safe mobility, particularly when older people are in unfamiliar or institutional environments. Because two chapters in this text have been devoted to hearing and vision (Chapters 6 and 7,

respectively), these changes will not be discussed in this chapter. However, they must be considered in any discussion of safe mobility.

Postural hypotension, discussed in Chapter 10, is another negative functional consequence that can interfere with safe mobility. Other age-related changes, primarily involving the autonomic and central nervous systems, also may affect gait, balance, body sway, and reaction time. Any of these changes can, in turn, influence safe ambulation. These changes have not been discussed in other chapters and, therefore, are briefly reviewed here as they affect mobility and safety.

Gait changes, which differ in men and women, are one of the more noticeable functional consequences that occur after the age of 75 years. A waddling gait and a narrower base of walking and standing develop in older women. In addition, women have less muscular control, and bowlegged-type changes develop that affect the lower extremities and alter the angle of the hip. In contrast to the narrower gait of older women, the walking and standing gait of older men becomes wider with age. The walking pattern of older men is characterized by less arm swing, a shorter stride, decreased steppage height, and a more flexed position of the head and trunk. The overall impact of these changes is that older men and women have a slower walking speed and spend more time in the support phase of gait than in the swing phase. These changes are thought to contribute to the increased susceptibility of older adults to falls. For example, studies indicate that elderly persons who fall tend to have a slower walking speed, shorter stride length, and a greater variability in step length (Tideiksaar, 1997).

Maintenance of balance in an upright position is a complex skill that is affected by the following age-related changes: a decline in the righting reflex; impaired proprioception, particularly in women; and diminished vibratory sensation and joint position sense in the lower extremities. Body sway is a measure of the motion of the body when a person is standing still. The following conclusions have been drawn from studies of age-related changes in body sway: (1) impaired vision may increase sway; (2) people who fall have a greater degree of sway than do those who do not fall; (3) body sway increases more significantly with age in women than in men; and (4) age-related changes result in increased sway and impaired postural control, which may contribute to the risk of falls (Alexander, 1994; Hu and Woolacott, 1994; Maki et al., 1994; Tideiksaar, 1997).

Finally, age-related decreases in reaction time and speed of performance can influence mobility and safety. Diminished reaction time is one of the most widely acknowledged age-related changes, but there is disagreement about the mechanisms underlying this change. Regardless of the causative factors, the end result is slowed performance in walking and other ADL. Also, decreased reaction time may interfere with cognitive and perceptual processes; indeed, older people have been found to respond more slowly to unexpected environmental stimuli than their younger counterparts. Therefore, in unfamiliar environments, or when encountering the unexpected, older adults are at an increased risk for falls.

Osteoporosis

Definitions of osteoporosis generally cite all of the following characteristics: it is a process of gradual loss of bone mass, it affects all adults to some degree, and it predisposes older adults to fractures. When described in this way, osteoporosis is the only age-related condition that is defined in terms of its potential for negative functional consequences. The close association between increased age and osteoporotic fractures is apparent in the fact that 97% of hip fractures in American women occur after the age of 65 years (Gordan and Genant, 1985). Moreover, many of these fractures are not the result of the type of trauma that generally causes fractures. Of all the age-related changes, therefore, osteoporosis is the one that is most likely to cause serious negative functional consequences, even in the absence of additional risk factors.

Theories Regarding Osteoporosis

Primary care providers have been aware of the increased frequency of hip and forearm fractures in older women since the 1880s. However, the underlying risk factors did not begin to be identified until 6 decades later, when estrogen deficiency was identified as a cause of osteoporosis and fractures in older women. By the 1960s, primary care providers suspected that many fractures in older women were associated with moderate or no trauma. During the 1970s and 1980s, the use of noninvasive methods for measuring bone density allowed much progress to be made in our understanding of osteoporosis. As understanding increased, so did the recommendations for preventing and treating this common condition of older adulthood. By the late 1990s, the medical literature was referring to an "osteoporosis revolution," which came about largely because of the widespread availability and low cost of noninvasive measurements of bone density (Raisz, 1997). As a result of this revolution, attention is being focused on the prevention of fractures in older men, as well as in women, and new medications have been approved and are being developed for the prevention and treatment of osteoporosis. Findings on patterns of bone loss in adulthood are reviewed in the following sections and are summarized in Display 12-1. Treatment approaches are discussed in the section entitled Interventions.

Gender differences account for the relatively higher rate of osteoporosis among women compared to men. Specifically, women have less cortical bone and experience bone loss at an earlier age and at a more rapid pace than do men, with the result that women have a much greater percentage of bone loss over their lifetime. Men

---

DISPLAY 12-1
Patterns of Bone Loss in Adults

Cortical Bone

- Beginning around the age of 40 years, age-related changes decrease the amount of cortical bone by 3% per decade in both men and women.
- Age-related decreases in cortical bone (i.e., 3% per decade) in men and women continue throughout later adulthood.
- After menopause, women experience an additional loss of cortical bone, so their total rate of decrease is 9% to 10% per decade between the ages of 45 and 75 years.
- The menopause-related decrease in cortical bone ends around the age of 70 to 75 years.
- The end result of these changes is approximately a 35% and 23% lifetime loss of cortical bone for women and men, respectively.

Trabecular Bone

- The onset of trabecular bone loss is about a decade earlier than the onset of cortical bone loss in both men and women.

- The rate of bone loss for both men and women is about 6% to 8% per decade.
- After menopause, women may experience an accelerated rate of trabecular bone loss.
- The end result is approximately a 50% and 33% lifetime loss of trabecular bone for women and men, respectively.

Factors That Influence the Rate of Bone Loss

- Bed rest and immobility increase trabecular bone loss.
- The rate of menopause-related bone loss is greater in thin women than in overweight women.
- The rate of bone loss can be slowed by using interventions and preventive strategies.

---

first show significant loss of peripheral cortex around the age of 70 years, and they lose cortical bone only in proportion to a loss of lean body mass. Osteoporosis involves a biphasic pattern of bone loss affecting both cortical and trabecular bone, as described in Display 12-1. This pattern involves a prolonged slow phase in both men and women, as well as a transient, accelerated phase that occurs in women after menopause. Many studies of cortical and trabecular bone changes support this theory, but some findings are inconsistent, primarily with regard to the onset and rate of change in trabecular bone. Although there is little controversy about the two phases or the changes in cortical bone, the differences between longitudinal and cross-sectional studies appear to account for many of

these inconsistencies. For instance, the results of cross-sectional studies have been questioned because people who today are 75 years of age were an average of 4 cm shorter at the age of 25 years than the present cohort of younger adults.

Types of Osteoporosis

Traditionally, osteoporosis has been classified as primary when it is associated with age- and menopause-related changes, and as secondary when it is caused by medications or pathophysiologic disturbances, such as endocrine disorders. Based on this classification system, only 5% of all cases of osteoporosis are of the secondary type (Meier, 1988). In the 1940s, Albright proposed that involutional osteoporosis was the major type of primary osteoporosis, and he suggested that it could be further categorized as either postmenopausal or senile (Albright, 1947). Albright identified estrogen deficiency as the underlying cause of postmenopausal osteoporosis, and he was the first physician to advocate the use of estrogen to correct negative calcium and phosphorus balances (Gordan and Genant, 1985).

In the 1980s, a similar but more detailed classification scheme was proposed by Riggs and Melton (1983), based on numerous studies of bone changes. Their classification system of types I and II osteoporosis has become widely accepted as a basis for evaluating, preventing, and treating osteoporosis. Type I (postmenopausal) osteoporosis affects women within 15 to 20 years after menopause, whereas type II (senile) osteoporosis affects both men and women and is attributable to age-related processes. Type I osteoporosis is associated with the following menopausal sequence of events: accelerated bone loss, increased secretion of parathyroid hormone and increased secretion of calcitonin, impaired function of vitamin D metabolites with a concomitant decrease in calcium absorption, and acceleration of bone loss from decreased calcium absorption. Type II osteoporosis is associated with the factors described in the earlier section on age-related bone changes. According to Riggs and Melton, the most important of these age-related changes are the decreases in osteoblast function and calcium absorption.

In addition to identifying different causative factors for types I and II osteoporosis, Riggs and Melton (1986) also suggested that the consequences of these two processes differ. For instance, as a consequence of the greatly accelerated trabecular bone loss associated with type I osteoporosis, vertebral fractures and Colles' fractures of the distal forearm are common. By contrast, the most common fractures occurring in those with type II osteoporosis, in which the rate of loss of cortical and trabecular bone is about equal, are hip and wedge-type vertebral fractures. Type II osteoporosis is responsible for dorsal kyphosis and the gradual loss of height with increased age. Table 12-1 summarizes the characteristics of types I and II osteoporosis.

Risk Factors

The risk factors that are of greatest concern with regard to safe mobility are those that contribute to falls, fractures, and osteoporosis. These risks are of particular importance to gerontological

TABLE 12-1
Comparison of Types I and II Osteoporosis

Characteristic	Type I	Type II
Age of onset	Postmenopause	30 to 40 years
Age at which consequences occur	10 to 20 years postmenopause	>70 years
Type of bone affected	Mostly trabecular	Cortical and trabecular
Causative factors	Menopause-related estrogen depletion and other changes	Age-related changes that affect calcium absorption and bone remodeling
Most common consequences	Vertebral (crush) and distal radius fractures; increased tooth loss	Hip and vertebral (wedge) fractures; kyphosis

nurses because many of them can be alleviated through nursing interventions. In addition, when the risks are eliminated or minimized, the serious functional consequences are likely to be prevented.

Risks for Osteoporosis

Although prevention of osteoporosis ideally begins in childhood, interventions that address the risk factors for this condition can be beneficial at any age. Some of the risks for osteoporosis, such as heredity, cannot be changed; however, determining the number of risk factors that exist for an older adult can be helpful in deciding on medical interventions and in weighing factors associated with cost, convenience, and possible adverse effects. Knowledge about the risks for osteoporosis has grown during the past 3 decades, but questions about some of the risks remain unanswered. Many of the questions are related to the degree to which the factor must be present before it becomes a risk factor. For example, it has been shown that bed rest can result in an average loss of vertebral bone of 0.9% per week (Krolner and Toft, 1983). Also,

there is abundant evidence that weight-bearing exercise is beneficial in preventing bone loss. What is not known, however, is the relative benefit or risk of the levels of activity that lie between the extremes of bed rest and a regular program of weight-bearing exercise 3 to 4 hours per week. Similarly, there is a strong association between excessive alcohol ingestion and osteoporotic fractures, but less is known about the effects of moderate alcohol consumption on osteoporosis. The most widely acknowledged risks are summarized in Display 12-2. Also listed in the display are the few factors that have been found to decrease the risk of osteoporosis.

Risks for Unsafe Mobility

Falling is an age-related functional consequence that has been the focus of a great number of studies in Great Britain and the United States. Four decades ago, an article entitled "On the Natural History of Falls in Old Age" began with the following declaration: "The liability of old people to tumble and often to injure themselves is such a commonplace of experience that it has been tacitly accepted as an inevitable aspect of

---

DISPLAY 12-2
Factors Influencing the Risk of Osteoporosis

Factors That Increase the Risk of Osteoporosis

Female gender

Increased age

White or Asian race

Estrogen deficiency (women)

Decreased testosterone levels (men)

Low calcium intake, both past and current

Prolonged immobility

Absence of menstruation, secondary to natural or surgical menopause, or to any other reason

Small bones

Thinness or less-than-normal weight

Excessive alcohol intake

Genetic predisposition

Excessive use of antacids, particularly those that contain aluminum

Inadequate vitamin D intake

Cigarette smoking

Long-term use of certain medications (e.g., corticosteroids, anticonvulsants, thyroid hormones)

Factors That Reduce the Risk of Osteoporosis

Obesity

Thiazide diuretics

Long-term use of estrogens

Black or Hispanic race

ageing, and thereby deprived of the exercise of curiosity" (Sheldon, 1960). In the last decade, geriatricians and gerontologists have challenged this view that falls are a normal consequence of aging or are accidental or random events. Falls are now considered to be predictable events that are caused by a complexity of environmental and intrinsic factors, many of which are amenable to interventions. In fact, the phrase "accidental falls" has been replaced by the phrase "unintentional injuries" in an atempt to reflect more accurately the etiology of falls (Tideiksaar, 1997).

Risk factors for falls can be categorized, according to their origin, as follows: age-related changes, medical conditions and functional impairments, medication effects, psychosocial impairments, and extrinsic factors. Like other negative functional consequences, falls are the result of a combination of these factors, rather than one isolated risk factor. Because so many studies have been conducted to identify the underlying causes of falling in older adults, conclusions have been drawn regarding different underlying causes according to age group. Falls in older adults younger than 75 years of age are predominantly attributable to a combination of age-related changes, such as vision changes, and unfavorable environmental conditions, such as poor lighting. As a result, falls in young-old adults are often the consequence of trips and slips. By contrast, falls in people older than 75 years of age are predominantly the result of a combination of disease- and medication-related factors (Tideiksaar, 1997). Similarly, it has been concluded that risks for falls differ according to the environment in which the older person lives. For example, falls in institutionalized older people are most often associated with weakness, dizziness, confusion, and gait disorders, whereas falls in community-living populations tend to be associated with environmental factors (Rubenstein et al., 1996).

Age-related changes that can contribute to falls have been discussed throughout this text

and were reviewed in the first section of this chapter. Specifically, nocturia, osteoporosis, vision changes, gait changes, postural hypotension, and central nervous system changes, such as decreased reaction time, may increase the risk of falls in older adults. Also, osteoporosis may increase the risk of serious injury when falls occur. It is important to keep in mind that age-related changes alone rarely cause falls; rather, falls are usually attributable to interactions between multiple risk factors that commonly affect older adults. A recent study found an association between a history of falling and the age-related changes of decreased muscle endurance and increased recovery time from fatiguing exercise in older women (Schwendner et al., 1997).

Some environmental hazards were discussed in Chapter 7, but additional environmental influences must be considered specifically in relation to falls. Studies have identified different environmental influences according to the type of setting. In hospitals and nursing homes, for example, the first and second most common sites of falls are the bedroom and bathroom, respectively. In the bedroom, most falls occur while the person is getting in or out of bed, and some falls are related to climbing over side rails or footboards. In the bathroom, falls generally occur while transferring on or off toilet seats or while hurrying to urinate or defecate. In community settings, most falls occur in the home, particularly in stairways, bedrooms, and living rooms. Activities that have been associated with falling in home settings include slipping on wet surfaces, slipping while descending stairs, getting in and out of beds and chairs, and tripping over floor coverings or objects on the floor. Studies have also revealed that the influence of some environmental factors differs depending on the setting. For example, assistive devices have been associated with falls in hospitals and nursing homes, but not in community settings (Tideiksaar, 1997). A recent nursing study of rural older adults found an association between a rural lifestyle and episodes of falling. For example, more than 50% of the falls occurred outdoors, and 44% of the falls occurred during tasks related to support or maintenance of the home (Baldwin et al., 1996).

Since the mid-1960s, physical restraints have commonly been used in institutional settings for the purpose of protecting impaired people from injury. Since the mid-1980s, however, many questions have been raised about the validity of the assumption that restraints are effective in protecting people from falls. In the past decade, numerous studies of nursing home residents have concluded that restraints do not reduce the risk of falls, and that when they are used, older adults are more likely to experience serious injury from falls (Tinetti et al., 1992; Tideiksaar, 1997; Capezuti et al., 1998). More recently, attention has been focused on the detrimental effects of physical restraints on hospitalized patients. Currently, there are many questions about the benefits versus the risks of physical restraints, and there is some evidence that restraints cause more problems, disabilities, and deaths than they prevent.

Medical conditions are associated with falls in older adults in all of the following ways:

1. Medical conditions may be treated with medications that create risks for falling;
2. Illnesses can cause functional impairments, such as vision or mobility limitations;
3. Illnesses may cause metabolic or other physiologic disturbances that create risks for falls;
4. Falls may be one manifestation of an acute illness or a change in a chronic illness; and
5. Chronic illnesses interfere with optimal exercise and other health practices that are important in promoting safe mobility.

Considering all of these possible associations, it is not surprising that most falls resulting in unintentional injuries occur in people who have functional impairments and multiple, chronic, medical problems. One recent nursing study found that an acute change in health status was a strong predictor of falls in nursing home residents (Kuehn and Sendelweck, 1995). Another recent study emphasized the important role of acute medical conditions and other intrinsic factors as risk factors for hip fractures in older adults (Norton et al., 1997).

Studies have identified hundreds of medications that can contribute to falls, and some studies have looked at the relationship between falls, medications, and diagnosis. Not all conclusions are consistent with regard to specific medications or diagnoses. Instead, the key to identifying an association between medications and falls is to consider the underlying mechanism, as well as the medical condition and the potential interactions between various factors. For example, postural hypotension can be caused by medical conditions, age-related changes, or adverse medication effects. If an 80-year-old person has a medical condition (e.g., hypertension) that may cause postural hypotension, and if the person is taking a medication (e.g., a vasodilator) that causes postural hypotension, the risk for falls is significantly increased. Therefore, rather than memorizing all of the medications that have been found to increase the risk for falls, gerontological nurses can focus their attention on the underlying mechanisms that increase the risk for falls.

The following medication effects can increase the risk for falls: confusion, depression, sedation, arrhythmias, hypovolemia, postural hypotension, delayed reaction time, diminished cognitive function, and changes on gait and balance (e.g., ataxia, decreased proprioception, and increased body sway). Thus, any medication that has one or more of these adverse effects may increase the risk of falls. A recent study suggests that one of the ways that benzodiazepines increase the risk of falls is by their effect on neuromuscular processing, which can affect balance control (Cutson et al., 1997). This effect is just one adverse effect of benzodiazepines, which also include sedation and impaired cognitive function. In addition to these actions, other medication-related considerations that influence the risk of falls include medication-disease interactions, medication-medication interactions, and medication-alcohol interactions. Also, the risk of falls can be affected by the dose, half-life, and administration time of the medication. For example, an association has been found between benzodiazepines with long half-lives (e.g., flurazepam) and an increased risk for falls and fractures.

Studies have focused primarily on prescription medications, but over-the-counter medications also can create risks for falls, particularly as a result of interactions with other medications. For example, many over-the-counter preparations for pain, colds, and insomnia contain alcohol or anticholinergics. These ingredients may themselves pose risks, or they may interact with other medications to increase the risk for falls. Some of the types of medications that are likely to increase the risk for falls are listed in Display 12-3.

Finally, impairments in cognition or other areas of psychosocial function can increase the risk for falls in older adults. Both dementia and depression may contribute to falls in that they diminish a person's awareness of the environment. Dementia can also interfere with the per-

---

DISPLAY 12-3
Examples of Risk Factors for Falls

Age-Related Changes

Vision and hearing changes
Osteoporosis
Slowed reaction time
Altered gait, increased sway
Postural hypotension
Nocturia

Medical Problems

Dementia, confusion
Cardiovascular diseases (e.g., arrhythmias or myocardial infarction)
Respiratory diseases (e.g., chronic obstructive pulmonary disease)
Neurologic disorders (e.g., parkinsonism, stroke)
Metabolic disturbances (e.g., dehydration, electrolyte imbalances)
Musculoskeletal problems (e.g., osteoarthritis)
Transient ischemic attack
Cataracts, macular degeneration, glaucoma

Psychosocial Factors

Depression
Anxiety
Distractions
Agitation

Medications

Anticholinergics
Diuretics
Antianxiety and hypnotic agents, especially those with long half-lives
Antipsychotics
Antidepressants (e.g., tricyclics)
Antihypertensives (e.g., beta-blockers)
Vasodilators
Nonsteroidal anti-inflammatory agents
Alcohol
Medication interactions

Extrinsic Factors

Physical restraints
Glare or poor lighting
Lack of handrails
Slippery floors
Throw rugs
Unfamiliar environments
Highly polished floors
Improper height of beds, chairs, or toilets

Any Combination of the Preceding Factors

son's ability to process information regarding environmental stimuli. Numerous studies of people with Alzheimer's disease and other dementias suggest that the following combination of factors significantly increase the risk for falls: medications, concurrent conditions, decreased level of awareness, diminished ability to cope with environmental surroundings; and the severity of associated functional disabilities, such as mobility impairments. Older adults who are depressed are at increased risk for falls secondary to gait changes, medication effects, and a diminished ability to concentrate on and respond to environmental factors. Display 12-3 summarizes some of the risk factors that may cause or contribute to falls in older adults. This list is not all-inclusive; rather it is intended to provide examples of the hundreds of possible risk factors, organized by categories.

Functional Consequences

Age-related changes affect muscle function, but the functional consequences do not significantly affect the quality of life and can be compensated for, at least in part, through exercise. Age-related changes in joint function can interfere with mobility and full range of motion, but in the absence of osteoarthritis and other disease-related processes, these functional consequences are not serious. The functional consequences of osteoporosis, however, are quite serious, as are the functional consequences that occur as a result of the combination of age-related changes and the hundreds of risk factors that contribute to falls in older adults.

Muscle and Joint Function

Muscle strength, endurance, and coordination are affected to some extent by age-related changes, even in the absence of risk factors. Beginning around the age of 40 years, muscle strength declines gradually, resulting in an overall decrease of 30% to 50% by the age of 80 years. There is a greater decline in muscle strength in the lower extremities than in the upper extremities. Diminished muscle strength is attributed primarily to age-related loss of muscle mass. In addition, a person's current level of activity and lifelong patterns of exercise can influence muscle strength at any age. Muscle endurance and coordination diminish as a result of age-related changes in the muscles and central nervous system. As a consequence of these changes, compared to their younger counterparts, older adults experience muscle fatigue after shorter periods of exercise.

Joint function begins to decline in the 3rd decade and diminishes gradually throughout one's lifetime. The outcome of these degenerative changes is a diminished range of motion, resulting, in particular, in the following changes: (1) decreased motion in the upper arms, potentially causing difficulty with activities such as writing, eating, and grooming; and (2) decreased lower back flexion, hip flexion and external rotation, knee flexion, and foot dorsiflexion, causing potential difficulties with putting shoes and socks on and climbing stairs and curbs. The overall impact of diminished joint function is that older people's ability to respond to environmental stimuli and perform ADL is slowed.

Increased Susceptibility to Fractures

One of the most significant of all age-related functional consequences is the increased susceptibility to fractures that is the direct result of osteoporosis. Even in the absence of additional risk factors, this age-related change contributes to the high incidence of fractures in older adults. Fractures are not unique to older adults, but they do differ in many respects from those that occur in younger populations. First, bones of older adults may be fractured with little or no trauma, whereas bones of children and younger adults are fractured only in response to a forceful impact. Fractures are defined as osteoporotic, or fragility fractures, when they occur as the result of even minimal trauma—that is, trauma that is no more severe than that resulting from falling to the floor from a standing position. Second, the risk of fractures increases in direct relation to age; however, in older women, the number of years since menopause may be a more accurate risk indicator than chronologic age. Third, poor recovery after a fractured hip has been associated with all of the following factors: age of 75 years or older, female gender, prefracture dependency, cognitive impairment, postsurgical delirium, lengthy hospital stays, and lack of social supports (Tideiksaar, 1997).

Gender and Racial Differences with Regard to Susceptibility to Fractures

There is little doubt that the functional consequences of age-related changes affecting the musculoskeletal system differ between men and women. Vertebral compression fractures, for example, occur 8 times more frequently in women than in men (Meier, 1988). There is controversy, however, about the extent to which the differences are attributable to menopausal changes or to other gender differences. It is well known that there is a perimenopausal increase in cortical bone loss, and that this is associated with decreased estrogen levels. Additional gender differences, however, may have equal significance in contributing to the increased risk of fractures in older women.

Much attention has been focused on the gender differences in bone size at the time of maturity. At the age of 18 years, women have a 20% lower bone mass in relation to body weight than do men. Several researchers have pointed out that, because women have a smaller bone mass at skeletal maturity, they are less able to compensate for age-related bone loss. According to this theory, women reach the so-called theoretical fracture threshold at an earlier age than men, and are thus more prone to fractures because of the smaller size of their bones (Cummings et al., 1985; Meier, 1988).

Whites and Asians have a much higher rate of osteoporotic fractures than do Blacks, but the reasons for this are not clear. Factors that may contribute to this discrepancy include the higher bone mass of Blacks at skeletal maturity, the greater bone density and thicker bone cortex of Blacks, and the slower rate of age- or menopause-related bone loss in the Black population (Cummings et al., 1985; Meier, 1988). Additional cultural variations in bone mass and incidence rates for fractures are highlighted in the Culture Box.

Increased Susceptibility to Falls

Numerous age-related changes and risk factors contribute to the high incidence of falls among older adults, particularly older women. A review of studies regarding the frequency of falls in

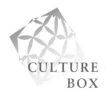

CULTURE BOX

Cultural Variations in Bone Mass and Incidence Rates for Fractures

- Cultural variations in bone density, ranging from highest density to lowest, are as follows: African American men, White men and African American women, White women, Asian Americans, and Eskimos (Overfield, 1996).
- White races, particularly those of Scandinavian origin, have relatively low bone mass and high rates of fractures (Kalu and Bauer, 1996).
- African Americans have only one third to one half the risk of fractures of Whites, and they have bone masses that are 10% greater (Kalu and Bauer, 1996).

older adults revealed the following (Tideiksaar, 1997):

1. In community settings, 25% of people aged 65 to 74 years, and 33% of those aged 75 years and older fall every year. Fifty percent of these older adults experience multiple falls.
2. In acute care settings, approximately 20% of older patients fall during their hospital stay, with as many as 50% of these patients experiencing multiple falls.
3. In nursing homes, up to 50% of residents fall each year, with at least 40% of these experiencing multiple falls.

Psychosocial Consequences of Falls

The term "fallaphobia" was suggested by Tideiksaar and Kay (1986) to describe the following sequence of events: (1) older people fall, lose their balance, or feel at risk for falling; (2) they lose confidence in their ability to perform the activity that led to or created a risk for falling; (3) they stop performing the activity; and (4) they eventually become homebound or chairbound. Fallaphobia can have a protective effect when it helps older adults avoid hazards. More often, however, it is detrimental, contributing to shame, anxiety, depression, loss of confidence and diminished quality of life, and leading to the avoidance of activities (Tinetti and Powell, 1993; Tideiksaar, 1997; Lachman et al., 1998). Even in the absence of these events, fallaphobia may arise in older people whose friends have experienced serious fall-related consequences. One study found that one-third of the older adults who had not fallen reported that they limited their activity owing to fear of falling (Downton and Andrews, 1990).

Another serious psychosocial impact of falls has been called the "postfall syndrome" (Murphy and Isaacs, 1982). This phrase describes a distinct gait pattern that is adopted by older people who have fallen and have been admitted to the hospital for postfall injuries. The people who have this syndrome do not have any neurologic or orthopedic problems that could account

for the gait, and the characteristic gait pattern was not present before the fall. People with the postfall syndrome have the following characteristics: an expressed fear of falling when standing erect, a tendency to grab and clutch at objects within their view, and marked hesitancy and irregularity in their walking attempts (Murphy and Isaacs, 1982). A recent study found that some gait changes, such as prolonged double support and reduced speed and stride length, are more common in older people who are afraid of falling than those who are not. The authors of this study suggested that these fear-related gait changes may increase stability and serve to protect against falls (Maki, 1997).

Family caregivers of older adults also may be quite anxious about potential falls, and they may experience a sort of "what-if" phobia. This fear can lead to decisions that restrict an older adult's activities unnecessarily or that involve a move to a setting that provides a greater level of assistance or supervision than the older person desires. Although a move to an unfamiliar environment may lead to falls, the caregivers who encourage or make such a decision may derive some peace of mind, at least initially. Nurses, primary care providers, nursing home administrators, and other people with responsibility for the care of older people in institutional settings may adopt a protectionist approach regarding falls. This perspective is attributable, at least in part, to a fear of lawsuits and the demands of family members who insist that the older person be restrained and that their activities be restricted in order to minimize the chance of falls. The end result may be that dependent older adults are restrained or restricted to a degree that is just as detrimental as the effect of a fall. In fact, bed rails and physical restraints may contribute to falls in some cases (Tideiksaar, 1997). It is an unfortunate reflection on our medicolegal system that lawsuits are initiated more often because of falls than because of restricted activity. Older adults, therefore, are not only subject to their own fallaphobia, but also to the fall-related anxieties of their caregivers.

Economic Impact of Falls, Fractures, and Osteoporosis

One of the reasons that falls, fractures, and osteoporosis have been the focus of so many studies is that these age-related events have a tremendous impact on health care expenditures for older adults. Much of this impact is borne by society at large and the health care system. The following statistics can be translated into health care dollars to reflect the economic impact of falls, fractures, and osteoporosis (Tideiksaar, 1997):

- Twenty percent of hospital admissions and up to 40% of nursing home admissions of older adults are related to falling.
- The average length of hospital stay for an individual who has fallen is nearly twice that of an individual who has not fallen.
- Approximately 50% of patients hospitalized for falling are admitted to long-term care facilities.
- By the age of 90 years, hip fractures affect 33% and 17% of women and men, respectively.
- The annual incidence rate of hip fractures doubles during each decade beyond the age of 50 years.

A recent study found a strong independent relationship between falls and functional decline in community-living older adults (Tinetti and Williams, 1998). Recent studies also have shown that postfall assessment and interventions can significantly reduce the number of future hospitalizations and hospital days (Rubenstein et al., 1996).

Table 12-2 summarizes the age-related changes and functional consequences that affect safe mobility, and Figure 12-1 illustrates the factors that influence mobility of older adults.

Nursing Assessment

Nursing assessment of mobility and safety focuses on identifying the risk factors for falls and

TABLE 12-2
Age-Related Changes Affecting Mobility and Safety

Change	Consequence
Diminished muscle mass and central nervous system changes	Diminished muscle strength, endurance, and coordination
Degenerative changes in connective tissue and other joint structures	Limited range of motion in all joints; increased difficulty in performing ADL
Osteoporosis	Increased susceptibility to fractures
Functional changes in vision, gait, balance, mobility, and nervous system	Increased susceptibility to falls

osteoporosis, as well as the functional consequences of age-related musculoskeletal changes that affect ADL. It is particularly important to identify the risks for falls and osteoporosis that can be modified or alleviated through nursing interventions. Assessment of these three aspects of mobility and safety is discussed in the following sections, and guidelines for assessment are summarized in Displays 12-4 and 12-5.

Overall Musculoskeletal Performance

For healthy older adults, the primary effects of age-related changes on musculoskeletal performance are a change in gait and a slowing in performance of some ADL. To assess overall musculoskeletal performance, therefore, nurses should observe the person's mobility and activities and ask questions about their ability to perform ADL. In addition, when any limitations are identified, it is important to find out whether older adults are using assistive devices to improve function, or if they are aware of the availability of such devices. The nurse, therefore, can include a question to assess the older person's knowledge about and use of assistive devices in performing ADL. Criteria for the functional

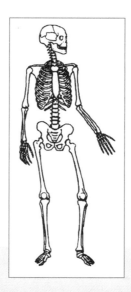

AGE-RELATED CHANGES

- Diminished muscle mass
- Degenerative connective tissue changes
- Osteoporosis
- Changes in central nervous system

NEGATIVE FUNCTIONAL CONSEQUENCES

- Diminished muscle strength, endurance, and coordination
- Limited range of joint motion
- Increased susceptibility to falls
- Increased susceptibility to fractures

RISK FACTORS

- *Risks for Osteoporosis*: Female gender, advanced age, immobility, inadequate calcium intake, small bones, thinness, estrogen deficiency, genetic predisposition
- *Risks for Falls and Fractures*: Osteoporosis, age-related changes in sensory function and in central nervous system, medical conditions, medications, depression, dementia, environmental factors

FIGURE 12-1. Mobility in older adults.

assessment of all ADL are provided in Chapter 17 and can be used in conjunction with the assessment information in this chapter.

In addition to experiencing minor changes in performance of ADL, older adults experience changes in posture, and their height will diminish. Older adults may be concerned about loss of height, or they may not even be aware of this change; in any case, height changes do not significantly affect the usual activities of older adults. A height loss of about 2 to 4 cm per decade is normal, owing to osteoporosis and other age-related changes. Including a question about the person's usual height and any noticeable loss of height will give the nurse an opportunity to assess the older adult's awareness of this change. Although the functional consequences of decreased height are minimal, older people who never were very tall may experience increased difficulty performing activities that depend on height. In these situations, they may find that it is safer and more effective to use assistive devices, such as long-handled reachers.

Risks for Osteoporosis

An assessment of risks for osteoporosis should be undertaken in all older men and women because preventive and protective measures are important at any age. Several risk factors can be alleviated through lifestyle interventions that may have positive effects that extend beyond their impact on osteoporosis. For all older adults, these interventions include adequate intakes of calcium and vitamin D and participation in regular weight-bearing exercise to the extent of their ability. Older adults who smoke cigarettes or consume excessive amounts of alcohol can benefit in many ways from eliminating or limiting these practices. If an assessment identifies risk factors that cannot be modified (e.g., small bones), this information may be used to motivate the person to take action to eliminate the risks that can be addressed. Much of the

information regarding risks for osteoporosis is obtained during an overall assessment or health history, and this information should be considered in relation to mobility and safety. Assessment questions and considerations relating to osteoporosis are listed in Display 12-4.

Risks for Falls

Assessment of an individual's risks for falls is multidimensional and ideally includes observations of the person in their usual environment. Although nurses in institutional settings are naturally most concerned about the person's immediate environment, they also must be concerned about the person's home environment as part of their discharge planning for people who are at risk for falls. The same assessment criteria are used for environmental safety, regardless of the setting. The best assessment information is obtained by observing the person in the environment and paying particular attention to the person's awareness of and attention to the environment. Observations are especially helpful in identifying discrepancies between the person's perception of his or her abilities and his or her actual performance. Observations also provide information about adaptive behaviors that otherwise might not be acknowledged. For example, a person might state that he or she has no difficulty with stair climbing, but observations might reveal that the person performs this activity in a highly unsafe manner. Nurses in institutional settings generally do not have opportunities to observe home environments directly, but they can observe the person in the immediate environment and ask questions about the home setting. They can also ask caregivers of dependent older adults about home environments and the person's ability to function safely in that setting. The guidelines summarized in Display 12-5 can be used to assess the safety of any environment, and can be applied to all older adults, particularly those who are older than 75 years of age.

DISPLAY 12-4
Guidelines for Assessing Mobility and Risks for Osteoporosis

Interview Questions to Assess Overall Musculoskeletal Performance

- Do you have any trouble performing your usual activities because of joint limitations?
- Do you have any pain or discomfort in your joints?
- Do you ever feel like you're losing your balance?
- Do you have any trouble walking or getting around?
- Have you had any falls in the past few years? (If yes, what were the circumstances?)
- Are you afraid of falling?
- Do you use any assistive devices to help you do things (e.g., a walker, quad cane, or reaching devices)?
- Are there any activities you would like to do, but don't do, because of any difficulty moving or getting around or because you are afraid of falling?

Observations Regarding Overall Musculoskeletal Performance

- Measure and record the person's present height and stated peak height.
- Observe the individual's walking and gait pattern.
- Observe and document information regarding ADL (as described in Chapter 17).

Interview Questions to Assess Risks for Osteoporosis

- Do you know of any blood relatives who have had osteoporosis or who have sustained fractures late in life?
- Have you sustained any fractures during your adult years? (If yes, ask additional questions regarding age at the time, type, location, circumstances, treatment, and so on.)

- Do you take any calcium or vitamin D supplements?
- Have you ever had your bone density measured?
- Do you take any medications for osteoporosis?

Interview Questions for Women Only

- When did you begin menopause?
- Do you take estrogen, or have you ever taken it? (If yes, ask additional questions regarding type, dose, duration, and so on.)

Observations Made During Other Portions of an Overall Assessment That Are Also Useful in Assessing Mobility and Risks for Osteoporosis

- How much exercise does the person get on a regular basis? (In particular, how much weight-bearing exercise?)
- Does the person smoke cigarettes?
- How much alcohol does the person consume?
- What is the person's usual daily intake of calcium and vitamin D?
- Does the person have any medical conditions that are associated with falls or osteoporosis?
- Is the person taking any medications that might create risks for falls (including over-the-counter medications)?
- Does the person have postural hypotension?
- Does the person have any cognitive impairments or other psychosocial impairments that diminish his or her attention to the environment or interfere with the ability to respond to environmental stimuli?

Nurses also should assess the older adult's attitude toward the use of assistive devices, as attitudes are likely to influence the acceptability of using recommended aids. One nursing study found that assessing a person's thoughts, feelings, and perceptions about mobility aids is as important as assessing the actual need for these aids (Rush and Ouellet, 1997).

For older adults who have already fallen, a more extensive assessment is required. A recent development in geriatric care has been the establishment of "Fall Clinics" or "Mobility Clinics."

Illumination and Color Contrast

- Is the lighting adequate but not glare-producing?
- Are the light switches easy to reach and manipulate?
- Can lights be turned on before entering rooms?
- Are night-lights used in appropriate places?
- Is color contrast adequate between objects such as a chair and floor?

Hazards

- Are there throw rugs, highly polished floors, or other hazardous floor coverings?
- If area rugs are used, do they have a nonslip backing and are the edges tacked to the floor?
- Are there cords, clutter, or other obstacles in pathways?
- Is there a pet that is likely to be running underfoot?

Furniture

- Are chairs the right height and depth for the person?
- Do the chairs have arm rests?
- Are tables stable and of the appropriate height?
- Is small furniture placed well away from pathways?

Stairways

- Is lighting adequate?
- Are there light switches at the top and bottom of the stairs?
- Are there securely fastened handrails on both sides of the stairway?
- Are all the steps even?
- Are the treads nonskid?
- Should colored tape be used to mark the edges of the steps, particularly the top and bottom steps?

Bathroom

- Are grab bars placed appropriately for the tub and toilet?
- Does the tub have skidproof strips or a rubber mat in the bottom?
- Has the person considered using a tub seat?

- Is the height of the toilet seat appropriate?
- Has the person considered using an elevated toilet seat?
- Does the color of the toilet seat contrast with surrounding colors?
- Is toilet paper within easy reach?

Bedroom

- Is the height of the bed appropriate?
- Is the mattress firm at the edges to provide enough support for sitting?
- If the bed has wheels, are they locked securely?
- Would side rails be a help or a hazard?
- When side rails are in the down position, are they completely out of the way?
- Is the pathway between the bedroom and bathroom clear of objects and adequately illuminated, particularly at night?
- Would a bedside commode be useful, especially at night?
- Does the person have sufficient physical and cognitive ability to turn on a light before getting out of bed?
- Is furniture positioned to allow safe use of assistive devices for ambulation?
- Is a telephone situated near the bed?

Kitchen

- Are storage areas used to the best advantage (e.g., are objects that are frequently used in the most accessible places)?
- Are appliance cords kept out of the way?
- Are nonslip mats used in front of the sink?
- Are the markings on stoves and other appliances clearly visible?
- Does the person know how to use the microwave safely?

Assistive Devices

- Is a call light available, and does the person know how to use it?
- What assistive devices are used?
- Would the person benefit from any assistive devices that are not being used?
- Are assistive devices being used safely and properly, or do they present additional hazards?

(continued)

DISPLAY 12-5
Guidelines for Assessing the Safety of the Environment (Continued)

Temperature

- Is the temperature of the room(s) comfortable?
- Can the person read the markings on the thermostat and adjust it appropriately?
- During cold months, is the room temperature high enough to prevent hypothermia?
- During hot weather, is the room temperature cool enough to prevent hyperthermia?

Overall Safety

- How does the person obtain objects from hard-to-reach places?
- How does the person change overhead light bulbs?
- Are doorways wide enough to accommodate assistive devices?

- Do door thresholds create hazardous conditions?
- Are telephones accessible, especially for emergency calls?
- Would it be helpful to use a cordless portable phone?
- Would it be helpful to have some emergency call system available?
- Does the person wear sturdy shoes with non-skid soles?
- Are smoke alarms present and operational?
- Is there a carbon monoxide detector (if the house has gas appliances)?
- Does the person keep a list of emergency numbers by the phone?
- Does the person have an emergency exit plan in the event of fire?

These types of programs are not yet widely available, but a growing attention to falls and their associated high medical care costs is sure to stimulate the development of additional programs. Rehabilitation programs, particularly geriatric rehabilitation programs, are another source for the comprehensive assessment of older adults who have fallen. These specialized programs use a multidisciplinary approach and generally include a direct assessment of the person's usual environment. Interdisciplinary geriatric assessment programs are yet another resource for fall assessment. Gerontological nurses can encourage older adults who have fallen or who are at increased risk for falls to take advantage of these specialized programs, rather than accepting falls as an inevitable consequence of aging.

Nursing Diagnosis

Nurses working with community-living older adults may identify risks for osteoporosis that can be addressed through health education. For example, postmenopausal women may express an interest in preventing osteoporosis because they are aware of the association between decreased estrogen and an increased likelihood of fractures. In these situations, a nursing diagnosis of Health-Seeking Behaviors may be applicable. This is defined as "the state in which an individual in stable health actively seeks ways to alter personal health habits and/or the environment in order to move toward a higher level of wellness" (Carpenito, 1997, p. 450).

If the nursing assessment identifies risks for falls, as well as factors that interfere with safe mobility, the nursing diagnosis of Risk for Injury would be applicable. This is defined as "the state in which an individual is at risk for harm because of a perceptual or physiologic deficit, a lack of awareness of hazards, or maturational age" (Carpenito, 1997, p. 509). Related factors common in older adults include all those factors listed in Display 12-3. The case example in this chapter addresses this nursing diagnosis.

Impaired Physical Mobility is a nursing diagnosis that is applicable when the assessment identifies limitations in mobility of an older adult. This is defined as "a state in which the individual experiences or is at risk of experiencing limitations of physical movement but is not immobile" (Carpenito, 1997, p. 565). Related factors common in older adults include arthritis, depression, chronic pain, and neurologic disorders (e.g., dementia or Parkinson's disease).

When older adults express feelings associated with fallaphobia, the nurse may address this concern by applying a nursing diagnosis of Fear. Related factors would be postural instability, gait or balance disorders, or history of falls. This diagnosis is applicable when the nursing assessment reveals that the older adult limits his or her activities because of fallaphobia to the point that quality of life is affected.

Nursing Goals

Nursing care of older adults who are at risk for osteoporosis is directed toward alleviating the factors that increase the risk of osteoporosis. This is accomplished through health education about osteoporosis, as summarized in the accompanying box. Most of these interventions are associated with lifestyle factors that a motivated older adult can address.

Care of older adults with a nursing diagnosis of High Risk for Injury focuses on addressing the factors that increase the risk of falls and fall-related injuries. This is accomplished through environmental modifications and interventions, such as fall prevention programs. When falls cannot be prevented, the goal is to prevent fall-related injuries. This goal is addressed by providing a safe environment and ensuring that the person receives quick assistance after a fall occurs. Nursing goals for older adults with impaired physical mobility are to restore their functional abilities and to prevent further loss of function. Interventions to accomplish this goal include the use of suitable adaptive and assistive devices and the implementation of appropriate exercise regimens.

Maintaining quality of life is a nursing goal for older adults with fallaphobia. This is accomplished by addressing the actual risk factors for falls and by educating the older adult about interventions to prevent falls. Also, such interventions as emergency response systems may be very reassuring to, as well as helpful for, older adults who spend much of their time alone.

Nursing Interventions

Preventing Osteoporosis

Prevention of osteoporosis is accomplished through medical, nutritional, and lifestyle interventions. Although studies on the prevention of osteoporosis have focused on postmenopausal women, men also are affected by osteoporosis. The only gender difference relating to risk factors for hip fractures is that men tend to be older than women when fractures occur. With the exception of estrogen deficiency, older men are probably affected by the same risk factors as women, although they may have more protection, such as that conferred by greater bone mass at maturity. The recent medical and nursing literature reflects the growing awareness of the need to include older men in efforts to prevent and treat osteoporosis (Kessenich and Rosen, 1996; Raisz, 1997). Thus, it is important to consider interventions for older men as well as postmenopausal women.

Medical Interventions

For the past 2 decades, studies have consistently found that oral or transdermal estrogen is effective in preventing bone loss and reducing the incidence of fractures in postmenopausal women. Postmenopausal women who take oral estrogen for 5 years or longer reduce their risk of hip fracture by 50% (National Institute of Arthritis and Musculoskeletal and Skin Diseases, 1991). Moreover, estrogen is effective in preventing further bone loss even when treatment is begun at a late age, but it is most effective when administered early in the postmenopausal period. Many questions regarding the safety of estrogen replacement therapy arose during the 1970s, but there is now much agreement that the risks are minimal, especially when estrogen is used in low doses and administered in combination with progesterone. The risks and benefits

ALTERNATIVE
AND
PREVENTIVE
HEALTH
CARE
PRACTICES

Preventing Osteoporosis

Herbs
- Sources of calcium: nettle, parsley, horsetail, dandelion leaf
- Sources of natural estrogen: sage, ginseng, licorice, motherwort, dong quai, black cohosh, chaste tree

Homeopathic Remedies
- Silica, calcaria phosphorica, calcarea carbonica

Nutritional Considerations
- Intake of optimal daily levels of boron, calcium* (1500 mg/d), selenium, magnesium, folate, and vitamins A,* B-complex, C, D,* E, and K
- Limiting consumption of beverages containing alcohol, caffeine, or phosphorus; avoiding phosphate food additives
- Intake of foods high in plant estrogen (e.g., tofu, soy foods)

Preventive Measures and Additional Approaches
- Weight-bearing exercise regimen for 1/2 hour daily, wearing of good support shoes, no cigarette smoking, maintenance of ideal body weight
- Yoga, rolfing, swimming, massage, acupressure, t'ai chi, chiropractic treatment
- Acupuncture for arthritis and/or joint and muscle disorders

Specific Information About Calcium
- Because the diet of older adults generally contains less than 800 mg of calcium per day, calcium supplements often are recommended so that the total intake is 1500 mg per day.
- Foods that are high in calcium include milk, cheese, yogurt, custard, ice cream, raisins, tofu, canned salmon or sardines, and broccoli and other dark green vegetables.
- Calcium carbonate, which is found in some antacids, is an effective and inexpensive source of elemental calcium.

Special Precautions
- Vitamin D in amounts greater than 400 to 600 IU per day, and vitamin A in amounts exceeding 5000 IU per day, can have detrimental effects.
- Calcium supplements are not recommended for people with poor kidney function or a predisposition for kidney stones.
- Because calcium may contribute to constipation, measures should be taken to promote bowel function (e.g., regular exercise and adequate fiber and fluid intake).
- Calcium supplements can interact with some medications (e.g., calcium decreases absorption of tetracycline).

*Further information on calcium and vitamins A and D supplements is included under Special Precautions.

of estrogen replacement therapy are discussed in greater detail in Chapter 16.

Although estrogen is known to be effective in preventing bone loss, it does not stimulate new bone growth. Sodium fluoride is a medical agent that can stimulate new bone formation, but there are many questions about its safety and effectiveness as a treatment for osteoporosis. Various regimens using sodium fluoride were still under investigation in 1998. Antiestrogens, such as tamoxifen, are also currently under investigation for the treatment of osteoporosis and the prevention of fractures.

In 1984, calcitonin became the first nonestrogen medication approved by the Food and Drug Administration (FDA) for the treatment of osteoporosis. The initial limitations of calcitonin therapy included its high cost, the need for subcutaneous injections, and questions about its long-term effectiveness. In 1995, a nasal spray form of calcitonin was approved as an option for the treatment of low mineral density of bone. One therapeutic advantage of calcitonin over estrogen is that it reduces the pain associated with vertebral fractures in some people.

In late 1995, alendronate became the first nonhormonal medication approved by the FDA for the prevention of fractures and bone loss. This medication prevents further bone loss and also increases bone mass. In 1998, a new class of medications, called selective estrogen receptor modulators, was approved for the prevention of osteoporosis in postmenopausal women.

Calcium and Vitamin D

Most medical experts on osteoporosis are currently recommending calcium intakes of 1200 to 1500 mg per day for men and women aged 51 year or older. A calcium intake of 1000 mg per day is adequate for women who are taking estrogen. Because the average American adult diet provides between 500 and 800 mg of calcium daily, calcium supplements are usually necessary. Calcium supplements, however, may have detrimental effects in older adults who take medications or in those who have renal impairments or any other physiologic disturbance. The most common adverse effects of daily calcium supplements of 1500 mg or less are constipation, flatulence, and rebound gastric acidity. Because vitamin D is necessary for the absorption of calcium, older adults should consume 400 to 800 IU of vitamin D daily. Older adults who have limited exposure to sunlight may not synthesize adequate amounts of vitamin D and are likely to require vitamin D supplements. Considerations regarding calcium and vitamin D intake are summarized with other alternative and preventive health care practices on page 366.

Lifestyle Interventions

Lifestyle interventions aimed at preventing osteoporosis should be encouraged for older adults because of the many overall benefits of these interventions. For example, quitting smoking, limiting alcohol intake, and engaging in regular weight-bearing exercise are lifestyle habits that may be beneficial in reducing the risk for osteoporosis, and they are definitely beneficial in other areas of function. The Alternative and Preventive Health Care Practices box can be used as a guide for teaching older adults about preventive interventions for osteoporosis.

Preventing Falls and Fall-Related Injuries

Interventions for preventing falls and fall-related injuries are directed toward correcting the environmental conditions that pose risks for safe mobility. Display 12-5 can be used as a guide for interventions that may eliminate or reduce environmental risks. Moreover, any interventions that prevent osteoporosis are beneficial in preventing fall-related injuries, such as fractures. In recent years, increased attention has been directed toward implementing exercise routines and gait training programs to prevent falls. For example, a nursing study found that t'ai chi exercises can be valuable in improving and maintaining balance (Schaller, 1996). Recent gerontological articles support the use of t'ai chi to improve strength, balance, and range of motion, and to preserve musculoskeletal function in older adults (Lumsden et al., 1998). Another study revealed that an exercise program was beneficial, in terms of gait and lower limb muscle strength, for women aged 60 to 83 years (Lord et al., 1996). Nurses can help identify and refer older people with gait and balance disorders who might benefit from a gait training program implemented by a physical therapist (Galindo-Ciocon et al., 1995). When older adults are likely to benefit from the use of mobility aids, nurses can facilitate a referral to a physical therapist for evaluation and teaching regarding the use of assistive devices.

Some nurses in home care and institutional settings have begun implementing fall awareness and prevention programs (e.g., Hollinger and Patterson, 1992; Brady et al., 1993). A recent nursing study found that almost 75% of older women who attended a community-based fall prevention program made at least one low-cost change to decrease the likelihood of their falling in their home environments (Ryan and Spellbring, 1996). Key aspects of fall prevention programs are the identification of people who are at risk for falls and the consistent implementation of preventive actions by all staff. Thus, an important part of these programs is education of all professional and nonprofessional staff members who have contact with the person who is at risk for falls. Education may involve strategies to heighten staff awareness of the importance of reducing the risks of falls. For example, posters and brochures may be used initially and periodically as reminders. Also, some form of patient/resident or chart identification can be used to draw attention to those people who have an increased risk for falls.

Fall prevention programs involve a focused assessment that is based on the risk factors found to occur most often in a particular setting. For example, home care nurses may assess an individual's home for the presence of slippery rugs, whereas nursing home staff might assess the use of restraints. In addition to focused assessment criteria, fall awareness and prevention programs address specific interventional strategies appropriate for the care setting. Interventions may include environmental modifications, decreased use of restraints, and the provision of assistance with ADL at specific times. One relatively simple and inexpensive intervention that has been applied successfully in special care units is for residents to wear terry cloth socks with anti-slip treads at night (Meddaugh et al., 1996). Display 12-6 describes a fall prevention program that could be adapted for use in institutional settings.

Monitoring devices can be very useful in alerting staff to potentially dangerous patient/resident activity, such as getting out of bed or a chair without assistance. Several types of devices are available, and they all have the ability to transmit a signal to a remote location (e.g., a nursing station) when activated by certain levels of patient/resident movement. Some devices, such as a pad, are applied to the bed, whereas others are used in conjunction with the person's clothing. Most movement detection devices are designed for institutional use, but some have been designed for home use by family caregivers.

A major limitation of movement detection devices is that their effectiveness depends on the timely response of someone who is able to prevent the fall. These devices are not useful for people living alone or for people without responsible caregivers. Several of the companies that manufacture movement detection devices are listed in the Educational Resources section of this chapter. In home settings, a room monitoring device may be useful when caregivers need to detect the sound of someone moving around in another room. These devices are widely available in stores where infant care supplies are sold.

DISPLAY 12-6
A Fall Prevention Program for Older Adults Being Cared for in Hospitals or Nursing Homes

Identification of Patients/Residents Who Are at Risk for Falling

- During the initial nursing assessment, identify any risks for falling (e.g., medications, medical conditions, history of falls, impaired cognition, diminished alertness, impaired mobility, age of 75 years or older).
- Document the risk factors on the designated fall assessment guide.
- Reassess the risks for falling at predetermined times (e.g., every shift, every day, whenever there is a change in the patient's/resident's functional status).
- Use color-coded items (e.g., brightly colored stickers for the chart, a brightly colored identification band for the person's wrist, and signs near the person's bed and outside the room) to identify those who are included in the program.

Education of the Staff, Patient/Resident, and Family

- Instruct the patient or resident and family about the fall prevention program using brochures that provide information about preventing falls and obtaining help if falls occur.

- Provide staff education about the fall prevention program and the risk factors for falls, especially those factors that the staff influences (e.g., use of restraints, selection of footwear).
- Use posters and fliers to heighten staff awareness of the fall prevention program.

Interventions to Be Implemented for All High-Risk Patients/Residents

- Keep the call light within reach at all times.
- Make sure the bed is in the lowest position possible and the wheels are locked.
- Consider the use of a movement detection monitor.
- If restraints are used, reevaluate their use every shift.
- If appropriate, orient the person to person, place, and time every shift and p.r.n.
- Offer assistance with ADL and try to anticipate the person's needs before help is needed.
- Encourage the patient or resident to call for help when needed.
- Document fall prevention interventions on the patient's or resident's chart.

When falling cannot be prevented, efforts should be directed toward preventing serious injury and providing assistance. For example, heavy furniture that is in a pathway where a fall is likely to occur can be moved out of the way, and sharp edges of furniture can be padded. In recent years, externally applied hip pads have been used as shock absorbers in an effort to prevent fractured hips. However, results of studies evaluating the effectiveness of these pads have been inconclusive (Tideiksaar, 1997).

An emergency call system can be useful in situations in which falls cannot be prevented. These devices involve the use of a remote control mechanism that is worn on the person's body or clothing. Examples of such devices are beeper-type devices worn on the belt or pendants worn as necklaces or bracelets. When the person falls, they can summon help by using the remote control mechanism to signal a receiver unit that is attached to the phone. In turn, a call is automatically made to a programmed number, such as a neighbor or an emergency rescue team. The effectiveness of these devices depends on the ability of the fallen person to signal for help and on the availability of a helping person. A major limitation of such devices is that they cannot be used by many people with cognitive impairments. Most hospitals and home care agencies can provide information about obtaining emergency call systems. Cordless phones may provide a practical alternative to such call systems for people who are able to use them.

Evaluating Nursing Care

The nursing care of older adults who are at high risk for osteoporosis is evaluated according to the degree to which the older adult incorporates preventive measures in their daily life. For example, older adults might begin a regimen of three half-hour periods of weight-bearing exercise weekly. The nursing care of older adults who are at high risk for falls and fall-related injuries is evaluated according to the extent to which falls and serious injuries are prevented. Nurses cannot measure the number of falls that do not occur, but they can measure the risk factors that have been addressed in the care plan. Evaluation of these risk factors is facilitated by careful documentation of interventions, such as environmental modifications and fall prevention programs. The nursing care for older adults with impaired physical function is evaluated by the degree to which the person achieves and maintains the highest possible level of independence.

Chapter Summary

Osteoporosis is an age-related loss of bone mass that predisposes older adults to fractures. Although osteoporosis cannot be totally prevented in older adults, many risk factors can be addressed. Age-related changes in the musculoskeletal and central nervous systems affect the mobility and safety of older adults, increasing their susceptibility to falls. Common risk factors for falls in older adults include medical problems, adverse medication effects, and environmental factors.

Nursing assessment focuses on identifying the risk factors for falls and osteoporosis that can be alleviated through nursing interventions, such as environmental modifications and health education. Relevant nursing diagnoses would be High Risk for Injury and Impaired Physical Mobility. Health-Seeking Behaviors is a nursing diagnosis that would be applicable to older adults who are motivated to prevent osteoporosis. Nursing goals are directed toward alleviating or eliminating factors that increase the risk of falls and osteoporosis. Interventions to decrease the risk of falls and fall-related injuries focus on environmental modifications and the implementation of fall prevention programs. Osteoporosis can largely be prevented through medications, adequate calcium intake, and lifestyle interventions. Nursing care is evaluated by documenting the use of fall prevention strategies and the implementation of interventions designed to prevent osteoporosis.

Critical Thinking Exercises

1. Identify factors that increase or reduce the risk for osteoporosis.
2. Describe how each of the following age-related or risk factors might increase an older person's risk for falls and fractures: nocturia, osteoporosis, medications, altered gait, pathologic conditions, sensory impairments, cognitive impairments, functional impairments, slowed reaction time.
3. Describe the environmental factors that you would assess, in both home and institutional settings, to identify potential risks for falls.
4. Describe how you would design and implement a fall prevention program in a nursing home.
5. What information would you include in health education about osteoporosis?
6. Contact an organization to request information about fall prevention products that you might use in your clinical practice.

Case Example and Nursing Care Plan

Pertinent Case Information

Mrs. M. is an 89-year-old woman who was admitted to the hospital for congestive heart failure. Additional medical problems include arthritis, depression, early-stage dementia, and remote fractured hip. Current medications include furosemide, 40 mg b.i.d.; digoxin, 0.125 mg q.d.; enalapril, 2.5 mg t.i.d.; and Zoloft, 50 mg q.h.s. Mrs. M. lives alone in an assisted living facility, where she receives help with her meals and medications.

Nursing Assessment

During your initial nursing assessment, Mrs. M. is quiet and withdrawn. When you ask about her living situation, she says she moved to the assisted living facility 2 years ago, after she was hospitalized for treatment of a fractured hip. At the time of the injury, she had been living alone. She had fallen while making her way to the bathroom at night, and she remained lying on the floor until her daughter came to visit her the next morning. During the past year, Mrs. M. reports that she has fallen twice in her room, but that she has been able to call for help and has not had any serious injuries. You determine that Mrs. M. will need help in ambulating to the bathroom and that she should be supervised whenever she gets out of bed.

Mrs. M. confides that she is worried that she will have to move to the nursing home section of her facility if she falls again. She's very depressed about her lack of energy and her hospitalization for congestive heart failure. A mental status assessment indicates that Mrs. M. is alert and oriented but that her short-term memory is impaired. She has a great deal of difficulty with abstract ideas, such as learning to use the call button. You check her vital signs, which are within normal range, with no evidence of postural hypotension.

Nursing Diagnosis

In addition to the nursing diagnoses related to Mrs. M.'s medical condition, you identify a nursing diagnosis of High Risk for Injury. Related factors include weakness, diuretic and cardiovascular medications, a history of falls, depression, and impaired cognition. You are concerned about preventing falls during her hospitalization.

Goals	Nursing Interventions	Evaluation Criteria
To ensure safe ambulation and the avoidance of falls during Mrs. M.'s hospital stay	Identify Mrs. M. as a participant in the fall prevention program by using an orange wrist bracelet, by posting a "Fall Alert" sign near her bed, and by placing an orange "Fall Alert" sticker on her chart.	Mrs. M. will receive assistance with ambulation every time she is out of bed. Mrs. M. will not fall during her hospitalization.

(continued)

Nursing Interventions

Provide Mrs. M. with a brochure that explains the fall prevention program.

Reassess fall risks every shift and document these on the "Fall Assessment" form included in Mrs. M.'s chart.

Keep the call light button within reach and review instructions for its use every shift.

Make sure that the bed is in the lowest possible position with the wheels locked.

Use a movement detection bed pad and explain to Mrs. M. that the purpose of the pad is to ensure that the staff knows when she needs to get out of bed.

Every 2 hours, when Mrs. M. is awake, the nursing staff will ask Mrs. M. if she needs to go to the bathroom.

Educational Resources

American Menopause Foundation, Inc.
350 Fifth Avenue, Suite 2822, New York, NY 10118
(212) 714–2398

Arthritis Foundation
P.O. Box 7669, Atlanta, GA 30357–0669
(800) 283–7800
www.arthritis.org

National Arthritis and Musculoskeletal and Skin Diseases Information Clearinghouse
NAMSIC AMS Circle, National Institutes of Health, Bethesda, MD 20892–3675
(301) 495–4484
www.nih.gov/niams

National Osteoporosis Foundation
Osteoporosis and Related Bone Diseases National Resource Center
1150 17th Street, NW, Suite 500, Washington, DC 20036–4603
(800) 624–2663
www.nof.org

National Safety Council
1121 Spring Lake Drive, Itasca, IL 60143
(800) 621–7619

North American Menopause Society
P.O. Box 94527, Cleveland, OH 44101
(216) 844–8748
www.menopause.org

References

Albright, F. (1947). Osteoporosis. *Annals of Internal Medicine, 27,* 861–882.

Alexander, N. B. (1994). Postural control in older adults. *Journal of the American Geriatrics Society, 42,* 93–108.

Baldwin, R. L., Craven, R. F., & Dimond, M. (1996). Falls: Are rural elders at greater risk? *Journal of Gerontological Nursing, 22*(8), 14–21.

Brady, R., Chester, F. R., Pierce, L. L., Salter, J. P., Schreck, S., & Radziewicz, R. (1993). Geriatric falls: Prevention strategies for the staff. *Journal of Gerontological Nursing, 19*(9), 26–32.

Capezuti, E., Strumpf, N. E., Evans, L. K., Grisso, J. A., & Maislin, G. (1998). The relationship between physical restraint removal and falls and injuries among nursing home residents. *Journal of Gerontology: Medical Sciences, 53A,* M47–M52.

Carpenito, L. J. (1997). *Nursing diagnosis: Application to clinical practice* (7th ed.). Philadelphia: J. B. Lippincott.

Cummings, S. R., Kelsey, J. L., Nevitt, M. C., & O'Dowd, K. J. (1985). Epidemiology of osteoporosis and osteoporotic fractures. *Epidemiological Reviews, 7,* 178–208.

Cutson, T. M., Gray, S. L., Hughes, M. A., Carson, S. W., & Hanlon, J. T. (1997). Effect of a single dose of diazepam on balance measures in older people. *Journal of the American Geriatrics Society, 45,* 435–440.

Downton, J. H., & Andrews, K. (1990). Postural disturbance and psychological symptoms amongst elderly people living at home. *International Journal of Geriatric Psychiatry, 5,* 93–98.

Galindo-Ciocon, D. J., Ciocon, J. O., & Galindo, D. J. (1995). Gait training and falls in the elderly. *Journal of Gerontological Nursing, 21*(6), 10–17.

Gardner, D. L. (1983). The nature and causes of osteoarthrosis. *British Medical Journal, 286,* 418–424.

Gordan, G. S., & Genant, H. K. (1985). The aging skeleton. *Clinics in Geriatric Medicine, 1,* 95–118.

Hamerman, D. (1993). Aging and osteoarthritis: Basic mechanisms. *Journal of the American Geriatrics Society, 41,* 760–770.

Hollinger, L. M., & Patterson, P. A. (1992). A falls prevention program for the acute care setting. In S. G. Funk, E. M. Tornquist, M. T. Champagne, & R. A. Wiese (Eds.), *Key aspects of elder care* (pp. 110–117). New York: Springer.

Hu, M-H., & Woolacott, M. H. (1994). Multisensory training of standing balance in older adults: I. Postural stability and one-leg stance balance. *Journal of Gerontology: Medical Sciences, 49*(2), M52–M61.

Kalu, D. K., & Bauer, R. L. (1996). Bone and osteoporosis. In J. E. Birren (Ed.), *Encyclopedia of gerontology: Age, aging, and the aged,* Vol. 1 (pp. 203–215). San Diego: Academic Press.

Kessenich, C. R., & Rosen, C. J. (1996). Osteoporosis: Implications for elderly men. *Geriatric Nursing, 17*(4), 171–174.

Krolner, B., & Toft, B. (1983). Vertebral bone loss: An unheeded side effect of therapeutic bed rest. *Clinical Science, 64,* 537–540.

Kuehn, A. F., & Sendelweck, S. (1995). Acute health status and its relationship to falls in the nursing home. *Journal of Gerontological Nursing, 21*(7), 41–49.

Lachman, M. E., Howland, J., Tennstedt, S., Jette, A., Assmann, A., & Peterson, E. W. (1998). Fear of falling and activity restriction: The Survey of Activities and Fear of Falling in the Elderly (SAFE). *Journal of Gerontology: Psychological Sciences, 53B,* P43–P50.

Lord, S. R., Lloyd, D. G., Nirui, M., Raymond, J., Williams, P., & Stewart, R. A. (1996). The effect of exercise on gait patterns in older women: A randomized controlled trial. *Journal of Gerontology: Medical Sciences, 51A*(2), M64–M70.

Lumsden, D. B., Baccala, A., & Martire, J. (1998). T'ai chi for osteoarthritis: An introduction for primary care physicians. *Geriatrics, 53*(2), 84–88.

Maki, B. E. (1997). Gait changes in older adults: Predictors of falls or indicators of fears? *Journal of the American Geriatrics Society, 45,* 313–320.

Maki, B. E., Holliday, P. J., & Topper, A. K. (1994). A prospective study of postural balance and risk of falling in an ambulatory and independent elderly population. *Journal of Gerontology: Medical Sciences, 49*(2), M72–M84.

Meddaugh, D. I., Friedenberg, D. L., & Knisley, R. (1996). Special socks for special people: Falls in Special Care Units. *Geriatric Nursing, 17,* 24–26.

Meier, D. E. (1988). Skeletal aging. In B. Kent & R. N. Butler (Eds.), *Human aging research: Concepts and techniques* (pp. 221–244). New York: Raven Press.

Murphy, J., & Isaacs, B. (1982). The post-fall syndrome. *Gerontology, 28,* 265–270.

National Institute of Arthritis and Musculoskeletal and Skin Diseases. (1991). *Osteoporosis research, education, and health promotion* (NIH Publication No. 91–3216). Washington, DC: U.S. Department of Health and Human Services.

Norton, R., Campbell, A. J., Lee-Joe, T., Robinson, E., & Butler, M. (1997). Circumstances of falls resulting in hip fractures among older people. *Journal of the American Geriatrics Society, 45,* 1108–1112.

Overfield, T. (1996). *Biologic variation in health and illness: Race, age, and sex differences.* Boca Raton, FL: CRC Press.

Quinet, R. J. (1986). Osteoarthritis: Increasing mobility and reducing disability. *Geriatrics, 41*(2), 36–50.

Raisz, L. G. (1997). The osteoporosis revolution. *Annals of Internal Medicine, 126*(6), 458–462.

Riggs, L. B., & Melton, L. J. (1983). Evidence for two distinct syndromes of involutional osteoporosis. *American Journal of Medicine, 75,* 899–901.

Riggs, L. B., & Melton, L. J. (1986). Involutional osteoporosis. *The New England Journal of Medicine, 314,* 1676–1685.

Rubenstein, L. Z., Josephson, K. R., & Osterweil, D. (1996). Falls and fall prevention in the nursing home. *Clinics in Geriatric Medicine, 12*(4), 881–902.

Rush, K. L., & Ouellet, L. L. (1997). Mobility aids and the elderly client. *Journal of Gerontological Nursing, 23*(1), 7–15.

Ryan, J. W., & Spellbring, A. M. (1996). Implementing strategies to decrease risk of falls in older women. *Journal of Gerontological Nursing, 22*(12), 25–31.

Schaller, K. J. (1996). Tai Chi Chih: An exercise option for older adults. *Journal of Gerontological Nursing, 22*(10), 12–17.

Schwendner, K. I., Mikesky, A. E., Holt, W. S., Peacock, M., & Burr, D. B. (1997). Differences in muscle endurance and recovery between fallers and nonfallers, and between young and older women. *Journal of Gerontology: Medical Sciences, 52A*(3), M155–M160.

Sheldon, J. H. (1960). On the natural history of falls in old age. *British Medical Journal, 2,* 1685–1690.

Tideiksaar, R. (1997). *Falling in old age: Prevention and management* (2nd ed.). New York: Springer.

Tideiksaar, R., & Kay, A. D. (1986). What causes falls? A logical diagnostic procedure. *Geriatrics, 41*(12), 32–50.

Tinetti, M. E., Liu, W. L., & Ginter, S. F. (1992). Mechanical restraint use and fall-related injuries among residents of skilled nursing facilities. *Annals of Internal Medicine, 116,* 369–374.

Tinetti, M. E., & Powell, L. (1993). Fear of falling and low self-efficacy: A cause of dependence in elderly persons. *The Journals of Gerontology, 48* (special issue), 35–38.

Tinetti, M. E., & Williams, C. S. (1998). The effect of falls and fall injuries on functioning in community-dwelling older persons. *Journal of Gerontology: Medical Sciences, 53A,* M112–M119.

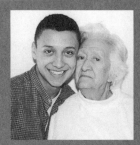

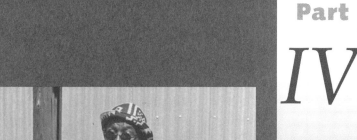

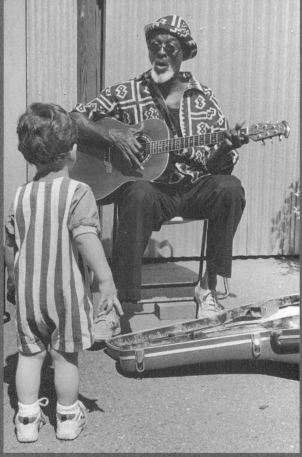

*Changes, Consequences,
and Care Related to
Comfort and Pleasure*

Skin and Its Appendages

Chapter

13

Learning Objectives

1. *Delineate age-related changes that affect the skin and its appendages.*

2. *Examine risk factors that can affect the skin of older adults.*

3. *Discuss the functional consequences of age-related changes and risk factors that affect the skin and its appendages.*

4. *Describe interview questions, inspection techniques, and observations that apply to the assessment of skin and its appendages in older adults.*

5. *Identify interventions that address the following aspects of skin care: maintenance of healthy skin, prevention of xerosis, detection and treatment of harmful skin lesions, and prevention of pressure sores.*

The skin, hair, and nails have many physiologic and social functions. The skin participates in the following physiologic processes: (1) thermoregulation; (2) excretion of metabolic wastes; (3) protection of underlying structures; (4) maintenance of fluid and electrolyte balance; and (5) sensation of pain, touch, pressure, temperature, and vibrations. The social functions of the skin include facilitating communication and serving as an indicator of age, race, gender, work status, and other personal characteristics. The common perception that skin is an indicator of age has been confirmed by researchers. A study of 1086 men revealed that the subjects who looked old for their age were biologically older on 19 of 24 age-related variables (Borkan and Norris, 1980).

Hair serves to protect underlying organs, primarily the skin, from injury and adverse temperatures. In addition, in social contexts, the length and style of one's hair can reflect certain characteristics, such as age, gender, and personality. Hair is one of the most visible manifestations of aging, and gray hair is the age-related characteristic that is most readily altered when it is viewed as an undesirable indicator of age.

Like the skin and hair, nails also have both a physiologic and social capacity. Physiologically, nails protect the underlying tissue from injury. In social contexts, nails can reflect personal characteristics, such as grooming and occupational activities.

Age-Related Changes

The skin is the largest, as well as the most visible, body organ. Structurally, the skin is composed of three layers: the epidermis, the dermis, and the subcutaneous tissue. Hair, nails, and sweat glands are considered to be skin appendages. As with other changes that affect older adults, it is difficult to distinguish between those changes in the skin and its appendages that are strictly attributable to aging and those that occur because of risk factors. Many skin changes in older adults are the result of the cumulative effects of exposure to sunlight, rather than to inherent age-related changes. With regard to baldness and gray hair, the influence of genetic factors is stronger than that of age-related changes.

Epidermis

The epidermis is the relatively impermeable outer layer of skin that serves as a barrier, preventing both the loss of body fluids and the entry of substances from the environment. The epidermis consists of layers of cells that undergo a continual cycle of regeneration, cornification, and shedding. Corneocytes and melanocytes, respectively, account for approximately 85% and 3% of epidermal cells; both develop in the innermost layer of the epidermis, called the basal layer, or stratum germinativum. Corneocytes continually migrate to the surface of the skin, where they are shed. With increasing age, corneocytes become larger and more variable in shape; these changes are more marked in sun-exposed skin as compared to sun-protected skin. In addition, the rate of epidermal proliferation slows, with a sharp decline beginning in the 5th decade.

Density of the epidermis varies, depending on the part of the body it covers. Papillae serve to give the skin its texture and connect the epidermis to the underlying dermis at the dermal-epidermal junction. With increased age, the papillae retract, causing a flattening of the dermal-epidermal junction. Because of this, the epidermis appears to be thinner. In contrast to other epidermal changes that are more prominent on exposed skin surfaces, this change is found to some degree on all skin surfaces.

Melanocytes, located in the basal layer of the epidermis, give the skin its color. The primary age-related factor affecting melanocytes is a decrease of 8% to 20% in the number of active cells each decade. Although this decline occurs in both sun-exposed and sun-protected skin, the density of melanocytes in exposed skin is double or triple that in unexposed skin. With increased age, there is a decrease in the number of Langerhans cells, which serve as macrophages, in both sun-exposed and sun-protected skin; the decrease ranges from 50% to 70% in sun-exposed skin. Another age-related change that has been identified is a decrease in the moisture content of the outer epidermal layer, also known as the stratum corneum.

Dermis

The primary functions of the dermis are the provision of support for structures within and below this layer and the nourishment of the epidermis, which has no blood supply of its own. In addition, the dermis has a role in skin coloration, sensory perception, and temperature regulation. Collagen, which constitutes 80% of the dermis, confers elasticity and tensile strength, which help to prevent tearing and overstretching of the skin. Elastin, which constitutes 5% of the dermis, functions to maintain skin tension and to allow for stretching in response to movement. The dermal ground substance, which has a water-binding capacity, determines skin turgor and elastic properties. Blood vessels in the deep plexus play a role in thermoregulation, and those in the superficial plexus supply nutrients to the epidermal layer. Cutaneous nerves in the dermis receive information from the environment for pain, pressure, temperature, and deep and light touch.

Beginning in the 3rd decade, dermal thickness gradually diminishes, with collagen thinning at a rate of 1% per year. The fact that the dermis of women is thinner than that of men may explain the more rapid age-related deterioration of female facial skin (Kligman et al., 1985). Elastin increases in quantity and decreases in quality because of age-related and environmentally induced changes. The dermal vascular bed is decreased by about one third with increased age; this contributes to the atrophy and fibrosis of hair bulbs and sweat and sebaceous glands.

Subcutaneous Tissue and Cutaneous Nerves

The subcutis is the inner layer of fat tissue that protects the underlying tissues from trauma. Additional functions of the subcutis are storage of calories, insulation of the body, and regulation of heat loss. With increased age, some areas of subcutaneous tissue atrophy, particularly in the plantar foot surface and in sun-exposed areas of the hands, face, and lower legs. Other areas of subcutaneous tissue hypertrophy, however, with the overall effect being a gradual increase in the proportion of body fat between the 3rd and 8th decades. This increased body fat is more pronounced in women than in men, and it is most noticeable in the waists of men and the thighs of women.

Although cutaneous nerve endings responsible for pain perception are not affected by age-related changes, the cutaneous end organs responsible for sensations of pressure, vibration, and light touch are affected by age-related changes. The number and structure of Meissner's and pacinian corpuscles gradually decline in density beginning in the 3rd decade.

Sweat and Sebaceous Glands

Eccrine and apocrine sweat glands originate in the dermal layer and are most abundant in the palms of the hands, soles of the feet, and axillae. Eccrine glands open directly onto the skin surface and are most abundant on the palms, soles, and forehead. Apocrine glands are larger than eccrine glands and open into hair follicles, primarily in the axillae and genital area. Although eccrine glands are important in thermoregulation, apocrine glands function solely in the production of secretions that are decomposed by skin bacteria to create a distinctive odor. It is generally agreed that both eccrine and apocrine glands decrease in both number and functional ability with increased age.

Sebaceous glands are present in the dermal skin layer over every part of the body except the palms of the hands and the soles of the feet. These glands continually secrete sebum, which combines with sweat to form an emulsion. Functionally, sebum prevents the loss of water and serves as a mild retardant of bacterial and fungal growth. One study of age-related variations in the rate of sebum secretion found that sebum secretion peaks at around 20 years of age and declines steadily thereafter (Jacobsen et al., 1985). Jacobsen and associates found that the rates of decline for men and women were 23% and 32%, respectively, per decade. In younger adults, sebum production is closely related to the size of the sebaceous glands. However, in older adults, there is an increase in the size of the sebaceous glands, but a decrease in the amount of sebum produced.

Nails

The rate of nail growth is influenced by many factors, including age, climate, state of health, circulation to and around the nails, and activity of the fingers and toes. Nail growth begins to slow in early adulthood, with a gradual decrease of 30% to 50% over the life span. Other age-related changes affecting the nails include the development of longitudinal striations and a decrease in lunula size and nail plate thickness. Because of these changes, the nails become increasingly soft, fragile, and brittle, and are increasingly likely to split. In appearance, the older nail is dull, opaque, longitudinally striated, and yellow or gray in color.

Hair

Hair color and distribution are altered to some degree in all older adults, with the most noticeable changes being baldness and gray hair. By the age of 50 years, about 50% of people have graying hair and about 60% of White men have a noticeable degree of baldness. Graying of the hair is caused by a decline in melanin production and the gradual replacement of pigmented hairs by nonpigmented ones. Hair distribution is also affected by age-related changes, with patches of coarse terminal hair developing over the upper lip and lower face in older women, and in the ears, nares, and eyebrows of older men. Most older adults experience an age-related, progressive loss of body hair, initially in the trunk, then in the pubic area and axillae. In addition, some men are genetically predisposed to baldness, which is attributable to a change in production from coarse terminal hair to fine vellus hair.

Risk Factors

The risk factors that influence the skin and appendages of older adults include heredity, pathologic conditions, adverse medication effects, and lifestyle and environmental factors. Genetic influences, which are irreversible, have only a small impact on the skin and its appendages, whereas lifestyle and environmental factors, which are the most amenable to interventions, have a significant impact. Thus, it is important to identify those risk factors, such as exposure to ultraviolet radiation (UVR), that can be alleviated through relatively simple interventions.

Genetic Influences

Heredity plays an important role in the development of pathologic and age-related skin and hair changes. People with fair skin, light hair, and light eyes are more sensitive to the effects of UVR than people with dark skin, as evidenced by the fact that skin cancers are common in light-skinned people of northern European ancestry but are rare in Blacks.

Environmental and Lifestyle Influences

The skin changes that occur as a result of exposure to UVR are referred to as photoaging. Although these skin changes have been viewed as premature or accelerated aging, UVR-related skin changes are distinct from age-related changes. One reason for this common misconception is that the cumulative effects of UVR may not be evident until later adulthood. Some of the distinct characteristics of UVR-damaged skin are a thickened epidermis, enlarged sebaceous glands, dilated and tortuous blood vessels, decreased amounts of mature collagen, greatly increased amounts of dermal ground substance, large quantities of thickened and tangled elastic fibers, and the presence of pathologic lesions and seborrheic and actinic keratoses. Photoaged skin looks ruddy and feels coarse and leathery. Also, it has a marked decrease in elasticity and many deep wrinkles, particularly on the face and neck.

Although these characteristics of UVR-damaged skin are distinct from age-related changes, other manifestations, such as slowed wound healing and diminished immune responsiveness, are thought to be accelerations of age-related changes. Questions have also been raised about the degree to which environmentally induced damage is superimposed on intrinsic aging. In the absence of clear research conclusions, the most accurate statement about the relationship between UVR-induced skin changes and age-related changes is that some characteristics of UVR-damaged skin are distinct from age-related changes, whereas some characteristics represent exacerbations or accelerations of age-related changes.

In addition to the effects of exposure to sunlight, negative consequences may be caused by other environmental factors, such as an adverse climate. For example, because the water content of the stratum corneum is influenced by relative humidity, xerosis is exacerbated when the relative humidity is below 30%. Cigarette smoking is another factor that has been associated with detrimental skin changes, as well as with hair changes, such as balding and gray hair.

Adverse Medication Effects

Common adverse medication effects involving the skin include pruritus, dermatoses, and photosensitivity reactions. Less common adverse medication effects on the skin and hair include alopecia and pigmentation changes of the skin or hair. Age-related skin changes also may be exacerbated by medications. For example, fluid loss from diuretics can exacerbate xerosis and cause further discomfort or skin problems for the older adult.

Dermatoses, or rashes, are the most frequently cited adverse medication effect, and they can be caused by virtually any medication. Medication-related skin eruptions vary widely in their manifestations and have no specific characteristics. In contrast to dermatoses arising from other causes, however, medication-related dermatoses tend to be redder in appearance, more abrupt in onset, and more widespread and symmetrical in distribution. Although adverse dermatologic reactions frequently occur early in the course of treatment with a new medication, they can occur at any time during an initial or subsequent treatment course. Penicillin and penicillin-based medications are the medications most often associated with skin eruptions. Other medications that are commonly associated with dermatoses include sulfonamides, cephalosporins, barbiturates, and salicylates.

Photosensitivity is an adverse medication effect that causes an intensified response to UVR and that is widely distributed over sun-exposed areas. Photosensitivity may begin during a seasonal exposure to bright sun or during a vacation in an unusually hot climate, and it may persist even after a medication is discontinued. Thiazides, phenothiazines, tetracyclines, and sulfonamides are the medications most often associated with photosensitivity reactions. Some herbal preparations also may increase the risk of photosensitivity.

Personal Habits

Cultural factors, societal attitudes, and advertising trends influence hygiene and skin care practices. People in industrialized societies place a high value on frequent bathing and the use of commercial products for hygienic and cosmetic purposes. Although most of the personal practices arising from these values are desirable or harmless in younger adults, they may create risks for negative functional consequences in older adults. For example, frequent bathing with harsh deodorant soaps may cause or exacerbate dry skin problems in an older person.

Limited Activity

Most older adults do not have mobility or activity limitations that are serious enough to cause skin problems. For the small percentage of older people with mobility or activity limitations, however, the risk of skin breakdown is a serious problem with far-reaching negative functional consequences. Prevention and treatment of decubiti (pressure sores) are the foci for much of the nursing care for dependent older adults in any setting. Other risk factors that combine with activity limitations to cause pressure sores are moisture, friction, poor hydration or nutrition, and certain pathologic conditions, especially those that alter level of consciousness.

Functional Consequences

Age-related changes and risk factors negatively affect many functions of the skin, including thermoregulation, tactile sensitivity, and response to injury. Psychosocial consequences may occur when changes in the appearance of the skin and hair are associated with negative attitudes about visible indicators of aging.

Response to Injury and Adverse Environmental Temperatures

Under most circumstances, age-related changes in the dermis and epidermis do not cause negative functional consequences. In the presence of any threat to skin integrity, however, age-related changes interfere with the protective function of the skin. Because of the flattened dermal-epidermal junction, older skin is less resistant to shearing forces than younger skin and is, therefore, more susceptible to bruises and shear-type injuries. Older skin is also more likely to develop blisters in response to disease processes. The age-related decrease in dermal thickness compounds the effects of the flattened dermal-epidermal junction, further increasing the susceptibility of older skin to injury and the effects of mechanical stress and UVR. Collagen changes also interfere with the tensile strength of the skin, causing it to be less resilient and more susceptible to damage from abrasive or tearing forces. One study found that 16% of nursing home residents sustained at least one skin tear each month (White et al., 1994).

Regeneration of healthy skin takes twice as long for an 80-year-old person than for a 30-year-old person. In perfectly intact skin, this slowed regeneration will not have any noticeable effects. When skin integrity is compromised, however, this age-related change contributes to delayed wound healing. A summary of age-related changes affecting the healing of deep wounds cited studies indicating that postoperative wound disruption increased with aging, and that the tensile strength of healing wounds was decreased after the age of 70 years (Fenske and Lober, 1986). This summary concluded that the age-associated delay in wound healing increased the risk of secondary infections in the elderly.

Thermoregulation in older adults is altered by age-related reductions in eccrine sweat, subcutaneous fat, and dermal blood supply. These age-related skin changes interfere with sweating, shivering, peripheral vasoconstriction and vasodilation, and insulation against adverse environmental temperatures. Thus, they increase the vulnerability of older adults to hypothermia and heat-related illnesses, as discussed in Chapter 15.

Response to Ultraviolet Radiation and Immune Response

Because of the age-related decrease in the number of melanocytes, the older adult tans less deeply and more slowly when exposed to UVR. Because there is a wider variability in the melanocyte density in exposed and unexposed skin, however, overall pigmentation in older adults may be mottled and irregular. A positive functional consequence of age-related melanocyte changes is a decrease in the occurrence of melanocytic nevi beginning around the 4th decade.

In addition to these cosmetic effects, a more serious functional consequence of the age-related decrease in melanocytes is the increased incidence of skin cancers in older adults. Another age-related skin change that contributes to the increased incidence of skin cancer is the decreased number of Langerhans cells. Many other factors, including increased age and cumulative exposure to UVR, contribute to the increased susceptibility of older adults to skin cancers.

Age-related changes also compromise immunologic responses and dermal clearance of foreign materials in older adults. The reduced number of Langerhans cells is a significant factor in altered immunologic responses, and reduced microcirculation is a significant factor in altered clearance. In the absence of any risk factors, these age-related changes would have little or no functional impact; however, alterations in dermal clearance and absorption may prolong the course of allergic dermatoses and alter the absorption of topical medications. In addition, compromised immunologic responses increase the susceptibility of older adults to skin infections and may interfere with skin test reactivity.

Comfort and Sensation

Dry skin, or xerosis, is one of the most universal complaints of older adults; indeed, it has been observed in up to 85% of noninstitutionalized older people. Age-related changes, such as diminished output of sebum and eccrine sweat, contribute to a decrease in the moisture content of the skin. Risk factors that may contribute to xerosis include stress, smoking, sun exposure, dry environments, excessive perspiration, adverse medication reactions, the excessive use of soap, and certain medical conditions (e.g., hypothyroidism).

Although it is a common belief that decreased pain sensitivity is a normal, age-related change, this conclusion has been challenged in recent years owing to conflicting results of studies on the effect of age on pain sensitivity. A recent review of the topic concluded that age has no significant effect on the perceived intensity of acute superficial pain, and that the intensity and frequency of chronic pain in fact increases with advanced age (Harkins and Scott, 1996). This same review also concluded that older adults are more likely to have atypical presentations of pain and that assessment of pain is complicated by the fact that many factors —including sensory, cognitive, affective, and behavioral components—influence the perception and expression of pain.

Studies consistently show an age-related decline in tactile sensitivity, which, in fact, begins before the age of 20 years. This decline is attributable, at least in part, to age-related changes in pacinian and Meissner's corpuscles. The effects of an age-related reduction in the number of pacinian corpuscles may be compounded by the fact that the sensitivity of these receptor cells is diminished by lower body temperatures, which are common in older adults (Weisenberger, 1996). A negative functional consequence of decreased tactile sensitivity is the increased susceptibility of older adults to scald burns because of their diminished ability to feel dangerously hot water temperatures.

Nails

Under normal circumstances, age-related changes do not interfere with the protective function of the nails, and the primary consequences are generally cosmetic. Because the nails in older persons are fragile and brittle, however, they are more likely to split. Moreover, if the nail has been injured, or if onychomycosis (a fungal infection of the nail) occurs, these age-related changes are likely to prolong the healing process. In appearance, the older nail looks dull, opaque, longitudinally striated, and yellow or gray in color.

Psychosocial Consequences and Changes in Appearance

The overall cosmetic effect of age-related skin changes is that the skin looks paler, thinner, more translucent, and irregularly pigmented. Additional indicators of age-related skin changes include sagging, wrinkling, and various growths and lesions. Skin coloration changes are attributable to decreased melanocytes and dermal circulation. Wrinkling and sagging of the skin are caused by age-related changes in the epidermis and dermis, particularly those changes that affect the collagen fibers. The age-related decrease in subcutaneous tissue contributes to sagging of the skin, especially over the upper arms, by allowing the skin to be pulled downward by gravity.

Although these changes in appearance are gradual and do not interfere significantly with physiologic function, the psychosocial consequences of these changes can be significant because of the social value placed on personal appearance and the negative attitudes that may be held about growing old. Regardless of age, one's physical appearance has been shown to be an important determinant of self-perception. A study of the effect of physical appearance on the self-perceptions of women aged 60 to 96 years revealed that women were categorized as unattractive because they showed signs of aging (Kligman and Graham, 1986). Kligman and Graham concluded that "attractiveness ratings were strongly dependent on the physical stigmata typically associated with the aged, namely wrinkling, sagging, blotches, growths, and yellowing" (1986, p. 504). Thus, age-related cosmetic changes will have psychosocial consequences in proportion to the prevalence of negative societal attitudes about aging and the extent to which the older adult adopts these attitudes.

Because of the high visibility of the face and neck, any signs of increased age that are prominent around the eyes and mouth may be especially bothersome to the person who wants to avoid visible indications of age. Characteristic signs of advanced age that are evident around the eyes include increased pigmentation, "crow's-feet" wrinkles, and fat and fluid accumulation in the upper lid and under the eye. Also, because of diminished skin elasticity and loss and shifting of subcutaneous fat, the neck skin sags and a "double chin" may be evident.

Table 13-1 summarizes the age-related changes of the skin and its appendages, as well as the associated functional consequences. Figure 13-1 illustrates the age-related changes, risk factors, and negative functional consequences affecting the skin and its appendages.

Nursing Assessment

Because the skin is the largest and most visible organ of the body, it is relatively easy to identify problems that affect functional aspects of the skin and its appendages. In addition, the skin may yield clues to other areas of physiologic and psychosocial function, such as nutrition, hydration, and personal care. Nurses collect information about the skin and its appendages during an assessment interview and through physical examination procedures. Opportunities for direct examination also arise during routine nursing care activities, such as assisting with personal care or listening to the lungs and apical heart rate. Information about other areas of function may be obtained by noting the characteristics of the skin and its appendages and using this information to validate or raise questions about other clinical impressions. For example, the observation that an older man has a beard of several days' growth, when combined with

TABLE 13-1
Age-Related Changes Affecting Skin and Appendages

Change	Consequence
Decreased rate of epidermal proliferation	Delayed wound healing; increased susceptibility to infection
Flattened dermal-epidermal junction; thinning of dermis and collagen; increased quantity, but decreased quality, of elastin	Decreased resiliency; increased susceptibility to injury, bruising, mechanical stress, UVR, and blister formation
Reductions in dermal blood supply and the number of melanocytes and Langerhans cells	Decreased intensity of tanning; irregular pigmentation; increased susceptibility to skin cancer; diminished dermal clearance, absorption, and immunologic response
Reductions in eccrine sweat, subcutaneous fat, and dermal blood supply	Decreased sweating and shivering; increased susceptibility to hypothermia or hyperthermia
Decreased moisture content	Dry skin; discomfort
Decreased number of Meissner's and pacinian corpuscles	Diminished tactile sensitivity; increased susceptibility to burns
Slowed nail growth	Increased susceptibility to cracking and injury; delayed healing
Changes in hair color, quantity, and distribution	Negative impact on self-esteem in proportion to negative attitudes

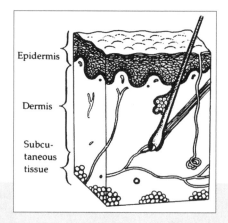

AGE-RELATED CHANGES

- Decreased rate of epidermal proliferation
- Decreased moisture
- Thinner dermis
- Flattened dermal-epidermal junction
- Decreased dermal blood supply
- Decreased melanocytes
- Decreased number of sweat and sebaceous glands

NEGATIVE FUNCTIONAL CONSEQUENCES

- Dry skin
- Skin wrinkles
- Delayed wound healing
- Increased susceptibility to burns, injury, infection, and altered thermoregulation
- Increased susceptibility to skin cancer
- Increased susceptibility of nails to cracks and injury

RISK FACTORS

- Exposure to ultraviolet rays (sunlight)
- Adverse medication effects
- Personal hygiene habits (e.g., too frequent bathing)
- Limited activity
- Heredity

FIGURE 13-1. Skin of older adults.

assessment information about his overall function, may support conclusions about possible depression or the need for assistance with personal care activities.

Interview Questions

Interview questions are aimed at identifying the person's perception of any problems, any risk factors that may contribute to skin problems, and the person's personal care behaviors that influence hair and skin status. Older adults often initiate questions about "age spots" or other noticeable skin changes, and they are usually very receptive to information about skin and hair care. During a comprehensive assessment interview, it may be advisable to ask questions about the skin early on, as most people feel quite comfortable discussing this topic. Information about medications and other risk factors can be obtained as part of the overall assessment, and this information is incorporated into the skin assessment. Likewise, other pertinent information obtained during a comprehensive assessment, such as information about fluid intake, nutritional status, and mobility and safety, is applicable to the assessment of the skin and its appendages. Assessment questions about skin and its appendages are summarized in Display 13-1.

Inspection and Observations

Close inspection of the skin and its appendages in a warm, private, and well-lit environment is an essential component of skin assessment. Examination of the skin is especially important in older adults because benign conditions, such as xerosis, may be the focus of complaints, whereas more serious conditions, such as skin cancer, may go unnoticed. The skin should be inspected for color, turgor, dryness, overall condition, and any growths or pathologic conditions. Cultural variations should be observed and documented. For example, older adults of Latin, Asian, or African ancestry may have faded Mongolian spots (i.e., irregular areas of blue coloration) that might be mistaken for bruises. Also, when assessing for erythema or pressure areas, nurses should keep in mind that early skin changes may be difficult to detect in people with darkly pigmented skin. Display

---

DISPLAY 13-1
Guidelines for Assessing the Skin and Its Appendages

Interview Questions to Assess Risk Factors and Abnormal Conditions

- Do you have any concerns about or trouble with your skin?
- Do you have any sores that won't heal?
- Do you bruise easily?
- Have you ever been treated for skin cancer or any other skin problems?
- How much time do you spend in the sun?
- Do you spend time in tanning booths?
- Do you do anything to protect yourself from the effects of the sun?
- Do you have any problems with rashes, itching, or swelling?

Interview Questions to Assess Personal Care Practices

- How do you manage your bathing?
- How often do you take a bath or shower?
- Do you use soap every time you bathe? What kind of soap do you use?
- Do you use any kind of skin lotion? What kind do you use and how frequently do you use it?
- Are you able to care for your fingernails and toenails?
- Do you get or need any help with nail care?

DISPLAY 13-2
Observations Regarding the Skin and Its Appendages

Examination of the Skin

- What is the color?
- Are there any areas of irregular pigmentation?
- Are there any areas of sunburn or tan?
- Are there areas that are discolored in any way?
- Are there any indications of poor circulation, especially in the extremities (e.g., varicosities, or areas of red, blue, or brown discoloration indicative of chronic stasis problems in the lower extremities)?
- What is the skin temperature?
- Is there a marked difference between the temperature of the extremities and that of the rest of the body?
- How does the skin feel in terms of moisture? Is it dry? Clammy? Oily?
- What is the skin's texture? Is it smooth or rough?
- Does the skin look tissue paper–thin?
- What is the turgor of the abdominal skin?
- Are scars present? (If so, describe their location and appearance.)
- Are there any signs of falling or physical abuse?
- Are any of the lesions described in Table 13-2 present?

Examination of the Hair and Nails

- What is the color, texture, and general condition of the hair?
- What is the distribution pattern of the hair?
- Is there any evidence of dandruff, scaling, or other problems with the hair?
- What is the color, length, cleanliness, and general condition of the toenails and fingernails?
- What is the color and general condition of the nail beds of the toes and fingers?

Personal Care Practices

- What is the person's overall appearance with regard to grooming and attention to personal attractiveness?
- If grooming is poor, does the person express concern about this or provide an explanation?
- Are there any psychosocial factors that influence personal care practices (e.g., is the person socially isolated or overburdened with caregiving responsibilities and, therefore, inattentive to personal care)?
- Are any of the following signs of neglect evident: presence of a body odor; unkempt, uncut, or matted hair; unusually long and unkempt fingernails or toenails; patches of brown crust on the skin; bruises or any pathologic skin conditions?

13-2 summarizes additional observations that may be made during an examination of the skin of older adults.

The skin and its appendages may provide clues to a broad spectrum of physiologic functional characteristics, particularly when nursing observations are combined with additional assessment information. For example, brown-stained fingertips are an indication of cigarette use, and brown material under the fingernails and around the cuticle may be a clue to constipa-tion. In some circumstances, toenails provide clues to mobility difficulties, especially when extremely long nails curl under the toes. Observations of the skin may provide the only objective evidence of serious functional problems, such as those stemming from falls, neglect, or abuse, that the older person might not otherwise acknowledge. For example, multiple bruises, especially in various stages of healing, may be a significant clue to falls, alcoholism, self-neglect, or physical abuse. Observation and documentation of these signs are especially important when neglect or abuse are suspected and the older adult or caregiver denies any such problems.

In assessing the skin and its appendages for clues to broader aspects of function, it is important to understand that some of the usual manifestations may be altered in older adults. For example, nurses often assess skin turgor on the hands or arms as an indication of hydration status. Because of xerosis and decreased elasticity in the skin of older adults, however, skin turgor is not necessarily a reliable indicator of hydration status in this population. Although the hands or arms may be convenient and socially acceptable sites of inspection, the skin over protected areas, such as the sternum or abdomen, is a more accurate indicator of hydration status in older adults. In nonmedicated, older adults, the oral mucous membranes usually are reliable indicators of hydration. However, many medications, including over-the-counter preparations containing anticholinergic ingredients, cause dry mouth. Another age-related change that complicates assessment of the skin is delayed wound healing. This change makes it difficult to assess patterns of wound healing using the same standards that are applied to younger adults.

Observations of the hair, skin, and nails provide multiple clues to self-esteem and other aspects of psychosocial function. Physical limitations can interfere with personal grooming, as can psychosocial influences, such as lack of motivation or awareness. Thus, evidence of self-neglect in grooming may indicate depression, dementia, or social isolation. The use of hair coloring may reflect the person's attitudes about aging, and unusually deep hues of hair coloring or facial cosmetics may be indicative of impaired color perception. Display 13-2 summarizes observations that are made in the assessment of skin and its appendages. The Culture Box summarizes some cultural aspects of skin and its appendages.

Common Skin Lesions in Older Adults

The common occurrence of various skin lesions complicates the assessment of skin in older adults. Although most of these changes are harmless except in terms of their cosmetic consequences, some are cancerous or precancerous. The challenge for the nurse is to reassure the older adult about the harmless changes and to encourage medical evaluation of the questionable ones. In general, a skin change with any of the following characteristics should be evaluated further: redness, swelling, dark pigmentation, moisture or drainage, pain or discomfort, and

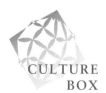

CULTURE BOX

Cultural Aspects of Skin and Its Appendages

- Whites develop wrinkles and gray hair at an earlier age than do other ethnic groups in the United States.
- Mongolian spots are common on the buttocks and lower back, and, sometimes, on the arms, thighs, and abdomen. In adults, they appear as irregular, faded blue areas. They occur in 90% of Blacks, 80% of Asians and American Indians, and 9% of Whites. They should not be mistaken for bruises.
- Assessment of stage I pressure ulcers in people with darkly pigmented skin should include broader criteria than the commonly used criterion of the presence of "nonblanchable erythema" (Henderson et al., 1997).

TABLE 13-2
Common Skin Lesions in Older Adults

Common Term(s)	Description
Age spots, liver spots, senile lentigines, senile freckles	Pale to dark brown macules, occurring most frequently on exposed areas
Actinic keratosis, solar keratosis	Red, yellow, brown, or flesh-colored papules or plaques; gritty texture; surrounded by erythema; *premalignant*
Seborrheic keratosis	Brown or black papules or plaques with sharp edges and a waxy or wart-like texture; appearing most frequently on trunk and face
Sebaceous hyperplasia	Yellowish, doughnut-shaped elevations; common on face, especially in men
Senile angiomas, cherry or ruby angiomas, telangiectasia	Bright, ruby-red, pinpoint, superficial elevations of small blood vessels
Spider angiomas	Tiny, red papules with radiating arms; *may indicate a pathologic condition*
Venous stars	Bluish, irregular, sometimes spider-shaped lesions, appearing mainly on legs or chest
Venous lakes	Bluish papules with sharp borders, appearing mainly on lips or ears
Acrochordons, skin tags	Flesh-colored, pedunculated, or stalk-like lesions
Corns, calluses	Hard masses of keratin caused by repeated pressure or irritation
Xanthelasma	Fatty deposits, usually around the eyes; *may be related to a pathologic condition*, especially if large or numerous

raised or irregular edges around a flat center. Also, any lesion that undergoes change, or any sore that does not heal within a reasonable period of time, should be evaluated further. Evaluation is also indicated when, because of its location, a mole or other skin lesion is subject to frequent rubbing or irritation. When a questionable skin lesion is observed, the following characteristics should be assessed and documented: size, shape, color, location, macular (flat) versus papular (raised), superficial versus penetrating, discrete versus diffuse borders, and the presence or absence of inflammation, redness, or of discharge.

Terminology related to various skin lesions in older adults is confusing, and many terms are used interchangeably for the same changes. Table 13-2 describes some of the terms used in conjunction with skin lesions that are common in older adults.

Nursing Diagnosis

Altered Comfort is a nursing diagnosis that may be applicable to older adults who complain of itching or dry skin. Carpenito defines altered comfort as "the state in which an individual experiences an uncomfortable sensation in response to a noxious stimulus" (1997, p. 181). Related factors commonly identified in older adults include dehydration, age-related skin changes, frequent bathing with harsh or perfumed soaps, and lack of environmental humidity.

For functionally impaired older adults, the nursing diagnosis of Impaired Skin Integrity (or High Risk for Impaired Skin Integrity) might be applicable. This is defined as "a state in which the individual experiences or is at risk for damage to the epidermal and dermal tissue" (Carpenito, 1997, p. 676). Some of the related factors that increase the risk for skin breakdown and are commonly found in functionally impaired older adults include incontinence, malnutrition, dehydration, limited mobility, prolonged bed rest, or a combination of these factors.

If the older adult has any suspicious-looking skin lesion, the nursing diagnosis of Altered Health Maintenance might be applicable. This is defined as "the state in which an individual or group experiences or is at risk of experiencing a disruption in health because of an unhealthy life-style or lack of knowledge to manage a condition" (Carpenito, 1997, p. 427). This diagnosis also would be applicable for people who are exposed to UVR (from sunlight or tanning booths) and who do not use protective measures.

Nursing Goals

A nursing goal for older adults with a nursing diagnosis of Altered Comfort related to such factors as age-related changes is to provide for skin comfort. This is achieved through interventions that promote healthy skin and prevent xerosis, as discussed in the Nursing Interventions section of this chapter. For older adults with a nursing diagnosis of Altered Health Maintenance, the nursing goal would be to detect and treat harmful skin lesions. Table 13-2 provides guidelines for assessing skin lesions and detecting potentially harmful ones. Because most

independent older adults perform skin care with little or no assistance from health care professionals, nursing goals are achieved through education about effective self-care methods.

The nursing goal for older adults with risk factors for Impaired Skin Integrity is to prevent skin breakdown. Nurses who care for dependent older adults are directly responsible for providing skin care or for supervising caregivers in the provision of skin care. Interventions directed toward this goal are discussed in the following sections.

Nursing Interventions

Maintaining Healthy Skin and Preventing Xerosis

Because the condition of the skin depends largely on the overall health of the person, the maintenance of optimal nutrition and hydration is an important intervention in the skin care of older adults. Because environmental conditions and personal care practices also influence the health of the skin, interventions are directed toward education of the older adult about these factors. Display 13-3 summarizes the teaching points that should be included in the education of older adults, or caregivers of dependent older adults, regarding skin health. Although much of the gerontological nursing literature advocates limiting the number of baths or showers to 1 to 3 times weekly, a recent nursing study has suggested that five or more baths or showers per week may be an effective intervention for skin dryness, as long as the soap is superfatted, nonperfumed, and does not contain hexachlorophene (Hardy, 1996).

The best method of preventing skin wrinkles is avoidance of exposure to sunlight and the use of sunscreen with a sun protection factor (SPF) of 15 or higher when exposure to the sun is unavoidable. In recent years, some evidence has indicated that topical products containing

DISPLAY 13-3
Tips on Skin Care for Older Adults

Maintaining Healthy Skin
- Include adequate amounts of fluid and vitamins A and C in the daily diet.
- Use humidifiers to maintain environmental humidity levels of 40% to 60%.
- Apply emollient lotions twice daily or more often.
- Use emollient lotions immediately after bathing, when the skin is still moist.
- Avoid massaging over bony prominences when applying lotions.
- Do not use rubbing alcohol.
- Avoid skin care products that contain alcohol or perfumes.
- Avoid multi-ingredient preparations because unnecessary additives may cause allergic responses.

Personal Care Practices
- When bathing or showering, use soap sparingly or use a mild, superfatted, nonperfumed soap (e.g., Castile, Dove, Tone, Basis).
- Maintain water temperatures for bathing at about 90°F to 100°F.
- Make sure skin is well rinsed after soap use.
- Whirlpool baths stimulate circulation, but moderate temperatures should be maintained.
- Apply emollient products after bathing, rather than using them in the bath water, to minimize the risk of falls on oily surfaces and to maximize the benefits of the emollient.
- Use emollient products containing petrolatum or mineral oil (e.g., Keri, Eucerin, Aquaphor).
- If you use bath oils, take extra safety precautions to prevent slipping.
- If emollient products are applied to the feet, don nonskid slippers or socks before walking.

- Make sure your skin is dried thoroughly, especially between your toes and in other areas where your skin rubs together.
- When drying your skin, use gentle, patting motions rather than harsh, rubbing motions.
- Obtain regular podiatric care.

Avoiding Sun Damage
- Wear wide-brimmed hats, sun visors, sunglasses, and long-sleeved garments when exposed to the sun.
- Wear clothing made of cotton, rather than polyester fabrics, because ultraviolet rays can penetrate polyester.
- Apply sunscreen lotions frequently, beginning 1 hour before sun exposure.
- Use sunscreen lotions with an SPF of 15 or higher.
- Avoid exposure to the sun between 10:00 A.M. and 3:00 P.M.
- Protect yourself from ultraviolet rays even on cloudy days and when you're in the water.
- Artificial tanning booths use ultraviolet type A rays, which are advertised as harmless, but which have been found to cause damage in high doses.

Preventing Injury from Abrasive Forces
- Do not use starch, bleach, or strong detergents when laundering clothing or linens.
- Use percale rather than muslin bed linens.
- Use soft terry or cotton washcloths.
- If plastic-lined pads are necessary, make sure that an adequate amount of soft, absorbent material is placed over the plastic.

---

alpha- or beta-hydroxy acids may be beneficial in reversing wrinkles and promoting the regression of solar keratoses. There is also recent evidence that estrogen replacement therapy may be helpful in preventing dry skin and wrinkles in postmenopausal women (Dunn et al., 1997).

Nurses can encourage women who are concerned about wrinkles and dry skin to discuss these interventions with their primary care provider.

Dry skin discomfort may be alleviated with emollients. Because the effectiveness of an emol-

ALTERNATIVE
AND
PREVENTIVE
HEALTH
CARE
PRACTICES

Promoting Healthy Skin

Herbs for Topical Use
- Emollients: aloe vera, calendula
- Itching and inflammation: burdock, chickweed, marigold, chamomile, purslane, pineapple, marshmallow, peppermint oil, witch hazel, walnut leaves, evening primrose oil

Herbs for Ingestion
- Evening primrose oil supplements

Homeopathic Remedies
- Petroleum, graphites, natrum muriaticum

Nutritional Considerations
- Zinc; magnesium; vitamins A, B-complex, C, and E

Preventive Measures and Additional Approaches
- Imagery, acupuncture, biofeedback, reflexology, relaxation for dermatologic problems
- Aromatherapy: bergamot, chamomile, lavender, geranium

lient is based on its ability to prevent water evaporation, its beneficial effects will be enhanced when it is applied to skin that already has some degree of moisture. Thus, an emollient applied to moist skin immediately after bathing will trap moisture and be more effective than an emollient that is added to the bath water. Display 13-3 includes information on the use of emollients and other interventions designed to prevent or care for dry skin in older adults. Alternative and preventive health care practices, as summarized in the box on this page, also may be used to treat or prevent skin problems.

Detecting and Treating Harmful Skin Lesions

Early detection and treatment of cancerous or precancerous skin lesions are key factors in the prevention of negative functional consequences because the cure rate for most skin cancers approaches 100% with early excision. The role of the nurse is to detect any suspicious-looking lesions and to encourage or facilitate further evaluation. If the older adult or caregiver has avoided medical evaluation because of fears about cancer, the nurse can provide assurance about the high cure rate and the minimal chance of long-term problems if early treatment is sought. Older adults, and caregivers of dependent older adults, will often respond to a nurse's encouragement to obtain medical care for skin lesions, especially if any unreasonable fears are allayed.

Preventing Pressure Sores

Prevention of pressure sores is one of the most important responsibilities of any nurse caring for dependent older adults who have activity or mobility limitations. Because skin tissue breakdown is attributable to both impaired circulation and external pressure to an area, the key intervention for preventing skin breakdown is to ensure adequate circulation and minimal external pressure. Thus, the nurse should make sure that older adults with mobility limitations change position at 2-hour intervals, and that pressure-relieving measures are instituted to relieve any external pressure areas. Also, it is important to avoid any friction or shearing forces and to ensure that the skin is free of excess moisture. The nurse also should promote good skin circulation by applying moisturizing agents at frequent intervals, avoiding massage over bony prominences. Good personal hygiene and the quick removal of irritants, such as urine, are important interventions, as are any measures aimed at promoting optimal hydration and nutrition. Also, many of the interventions summarized in Display 13-3 are effective in preventing pressure sores as well.

Evaluating Nursing Care

Nursing care for older adults with dry or itching skin is evaluated by determining the degree to which the interventions alleviate the person's complaints. It may take several weeks for older adults to feel the full effects of skin care interventions because of an age-related delay in dermal response to external stimuli. Also, there is a great deal of individual variation among older adults in their response to interventions. Thus, it may be necessary to evaluate the effects of one type of soap or lotion for several weeks before trying a different brand if the problem does not resolve. Because environmental humidity affects skin comfort, the evaluation of interventions may be influenced by environmental conditions.

Chapter Summary

Gray hair and skin wrinkles are the most visible signs of aging. Less visible changes in the skin and its appendages include slowed nail growth, decreased moisture content, a slowed rate of epidermal proliferation, and reductions in sweat glands and subcutaneous fat tissue. Although some skin changes are inevitable consequences of aging, most are associated with heredity and the cumulative effects of exposure to UVR. Like-

wise, balding and graying hair are strongly associated with heredity. Functionally, the age-related changes that affect the skin and its appendages have few significant physiologic consequences for healthy older adults. Negative functional consequences include dry skin, delayed wound healing, and increased susceptibility to altered thermoregulation and to shear-type injury. Because of negative stereotypes about old age, older adults with gray hair and skin wrinkles may experience negative psychosocial consequences, particularly if they have not challenged these stereotypes.

Nursing assessment of the skin and its appendages focuses on identifying factors that increase the risk of negative functional consequences (e.g., increased susceptibility to injury or altered thermoregulation). In addition, the nursing assessment might identify factors that cause physical or psychosocial discomfort for the older adult (e.g., dry skin or embarrassment about skin wrinkles). Nurses also assess any skin lesions to determine the need for medical evaluation of potentially harmful ones. Relevant nursing diagnoses are Impaired Skin Integrity and Altered Comfort related to dry skin. Nursing care focuses on alleviating uncomfortable skin conditions, addressing risk factors that contribute to skin problems, and referring older adults with questionable skin lesions for further evaluation. The risk factors that are most amenable to interventions are exposure to UVR and personal care habits that contribute to dry skin. Nursing care is evaluated according to the degree to which the interventions alleviate risk factors or relieve the person's complaints.

Critical Thinking Exercises

1. What would a healthy 85-year-old person notice with regard to his or her skin, hair, and nails?
2. Describe the questions you would ask and the observations you would make to assess

the skin, hair, and nails of an 82-year-old person.

3. Describe at least eight skin lesions that are normal and three skin lesions that require further evaluation.

4. You are asked to give a 20-minute presentation on "Maintaining Healthy Skin" at a senior center. Outline the content of your health education program.

5. What would you teach the family caregivers of a 74-year-old woman who is confined to a wheelchair with regard to the prevention of pressure sores?

Case Example and Nursing Care Plan

Pertinent Case Information

Ms. S. is a 92-year-old white woman who lives in an assisted living facility in Florida. She ambulates with a walker and needs assistance with meals, medications, and personal care. Three months ago, her doctor prescribed hydrochlorothiazide, 25 mg, every morning for isolated systolic hypertension. She has a history of arthritis but does not take any medication for it. Ms. S. attends your monthly nursing clinic for health education and blood pressure monitoring. When she comes to see you in January, she complains of dry skin and discomfort.

Nursing Assessment

You interview Ms. S. about her personal care practices and find out that she soaks in the tub in lukewarm water three times weekly. She enjoys using bath salts and perfumed skin lotions; she spends much of her leisure time outdoors on the patio or in the air-conditioned solarium. She does not use sunscreens because she thinks they are unnecessary and too oily. She states that she has not had a sunburn for several years, and that she's built up a good tolerance to the sun. She does not wear sunglasses or sun hats. She reports that she has had two skin cancers removed in the past 5 years, one from her cheek and the other from her ear lobe. She says she does not worry about recurrent skin cancer because she no longer swims outside or sits by the swimming pool. Also, because she doesn't get sunburned, she believes she is not at risk for skin cancer.

Inspection of Ms. S.'s skin reveals dry, wrinkled skin on her face and arms, and unevenly tanned skin on her face, neck, and extremities. She has many age spots over the exposed skin areas but no suspicious-looking lesions. Ms. S. has blue eyes and fair skin.

Nursing Diagnosis

Your nursing diagnoses are Altered Comfort related to dry skin and Altered Health Maintenance related to excessive sunlight exposure and insufficient knowledge of the effects of ultraviolet light. Evidence for the nursing diagnosis

(continued)

of Altered Comfort comes from Ms. S.'s complaints of dry skin and the risk factors related to her personal care practices and unprotected exposure to sunlight. Evidence for the diagnosis of Altered Health Maintenance comes from her misconceptions about risk factors for skin cancer. Also, you identify her lack of knowledge about the potential photosensitivity of hydrochlorothiazide as a factor that contributes to altered health maintenance.

Goals	Nursing Interventions	Evaluation Criteria
To alleviate Ms. S.'s discomfort from dry skin	Discuss and describe age-related skin changes. Discuss risk factors that contribute to skin discomfort (e.g., bath salts, perfumed lotions, unprotected exposure to sunlight). Use Display 13-3 to teach Ms. S. about skin care practices directed toward alleviating dry skin.	Ms. S. will report that she no longer experiences skin discomfort and dryness.
To increase Ms. S.'s knowledge about risk factors for skin cancer	Discuss the relationship between skin cancer and exposure to ultraviolet rays. Explain that any exposure to ultraviolet rays is a risk factor for skin cancer. Emphasize that a history of skin cancer increases the chance of recurrent skin cancer.	Ms. S. will verbalize an awareness of the risk factors for skin cancer.
To eliminate factors that increase the risk of skin problems and skin cancer	Inform Ms. S. that hydrochlorothiazide may increase the risk of photosensitivity, making protective measures increasingly important. Use Display 13-3 as a guide for discussing measures to avoid sun damage. Emphasize the importance of using sunscreens and wearing wide-brimmed hats when in the solarium or outside.	Ms. S. will use measures to reduce the risk of skin cancer and sun damage.

Educational Resources

American Cancer Society
1599 Clifton Road, NE, Atlanta, GA 30329
(800) 227–2345
www.cancer.org

National Arthritis and Musculoskeletal and Skin Diseases Information Clearinghouse
NAMSIC AMS Circle, National Institutes of Health, Bethesda, MD 20892–3675
(301) 495–4484
www.nih.gov/niams

Agency for Health Care Policy and Research
U.S. Department of Health and Human Services,
AHCPR Publications Clearinghouse, P.O. Box
8547, Silver Spring, MD 20907
(800) 358–9295
www.ahcpr.gov
• Clinical practice guide, quick reference guide, and patient's guide to preventing pressure ulcers

Consumer Information Center
Pueblo, CO 81009
(888) 878–3256
www.pueblo.gsa.gov
• Brochures about the effects of sun on the skin

References

Borkan, G. A., & Norris, A. H. (1980). Assessment of biological age using a profile of physical parameters. *Journal of Gerontology, 35*, 177–184.

Carpenito, L. J. (1997). *Nursing diagnosis: Application to clinical practice* (7th ed.). Philadelphia: J. B. Lippincott.

Dunn, L. B., Damesyn, M., Moore, A. A., Reuben, D. B., & Greendale, G. A. (1997). Does estrogen prevent skin aging? *Archives of Dermatology, 133*, 339–342.

Fenske, N. A., & Lober, C. W. (1986). Structural and functional changes of normal aging skin. *Journal of the American Academy of Dermatology, 15*(4), 571–585.

Hardy, M. A. (1996). What can you do about your patient's dry skin? *Journal of Gerontological Nursing, 22*(5), 10–18.

Harkins, S. W., & Scott, R. B. (1996). Pain and presbyalgos. In J. E. Birren (Ed.), *Encyclopedia of gerontology: Age, aging, and the aged*, (Vol. 2, pp. 247–260). San Diego: Academic Press.

Henderson, C. T., Ayello, E. A., Sussman, C., Leiby, D. M., Bennett, M. A., Dungog, E. F., et al. (1997). Draft definition of Stage I pressure ulcers: Inclusion of persons with darkly pigmented skin. *Advances in Wound Care, 10*(5), 16–19.

Jacobsen, E., Billings, J. K., Frantz, R. A., Kinney, C. K., Stewart, M. E., & Downing, D. T. (1985). Age-related changes in sebum secretion rate in men and women. *Journal of Investigative Dermatology, 85*, 483–485.

Kligman, A. M., & Graham, J. A. (1986). The psychology of appearance in the elderly. *Dermatologic Clinics, 4*, 501–507.

Kligman, A. M., Grove, G. L., & Balin, A. K. (1985). Aging of human skin. In C. E. Finch & E. L. Schneider (Eds.), *Handbook of the biology of aging* (pp. 820–841). New York: Van Nostrand Reinhold.

Weisenberger, J. M. (1996). Touch and proprioception. In J. E. Birren (Ed.), *Encyclopedia of gerontology: Age, aging, and the aged* (Vol. 2, pp. 591–603). San Diego: Academic Press.

White, M. W., Karan, S., & Cowell, B. (1994). Skin tears in frail elders: A practical approach to prevention. *Geriatric Nursing, 15*(2), 95–99.

Sleep and Rest

Chapter

14

Learning Objectives	1. *Delineate age-related changes that affect sleep and rest patterns in older adults.*
	2. *Examine psychosocial, environmental, attitudinal, and physiologic risk factors that influence sleep and rest in older adults.*
	3. *Discuss the functional consequences of age-related changes and risk factors that affect sleep and rest.*
	4. *List interview questions that are applicable to the assessment of actual sleep patterns, perceived adequacy of sleep, and risks that interfere with sleep.*
	5. *Identify interventions that can be implemented to promote optimal sleep and to address risks that interfere with sleep in older adults.*

Approximately one third of a person's lifetime is spent in sleep and rest activities, yet little attention is paid to the essential physiologic and psychosocial functions accomplished through these activities. During periods of sleep and rest, many metabolic processes decelerate, production of growth hormone increases, and tissue repair and protein synthesis accelerate. During the deeper stages of sleep, cognitive and emotional information is stored, filtered, and organized. Thus, physiologic function and psychosocial well-being are affected by the quality and quantity of sleep.

Prior to the 1930s, research on sleep was nonexistent, and nocturnal sleep was viewed as the absence of daytime activity, rather than an activity in its own right. In the 1950s, through the use of polygraphic measurements, sleep cycles were identified, greatly improving our understanding of sleep. By the 1960s, rapid eye movement (REM), nonrapid eye movement (NREM), and waking stages were recognized as three distinct states of consciousness. In the 1970s, sleep disorders centers were established for the purposes of conducting research on sleep and offering comprehensive evaluation and treatment programs for persons suffering from sleep disorders. In 1998, there were more than 2000 members of the American Sleep Disorders Association, a professional membership organization of primary care providers involved in the diagnosis and treatment of sleep disorders.

Age-Related Changes

Sleep research initially focused on identifying the characteristics of each phase of the sleep cycle across the life span, with some attention directed to the unique aspects of the sleep structure and patterns of older adults. Age-related changes in the sleep cycle are now fairly well understood, but many questions remain to be answered about sleep-related phenomena, such as apnea, that often affect older adults. A sleep cycle is characterized according to the quantity of time spent in bed while awake or asleep, and the depth and quality of sleep. Age-related changes have little impact on the overall quantity of sleep of older adults, but they have a significant impact on the quality of sleep and the quantity of rest. Complaints about sleep disturbances rank high among the problems for which older adults medicate themselves or seek medical care. Although some complaints about the quality of sleep may be attributable to age-related changes, most sleep disturbances are the result of risk factors and external influences. A recent study emphasizes that sleep disturbances in older adults are associated with a combination of age-related changes and multiple other causes (Campbell and Murphy, 1998).

Time in Bed and Total Sleep Time

Researchers agree that older adults spend increasing amounts of time in bed, with and without attempting to sleep, and a decreasing proportion of time in actual sleep. Disagreement arises, however, about changes in the total sleep time of older adults. One review of research on total sleep time in noninstitutionalized older adults concluded that studies using polygraphs in sleep laboratories demonstrated a reduction of total sleep time in older subjects, whereas surveys using subjective data showed an age-related increase in total sleep time over a 24-hour period (Dement et al., 1985).

When daytime naps are included, the mean diurnal sleep duration for both older and younger adults is 6.5 to 7.5 hours, but the mean duration of sleep and rest for older adults is 10 to 12 hours. A study of sleep patterns in more than 200 healthy older adults revealed a significant increase in the occurrence of daytime napping beginning at the age of 75 years, and a significant increase in the amount of time spent napping beginning at the age of 85 years (Hayter, 1985). Studies of healthy older and younger adults have found that older subjects report a greater number of daytime naps, a shorter period of nighttime sleep, and less daytime sleepiness than their younger counterparts (Reynolds et al., 1991; Buysse et al., 1992). The results of a more recent study did not support the finding that nap frequency increases with age, but it did support the conclusion that there is little or no relationship between napping and nighttime sleep behaviors (Floyd, 1995).

Sleep Efficiency and Number of Arousals

Sleep efficiency, or the percentage of time asleep during time in bed, influences the perception of the quality of sleep. Sleep efficiency ranges from 80% to 95% for younger people and is about 70% for older people. This diminished sleep efficiency is attributed both to prolonged sleep latency, which is the time required to fall asleep, and an increased number of awakenings during the night. Beginning in the 4th decade, the number of awakenings during the night gradually increases to the point that, by later adulthood, as much as one fifth of the night may be spent in periods of wakefulness.

As with many other changes that commonly occur in older adults, there is much controversy about whether the changes are attributable to pathologic conditions or to nonpathologic, age-related phenomena. The increased number of awakenings in older adults may be the result of any of the following factors: sleep apnea, physical discomfort, dementia or depression, periodic limb movements, lower auditory arousal threshold, and increased levels of plasma norepinephrine. Whether these conditions are age-related or pathologic, they occur with increased frequency in older adults and must be considered as risk factors for disturbed sleep.

Sleep Stages

Sleep stages are classified according to electroencephalogram characteristics and the presence or absence of REM. A sleep cycle consists of four stages of NREM and one stage of REM sleep. Nocturnal sleep typically occurs in four to six cycles of NREM/REM stages, each lasting 70 to 120 minutes. During the NREM stages, muscles gradually relax, body systems function at low levels, and heart and respiratory rates are slower and more regular than during REM or waking periods. Typically, in adults, stage I begins the sleep cycle and recurs for brief periods, and stages II through IV occur intermittently throughout the cycle. Stages III and IV are slow-wave stages, and essential restorative functions and the release of hormones take place during the fourth stage. REM periods occur at intervals after a change from slow-wave sleep to stage II.

Although some dreaming takes place in NREM stages, most active and vivid dreaming takes place during REM sleep, which is considered the primary dream stage. The first REM period is very brief and usually occurs about 90 minutes after sleep onset. As the sleep cycle progresses, REM periods occur more frequently, and their duration increases to a 1/2 hour or longer. REM sleep is characterized by the following physiologic changes:

- Flaccid muscles
- Fluctuating blood pressure values
- Diminished thermoregulatory functions
- REM
- Increased gastric acid secretions
- Production of more highly concentrated urine by the kidneys
- Approximately a 40% increase in cerebral blood flow
- Irregular and increased rate and rhythm of pulse and respirations
- Penile tumescence (in men)

During REM sleep, these physiologic alterations may exacerbate some medical problems. For example, increased gastric acid secretion during REM sleep may precipitate gastrointestinal pain for people with peptic ulcer disease. Likewise, people with chronic obstructive pulmonary disease (COPD) may experience dyspnea or even a respiratory crisis because of decreased oxygen saturation during REM periods.

Throughout adulthood, the duration of stage I sleep increases gradually, from 5% of a younger adult's sleep to 7% to 12% of an older adult's sleep. In the early part of the night, older adults experience longer periods of drowsiness without actual sleep in comparison to younger

adults. Moreover, during the night, older adults have more frequent shifts in and out of stage I sleep than do younger adults. The length of stage II sleep does not change significantly in older adulthood.

Studies of stage III sleep changes are inconsistent, with agreement only on the fact that there is a greater degree of variability in this sleep stage in older adults as compared to younger adults. Although stage IV sleep decreases to the point that it is absent in many older adults, stage IV sleep increases significantly during the night after sleep loss.

REM sleep diminishes in proportion to the decrease in nocturnal total sleep time, but the relative amount of REM sleep does not change significantly until extreme old age, when it shows some decline. In older adults, REM sleep tends to occur in the same number of episodes as in younger adults, but the length of each episode diminishes. In early childhood, more than 40% of sleep time is spent in dream stages, but this decreases to about 25% by the age of 70 years (Blazer, 1998). Also, in older adults, REM sleep occurs more uniformly throughout the night, rather than occurring more predominantly during the second half of the night, as occurs in young adults.

Table 14-1 summarizes the usual adult sleep cycle and typical age-related changes in sleep patterns. Typical sleep cycles for younger and older adults are illustrated in Figure 14-1 (p. 408).

Gender-Related Differences in Sleep Patterns

Beginning at puberty, sleep patterns of men and women differ, with men having a relatively higher percentage of stage I sleep and more awakenings during the night. The gender differences in stage I sleep remain consistent throughout adulthood, but by the 8th decade, men and women have an equivalent number of awakenings during the night. Studies of gender effects

TABLE 14-1
Age-Related Changes in Sleep

Sleep Stage	Young Adults	Older Adults
NREM: slow eye movements, normal muscle tension		
Stage I	5% TST	Increased number of shifts into NREM sleep; steady increase to 7% to 11% of TST
Stage II	50% TST	Generally unchanged
Stage III	10% TST	Little or no change
Stage IV	10% TST	Very short or absent, especially in men
REM: rapid eye movements, weak muscle tension, vivid dreams	25% TST	Shorter, less intense, more evenly distributed
Overall changes		Longer time required to fall asleep
		More frequent arousals
		Different quality of sleep, with less time in deep sleep
		More time in bed
		Same quantity of sleep during a 24-hour period

NREM, nonrapid eye movement; *REM,* rapid eye movement; *TST,* total sleep time.

on sleep patterns of healthy older subjects have demonstrated that older men have shorter but more frequent REM episodes and decreased amounts of both total sleep time and stages III and IV sleep compared to women (Wauquier et al., 1992). In contrast to the results of these studies, which were obtained using monitoring devices, studies of sleep complaints have revealed that women are more likely than men to report sleep problems, such as difficulty falling asleep and not feeling rested in the morning (Blay and Mari, 1990; Frisoni et al., 1993).

Risk Factors

More than 50% of older adults complain about sleep problems that arise from primary sleep disorders (i.e., apnea and periodic limb movements in sleep), altered circadian rhythms, and other risk factors (Ancoli-Israel, 1997). This conclusion is confirmed by the clinical experi-

ences of nurses working evening and night shifts, who spend much of their time dealing with sleep-related problems. Risk factors contributing to disturbed sleep may be psychosocial, environmental, attitudinal, or physiologic.

Psychosocial and Environmental Influences

Beliefs about sleep and medications may be detrimental to sleep patterns and bedtime behaviors (Morin et al., 1993). Likewise, worrying, negative thoughts, and anxious thoughts about awakening may add to distress about insomnia for older adults (Libman et al., 1997). A recent study found that anxiety and other psychological factors account for most reported difficulties falling asleep (Maggi et al., 1998). If the older adult believes that arousals during the night are abnormal and unhealthy, this pattern may be labeled as insomnia and treated with medications. Rigid beliefs about the amount of sleep required during the night, or the need for the same amount of sleep every night, may also lead to false definitions of insomnia and inappropriate treatment.

Sleep patterns are also influenced by social and environmental circumstances. For people who do not live alone, the actions and demands of other people in the home or institutional setting, especially those sharing the same sleeping area, influence sleep patterns. For adults at any age, a change in the sleeping environment usually requires a period of adjustment before optimal sleep patterns are established. Older adults may have a particularly difficult time sleeping in institutional settings, especially during the first few nights in a new environment.

Anxiety, dementia, depression, and sensory impairments are psychosocial disorders associated with disrupted sleep. Anxiety and dementia are likely to be manifested by difficulty falling asleep, and they may lead to frequent arousals during the night, after which it may be difficult to return to sleep. Compared to people unaffected by depression, people who are depressed typically take longer to fall asleep, have less deep sleep and more light sleep, awaken more frequently during the night and earlier in the morning, and feel less rested in the morning. People with dementia have been found to have the following sleep alterations: no stage IV sleep, very little REM or stage III sleep, and frequent nighttime arousals and daytime napping. In addition, the presence of dementia, depression, or sensory impairments may interfere with the person's ability to respond to time cues and environmental stimuli, thereby disrupting the overall sleep-wake pattern.

Daytime boredom and lack of social demands or environmental stimulation can also interfere with sleep habits. Older adults with little or no structured activities, work responsibilities, or social responsibilities may find it particularly difficult to establish healthy sleeping patterns. Older adults with dementia or depression who are living alone are particularly susceptible to disturbed sleep patterns because of the tendency to stay in bed during the day out of boredom, lack of motivation, an inability to concentrate on stimulating activities, or a desire to withdraw from stressful situations.

In institutional settings, lack of quiet and privacy, conflicting needs of various people, and sleeping in close proximity to others are all factors that can interfere with sleep. Older adults who are accustomed to sleeping alone or with family members may feel their privacy is being violated in institutional settings where they are required to wear nightclothes, remove their dentures, and share a room with people from outside their family. Difficulty falling asleep also may arise if environmental circumstances do not allow the performance of usual pre-bedtime activities, such as listening to music or reading a book. Schedules of caregivers also may interfere with the sleeping habits of the older adult. For example, in institutional settings, the time for awakening patients/residents is often based on the most efficient use of nursing and dietary time, and patients/residents are expected to adjust their sleep routines accordingly. Likewise, in home settings, dependent older adults may have to adjust their sleep routines to the schedule of their caregivers, who may have work and other responsibilities.

In a study of sleep patterns of hospitalized and nonhospitalized older adults, the hospitalized subjects reported less nocturnal sleep time, more daytime sleep, and earlier bedtimes and rising times (Pacini and Fitzpatrick, 1982). Factors identified as having a significant impact on sleep patterns included environmental influences, health status, state of mind, and state of fatigue. A study of sleep patterns in nursing home residents identified the following changes after admission to the facility: earlier bedtimes, increased midsleep awakening, and increased daytime napping (Clapin-French, 1986). In this study, the most frequent causes of disturbed sleep were use of the bathroom, proximity of other people, and symptoms of pain.

Noise is a disturbing environmental influence that interferes with sleep and often can be modified, especially in institutional settings. Beginning around the age of 40 years, people become more sensitive to noise when they are sleeping and can be awakened by less intense auditory stimuli. A study of nursing home residents found that noise and light changes were associated with 50% of all waking episodes lasting 4 minutes or longer and 35% of all waking episodes lasting 2 minutes or shorter (Schnelle et al., 1993). Another recent study of nursing home residents found a strong association between sleep disruption and noise and incontinence care practices (Cruise et al., 1998). Uncomfortably low or high temperatures, perhaps caused by inadequate heating or cooling systems, also contribute to decreased sleep efficiency.

Despite these findings, institutional settings are not necessarily detrimental to the sleep of older adults. In fact, they may be more conducive to sleep than home environments. If the older adult lives in a household with dependent or disruptive family members who demand attention during the night, an institutional environment may be an improvement over the home environment in terms of sleep efficiency. Likewise, if an older adult lives alone and is quite fearful at night, an institutional environment may provide the security needed for more peaceful sleeping. In Clapin-French's study (1986) of the sleep patterns of older adults, traffic noise as a cause of sleep disturbances was one influence that decreased after admission to a nursing home. If the older adult spends sleeping and waking hours in the same room, either in a home or institutional setting, sleeping difficulties may arise from the lack of differentiation between space for waking and sleeping activities.

Physiologic Disturbances

Pathologic processes, physical pain or discomfort, and adverse effects of chemicals and medications are physiologic factors that can interfere with sleep. As with many other risk factors, these are not unique to older adults, but they are increasingly likely to occur in older adults, and they are more detrimental in the presence of age-related changes and other risk factors.

Pathologic Processes

Disease processes and physical discomfort interfere with sleep patterns in many ways, with some pathologic conditions being exacerbated during sleep, particularly during REM sleep stages. Specific disease conditions that may be exacerbated during sleep, especially REM stages, include angina, hypertension, duodenal ulcers, coronary artery disease, and COPD. Acute and chronic pain and discomfort are significant factors contributing to sleep disturbances. Cramps in the calf or foot muscles are a nighttime problem for some older adults and may interrupt sleep patterns. Table 14-2 lists specific pathologic processes and their effects on sleep.

Sleep Apnea

Although 19th century medical literature referred to syndromes in which sleep disorders were associated with brief interruptions in respirations, this phenomenon received little attention until the mid-1970s. Largely because of research in sleep disorders centers, sleep apnea syndromes have received widespread attention in the literature, to the point that they are a dominant focus of sleep disorders programs.

Sleep apnea is defined as the involuntary cessation of airflow for 10 seconds or longer; the occurrence of more than five to eight of these episodes per hour is considered to be pathologic. In addition to being associated with increased age, sleep apnea is associated with snoring, obesity, dementia, depression, hypothyroidism, kyphoscoliosis, and the use of nicotine, alcohol, and medications that depress the respiratory center. The prevalence of apnea increases with advancing age, beginning around the 5th decade, and is higher in men than in women. Although studies vary, it is generally agreed

TABLE 14-2
Physiologic Factors Affecting Sleep

Risk Factor	Sleep Alteration
Arthritis	Chronic pain and discomfort that interfere with sleep
COPD	Awakening as a result of apnea and respiratory distress
Diabetes mellitus	Awakening secondary to nocturia or poorly controlled blood glucose levels
Gastrointestinal disorders, ulcers	Nocturnal pain secondary to increased gastric secretions during REM sleep
Hypertension	Early morning awakening
Hyperthyroidism	Increased difficulty falling asleep
Nocturnal angina	Awakening without perception of pain, especially during REM sleep
PLMS ("restless leg syndrome")	Awakening caused by periodic, involuntary leg movements
Altered circadian rhythm	Earlier sleep time; earlier awakening in the morning; difficulty returning to sleep after arousals
Parkinsonism	Increased time awake; decreased amount of sleep

COPD, chronic obstructive pulmonary disease; *PLMS,* periodic limb movements in sleep; *REM,* rapid eye movement.

that between one third and two thirds of adults aged 60 years or older experience five or more brief sleep interruptions per hour because of respiratory disturbances. There is unanimous agreement about the common occurrence of sleep apnea, but there is little agreement and much speculation about the extent to which apnea contributes to complaints about sleep or

interferes with sleep or daytime activities. Because studies of the functional consequences of sleep apnea have shown contradictory results, the association between apnea and sleep complaints or disorders remains unclear.

Periodic Limb Movements in Sleep
Along with sleep apnea, periodic limb movements in sleep (PLMS) have been a topic of interest and research in sleep disorders centers since the mid-1970s. PLMS is the occurrence of brief muscle contractions, spaced at intervals of about 30 seconds, that cause leg jerks and brief arousals. They may occur several times to a couple hundred times nightly, and their prevalence increases with increasing age. Although there is little controversy about the increased prevalence of PLMS in older adults, there are no consistent findings about the impact of this phenomenon on sleep satisfaction. Caffeine, alcohol, and certain medications (i.e., benzodiazepines and antidepressants) may increase the chance of having PLMS (Blazer, 1998).

Altered Circadian Rhythm
Sleep patterns are determined, in part, by an individual's circadian rhythm, also known as one's biologic clock. With increasing age, the circadian rhythm may advance, causing older adults to become sleepy early in the evening and to awaken earlier in the morning. Alterations in circadian rhythm may also account for difficulties maintaining sleep, as well as difficulty returning to sleep after awakening during the night. Sleep disturbances associated with altered circadian rhythm may be exacerbated by lack of exposure to sunlight. One study found that exposure to bright light during evening hours significantly improved sleep quality in older adults with sleep maintenance insomnia (Campbell et al., 1993).

Chemical Effects and Adverse Medication Effects
Adverse effects of medications and chemicals, such as caffeine, alcohol, and nicotine, can inter-

fere with sleep in a number of ways. Caffeine and nicotine are central nervous system stimulants that lengthen the sleep latency period and cause awakening during the night. Although alcohol may induce drowsiness as an initial effect, it suppresses REM sleep and increases the number of awakenings, especially during the latter half of the sleep period. The end result of alcohol consumption is a decrease in total sleep time and an increase in daytime sleepiness. Moreover, people who have consumed alcohol over many years may experience alcohol-related insomnia for a couple of years after withdrawing from it. If sleep apnea is an underlying causative factor of insomnia, the use of alcohol, hypnotics, or other central nervous system depressants may exacerbate the sleep disorder and lead to increased doses of medication and further detrimental effects. These chemical effects are not unique to older adults; however, sensitivity to caffeine and hypnotics increases because of age-related changes.

Contrary to their primary purpose, hypnotic medications often cause or contribute to sleep disturbances in the following ways:

1. Although the initial response to hypnotics may be good, tolerance to these medications usually develops, sometimes within several days.
2. Because of central nervous system depression and the increased sensitivity of older adults to these medications, adverse effects are likely to occur, especially if the dose is increased to compensate for tolerance.
3. Hypnotics tend to have paradoxical effects, including nightmares and agitation.
4. Hypnotics interfere with REM and deep sleep stages.
5. Rebound insomnia and nightmares occur after the withdrawal of many hypnotics.
6. Many hypnotic medications, particularly those that have been in use for many years, tend to have very long half-lives, interfering with nighttime sleep by causing daytime drowsiness. For example, flurazepam is broken down to an active metabolite with an average half-life of 47 to 100 hours. When used nightly for 1 week, the blood level of flurazepam reaches a level 5 to 6 times that of the initial dose.

Other medications that have been associated with disturbed sleep include steroids, antidepressants, aminophylline preparations, thyroid extracts, antiarrhythmic medications, and centrally acting antihypertensives. Table 14-3 summarizes the effects of various medication on sleep in older adults.

TABLE 14-3
The Effect of Various Medications/Chemicals on Sleep

Medication/Chemical	Sleep Alteration
Alcohol	Suppression of REM sleep; early morning awakening
Alcohol or hypnotic withdrawal	Sleep disturbances; nightmares
Anticholinergics	Hyperreflexia; overactivity; muscle twitching
Barbiturates	Suppression of REM sleep; nightmares; hallucinations; paradoxical responses
Benzodiazepines	Awakening secondary to apnea
Beta-blockers	Nightmares
Corticosteroids	Restlessness; sleep disturbances
Diuretics	Awakening for nocturia; sleep apnea secondary to alkalosis
Theophylline, levodopa, isoproterenol, phenytoin	Interference with sleep onset and sleep stages
Antidepressants	PLMS; suppression of REM sleep

PLMS, periodic limb movements in sleep; *REM,* rapid eye movement.

Functional Consequences

The overall impact of age-related sleep changes can be summarized as follows: in comparison to younger adults, older adults have more difficulty falling asleep, awaken more readily and more frequently, and spend more time in the drowsiness stage and less time in deep sleep. Functionally, these changes alone have little impact on the daily life of the older adult, especially because the total amount of sleep time is not significantly changed. However, the prevalence of risk factors that make the older adult more vulnerable to sleep disorders often gives rise to complaints of insomnia and feelings of daytime fatigue. One survey of self-reported sleep patterns in older adults revealed that 70% of the respondents believed they had insomnia, too little sleep, or both (Friedman et al., 1991/1992). Another study revealed that older men were most likely to complain of excessive daytime sleepiness. This was in contrast to the experience of older women, who reported longer sleep latencies, more nighttime awakenings, less frequent napping, poorer quality of sleep, and more frequent use of hypnotics (Middelkoop et al., 1996). In addition to female gender, other factors that increased the likelihood of sleep complaints in older adults included angina, depression, White race, low educational level, cognitive impairment, poor self-rated health, and the presence of chronic health conditions (Blazer at al., 1995; Newman et al., 1997).

Older adults in institutional settings experience significantly increased functional consequences as a result of age-related changes and additional risk factors. An analysis of recordings of sleep patterns in 200 nursing home residents demonstrated that these subjects were asleep for almost 8 hours and awake for almost 7.5 hours of the recorded 15-hour period (Ancoli-Israel et al., 1989). In addition, the subjects reported spending an average of 17.5 hours in bed during a 24-hour period, and they averaged no more than 39.5 minutes of sleep in any hour of the night.

In the late 1970s, sleep disorders were classified systematically, and standards were established to diagnose these disorders. Insomnia is classified as a disorder of initiating and maintaining sleep and is one of the most common sleep disorders of older adults. At least one third of older adults complain of some type of sleep disturbance, usually involving primary symptoms of daytime sleepiness, difficulty falling asleep, and frequent arousals during the night.

Excessive daytime sleepiness is classified as hypersomnia and can be measured objectively with the Multiple Sleep Latency Test (MSLT). This test is based on polygraphic recordings of the speed of falling asleep at periodic intervals during a 24-hour period. A review of studies that compared the MSLT results of older and younger subjects concluded that older adults experienced more daytime sleepiness in proportion to the number of very brief arousals, many of which were associated with sleep apnea or PLMS (Dement et al., 1985).

Although sleep deprivation is not a normal consequence of age-related changes, it may arise from a combination of age-related changes and risk factors in older adults. Psychosocial manifestations of short-term sleep loss include fatigue, confusion, irritability, an inability to concentrate, and poor performance on psychometric tests. Manifestations of prolonged sleep deprivation include fatigue, irritability, disorientation, persecutory feelings, attention deficits, perceptual disturbances, and transient neurologic symptoms, such as hand tremors. When these manifestations occur in older adults, especially if they are superimposed on dementia or depression, they may mistakenly be attributed to pathologic processes, such as dementia.

Figure 14-1 illustrates the age-related changes, risk factors, and negative functional consequences that affect sleep and rest in older adults.

AGE-RELATED CHANGES

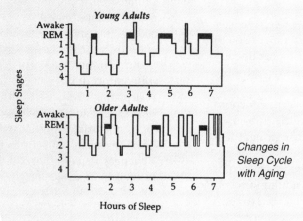

Changes in Sleep Cycle with Aging

NEGATIVE FUNCTIONAL CONSEQUENCES

- Longer time required to fall asleep
- Frequent arousals
- Poor quality of sleep
- Longer time in bed
- Same or shorter amount of sleep over 24-hour period

RISK FACTORS

- Pain, discomfort
- Alcohol
- Medications (e.g., aminophylline, antidepressants, hypnotics)
- Sleep apnea
- Periodic leg movements
- Environmental factors (e.g., noise)
- Lack of daytime activity or stimulation
- Systemic disease (e.g., dementia, arthritis)
- Nocturia

FIGURE 14-1. Sleep patterns in older adults. *Source of graph:* A. Kales & J. Kales. (1974). Sleep disorders: Recent findings in the diagnosis and treatment of disturbed sleep. *The New England Journal of Medicine, 290,* 487–499. Used with permission.

Nursing Assessment

The purposes of nursing assessment of sleep are to determine the perceived adequacy of the usual sleep and rest pattern for a person and to identify factors that may contribute to or interfere with the quality and quantity of sleep. In long-term care facilities, sleep histories may be used to assess normal sleep patterns and to plan interventions. For older adults in independent settings, a sleep-wake diary may help them identify problem areas and plan appropriate interventions. During the assessment, the nurse should listen for any indications of attitudes that are based on misinformation or lack of knowledge and that might contribute to sleep disorders. It is especially important to identify any detrimental behaviors, such as the prolonged use of hypnotics, that may be based on myths or misinformation.

In addition to obtaining subjective information from the older adult and from caregivers of the dependent older adult, the nurse should observe behavioral cues of nighttime and daytime rest and activities. This is especially important when objective observations are contrary to subjective complaints. For example, older adults may complain of "not sleeping at all," but when observed by caregivers, they may appear to be sleeping during the entire night. By contrast, older adults who deny any problems sleeping may nap frequently and readily fall asleep during daytime activities.

Recent nursing articles provide guidelines for the assessment and management of sleep disorders in older adults (e.g., Beck-Little and Weinrich, 1998). Display 14-1 summarizes interview questions that can be used to assess sleep and rest activities in older adults.

Nursing Diagnosis

When older adults report dissatisfaction with their sleep or when nursing staff find that pa-tients or residents have difficulty initiating or maintaining sleep, a nursing diagnosis of Sleep Pattern Disturbance would be applicable. This is defined as "the state in which the individual experiences or is at risk of experiencing a change in the quantity or quality of his rest pattern that causes discomfort or interferes with desired life-style" (Carpenito, 1997, p. 831). Related factors common in older adults include pain, anxiety, depression, nocturia, incontinence, medication effects, menopausal hormonal changes, environmental changes or conditions, and pathologic conditions, such as dementia.

Nursing Goals

A nursing goal for older adults with Sleep Pattern Disturbances is to improve the quantity and quality of sleep patterns. This goal is achieved by addressing the risk factors that interfere with sleep through health education and direct interventions, such as environmental modifications and comfort and relaxation strategies. When older adults have serious sleeping disturbances that do not respond to interventions, a comprehensive evaluation and treatment at a sleep disorders clinic may be warranted. A list of accredited sleep disorders centers can be obtained from the American Sleep Disorders Association (see the list of Educational Resources at the end of this chapter). Another goal for older adults who are dissatisfied with their sleep pattern would be to maintain their quality of life. This is achieved through all the interventions that improve the quality and quantity of sleep.

Nursing Interventions

Nurses in community and long-term care settings have numerous opportunities to teach older adults and their caregivers about interventions that can improve the sleep and quality of life of older adults. In hospital settings, the nursing focus is primarily on acute medical

---

DISPLAY 14-1
Guidelines for Assessing Sleep and Rest

Interview Questions to Assess Perception of Quality and Adequacy of Sleep

- On a scale of 1 to 10, with 10 as the highest, how would you rate your sleep?
- When you awaken in the morning, do you feel like you've had adequate sleep?
- Do you feel drowsy or sleepy during the day or early evening?
- Does fatigue interfere with your desired daytime activity level?

Interview Questions to Assess Pre-Bedtime Activities That Influence Sleep and Rest

- Describe your usual activities during the evening hours before you fall asleep.
- What is your usual time for getting into bed?
- What are the factors that help you fall asleep (e.g., food or drink, relaxation strategies, environmental influences)?
- Do you take any medicines to help you sleep? Do you take medicines to help you stay awake during the day?
- Do you drink alcoholic beverages, or take medicines that contain alcohol, during the late afternoon or evening? (If yes, how much and what kind?)

- What kind of activities do you engage in during the day and evening?

Interview Questions to Assess Nighttime Sleep Pattern

- Where do you sleep at night (e.g., bed, couch, recliner chair)?
- How long does it usually take to fall asleep after you get into bed?
- Do you think you lie awake too long before falling asleep?
- After you fall asleep, do you wake up during the night? (If so, how many times?)
- What kinds of things disturb your sleep during the night (e.g., getting up to urinate; activities of roommates or other people in the setting; environmental factors, like noise or lighting)?
- (If changes in living arrangements have occurred in the past few months) Has your sleep pattern changed since . . . (e.g., since you came to this nursing home; since your spouse passed away)?

---

problems, but quality of life concerns, such as sleep disturbances, should not be overlooked. Nursing practice guidelines have been developed to improve the quality of care and decrease the poorer outcomes of care associated with sleep disturbances of hospitalized older adults (Foreman and Wykle, 1995).

Educating Older Adults About Measures to Promote Good Sleep Patterns

Nursing interventions should begin with the education of independent older adults and caregivers of dependent older adults about age-related sleep changes. These changes can be summarized

as follows: older adults may need more time to fall asleep, may awaken more readily and more often during the night, and may have greater difficulty falling back to sleep after awakening. Also, nurses can emphasize the importance of establishing good sleep habits, as summarized in Display 14-2. Certain alternative and preventive health care practices, as summarized in the box on page 412, also may be used to promote sleep and rest.

Hypnotic Medications

Hypnotics may be effective for short-term management of sleep disorders, especially in temporary circumstances, such as in acute care set-

DISPLAY 14-2
Measures to Promote Healthy Sleep

- Establish a bedtime ritual that is effective for you, and try to follow it every night.
- Take a warm, relaxing bath in the afternoon or early evening.
- After 1:00 PM avoid foods, beverages, and medications that contain caffeine, including tea, cocoa, coffee, chocolate candy, hot chocolate, and some over-the-counter pain relievers and cold preparations.
- Avoid alcohol entirely, or use it only in small amounts (e.g., 4 ounces of wine per day). Do not drink alcohol before bedtime because it may cause early morning awakening.
- Avoid smoking cigarettes in the evening because nicotine is a stimulant.
- Drinking milk or chamomile tea and consuming a light carbohydrate snack prior to bedtime may be beneficial.
- Any of the following relaxation methods may be helpful: imagery, meditation, deep breathing, progressive relaxation, passive exercise, soothing music, body or foot massage, rocking in a chair, reading nonstimulating materials, or watching nonstimulating television.

- Perform daily moderate aerobic exercise, preferably before the late afternoon, but avoid vigorous exercise in the evening.
- Maintain the same daily schedule for waking, resting, and sleeping.
- Avoid staying in bed beyond your usual waking time.
- If your bedtime is temporarily changed, try to keep your waking time as close to the usual time as possible.
- Don't use your bed for reading or other activities not associated with sleeping.
- If you awaken during the night and cannot return to sleep, get out of bed after 30 minutes and engage in a nonstimulating activity, such as reading, in another room.
- Arise at your usual time, even if you have not slept well.

tings. In any community or long-term care setting, however, the adverse effects of hypnotics usually outweigh their advantages. A National Institute of Aging Consensus Statement on the treatment of sleep disorders in older people (National Institutes of Health Consensus Development Conference, 1990) advises that hypnotic medications should not be the primary mode of management for most people with disturbed sleep. The consensus statement also reports that there are no studies demonstrating the long-term effectiveness of hypnotic medications.

If a hypnotic agent is used for older adults, special attention should be paid to its half-life. There is a great variability in half-life among the benzodiazepines, and some have an extremely long half-life in older adults. Table 14-4 provides information about the half-life of

hypnotics in younger and older adults. Nurses can educate older adults and their caregivers about the effects of alcohol, medications, and certain chemicals on sleep. Display 14-3 summarizes the pertinent teaching points for older adults.

Direct Nursing Actions

Nursing actions are directed toward eliminating risk factors and promoting sleep when risk factors cannot be eliminated. Nurses who work evening or night shifts in institutional or home care settings have many opportunities to engage in activities that promote good nighttime sleep. For dependent older adults, nursing responsibilities include assisting with positioning in bed and ensuring the most comfortable environment possible. If dementia or depression interfere

ALTERNATIVE
AND
PREVENTIVE
HEALTH
CARE
PRACTICES

Promoting Sleep and Rest

Herbs
- Hops, skullcap, chamomile, valerian, rose hips, lemon balm, passion flower

Homeopathic Remedies
- Oat, arnica, aconite, coffea, arsenicum, chamomile, pulsatilla, rhus tox, nux vomica

Nutritional Considerations
- Foods and substances to avoid: caffeine, alcohol, sugar, refined carbohydrates, food additives and preservatives
- Pre-bedtime foods to consume: milk (warm), complex carbohydrates (e.g., whole grains)
- Zinc, calcium, magnesium, manganese, and vitamins B-complex and C
- For restless leg syndrome: vitamin E and folic acid

Preventive Measures and Additional Approaches
- Aerobic exercise for 30 minutes a day at least 3 times/week
- Avoidance of nicotine
- Yoga, meditation, acupuncture, imagery, hypnotherapy, light therapy, warm bath, warm footbath, progressive relaxation (refer to Display 14-4)
- Aromatherapy: chamomile, coriander, lavender, marjoram

Special Precautions
- Although widely promoted as sleep aids, tryptophan and melatonin should be used with caution in older adults because of their possible adverse effects, and only under the supervision of a qualified health care provider
- Melatonin: may cause drowsiness, hypothermia, loss of libido

TABLE 14-4
Half-Life of Benzodiazepines

Medication	Half-Life in Average Adult (hours)	Half-Life in Older Adult (hours)
Flurazepam (Dalmane)	47–100	120–160
Diazepam (Valium)	20–50	36–98
Estazolam (ProSom)	10–24	10–24*
Lorazepam (Ativan)	10–20	10–20*
Chlordiazepoxide (Librium)	5–20	15–30
Temazepam (Restoril)	9–13	8–20
Oxazepam (Serax)	5–20	5–20*
Alprazolam (Xanax)	6–20	6–20*
Triazolam (Halcion)	2–5	2–6

*Insufficient data available to determine a difference in younger and older adults.

DISPLAY 14-3
Information About Medications and Sleep

- Hypnotic medications are not effective for long-term use because of increasing tolerance, which often develops within the first week and inevitably develops after a month of regular use.
- Hypnotics should not be used for more than 3 nights in a row.
- Sleeping medications, even over-the-counter ones, are likely to have adverse effects that interfere with daytime function and with the quality of nighttime sleep.
- Older adults are more susceptible than younger adults to the adverse effects of sleeping medications.
- Most hypnotics interfere with REM sleep.
- When hypnotics are discontinued, a rebound effect, characterized by nightmares and excessive dreaming, may occur.

- Over-the-counter sleeping preparations generally contain antihistamines and can have adverse effects, such as confusion, constipation, or blurred vision, either alone or in combination with other medications.
- Alcohol, in any amount, is likely to have detrimental effects on sleep, such as nightmares and awakenings during the latter part of the night.
- Medications that can interfere with sleep include steroids, diuretics, theophylline, anticonvulsants, decongestants, and thyroid hormone.
- Combining a sleeping medication with any other medication can be harmful and even fatal.
- L-tryptophan probably has some hypnotic effects; it occurs naturally in milk, eggs, meat, fish, poultry, beans, peanuts, and green leafy vegetables.

with sleep onset, the nurse may simply stay with the older person to provide reassurance until the person is able to fall asleep. In addition, relief of pain and anxiety are nursing responsibilities that directly influence the sleep of older adults. Older adults who do not request analgesics may give nonverbal cues that pain is interfering with sleep. An analgesic taken 30 minutes before bedtime may help induce sleep in people with chronic pain or discomfort.

Soft music and dim lighting also may be helpful. A study of the effects of afternoon baths, with bath water at a temperature of 41°C, revealed significant increases in bedtime sleepiness, slow-wave sleep, and the amount of stage IV sleep reported following the bath (Horne and Reid, 1985). Comfort and relaxation measures, such as backrubs and the use of therapeutic touch, are particularly helpful when emotional stress or physical pain interfere with sleep. One study found that use of relaxation techniques significantly improved the sleep of older women with insomnia who were not taking hypnotics, and substantially reduced the use of hypnotics in subjects who had been taking them (Lichstein and Johnson, 1993). A recent study of older adults who were caregivers found that stress management and other behavioral techniques are effective alternatives to medication for sleep problems (McCurry et al., 1998). Older adults and caregivers of dependent older adults can be taught to use relaxation techniques as an effective method of inducing sleep without any adverse effects. Cassette tape recorders with automatic shut-offs can be used to play soothing music or tapes of instructions for deep breathing, guided imagery, or relaxation exercises. These tapes are growing in popularity and can be purchased in many book and music stores or through the Internet. Display 14-4 summarizes simple instructions for relaxation and mental techniques designed to promote sleep.

DISPLAY 14-4
Relaxation and Mental Imagery Techniques That Promote Sleep

Deep Breathing
- Focus your attention on your breathing; extend your belly and draw in a deep breath as you count.
- Hold your breath for 3 or 4 counts.
- Exhale completely.
- Repeat this pattern, focusing your total attention on breathing.
- Phrases, such as "I am sleepy," or counting, using simple numbers, may be repeated during each exhalation to help keep your attention focused on breathing.

Progressive Relaxation
- Start by focusing your attention on the muscles in your toes.
- Flex or tense these muscles, and then relax them.
- Repeat 2 or 3 times.

- Focus your attention on the muscles in your foot.
- Flex or tense, then relax these muscles, 2 or 3 times.
- Repeat this process, progressively focusing on different muscle groups and proceeding from your feet to your head.

Mental Imagery
- Begin with deep breathing exercises to relax yourself.
- Focus your attention on a serene and peaceful scene, visualize the setting, and imagine the sounds (e.g., a beach with waves gently washing ashore).
- Imagine yourself in the setting, lying relaxed, enjoying the environment.
- Keep your attention focused on the scene.
- Imagine repetitive motions, such as waves on the beach or sheep jumping over a fence.

Environmental Modifications

Environmental modifications are among the simplest and most effective interventions to improve sleep, especially in institutional settings. Such activities as closing bedroom doors and adjusting bedroom lighting to meet the needs of a patient or resident may be quite effective in promoting adequate sleep for older adults. In long-term care settings, preferences for bedtime routines and measures that promote sleep can be documented on each resident's care plan and carried out by nursing staff. Elimination of unnecessary staff-initiated noise, especially conversations at the nursing station, is a helpful intervention for patients/residents located near the center of nursing activity. In long-term care settings, decisions about room assignments should be based partially on an assessment of sleep requirements and compatibility of individual needs. Once room assignments have been made, roommate behaviors that interfere with sleep may be addressed by a room change, if necessary.

If a noisy environment contributes to sleeping difficulties, and the noise cannot be controlled or eliminated, the older person may wish to use earplugs. Any person who lives alone, however, should be cautioned about the danger of blocking out protective noises, such as that of a smoke detector. Environmental noise that cannot be eliminated can be masked by "white noise" (e.g., using a fan, air conditioner, soft music, tape-recordings of such sounds as waves or rain, or white noise machines). If outside noise is bothersome, heavy draperies can be installed over windows to filter out neighborhood noise. The nighttime room temperature should be comfortable, and is usually slightly lower than during the day. In cooler environments, the older adult should wear a nightcap to prevent loss of heat through the head.

L-Tryptophan

L-tryptophan is an amino acid essential to the synthesis of serotonin in the brain. Approximately 0.5 to 2 g are consumed daily in the typical adult diet, primarily in protein and dairy products. L-tryptophan has natural sedative qualities, especially in its effect on sleep latency and slow-wave sleep. L-tryptophan, in doses of 1 g or less, shortens the sleep latency period for people who have difficulty falling asleep, but has no impact on the number of awakenings during the night. Although doses of 1 g or less were thought to be harmless in humans, the Food and Drug Administration (FDA) declared a recall of synthetic L-tryptophan in late 1989. This action was based on reports of an association between L-tryptophan and a rare, but potentially fatal, blood disorder. There is no contraindication to taking L-tryptophan in its natural form.

Evaluating Nursing Care

Nursing care for older adults with Sleep Pattern Disturbances is evaluated by measuring the extent to which nursing goals have been achieved. A subjective measurement would be that the older adult feels rested when he or she awakens in the morning. An example of objective measurements would be that the older adult is able to sleep for 6 to 8 hours at night with only brief interruptions, and that the person looks and acts rested during the day. Short-term goals are directed toward the immediate problem of sleep disturbance; long-term goals are directed toward lifestyle factors that promote good sleep habits.

Chapter Summary

Healthy older adults may experience the following changes in their sleep patterns: it may take longer to fall asleep, they may awaken more frequently, and they may spend a longer time in bed but sleep for the same or a shorter amount of time than when they were younger. Also, because they tend to awaken frequently and spend less time in the deep stages of sleep, they may feel that the quality of their sleep is unsatisfactory. Risk factors that may interfere with sleep patterns of older adults include sleep apnea; PLMS; adverse effects of hypnotics and other medications; physical pain, illness, or discomfort; and psychosocial disturbances, such as anxiety, dementia, or depression.

Nursing assessment of sleep focuses on identifying the older adult's perception of their sleep and rest pattern and on identifying the risk factors that interfere with the quality and quantity of sleep. The relevant nursing diagnosis is Sleep Pattern Disturbance. Nursing care is directed toward improving the quantity and quality of sleep. Interventions focus on eliminating risk factors and establishing routines that promote good sleep. Nursing care is evaluated by the extent to which the older adult feels rested when he or she awakens in the morning.

Critical Thinking Exercises

1. What is an older adult likely to experience with regard to sleep and rest patterns? How would you explain these changes to an older adult?
2. Identify three specific factors in each of the following categories that might interfere with sleep: environmental influences, physiologic disturbances, and psychosocial factors.
3. How would you assess a 79-year-old person who comes to the nursing clinic at the senior wellness center complaining of feeling tired all the time and not getting enough sleep?
4. What would you include in a half-hour presentation on "Tips for Good Sleep" for participants in a senior wellness program at a community-based center?

5. What information about sleep and rest would you include in an inservice program for evening and night shift nursing assistants employed at a nursing home?

Case Example and Nursing Care Plan

Pertinent Case Information

Mrs. S. is a 74-year-old woman who is being admitted to a nursing home for skilled care after a total hip replacement. Her diagnoses include osteoarthritis and osteoporosis. After a few weeks in the nursing home, she plans to return to her ranch-style home where she lives with her husband. Prior to surgery, she was independent in her ADL, and she expects to regain her independence and walk with a walker. The hospital transfer form has orders for nabumetone, 750 mg, every morning and temazepam, 15 mg, at bedtime as needed.

Nursing Assessment

During the admission interview, you ask Mrs. S. about her sleep patterns. She states that, for the past few years, she has been awakened frequently at night by her hip pain and other arthritic discomforts. Also, she reports that she would usually get up 3 or 4 times during the night to go to the bathroom. When questioned further, she explains that the pain and discomfort would wake her, and so she would go to the bathroom because she wanted to move around, not because she felt an urge to urinate that often. Although her primary care provider had advised her to take ibuprofen 4 times daily, she tried not to take this medication more than 2 times a day because the pills upset her stomach. She avoided taking any medications at night because she thought she shouldn't take the medications on an empty stomach.

During her 1-week hospitalization, she had taken a sleeping pill several times. She had also taken Darvon-N 100 mg every 4 hours while she was in the hospital, but she said her primary care provider wanted her to start taking a nonsteroidal, anti-inflammatory drug on a regular basis for her arthritis and hip pain. She said he had prescribed a new drug that wouldn't upset her stomach, but she had not yet begun to take it. Mrs. S. expressed anxiety about sleeping in the nursing home because she said the noise in the hospital was very disruptive to her sleep. She reports that she feels rested in the morning if she gets at least 6 hours of sleep during the 8 hours she spends in bed. During her hospitalization, she never felt rested in the morning, and she was unable to sleep for 6 hours except when she took sleeping pills. Mrs. S. says that listening to relaxing music helps her to fall asleep.

Nursing Diagnosis

In addition to nursing diagnoses related to Mrs. S.'s osteoarthritis and hip surgery, you identify a nursing diagnosis of Sleep Pattern Disturbance. Related factors are pain, age-related changes, and environmental conditions. You decide that you will not list nocturia as an associated factor because Mrs. S. does not feel an urge to void during the night. Rather, she wakes up with pain and then goes to the bathroom. You decide to list age-related changes as a related factor because it is important for Mrs. S. to understand that, even though she may not awaken with pain, she may awaken because of age-related changes.

Goals	Nursing Interventions	Evaluation Criteria
To educate Mrs. S. about the factors that interfere with her sleep pattern	Describe age-related changes in sleep patterns. Discuss the important role of pain-relieving measures in promoting good sleep.	Mrs. S. will be able to describe the age-related changes and other conditions that affect her sleeping pattern.
To enable Mrs. S. to consistently obtain 6 hours sleep per night without the aid of sleeping medications	Administer nabumetone as ordered and evaluate its effectiveness in controlling Mrs. S.'s pain. Explain that sleeping medications should be avoided, except for periodic use in short-term situations. Assign Mrs. S. to a room that is not close to the nursing station. Make sure Mrs. S.'s door is closed at night. Encourage Mrs. S. to use her tape recorder to play quiet music at bedtime. Give Mrs. S. a copy of Displays 14-3 and 14-4 and discuss additional nonpharmacologic methods for promoting sleep.	Mrs. S. will report that she feels rested upon awakening in the morning. Mrs. S. will report that she is not awakened by pain.

Educational Resources

American Sleep Apnea Association
2025 Pennsylvania Avenue, NW, #905, Washington, DC 20006
(202) 293–3650
www.sleepapnea.org

American Sleep Disorders Association
1610 14th Street, NW, Suite 300, Rochester, MN 55901
(507) 287–6006
www.asda.org

National Center on Sleep Disorders
NHLBI Information Center, P.O. Box 30105, Bethesda, MD 20892–0105
(301) 251–1222
www.nhlbi.nih.gov/nhlbi/sleep/sleep.htm

National Sleep Foundation
729 Fifteenth Street, NW, 4th Floor, Washington, DC 20005
www.sleepfoundation.org

References

Ancoli-Israel, S. (1997). Sleep problems in older adults: Putting myths to bed. *Geriatrics*, *52*(1), 20–30.

Ancoli-Israel, S., Parker, C., Sinaee, R., Fell, R. L., & Kripke, D. F. (1989). Sleep fragmentation in patients from a nursing home. *Journal of Gerontology*, *44*(1), M18–M21.

Beck-Little, R., & Weinrich, S. P. (1998). Assessment and management of sleep disorders in the elderly. *Journal of Gerontological Nursing*, *24*(2), 21–29.

Blay, S. L., & Mari, J. J. (1990). Subjective reports of sleep disorders in the community elderly. *Behavior, Health, and Aging*, *1*, 1990.

Blazer, D. G. (1998). *Emotional problems in later life: Intervention strategies for professional caregivers* (2nd ed.). New York: Springer.

Blazer, D. G., Hays, J. C., & Foley, D. J. (1995). Sleep complaints in older adults: A racial comparison. *Journal of Gerontology: Medical Sciences*, *50A*(5), M280–M284.

Buysse, D. J., Browman, K. E., Monk, T. H., Reynolds, C. F., Fasiczka, A. L., & Kupfer, D. J. (1992). Napping and 24-hour sleep/wake patterns in healthy elderly and young adults. *Journal of the American Geriatrics Society*, *40*, 779–786.

Campbell, S. S., Dawson, D., & Anderson, M. W. (1993). Alleviation of sleep maintenance insomnia with timed exposure to bright light. *Journal of the American Geriatrics Society*, *41*, 829–836.

Campbell, S. S., & Murphy, P. J. (1998). Relationships between sleep and body temperature in middle-aged and older subjects. *Journal of the American Geriatrics Society*, *46*, 458–462.

Carpenito, L. J. (1997). *Nursing diagnosis: Application to clinical practice* (7th ed.). Philadelphia: J. B. Lippincott.

Clapin-French, E. (1986). Sleep patterns of aged persons in long-term care facilities. *Journal of Advanced Nursing*, *11*, 57–66.

Cruise, P. A., Schnelle, J. F., Alessi, C. A., Simmons, S. F., & Ouslander, J. G. (1998). The nighttime environment and incontinence care practices in nursing homes. *Journal of the American Geriatrics Society*, *46*, 181–186.

Dement, W., Richardson, W., Prinz, P., Carskadon, M., Kripke, D., & Czeisler, C. (1985). Changes of sleep and wakefulness with age. In C. E. Finch & E. L. Schneider (Eds.), *Handbook of the biology of aging* (2nd ed., pp. 692–717). New York: Van Nostrand Reinhold.

Floyd, J. A. (1995). Another look at napping in older adults. *Geriatric Nursing*, *16*, 136–138.

Foreman, M. D., & Wykle, M. (1995). Nursing standard-of-practice protocol: Sleep disturbances in elderly patients. *Geriatric Nursing*, *16*, 238–243.

Friedman, L. F., Bliwise, D. L., Tanke, E. D., Salom, S. R., & Yesavage, J. A. (1991–1992). A survey of self-reported poor sleep and associated factors in older individuals. *Behavior, Health, and Aging*, *2*(1), 13–20.

Frisoni, G. B., De Leo, D., Rozzini, R., Bernardini, M., Buono, M. D., & Trabucci, M. (1993). Night sleep symptoms in an elderly population and their relation with age, gender, and education. *Clinical Gerontologist*, *13*(1), 51–68.

Hayter, J. (1985). To nap or not to nap? *Geriatric Nursing*, *6*, 104–106.

Horne, J. A., & Reid, A. J. (1985). Night-time sleep EEG changes following body heating in a warm bath. *Electroencephalography and Clinical Neurophysiology*, *60*, 154–157.

Libman, E., Creti, L., Amsel, R., Brender, W., & Fichten, C. S. (1997). What do older good and poor sleepers do during periods of nocturnal wakefulness? The Sleep Behaviors Scale: 60+. *Psychology and Aging*, *12*(1), 170–182.

Lichstein, K. L., & Johnson, R. S. (1993). Relaxation for insomnia and medication use in older women. *Psychology and Aging*, *8*(1), 103–111.

Maggi, S., Langlois, J. A., Minicuci, N., Grigoletto, F., Pavan, M., Foley, D. J., & Enzi, G. (1998). Sleep complaints in community-dwelling older persons: Prevalence, associated factors, and reported causes. *Journal of the American Geriatrics Society*, *46*, 161–168.

McCurry, S. M., Logsdon, R. G., Vitiello, M. V., & Teri, L. (1998). Successful behavioral treatment for reported sleep problems in elderly caregivers of dementia patients: A controlled study. *Journal of Gerontology: Psychological Sciences*, *53B*, P122–P129.

Middelkoop, H. A. M., Smilde-van den Doel, D. A., Neven, A. K., Kamphuisen, H. A. C., & Springer, C. P. (1996). Subjective sleep characteristics of 1,485 males and females aged 50–93: Effects of sex and age, and factors related to self-evaluated quality of sleep. *Journal of Gerontology: Medical Sciences*, *51A*(3), M108–M115.

Morin, C. M., Stone, J., Trinkle, D., Mercer, J., & Remsberg, S. (1993). Dysfunctional beliefs and attitudes about sleep among older adults with and without insomnia complaints. *Psychology and Aging*, *8*(3), 463–467.

National Institutes of Health Consensus Development Conference. (1990, March 26–28). Treatment of sleep disorders of older people. NIH Consensus Statement, *8*(3). Washington, DC: National Institutes of Health.

Newman, A. B., Enright, P. L., Manolio, T. A., Haponik, E. F., & Wahl, P. W. (1997). Sleep disturbance, psychosocial correlates, and cardiovascular disease in 5201 older adults: The cardiovascular health study. *Journal of the American Geriatrics Society*, *45*, 1–7.

Pacini, C. M., & Fitzpatrick, J. J. (1982). Sleep patterns of hospitalized and nonhospitalized aged individuals. *Journal of Gerontological Nursing*, *8*, 327–332.

Reynolds, C. F., Jennings, R., Hoch, C., Monk, T. H., Berman, S. R., Hall, F. T., Matzzie, J. V., Buysse,

D. J., & Kupfer, D. J. (1991). Daytime sleepiness in healthy "old old": A comparison with young adults. *Journal of the American Geriatrics Society, 39,* 957–962.

Schnelle, J. F., Ouslander, J. G., Simmons, S. F., Alessi, C. A., & Gravel, M. D. (1993). The nighttime environment, incontinence care, and sleep disruption in nursing homes. *Journal of the American Geriatrics Society, 41,* 910–914.

Wauquier, A., van Sweden, B., Lagaay, A. M., Kemp, B., & Kamphuisen, H. A. C. (1992). Ambulatory monitoring of sleep-wakefulness patterns in healthy elderly males and females (>88 years): The "Senieur" protocol. *Journal of the American Geriatrics Society, 40,* 109–114.

Thermoregulation

Chapter

15

Learning Objectives

1. Delineate age-related changes that affect the following aspects of thermoregulation: normal body temperature, febrile response to illness, and response to hot and cold environmental temperatures.

2. Examine risk factors that influence thermoregulatory function in older adults and that increase the potential for hypothermia or hyperthermia.

3. Discuss the functional consequences of age-related changes and risk factors that affect temperature regulation in older adults.

4. Describe the principles of assessing baseline temperature in older adults.

5. Describe signs of hypothermia and hyperthermia, as well as pertinent questions for identifying risks for altered thermoregulation in older adults.

6. Identify interventions for preventing hypothermia and hyperthermia in older adults.

The primary function of thermoregulation is to maintain a stable core body temperature in a wide range of environmental temperatures. In the presence of infections, thermoregulation also assists in maintaining homeostasis. With increased age, subtle alterations in thermoregulation occur, and these become important considerations in caring for healthy, as well as frail, older adults.

Age-Related Changes

Under normal circumstances, the core body temperature is maintained at 97°F to 99°F through complex physiologic mechanisms governing heat production and dissipation. Nervous system control over thermoregulation is centered in the hypothalamus and is affected by many internal and external influences. The following internal factors affect temperature regulation: metabolism rate; disease processes; muscle activity; peripheral blood flow; amount of subcutaneous fat; function of the cutaneous nerves; inges-

tion of fluid, nutrients, and medications; and temperature of the blood flowing through the hypothalamus. External factors that influence thermoregulation include the environmental temperature, humidity level, and air flow, as well as the type and amount of clothing and covering used.

Response to Cold Temperatures

In cold environmental temperatures, physiologic mechanisms are initiated to prevent loss of body heat and increase heat production. At the same time, protective behaviors are initiated, in response to central nervous system mechanisms, to warm the body and protect the person from adversely cold temperatures. The following physiologic mechanisms prevent heat loss and increase heat production: shivering, muscle contraction, increased heart rate, peripheral vasoconstriction, dilation of the blood vessels in the muscles, insulation of deeper tissues by subcutaneous fat, and the release of thyroxine and corticosteroid by the pituitary gland. The following actions can be initiated to protect the person in cold temperatures: seeking of shelter, ingestion of warm fluids, use of warm clothing or covering, and an increase in activity to stimulate circulation.

The age-related changes that interfere with an older person's ability to respond to cold temperatures include inefficient vasoconstriction, decreased cardiac output, decreased muscle mass, decreased subcutaneous tissue, and delayed and diminished shivering. Older adults are less able to retain heat owing to diminished peripheral circulation, particularly in the superficial microvasculature (Jennings et al., 1993). In one study of 104 women aged 61 to 100 years, the mean temperature gradient between the groin and toes was 8.8°C (Howell, 1982). Age-related changes affecting the response to cold usually begin during the 5th decade, but their impact is not felt until the 7th or 8th decade. The overall effect of these changes is a dulled perception of cold and a concomitant lack of stimulus to initiate protective actions, such as adding more clothing or raising the environmental temperature.

Response to Hot Temperatures

In hot environmental temperatures, or when metabolic heat production is high, the normal mechanisms for heat dissipation are the production of sweat to facilitate evaporation and the dilation of peripheral blood vessels to facilitate heat radiation. Healthy adults can produce about 2 L of sweat per hour, and cutaneous blood flow may increase to 20% of the total cardiac output (Olson and Benowitz, 1984). When exposed to hot climates or engaged in strenuous activity over a period of several days or weeks, healthy adults are able to acclimatize, or gradually increase their metabolic efficiency.

The older person's response to heat is altered primarily by age-related dermal changes affecting sweating and vasoconstriction. Older adults have an increased threshold for the onset of sweating, a diminished response when sweating

occurs, and a dulled sensation of warm environments. Impaired sweating mechanisms and decreased cardiac output can interfere with the older person's ability to acclimatize.

Normal Body Temperature and Febrile Response to Illness

Normal human body temperature is maintained at 98.6°F, plus or minus 1°F, with diurnal variations of 2°F. An elevated temperature, or fever, is the body's protective response to pathologic conditions, such as cancer, infection, dehydration, or connective tissue disease. Normal body temperature decreases with increased age, particularly in people older than 75 years of age. Mean body temperatures in older adults range from 96.9°F to 98.3°F orally and 98°F to 99°F rectally.

Questions have been raised about the accuracy of oral and axillary temperatures as a reflection of core temperature in older adults. One study comparing oral, rectal, and axillary measurements of body temperature in 73 subjects whose mean age was 80 years indicated that oral and axillary temperatures were significantly lower than rectal temperatures (Downton et al., 1987). Downton and colleagues concluded that oral and axillary temperature measures were unreliable estimates of core temperature in older adults because the difference between their core and skin temperatures is greater and more variable than in younger people. Other studies have suggested that rectal and auditory canal temperatures provide the most accurate indicators of body temperature in frail older adults (Darowski et al., 1991; Castle et al., 1992).

Risk Factors

Age alone predisposes people to both hypothermia and hyperthermia. Whereas hypothermia develops in healthy young adults only when they are exposed to adversely cold temperatures, older adults can become hypothermic even in moderately cool environments, especially in the presence of additional risk factors. Likewise, healthy young adults can tolerate hot environmental temperatures without adverse effects, whereas heat-related illnesses may develop in older adults in moderately hot temperatures. Any combination of environmental and other risk influences in the older adult is likely to lead to serious problems, and even death, because of impaired thermoregulatory mechanisms that increase the older adult's vulnerability to hypothermia and hyperthermia.

Environmental and Socioeconomic Influences

Environmental factors directly affect thermoregulation and are the factors that are most amenable to intervention. In addition to the obvious environmental influence of cold or hot temperatures, other environmental and socioeconomic factors that have been associated with hypothermia and hyperthermia include substandard living conditions and diets deficient in protein and calories. Because hypothermia and hyperthermia usually are not self-reported disorders, social isolation and living alone are additional risk factors. Thus, during periods of extremely hot or cold weather, lack of daily contact with other people increases the risk of not identifying progressive hypothermia or hyperthermia in an older adult.

Heat waves are especially hazardous for older adults living in environments with poor ventilation. The detrimental effects of heat waves are compounded when high temperatures are combined with high humidity levels and air pollutants. For older adults living in urban areas with high crime rates, ventilation may be restricted when windows are kept closed because of safety considerations. In Great Britain, the term ''urban hypothermia'' has been used to refer to older adults living alone in poorly heated dwellings. Likewise, the term ''urban hyperthermia'' could be applied to older adults living in poorly ventilated houses and apartments, particularly public housing, in cities where heat waves and air pollution are common.

Behaviors Based on Myths and Misunderstandings

Lack of knowledge about age-related vulnerability to hypothermia and hyperthermia may create risks secondary to inadequate protective measures. For example, when the use of heating or air conditioning is curtailed as a cost-saving measure, younger adults may be able to adjust to the moderately hot or cool temperature, whereas an older adult might become hyperthermic or hypothermic under the same circumstances. If older adults and their caregivers are not aware of the age-related decrease in the perception of environmental temperatures, appropriate measures to counteract hot or cold environments, such as removing or adding clothing, may not be taken.

In the presence of infection, lack of knowledge about age-related thermoregulatory changes may result in undetected illnesses. For example, if caregivers of older adults believe that an infectious disease is always accompanied by an elevated temperature, they may assume that no infection is present if there is no fever. This age-related lack of febrile response is one reason that pneumonia is the most frequently missed diagnosis in elderly patients (Fox, 1998).

Lack of knowledge about diurnal temperature variations, the age-related decrease in body temperature, and the age-related increase in the difference between core and skin temperature also may contribute to false expectations and undetected illness. For example, if body temperatures are recorded only in the morning, when they are normally lower, a slight or modest temperature elevation may not be detected.

Chemical Effects and Adverse Medication Effects

Chemical effects and adverse medication effects alter thermoregulation by predisposing people to hypothermia and hyperthermia and by interfering with the fever response in the presence of an illness. Antipsychotics, acetaminophen, steroid medications, and nonsteroidal anti-inflammatory agents may mask a fever. In usual doses, salicylates can predispose people to hypothermia and interfere with fever responses, and salicylate intoxication can induce hyperthermia by causing metabolic acidosis.

Medications may predispose a person to hypothermia through mechanisms that suppress shivering and increase vasodilation. Medications can also predispose a person to hyperthermia by inducing diuresis, increasing heat production, and interfering with sweating. Some medications, such as diuretics and phenothiazines, affect thermoregulation through several mechanisms, increasing the risk for both hypothermia and hyperthermia. Alcohol ingestion increases the risk of hyperthermia by inducing diuresis, and it increases the risk of hypothermia by inducing vasodilation and interfering with shivering. When excessive alcohol is consumed, the risks are increased even further because sensory perception is dulled and the person is less able to initiate protective behaviors. Table 15-1, which summarizes some of the risk factors for altered thermoregulation, identifies some of the medications that may predispose a person to hypothermia or hyperthermia. If combinations of these medications are taken, or if any medication is taken in combination with alcohol, the risk for altered thermoregulation is greatly increased.

Pathologic Influences

Thermoregulation can be compromised by any condition that interferes with cardiac output or peripheral circulation. Cerebrovascular and cardiovascular diseases increase the risk of both hypothermia and hyperthermia. Fluid and electrolyte imbalances, especially dehydration and hypernatremia or hyponatremia, increase one's susceptibility to both hyperthermia and hypothermia. Also, diminished renal function may

interfere with the febrile response of older adults.

Endocrine dysfunctions commonly associated with hypothermia in older adults include hypoglycemia, hypothyroidism, and hypopituitarism. Thyrotoxicosis and diabetic ketoacidosis also may cause or contribute to hyperthermia in older adults. Infections, particularly pneumonia and sepsis, are common causes of elevated body temperature in younger adults; however, in older adults, these conditions may predispose the person to hypothermia. Neurologic impairment secondary to parkinsonism or any type of dementia also can cause or contribute to hypothermia.

Inactivity secondary to chronic physical illness or psychosocial factors, such as depression or isolation, can increase the risk of hypothermia. Likewise, fatigue and hypoxia can increase the risk of hypothermia by suppressing shivering. An inability to rise after falling may precipitate hypothermia in cool environmental temperatures, and this risk is increased for people living alone. Postural hypotension also may cause or contribute to hypothermia. In acute care settings, older surgical patients are particularly prone to developing hypothermia owing to a combination of conditions, such as immobility, body exposure, low environmental temperatures, age-related changes, and anesthesia and other medication effects.

In older adults, heat-related illness may be precipitated by moderate exercise in hot weather, especially if fluid intake is not sufficient to replace fluid loss. If older adults rely solely on their sensation of thirst to signal the need for fluid intake, they may become underhydrated or dehydrated because the thirst mechanism becomes less efficient with advancing age. Additional risks for dehydration and heat-related illnesses arise from the diminished efficiency of the older adult's kidneys in concentrating urine. If adequate rehydration is not provided between periods of exercise or during prolonged exposure to a hot climate, a heat-related illness is likely to develop in the older adult.

TABLE 15-1
Risk Factors for Altered Thermoregulation

Risk Factor	Hypothermia	Hyperthermia
Age of 75 years or older	X	X
Slightly uncomfortable environmental temperatures	X	X
Dehydration	X	X
Electrolyte imbalances	X	X
Infections	X	X
Cardiovascular and cerebrovascular diseases	X	X
Peripheral vascular disease		X
Postural hypotension	X	
Diabetes	X	X
Hypoglycemia	X	
Hypothyroidism	X	
Hyperthyroidism		X
Parkinsonism	X	
Inactivity/immobility	X	
Hypertension		X
Obesity		X
Alcohol consumption	X	X
Phenothiazines	X	X
Anticholinergics		X
Barbiturates	X	X
Diuretics		X
Antidepressants	X	
Benzodiazepines	X	
Reserpine	X	
Cardiovascular drugs (e.g., sympatholytics, beta-blockers, calcium channel blockers)		X

Table 15-1 summarizes some of the important risk factors that predispose older adults to hypothermia and hyperthermia.

Functional Consequences

A healthy older adult in a comfortable environment will experience few, if any, functional consequences of altered thermoregulation. In the presence of any risk factor, however, hypothermia or hyperthermia may develop in an older adult. Even moderately adverse environmental temperatures may precipitate hypothermia or hyperthermia in an older adult, especially in the presence of additional predisposing factors, such as certain medications or pathologic conditions. In the United States, hypothermia and hyperthermia usually are seasonal hazards that occur during heat waves and cold spells, and these weather-related problems most often affect older adults who live in climates in which there are extremes of weather. For instance, a review of deaths from excessive heat in more than 2000 people, aged 60 years and older, during a 7-year period revealed that 57% of the deaths occurred during the heat wave of 1980 (Macey and Schneider, 1993). Older adults who live in climates where either hot or cold weather is the norm have been acclimatized to these conditions and usually live in housing environments that are suitable to the climate.

For older adults in whom hypothermia or hyperthermia develop, the risk of subsequent morbidity or mortality from this condition is greater than that for their younger counterparts. One study of deaths among the elderly from excessive heat and excessive cold found that three fifths of the preventable deaths were due to excessive cold (Macey and Schneider, 1993). The same study revealed that older men were more likely to die from excessive cold, whereas older women were more likely to die from excessive heat. Another finding of this investigation was that minority and rural elderly adults were disproportionately likely to suffer deaths from temperature-related causes.

Response to Cold Environments

Increased age is associated with an increased vulnerability to hypothermia because most older adults are less perceptive of cold environments, less aware of a low core body temperature, less efficient in their physiologic response to cold, and less apt to take corrective actions in cold environments. One study of the response of younger and older adults to environmental temperatures suggested that older adults are at greater risk of dysthermia because they may require a more intense thermal stimulus before they take appropriate actions (Taylor et al., 1995). Physiologic alterations, as well as behavioral factors, contribute to the increased risk of hypothermia in older adults.

Hypothermia is defined as a core body temperature of 95°F or lower. Low environmental temperatures usually contribute to hypothermia, and the term "accidental hypothermia" is used when an adversely low environmental temperature is the primary cause of the condition.

Even in normal environmental temperatures, however, the condition can result from serious alterations in homeostasis, such as endocrine or neurologic diseases. Accidental hypothermia can occur in older adults as a consequence of exposure to moderately cool temperatures, and it is thought to affect as many as 10% of older adults living in winter climates, such as Great Britain and the United States.

In the early stages of hypothermia, the older adult probably will not shiver or complain of feeling cold. In the absence of any protective measures, hypothermia will progress, clouding mental function. The effects of impaired thermoregulation are cumulative, and hypothermia progresses rapidly after the core body temperature falls to 93.2°F. The age-related diminished ability of the kidney to conserve water and the common occurrence of inadequate fluid intake in older adults exacerbate the effects of hypothermia. If the process is not reversed, death from hypothermia will ensue as a result of the myocardial effects of seriously impaired thermoregulation.

Response to Hot Environments

The functional consequences of age-related changes in the older adult's ability to respond to hot environments include delayed and diminished sweating and inaccurate perception of environmental temperatures. Because of these functional consequences, the older adult is more likely to have heat-related illnesses, including heat stroke and heat exhaustion. Although "hyperthermia" is the term often used to refer to heat-related illnesses in older people, this term more accurately refers to any condition in which the body temperature is elevated above normal. In addition to being caused by impaired thermoregulation and environmental factors, hyperthermia can be caused by pyrogens and other pathologic conditions.

Heat exhaustion is a condition that develops gradually from fluid and/or sodium depletion. It can occur in active or immobilized older people who are dehydrated or underhydrated and exposed to hot environments. Heat stroke is an even more serious condition that is likely to occur in active older adults because of a combination of age-related thermoregulatory changes and risk factors, such as overexertion and warm environments. Heat stroke can also occur in immobilized older adults in hot environments, either as a progression of untreated heat exhaustion or as a result of a combination of risk factors, such as diabetes and certain medications. The underlying mechanism in heat stroke is the inability to balance the rates of heat production and dissipation. This balance depends primarily on sweating and cardiac output.

In hot environments, the effects of altered thermoregulation are cumulative, and heat-related illnesses progress rapidly after the body temperature reaches 105.8°F. If fluid volume is not adequate to meet the requirements for effective sweating, then hyperthermia will progress even more rapidly. The age-related decrease in thirst sensation may contribute to inadequate fluid intake and diminished thermoregulation. If hyperthermia is not reversed, death will result from respiratory depression.

Increased morbidity and mortality of older people have been associated with heat waves in the United States and Great Britain. One study comparing reasons for hospitalization of older subjects during the summers of 1982 and 1983 found an association between increased environmental temperatures and hospital admissions for cerebrovascular accidents, subarachnoid hemorrhages, and transient ischemic attacks (Fish et al., 1985). An information paper published by the United States Senate Special Committee on Aging (1983) states that "heat waves claim more lives nationally than any other natural disaster, including floods, tornadoes, and hurricanes" (p. 1). This report cites a Centers for Disease Control study of the 1980 heat wave, which revealed that the rate of heat stroke was 12 to 13 times higher for persons 65 years

of age or older, as compared to that in the rest of the population (p. 1).

Thermoregulatory Response to Illness

A diminished febrile response to illness and infections, such as bacteremia, occurs in many older adults as a consequence of age-related changes in the thermoregulatory centers of the hypothalamus. A study of 25 older adults hospitalized for hypothermia revealed that 16 subjects had a definite infection and an additional six had a probable infection at the time of admission (Darowski et al., 1991a). Another study found that more than 50% of older patients admitted to the hospital with a febrile illness had a low or normal body temperature on admission (Darowski et al., 1991b).

Other studies indicate that infections in most older patients are accompanied by some degree of temperature elevation, but that the febrile response may be delayed or undetected (McAlpine et al., 1986; Berman et al., 1987; Castle et al., 1991). These studies suggest that infections in older adults often are accompanied by a decline in functional abilities and would be detected more accurately if temperatures were closely monitored at the earliest sign of functional decline. The study of nursing home residents conducted by Castle and associates (1991) revealed that about one fourth of the residents whose temperature did not reach 99°F did have an adequate change in their temperature, but had a low baseline temperature. The authors of this study concluded that early recognition of infections would be facilitated by lowering the definition of what temperature constitutes a fever, and by monitoring for changes from the baseline temperature for individual residents.

Altered Perception of Environmental Temperatures

A very common observation of nurses is that older adults frequently report feeling cool or cold, even in very warm environments. Also,

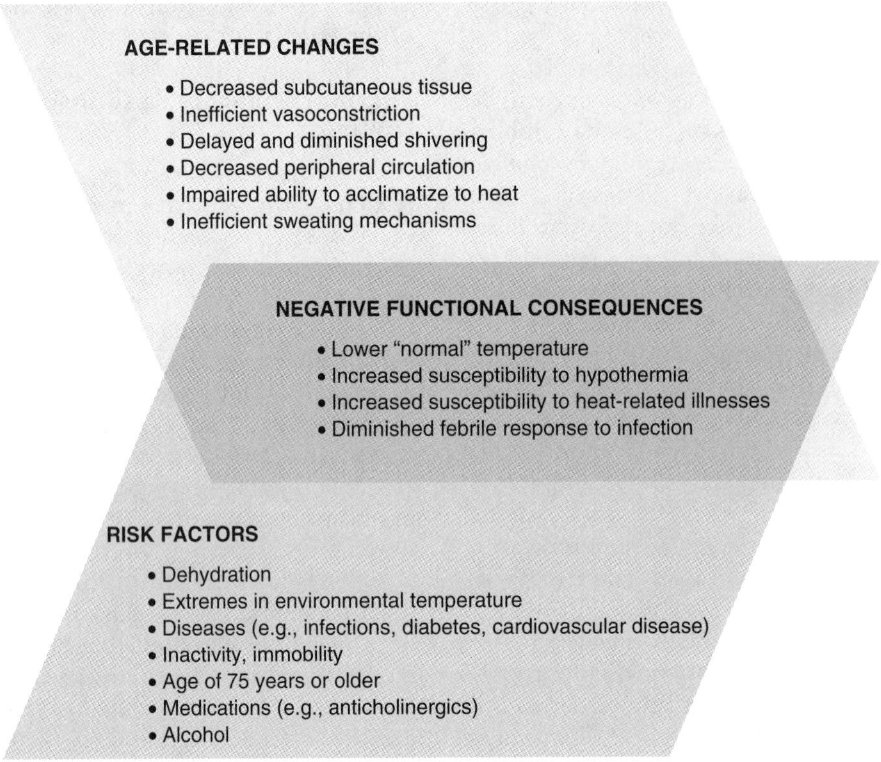

AGE-RELATED CHANGES

- Decreased subcutaneous tissue
- Inefficient vasoconstriction
- Delayed and diminished shivering
- Decreased peripheral circulation
- Impaired ability to acclimatize to heat
- Inefficient sweating mechanisms

NEGATIVE FUNCTIONAL CONSEQUENCES

- Lower "normal" temperature
- Increased susceptibility to hypothermia
- Increased susceptibility to heat-related illnesses
- Diminished febrile response to infection

RISK FACTORS

- Dehydration
- Extremes in environmental temperature
- Diseases (e.g., infections, diabetes, cardiovascular disease)
- Inactivity, immobility
- Age of 75 years or older
- Medications (e.g., anticholinergics)
- Alcohol

FIGURE 15-1. Temperature regulation in older adults.

older adults generally prefer environmental temperatures that are at least 75°F. These preferences are not the result of age-related changes in thermoregulation, but are probably related to impaired cardiovascular efficiency (Whitbourne, 1996). Misperceptions of environmental temperatures might also be associated with pathologic conditions, such as dementia or thyroid disorders.

Psychosocial Consequences

Psychosocial consequences do not arise from age-related thermoregulatory changes alone; however, they can be caused by hypothermia, hyperthermia, or diminished fever response. If hypothermia or hyperthermia is overlooked, or if interventions are not initiated at an early stage, the condition may progress to the point

of impairing cognitive function. Likewise, if a diminished or delayed febrile response to an infection is not recognized, a treatable condition may be overlooked and treatment may unintentionally be delayed or denied. Unrecognized infections are likely to progress in severity, and in older adults, they may manifest primarily as a functional decline, such as in cognitive function.

Figure 15-1 illustrates the age-related changes, risk factors, and negative functional consequences that affect thermoregulation.

Nursing Assessment

Assessment of thermoregulation is aimed at identifying the person's baseline body temperature, any risk factors for altered thermoregulation, and early manifestations of hypothermia or hyperthermia. Although much of the pertinent information about risk factors is collected as part of the overall assessment, specific information about thermoregulation is obtained by observing the environment, measuring the person's body temperature, and interviewing the older adult and the caregivers of dependent older adults.

Baseline Temperature

Body temperature measurements show a diurnal fluctuation of 1°F to 2°F, with a greater variation occurring during periods of fever-inducing illness. The highest temperature occurs in the evening, usually between 6:00 P.M. and 8:00 P.M, whereas the lowest temperature occurs between 2:00 A.M. and 3:00 A.M. Because older adults normally have a lower body temperature and may have a diminished febrile response to infection, it is especially important to determine the person's usual temperature, as well as to characterize the usual pattern of diurnal variation. Older adults in home settings should be encouraged to determine their usual temperature by recording their oral temperature at different times of the day for several days when they are feeling well. If this is done seasonally by people who live in fluctuating climates and annually by those who live in stable climates, there will be a good basis for comparison when symptoms of illness or functional decline occur. The same procedure can be followed in long-term care settings, with the results being recorded as baseline data on the chart.

Adult body temperature typically is measured by placing a thermometer under the tongue and having the person hold it in that position with the mouth closed until an accurate recording is obtained. For measurements of oral temperature to be accurate, the following precautions must be taken: an interval of 30 minutes should elapse following the smoking of tobacco or the ingestion of cold or hot liquids; the thermometer should be shaken so that the mercury is at the lowest possible point; the person's mouth should remain tightly closed; and the thermometer should be left in place until the temperature can accurately be recorded (7 minutes for a mercury thermometer; a shorter time for an electronic thermometer).

The advantages of oral measurements include convenience, social acceptability, and a standard degree of accuracy. A disadvantage of this technique, however, is that such measurements may not accurately reflect the core body temperature of older people because they tend to exhibit a wider difference between core and peripheral temperatures than do younger persons. Another disadvantage, if not controlled for, is the fact that cigarette smoking or ingestion of hot or cold liquids can interfere with the accuracy of oral temperature, and these effects may be prolonged in older adults. One study found that the effect of ice water on oral temperature measurements was likely to be exaggerated in older adults (Sugarek, 1986).

Tympanic thermometry is widely available as a method of assessing body temperature by measuring infrared energy emitted from the tympanic membrane. This method is quick, convenient, highly accurate, and unaffected by environmental factors. If the ear canal has impacted cerumen, the temperature may be inaccurately low (Hasel and Erickson, 1995). Because of the easy accessibility to the ear canal and the speed of temperature recording (within several seconds), this method can be used readily, even with uncooperative patients. Display 15-1 summarizes the principles underlying nursing assessment of thermoregulation in older adults.

Risks for Altered Thermoregulation

Anyone older than 75 years of age should be considered to be at risk for altered thermoregulation, as should any older adult who has one or more risk factors, such as those listed in Table 15-1. Risk factors involving medications and pathologic conditions usually are identified during the overall assessment, but they may be overlooked unless special attention is paid to their role in predisposing the person to hypothermia or hyperthermia. Although most nurses do not have the opportunity to assess the older adult's environment directly, nurses can ask pertinent questions and listen for clues to detect environmental risk factors. For example, older adults who live alone and express concern about paying utility bills or keeping the house warm in winter should be considered to be at risk for hypothermia. Likewise, older adults who live in poor housing conditions, or with family members who keep the house at low temperatures during winter months, should be considered to be at risk for hypothermia. Older people in urban environments who express fears about keeping windows open in houses that are not air-conditioned, or who live in poorly ventilated rooms, should be considered to be at risk for hyperthermia during heat waves. Interview questions aimed at identifying risk factors for altered thermoregulation are listed in Display 15-1.

Identification of Altered Thermoregulation

Older adults who have more than one risk factor for altered thermoregulation are likely to become hypothermic or hyperthermic in the presence of uncomfortable environmental temperatures. In addition, older adults who have a pathologic condition that normally causes a febrile response may not have the usual manifestations of the illness because of their inefficient thermoregulatory mechanisms. Manifestations of these three conditions that are likely to occur in older adults are discussed in the following sections.

Hypothermia

Hypothermia is best detected by measuring core body temperature with a thermometer that registers below 95°F. Cool skin in unexposed areas, such as the abdomen and buttocks, is a distinguishing characteristic of hypothermia. It is important to understand that the environmental temperature may be only moderately cool and that the older person will not necessarily shiver or complain of feeling cold. Even in environmental temperatures of 68°F or 69°F, an older person may become hypothermic, especially if other risk factors, such as immobility or hypothermia-inducing medications, are present. Early signs of hypothermia are subtle, and the most objective assessment tool is a comparison of the person's body temperature with their usual baseline temperature. As untreated hypothermia progresses, additional signs may include lethargy, slurred speech, mental changes, impaired gait, puffiness of the face, slowed or irregular pulse, low blood pressure, slowed tendon reflexes, and slow, shallow respirations. Severe stages of hypothermia are characterized by muscular rigidity, diminished urinary function, and a progression of all other manifestations to the point of stupor and coma. The skin will feel very cool, and, contrary to what might be expected, the color of the skin will be pink. Also contrary to what might be expected, a hypothermic person may not shiver, particularly if the body temperature is below 90°F.

Hyperthermia

Manifestations of heat-related illnesses range from mild headache to life-threatening respiratory and cardiovascular disturbances. In the early stages of heat-related illness, the person will feel weak and lethargic and may complain of headache, nausea, and loss of appetite. The skin will be warm and dry, and the sweating response may be absent, especially if the person's fluid intake is low. As the heat-related condition progresses, these manifestations will be exacerbated, and the following signs will become evident: dizziness, dyspnea, tachycardia, vomiting, diarrhea, muscle cramps, chest pain, mental impairment, and a wide pulse pressure.

Febrile Response to Illness

Manifestations of delayed or diminished febrile response to infections are very difficult to assess because they are subtle and variable. The most significant finding may be the absence of an expected elevation in temperature. Rather than emphasizing the presence or absence of temperature changes, however, the astute nurse understands the importance of observing for subtle changes in temperature and for other signs of illness, such as a decline in function. Nurses also should examine assumptions about temperature regulation that may apply to younger adults but not to older adults. For example, the expectation that pneumonia is accompanied by a temperature above 98.6°F is not necessarily applicable to older adults. A study of manifestations of infections in nursing home residents found that confusion was the only common sign in individuals with infections that were identified by health care providers (Hofland and Mort, 1994). Another study of fevers in nursing home residents revealed that 85% of the clinical manifestations were staff-detected rather than resident-reported (Pals et al., 1995). Thus, nurses in long-term care facilities need to be particularly vigilant about subtle temperature changes and other manifestations of fever. Some of these considerations are summarized in Display 15-1.

Nursing Diagnosis

If the nursing assessment identifies risks for impaired thermoregulation in an older adult, the nursing diagnoses of Risk for Altered Body Temperature, Hypothermia, or Hyperthermia may be applicable. Hypothermia, as a nursing diagnosis, is defined as "the state in which an individual has or is at risk of having a sustained reduction of body temperature of below 35.5°C (96°F) rectally because of increased vulnerability to external factors" (Carpenito, 1997, p. 148). The definition of Hyperthermia is "the state in which an individual has or is at risk of having a sustained elevation of body temperature of greater than 37.8°C (100°F) orally or 38.8°C (101°F) rectally due to external factors" (Carpenito, 1997, p. 146).

If several factors are identified that place the older person at risk of both hypothermia and hyperthermia, then the nursing diagnosis of High Risk for Altered Body Temperature may be appropriate. For example, an 83-year-old woman with diabetes, dementia, and hypertension who is taking a diuretic, haloperidol, and an oral hypoglycemic would have seven risk factors for both hypothermia and hyperthermia. Related factors that are common in older adults include immobility, advanced age, medication effects, adverse environmental conditions, and acute and chronic illnesses. For older adults living alone, social isolation may be a related factor that increases the risk for experiencing more serious consequences if hypothermia or hyperthermia occurs.

A common problem for older adults in institutional settings where they have little or no control over their room temperature is the perception of being too cold. For these older adults, nurses might identify a diagnosis of Altered Comfort, related to the perception of being cold. This nursing diagnosis would be appropriate when the older person is not necessarily at risk for hypothermia, but frequently complains of feeling cold. Nurses in long-term care settings have many opportunities to address this nursing diagnosis, particularly when it interferes with the sleep patterns and the quality of life of nursing home residents.

Nursing Goals

Nursing care for an older adult with a diagnosis of High Risk for Hypothermia or Hyperthermia is directed toward eliminating the risk factors and maintaining the older person's normal body

DISPLAY 15-1
Guidelines for Assessing Thermoregulation

Principles of Temperature Assessment

- Document the person's baseline body temperature and its diurnal and seasonal variations.
- Assume that even a small elevation above the baseline temperature is a clue to the presence of a pathologic process.
- Document actual temperature and deviations from the baseline, rather than using such terminology as "afebrile."
- Carefully follow all the standard procedures for accurate temperature measurement.
- Use a thermometer that registers lower than 95°F.
- Consider the influence of temperature-altering medications when evaluating a temperature reading (e.g., medications that mask a fever).
- Do not assume that an infection will necessarily be accompanied by an elevated temperature.
- Remember that, in the presence of an infection, a decline in function may be an earlier and more accurate indicator of illness than an alteration in temperature.
- Do not assume that an older adult will initiate compensatory behaviors or complain of discomfort when exposed to adverse environmental temperatures.

Interview Questions to Assess Risk Factors for Hypothermia or Hyperthermia

- Do you have any particular problems that occur in hot or cold weather?
- Are you able to keep your house or room at a comfortable temperature in both summer and winter months?
- Do you have any difficulty keeping up with your utility bills?
- What forms of protection against the cold do you use in the winter months (e.g., electric blanket, supplemental sources of heat)?

- Have you ever received medical care for exposure to heat or cold?
- Have you ever fallen and not been able to get up or get help?

Observations to Assess Risk Factors for Hypothermia or Hyperthermia

- Does the older person live in a house where low temperatures are maintained during the winter?
- Does the person drink alcohol or take temperature-altering medications (see Table 15-1)?
- Does the person live alone? If so, what is the frequency of outside contacts?
- Does the person have any pathologic conditions that predispose him or her to hypothermia (e.g., endocrine, neurologic, or cardiovascular disorders)?
- Is the person's fluid and nutritional intake adequate?
- Does the person have postural hypotension? (See Table 10-2 and Displays 10-1 and 10-2 for assessment criteria relating to postural hypotension.)
- Is the person immobilized or sedentary?
- Is the person's judgment impaired because of dementia, depression, or other psychosocial disorders?
- Does the person live in a poorly ventilated dwelling without air conditioning?
- Are atmospheric conditions very hot, humid, or polluted?
- Does the person engage in active exercise during hot weather?
- Does the person have chronic illnesses, such as diabetes or cardiovascular disorders, that predispose him or her to hyperthermia?
- Is the person at risk for hyponatremia or hypokalemia because of medications or chronic illnesses?

temperature. These goals are achieved by modifying the environment whenever possible and by addressing the socioeconomic factors that may contribute to the development of hypothermia or hyperthermia. When environmental tem-

peratures cannot be changed, then goals are addressed through the promotion of good health habits and actions that protect the older person from the detrimental effects of adverse temperatures. Goals are also achieved by educating older adults and their caregivers. Nurses working in areas of the country where extremes of climate are common have seasonal opportunities to teach about the prevention of hypothermia and heat-related illnesses.

A nursing goal for older adults with the diagnosis of Altered Comfort related to the perception of feeling cold is to maintain their quality of life. This is achieved through nursing measures that increase the person's feeling of being warm and comfortable. Also, any measures that reduce the risk factors for hypothermia will increase the comfort of older adults.

Nursing Interventions

Eliminating Risk Factors

Maintenance of an environmental temperature of around 75°F is the single most important intervention to prevent hypothermia or hyperthermia. In addition, relative humidity is an important consideration that can be altered to minimize the discomfort and detrimental effects associated with extremely warm or cool environments. With comfortable indoor temperatures, the ideal humidity is between 40% and 50%, and an acceptable range is between 20% and 70%. Older adults can be encouraged to humidify the air in their homes during the dry winter months by using humidifiers, either alone or in conjunction with their heating systems. Simpler measures, such as keeping wet towels near heating vents or using a vaporizer near the bed at night, may be appropriate if a humidifier is unavailable.

Interventions for the socially isolated older adult include establishing a system of social contact, such as a friendly phone call program, that ensures daily contact during periods of adversely hot or cold weather. In many areas of the United States in which cold winters are the norm, financial assistance for heating bills may be available through government-sponsored programs, such as the Home Energy Assistance Program (HEAP). Other government-sponsored programs provide financial assistance, such as low-interest loans, for home winterization and modernization measures to protect against adverse weather conditions. Older people and their family caregivers should be encouraged to take advantage of these programs, applications for which can be obtained from their local government offices or area agencies for the aging.

Maintaining Normal Body Temperature

In cool environmental temperatures, hypothermia can be prevented through the use of proper clothing and covering and the avoidance of risk factors. Older adults should be encouraged to wear several layers of warm clothing during the daytime, and caps and warm socks while sleeping. Electric blankets used during the night are a relatively inexpensive form of protection in cool environments, but proper safety precautions must be taken. Space heaters often are used to provide intense heat in a small area, but they can create serious fire and safety hazards. In addition to environmental considerations, special attention must be directed toward ensuring adequate nutrition, including fluid intake, and toward the treatment of any pathologic conditions.

During heat waves, hyperthermia can affect older adults living in their own homes or in long-term care settings that are not air-conditioned. Nurses in long-term care facilities without air conditioning must ensure that adequate fluids are provided. They must also observe for early signs of hyperthermia, especially in residents who are immobile or who have medical problems, such as endocrine or circulatory disorders, that predispose older adults to hyperthermia. If one part of the facility is air-conditioned, nurses can encourage residents to spend time in those areas and provide assistance for residents who have mobility limitations.

Older adults living in community settings can be instructed about measures to cool the environment, such as those summarized in Display 15-2. Older adults may be reluctant to use fans or air conditioners because of a desire to cut down on utility bills. If they understand the health risks associated with hyperthermia, however, they may be prompted to use these appliances judiciously. If the home setting cannot be cooled adequately during heat waves, older adults can be encouraged to spend time in air-conditioned public places. Older adults who have difficulty getting to these places can take advantage of transportation programs that are available through senior centers. Additional interventions to prevent hyperthermia during heat waves include the provision of adequate fluids and the avoidance of heavy meals and strenuous exercise. Display 15-2, which summarizes interventions for the prevention of hyperthermia, can be used as an educational tool for older adults.

DISPLAY 15-2
Tips for Preventing Hypothermia and Heat-Related Illnesses

Environmental and Personal Protection Considerations for Preventing Hypothermia

- Maintain a constant room temperature as close to 75°F as possible, with a minimum temperature of 70°F.
- Use a reliable, clearly marked thermometer to measure room temperature.
- Wear close-knit, but not tight, undergarments to prevent heat loss; wear several layers of clothing.
- Wear a hat and gloves when outdoors; wear a nightcap and socks for sleeping.
- Wear extra clothing in the early morning when your body metabolism is at its lowest point.
- Use flannel bed sheets or sheet blankets.
- Use an electric blanket set on low temperature.
- Take advantage of programs that offer assistance with utility bills and home weatherization.

Environmental and Personal Protection Considerations for Preventing Heat-Related Illnesses

- Maintain room temperatures at below 85°F.
- If your residence is not air-conditioned, use fans to circulate the air and cool the environment.
- During hot weather, spend time in public air-conditioned settings, such as libraries or shopping malls.

- Wear loose-fitting, lightweight, light-colored, cotton clothing.
- Wear a hat or use an umbrella to protect yourself against sun and heat when you are outside.
- Avoid outdoor activity during the hottest time of the day (i.e., between 10:00 A.M. and 3:00 P.M.); perform activities during the cooler hours of the morning or evening.
- Place an ice pack or cold, wet towels on your body, especially in the area of your groin and armpits.
- Take cool (about 75°F) baths or showers several times daily during heat waves, but do not use soap every time.

Health Habits for Maintaining Normal Body Temperature

- Maintain adequate fluid intake by drinking 8 to 10 glasses of non-caffeinated, non-alcoholic liquid daily.
- Do not rely on your thirst sensation as an indicator of the need for fluid.
- Eat small, frequent meals rather than heavy meals.
- Avoid drinking caffeinated beverages, such as cola and coffee.
- Avoid drinking alcohol.
- In cold weather, engage in moderate physical exercise and indoor activities to increase circulation and heat production.

ALTERNATIVE
AND
PREVENTIVE
HEALTH
CARE
PRACTICES

Preventing Infections

Herbs
• Garlic, ginger, thyme, sage, rosemary, Echinacea, goldenseal, licorice, ginseng

Nutritional Considerations
• Good hydration level (2000 cc of liquid daily)
• Vitamins A, C, and E; zinc; selenium

Preventive Measures and Additional Approaches
• Pneumonia and influenza immunizations (as discussed in Chapter 11)
• Tetanus and diphtheria vaccinations every 10 years
• Avoid melatonin and other bioactive substances that might alter temperature regulation (see Table 15-1)
• Exercise, massage, imagery, meditation

Maintaining Quality of Life

Nurses have many opportunities to improve the comfort of older adults who live in environments where they frequently feel cold. Interventions directed toward warming the hands, feet, and head are particularly effective because these areas of the body have the heaviest concentration of nerve endings that are sensitive to heat loss. Nurses can encourage older adults to wear caps, thermal socks, and leg warmers. These interventions are likely to increase the older adult's comfort level and their perception of warmth, even if they do not increase the core body temperature (Holtzclaw, 1993). Additional measures that can be used to increase comfort are summarized in Display 15-2. Alternative and preventive health care practices, as summarized in the box on this page, may improve quality of life with regard to preventing infections.

Evaluating Nursing Care

Nursing care of older adults who are diagnosed as being at High Risk for Hypothermia/Hyperthermia or Altered Body Temperature is evaluated according to the extent to which the goals have been achieved. A common nursing goal is the elimination of risk factors. For example, housing and financial factors that increase the risk of hypothermia and heat-related illnesses might be addressed by referring an older adult to HEAP. When the goal is to educate older adults and their caregivers about the prevention of hypothermia and heat-related illnesses, the nurse can use the information in Display 15-2 as a teaching tool. Evaluation of this intervention would be based on the person's ability to describe ways of decreasing the risk factors for hypothermia or heat-related illnesses. Nursing care of older adults with the diagnosis of Altered Comfort related to the perception of being cold can be evaluated according to the presence or absence of complaints about feeling cold.

Chapter Summary

Thermoregulation in older adults is altered by age-related changes that interfere with their ability to adapt effectively to environmental temperatures. Because of these changes, older adults are more likely to experience hypothermia or heat-related problems. In addition, even healthy older adults may have a lower normal body temperature and a diminished febrile response to illness. Risk factors that can further impair the thermoregulatory response of older adults include diseases, immobility, medication effects, and adverse environmental temperatures.

Nursing assessment of thermoregulation focuses on ascertaining the person's baseline body temperature and on identifying any risk factors for hypothermia or heat-related illnesses. Other aspects of the nursing assessment address the detection of illnesses in the absence of temperature elevations in the usual febrile range. Applicable nursing diagnoses include High Risk for Hypothermia, High Risk for Hyperthermia, High Risk for Altered Body Temperature, and Altered Comfort, related to the perception of being cold. Nursing goals are directed toward eliminating risk factors, maintaining the person's normal body temperature, and improving the comfort of older adults who frequently feel cold.

Nursing interventions focus on modifying environments, addressing socioeconomic factors, implementing measures to maintain normal body temperature, and educating older adults and their caregivers about the prevention of hypothermia and heat-related illnesses. Nursing care is evaluated according to the degree to which risk factors are eliminated. Another measure of nursing care is the absence of complaints about feeling cold.

Critical Thinking Exercises

1. Describe four major functional consequences that an older adult is likely to experience with regard to thermoregulation. How would you explain these changes to an older adult?
2. Explain how each of the following factors might affect an older person's thermoregulation: medications, pathologic conditions, environmental conditions, socioeconomic factors, and myths and misunderstanding.
3. What would you include in an assessment of thermoregulation in an older adult?
4. What would you teach older adults about hypothermia and its prevention?
5. What would you teach older adults about heat-related illnesses and their prevention?

Case Example and Nursing Care Plan

Pertinent Case Information

Mrs. T. is a 78-year-old woman who lives alone in her own home in a rural area of the northeastern United States. She has a history of hypertension and diabetic retinopathy, and she was recently hospitalized for uncontrolled diabetes. Upon discharge from the hospital in November, she was referred to the Visiting Nurses Association for teaching about insulin administration and monitoring of her diabetic care.

Nursing Assessment

During your initial visit, you observe that Mrs. T.'s house is poorly maintained and has no insulation or weatherization. Mrs. T. tells you she has lived in this house for 44 years and that, in recent years, she has had difficulty keeping up with the maintenance because of her poor eyesight and limited income. She has few social contacts, but her daughter visits her weekly and brings her groceries. A neighbor down the road also visits about every other week. Your assessment reveals that Mrs. T. has difficulty preparing meals because of her poor eyesight, but she is independent in all other activities of daily living.

During your initial visit, you identify several risk factors for hypothermia, so during subsequent visits, you follow up with further assessment. You learn that Mrs. T. was taken to the emergency room in January 2 years ago to be treated for hypothermia. She recalls that her daughter had come for her weekly visit and had found her in a very weak and confused state. Based on Mrs. T.'s statement that "they just warmed me up and sent me home again," it is apparent that she did not consider her condition to be of particular concern. In the winter, she keeps her utility bills low by using a small, portable heater in the living room during the day, moving it into the bedroom at night. Mrs. T. keeps her thermostat at 65°F during the day and 60°F at night. A neighbor told her that the county office on aging had a program to assist with utility bills, but she is embarrassed to ask her daughter to drive her to the county office to apply for this "welfare help."

Nursing Diagnosis

In addition to addressing the nursing diagnoses related to Mrs. T.'s diabetes, you identify a nursing diagnosis of High Risk for Hypothermia. Related factors include advanced age, diabetes, social isolation, poor housing conditions, low environmental temperatures, and a history of hypothermia.

Goals	Nursing Interventions	Evaluation Criteria
To increase Mrs. T.'s knowledge about risk factors for hypothermia	Discuss and describe risk factors for hypothermia, with emphasis on Mrs. T.'s diabetes, social isolation, environmental conditions, and history of hypothermia.	Mrs. T. will be able to state at least four factors that place her at risk for hypothermia.
To increase Mrs. T.'s knowledge about ways of preventing hypothermia	Use Display 15-2 to discuss interventions to prevent hypothermia and to explore ways of applying these interventions to Mrs. T.'s situation.	Mrs. T. will implement strategies aimed at reducing her risk of hypothermia.
To eliminate the risk factor of low temperatures in Mrs. T.'s house	Inform Mrs. T. that she is eligible for the Home Energy Assistance Program (HEAP) and can qualify for assistance with utility bills, as well as help with weatherization. Emphasize that HEAP is an important, health-related program aimed at preventing hypothermia in older adults. Ask Mrs. T.'s permission to arrange for a home assessment by a HEAP staff person.	Mrs. T. will accept assistance from the HEAP program. Mrs. T. will have her house weatherized. Mrs. T. will keep her thermostat at 70°F during the winter.

To eliminate the risk factor of social isolation	Suggest home-delivered meals to Mrs. T. as a means of providing prepared meals and daily contact.	Mrs. T. will accept home-delivered meals.
	Emphasize the fact that one of the purposes of such programs is to ensure that socially isolated older adults have daily contact with someone who can monitor their well-being.	Mrs. T.'s daughter will phone daily during cold spells.
	Ask Mrs. T. for permission to contact her daughter to suggest that she call her mother daily during cold spells to make sure she is OK.	

Educational Resource

National Institute on Aging (NIA), Age Pages
NIA Information Center, P.O. Box 8057,
Gaithersburg, MD 20898–8057
(800) 222–2225
www.senior.com/npo/nia-publications.htm/

References

Berman, P., Hogan, D. B., & Fox, R. A. (1987). The atypical presentation of infection in old age. *Age and Ageing, 16*, 201–207.

Carpenito, L. J. (1997). *Nursing diagnosis: Application to clinical practice* (7th ed.). Philadelphia: J. B. Lippincott.

Castle, S. C., Norman, D. C., Yeh, M., Miller, D., & Yoshikawa, T. T. (1991). Fever response in elderly nursing home residents: Are the older truly colder? *Journal of the American Geriatrics Society, 39*, 853–857.

Castle, S. C., Toledo, S. D., Daskal, S. L., & Norman, D. C. (1992). The equivalency of infrared tympanic membrane thermometry with standard thermometry in nursing home residents. *Journal of the American Geriatrics Society, 40*, 1212–1216.

Darowski, A., Najim, Z., Weinberg, J. R., & Guz, A. (1991a). Hypothermia and infection in elderly patients admitted to hospital. *Age and Ageing, 20*, 100–106.

Darowski, A., Najim, Z., Weinberg, J. R., & Guz, A. (1991b). The increase in body temperature of elderly patients in the first twenty-four hours following admission to hospital. *Age and Ageing, 20*, 107–112.

Darowski, A., Weinberg, J. R., & Guz, A. (1991). Normal rectal, auditory canal, sublingual and axillary temperatures in elderly afebrile patients in a warm environment. *Age and Ageing, 20*, 113–119.

Downton, J. H., Andrews, K., & Puxty, J. A. H. (1987). "Silent" pyrexia in the elderly. *Age and Ageing, 16*, 41–44.

Fish, P. D., Bennett, G. C., & Millard, P. H. (1985). Heatwave morbidity and mortality in old age. *Age and Ageing, 14*, 243–245.

Fox, R. A. (1988). Atypical presentation of geriatric infections. *Geriatrics, 43*(5), 58–68.

Hasel K. L., & Erickson, R. S. (1995). Effect of cerumen on infrared ear temperature measurement. *Journal of Gerontological Nursing, 21*(12), 6–14.

Hofland, S. L., & Mort, J. (1994). Infections in long-term care facilities: Issues for practice. *Geriatric Nursing, 15*, 260–264.

Holtzclaw, B. J. (1993). Keeping patients warm in bed [Letter to the editor]. *Geriatric Nursing, 14*, 180.

Howell, T. H. (1982). Skin temperature gradient in the lower limbs of old women. *Experimental Gerontology, 17*, 65–67.

Jennings, J. R., Reynolds, C. F., Houck, P. R., Buysse, D. J., Hoch, C. C., Hall, F., & Monk, T. H. (1993). Age and sleep modify finger temperature responses to facial cooling. *Journal of Gerontology: Medical Sciences, 48*(3), M108–M116.

Macey, S. M., & Schneider, D. F. (1993). Deaths from excessive heat and excessive cold among the elderly. *Gerontologist, 33*, 497–500.

McAlpine, C. H., Martin, B. J., Lennox, I. M., & Roberts, M. A. (1986). Pyrexia in infection in the elderly. *Age and Ageing, 15*, 230–234.

Olson, K. R., & Benowitz, N. L. (1984). Environmental and drug-induced hyperthermia. *Emergency Medicine Clinics of North America, 2*(3), 459–474.

Pals, J. K., Weinberg, A. D., Beal, L. F., Levesque, P. G., Cunningham, T. J., & Minaker, K. L. (1995). Clinical triggers for detection of fever and dehydration: Implications for long-term care nursing. *Journal of Gerontological Nursing, 21*(4), 13–19.

Sugarek, N. (1986). Temperature lowering after iced water: Enhanced effects in the elderly. *Journal of the American Geriatrics Society, 34,* 526–529.

Taylor, N. A. S., Allsopp, N. K., & Parkes, D. G. (1995). Preferred room temperature of young vs aged males: The influence of thermal sensation, thermal comfort, and affect. *Journal of Gerontology: Medical Sciences, 50A*(4), M216–M221.

United States Senate, Special Committee on Aging. (1983). *Heat stress and older Americans: Problems and solutions.* Washington, DC: U.S. Government Printing Office.

Whitbourne, S. K. (1996). *The aging individual: Physical and psychological perspectives.* New York: Springer.

Sexual Function

Chapter

16

Learning Objectives

1. *Delineate age-related changes that affect sexual function in men and women.*

2. *Examine the many risk factors that influence older adults' interest in, opportunities for, and performance of sexual activities.*

3. *Discuss the functional consequences of age-related changes and risk factors that affect reproduction, interest in sexual activity, and response to sexual stimulation.*

4. *Explain the reasons for, and the components of, an assessment of nurses' attitudes about sexual function in older adults.*

5. *Define the goals of assessment of sexual function in older adults.*

6. *Describe guidelines for interviewing older adults about sexual function.*

7. *Identify appropriate nursing interventions to address risk factors that influence sexual function in older adults.*

*S*exual function involves all the physiologic and psychosocial aspects of reproduction, interest in sexual activity, and response to sexual stimulation. Despite the complexity of this area of function, research on sexual function in older adults has been limited to the Masters and Johnson study (1966) of changes in physiologic response to sexual stimulation, and to a number of other studies of older adults' interest in and frequency of sexual activities. The psychosocial aspects of sexual function have not been addressed adequately, and sexual function in older women has not been studied as much as that in older men.

Age-Related Changes

A loss of reproductive ability at the onset of menopause in women is the age-related change in sexual function that is most easily delineated. Other, more subtle, age-related changes in sexual function include diminished reproductive abilities in older men and alterations in both male and female responses to sexual stimulation. In the absence of risk factors, these changes have little impact on sexual function because older adults generally do not desire high levels of reproductive ability and can readily compensate for any altered physiologic response to sexual stimulation. In the presence of risk factors, however, the sexual function of older adults may be severely compromised. This is because the risk factors, not the age-related changes, are the strongest determinants of sexual function.

Female Reproductive Function

Female reproductive function is governed by hormonally regulated cycles, called menses. With the onset of menses during adolescence, the cyclic release of ova marks the beginning of female reproductive abilities. Reproductive abilities decline around the 5th decade, when the frequency of ovulation diminishes and the menstrual cycle becomes shorter and more irregular. Menopause (the cessation of menses), which typically occurs around the age of 49 to 51 years, is a clear indicator that reproduction is no longer possible.

In addition to affecting reproductive ability, menopause influences other aspects of sexual function, predominantly as a result of the accompanying decline in endogenous estrogen levels. Before menopause, the primary source of estrogen is the production of estradiol by the ovaries. After menopause, the primary source of estrogen is the conversion of androstenedione to estrone in skin and fat tissue. Endogenous estrogen levels decline in all postmenopausal women, but the extent and manifestations of estrogen deficiency vary. Factors that may influence postmenopausal levels of endogenous estrogen include the interval since the onset of menopause; the production of hormones by the adrenal cortex; changes in the clearance rates of androgens and estrogens; and body weight, with higher body fat being positively correlated with higher levels of estrogen.

Because of a greatly diminished estrogen supply, the following changes occur, affecting sexual function:

1. The cervix, uterus, and Fallopian tubes atrophy.
2. The vaginal wall and mucosa become thinner.
3. The length and width of the vagina are reduced.
4. Bartholin's glands atrophy and secrete less fluid.
5. The amount of vaginal lubrication during periods of sexual excitement is diminished.
6. The labia lose their fullness owing to diminished subcutaneous fat.
7. Pubic hair becomes sparse.

Decreased estrogen levels also affect the breasts of older females, causing a gradual replacement of mammary gland tissue with fat tissue. In addition to this estrogen-related effect on the breasts, age-related connective tissue changes cause the breasts of older women to become less firm and more pendulous.

Male Reproductive Function

Male reproductive function depends on the secretion of hormones, the production and release of sperm, and the motility of sperm through the penile urethra. Luteinizing hormone and follicle-stimulating hormone are the two gonadotropins that regulate the production of testosterone and sperm in men. Controversy has persisted over the extent to which these hormones are affected by age-related changes. Some studies indicate that plasma gonadotropin concentration increases, but that the increase may be blunted when testosterone levels are low (Morley, 1991). Other studies have suggested that any reduction in testosterone can be attributed to pathologic conditions and decreased sexual activity, rather than to age-related changes. One review, however, concludes that circulating testosterone levels decline in most men as a result of age-related changes (Morley, 1991).

The seminiferous tubules, the site of sperm production, undergo the following degenerative changes: increased fibrosis; thinning of the epithelium; thickening of the basement membrane; and narrowing of the lumen, eventually to the point of obliteration of some of the tubules. It is generally thought that the number of normal, viable sperm gradually diminishes, beginning in the 6th decade. This reduced sperm count is probably associated with structural changes in the lumina of the seminiferous tubules. Questions have been raised, however, regarding the universality of these changes and the degree to which they are age-related or disease-related. Indeed, at least one study has challenged the assumption that an age-related decline in sperm occurs (Nieschlag et al., 1982). This study, which compared two groups of fathers having mean ages of 67 and 29 years, revealed an age-related decrease in sperm motility, but no differences in ejaculate volume, sperm morphology, or fertilizing capability. The authors concluded that age-related changes do not affect either the sperm count or the fertilizing capacity of sexually active men.

The seminal vesicles, prostate gland, and Cowper's glands are accessory structures that produce semen to facilitate the movement of sperm. The following degenerative changes affect the seminal vesicles: the mucosa becomes smoother, the epithelium becomes thinner, the muscle tissue is replaced with connective tissue, and the fluid-retaining capacity is reduced. The degenerative changes that affect the prostate gland include diminished secretions, atrophy of the gland cells, the formation of hard masses around the prostatic urethra, replacement of muscle tissue by connective tissue, and a change in the shape of epithelial cells from columnar to cuboidal and irregular. Age-related changes in Cowper's glands have not been documented.

Beginning around the 4th decade, the penis also undergoes age-related changes, but these degenerative changes do not affect reproductive function. The primary degenerative penile changes are venous and arterial sclerosis, and fibroelastosis of the corpus spongiosum. Studies investigating changes in the weight and volume of the testes have yielded contradictory results ranging from detection of no changes, to an age-related reduction in weight, to a weight reduction only in the presence of a pathologic condition.

Risk Factors

Risk factors interfere with the older adult's interest in, opportunities for, and performance of sexual activities. Attitudes, knowledge, stereotypes, social circumstances, pathologic conditions, and adverse effects of medications are risk factors that commonly interfere with sexual function in this population. A recent study of self-reported sexual function in older Blacks and Whites revealed that the significant predictors for sexual arousal problems included older age, decreased pulmonary function, physical disability, increased prescription drug use, and a fair or poor perception of health (Keil et al., 1992).

Attitudes, Knowledge, and Stereotypes of Older People

More than any other functional area, the sexual function of older adults is influenced by personal and societal attitudes. In America, sexuality typically is associated with physical attractiveness in very gender-specific ways. For example, male sexuality is associated with the image of a tanned, muscular, youthful man driving a truck or sports car. By contrast, female sexuality is associated with the image of a thin, but adequately endowed, young woman, smelling of perfume and wearing clothing that suggestively exposes parts of her body. These images are not consistent with evidence of fat deposits, skin wrinkles, sagging breasts, sensible shoes, gray or balding hair, or any other physical characteristics that typically are associated with middle or old age. Commercial advertising for the sensual and luxurious things in life, such as perfume, furs, liquor, and sport cars, reinforces these images to an extreme degree.

Because sex is so closely identified with youthfulness, the stereotype of "sexless seniors" is widely believed. It is not surprising, then, that almost 75% of the more than 4000 respondents polled in a Consumers Union report agreed with the statement, "Society thinks of older people as nonsexual" (Brecher, 1984, p. 19). For many older people, the belief that they are no longer sexy because they are no longer youthful becomes a self-fulfilling prophecy. Likewise, older adults who do not believe the stereotype may be embarrassed to acknowledge their sexual desires and activities for fear of being ridiculed or considered abnormal.

Sexual behaviors and personal values about the morality and appropriateness of specific sexual behaviors are based on both current and past societal attitudes. One study of sexual behaviors and attitudes in 106 cultures found that the continuation of sexual activity during old age was strongly influenced by social expectations (Winn and Newton, 1982). These researchers concluded that the full sexual expression of older people was affected by negative valuations of the sexual desirability of older persons. Another study, which examined changes in attitudes about sexual morality among cohorts between 1972 and 1982, indicated that attitudes about sexuality varied among cohorts but did not change significantly within each cohort during the 10-year period (Cutler, 1985). Cutler's data from nine national opinion surveys of 12,276 adults living in the United States suggested that older people did not become more conservative in their attitudes about sexual morality. Rather, attitudes of the older cohort, like those of younger cohorts, reflected the societal influences of their times. Thus, it is important to consider the societal context of attitudes about aging and sexuality to understand the related attitudes and behaviors of older adults.

People who today are in their seventies and eighties were strongly influenced in their childhood by the strict Victorian standards of morality that prevailed in Europe and America during the early 20th century. People who currently are in their 50s and 60s also have been biased by Victorian standards through the teaching of their parents and the continued dominance of these attitudes well into the mid-20th century. Unless these attitudes have been challenged, older adults are likely to base their sexual behaviors on these beliefs. From a historical perspective, sexuality of the older adult population "has been viewed as immoral, inappropriate, and negative" (Covey, 1989, p. 93). Indeed, Covey concludes that "Western cultural beliefs, at least from the Middle Ages onward, have held that sexual drive disappears with old age, that sex is perverse in old age, and that those elderly who attempt it practice self-deception. In addition, traditional concepts related to sexuality, such as beauty, attractiveness, sexual potency, and female orgasm, did not refer to elderly people, but excluded them" (p. 93).

In the Consumers Union survey, the respondents were judged as "Victorians" or "non-Victorians" based on answers to specific questions about sexual activity, homosexuality, masturba-

tion, and pornography. Victorian sexual views were positively correlated with the following characteristics: female, 70 years of age or older, income of less than $10,000, no education beyond high school, and low enjoyment and frequency of sex (Brecher, 1984). According to Victorian standards, masturbation, homosexual activity, public displays of affection, and sex with anyone except a marital partner were totally taboo. Moreover, masturbation was considered to be more detrimental than sex outside of marriage, as evidenced by the Victorian norm of tolerating prostitution for the purpose of obviating the need for men to practice masturbation (Brecher, 1984). In recent decades, sex outside of marriage and public displays of affection, including vivid media portrayals of sexual activity, have become increasingly prevalent and accepted. Masturbation and homosexuality, however, have not gained as much public acceptance, and any positive attitudes about these sexual activities are more likely to be acknowledged privately than publicly.

The current attitudes of Americans aged 50 years and older who participated in the Consumers Union report (Brecher, 1984) can be summarized as follows:

1. Of the 4149 respondents who expressed opinions about the statement, "Masturbation is not proper for older people," 63% disagreed with the statement (p. 234).
2. Personal attitudes about masturbation do not necessarily reflect one's own behavior, as evidenced by the responses of survey respondents regarding this practice. Respectively, 41% and 53% of the women and men who responded reported that they do engage in masturbation; 19% and 28% of the women and men who disapprove of masturbation reported that they engage in this activity (p. 234).
3. Respectively, 57% and 72% of the female and male respondents agreed that it was acceptable for older couples who are not married to have sexual relations (p. 242).

4. Seventy percent of the respondents agreed with the statement that "[Male] homosexual and lesbian relations between older people are nobody else's business" (pp. 259–260).

Attitudes, Knowledge, and Stereotypes of Caregivers

Attitudes of caregivers about sexual activities can be important determinants of the sexual function of dependent older adults. Most often, the sexual needs of dependent older adults are totally ignored by caregivers who do not have to address sexual needs as long as they believe the stereotype of the asexual older person. If caregivers do acknowledge sexual needs, it is usually because an older person displays sexual behaviors that are judged to be inappropriate by the caregivers.

Adult children of older people often find it difficult to deal with the sexuality of their parents, particularly with the sexual interests and activities of a parent who is widowed. In addition to being influenced by the usual stereotypes about older adults not being interested in sexual activities, children of older adults may be influenced by fears that a widowed parent may develop an intimate relationship that would threaten their inheritance. If the adult child can successfully deny the existence of their older parent's sexual needs, then the possibility of threatening relationships also can be ignored.

In long-term care settings, staff attitudes about the sexual activity of the residents often are based on Victorian standards, and these attitudes are conveyed through unwritten policies and staff approaches to residents. The sexual needs of residents usually are ignored by staff members unless a resident is discovered engaging in a sexual activity. If staff members do acknowledge sexual activities, they often judge these activities to be inappropriate, and they may punish the sexually active resident. Typically, the only expression of sexual needs by residents of long-term facilities that is considered to be appropriate and socially acceptable is a private, medically approved visit by a spouse. Any sexual activities in which a solitary resident or two unmarried people engage usually are not tolerated, even if done in private. When the staff of long-term care facilities become aware of sexual activities that are not considered to be acceptable, family members often are asked to intervene, even when the resident is a competent adult. Decisions regarding sexual activity, even between spouses, usually are dealt with as strictly medical matters. In addition to the prerequisite of medical approval for sexual activity, the permission of family members often is sought as part of the staff decision to allow or tolerate sexual activity. A study of attitudes about sexual activity in Canadian nursing homes concluded that "men and women in nursing homes and old-age homes are probably the most sexually deprived of the elderly" (Schlesinger, 1983, p. 267).

Social Circumstances

Sexual activity at any age is influenced by social circumstances, such as the response and availability of an acceptable and desirable partner. For older adults, particularly older women, social circumstances often are the strongest determinants of sexual activity. Studies consistently show that the level of sexual activity for older women is directly related to their marital status, whereas the level of sexual activity for older men is not as closely associated with marital status. Men at all ages report a higher frequency of extramarital sexual relationships, and older widowers have the advantage of a higher likelihood of remarriage in comparison with older widows. Statistics on the ratio of women to men provide one logical explanation for the gender differences in availability of sexual partners. With increasing age, the ratio of men to women gradually changes, from a ratio of 82 men per 100 women in the age group of 65 to 74 years to a ratio of 40 men per 100 women in the age group of 85 years and older (U.S. Bureau of the Census, 1996).

Past and present marital status and level of sexual interest and activity also influence current sexual activities. The importance assigned to sexual activity in the past has consistently been identified as a determinant of both frequency and enjoyment of sexual activities for older men and women (Bretschneider and McCoy, 1988). As a group, never-married women have the lowest rate of sexual activity compared to other categories of older adults. Although women of all ages are less sexually active than men in their cohort, the difference in their levels of sexual activity widens with increasing age.

Homosexuality is another social circumstance that significantly influences one's sexual activity and relationships. Prejudiced attitudes toward lesbians and gay men can seriously interfere with the freedom to cultivate and express satisfying sexual relationships. Only in recent years have lesbians and gay men become increasingly visible and felt somewhat accepted in American society. Thus, older adults who have lived for decades in a society where they were invisible and greatly stigmatized may find it particularly difficult to meet partners and enjoy satisfying sexual activities and relationships. One study identified the following problem areas for lesbians and gay men older than 50 years of age: loneliness, sexual preference discrimination, and health and financial concerns (Quam and Whitford, 1992). A model for a support and education group for older gay and lesbian individuals has been developed and can be used to address their needs (Slusher et al., 1996).

Pathologic Conditions

The negative impact of certain chronic illnesses on sexual performance has been well documented, especially regarding erectile dysfunction in men. Specifically, neurologic, endocrine, and cardiovascular illnesses are highly associated with sexual dysfunction. The probability of experiencing erectile dysfunction increases with age, as does the likelihood that the condition is associated with pathophysiologic causes, rather than psychological causes.

The physiologic conditions that most often cause erectile dysfunction in older men include vascular, neurologic, and endocrine disorders. The chronic illnesses most commonly associated with these pathophysiologic changes are diabetes mellitus and ischemic heart disease. Because nurses care for many older adults with these conditions, the effects of each of these conditions on the sexual function of older adults are discussed in detail. Other pathologic conditions that may cause erectile dysfunction include hypertension, atherosclerosis, hormonal insufficiencies, and injury from trauma, irradiation, or surgery.

Diabetes

Diabetes mellitus is a common cause of penile neuropathy in diabetic men at any age. The prevalence of erectile failure increases with advancing age, however, affecting between 50% and 95% of men with diabetes who are older than 70 years of age. Erectile dysfunction may be an early manifestation of uncontrolled diabetes, and the degree of sexual dysfunction may vary in accordance with the degree of diabetic control. The ability to ejaculate is not lost, although it may be retrograde, and libido and orgasm are not affected to the same degree that erection is affected. The sexual function of diabetic women does not seem to be affected to the same degree as that of men, but about one third of women with diabetes have difficulty achieving orgasm. Also, vaginal lubrication often is delayed and greatly diminished.

Cardiovascular Disease

Cardiovascular disease is associated with many aspects of sexual dysfunction, including decreased libido, impaired performance and pleasure, and decreased frequency of sexual activities. Within several months following a myocardial infarction, there usually is little or no physiologic basis for abstaining from sexual intercourse with a regular partner. It generally is agreed that sexual activity with a marital partner can be resumed when the affected person can perform moderate exercise—such as climbing two flights of steps—without experiencing harmful cardiac effects. A recent study concluded that there is a one in a million chance that sexual activity will trigger the onset of myocardial infarction, and even this small risk might be reduced by regular exercise (Muller et al., 1996). Thus, although some physiologic basis may exist for sexual dysfunction following myocardial infarction, the influence of psychological factors usually is most significant. Some of these psychological factors include fatigue, depression, partner's decision, fears and anxiety, diminished sexual desire, and symptoms of coronary disease.

Many psychosocial risk factors arise from lack of education regarding sexual activity and cardiac disease, particularly in persons who have a history of myocardial infarction. When people who have had heart attacks, or their sexual partners, believe that sexual activity is too risky and strenuous, their sexual interest, activities, or performance may be curtailed unnecessarily. Health professionals and patients often are uncomfortable discussing sexual function, and they may avoid initiating this topic because it is considered to be a private matter. Health professionals who care for older adults might further justify the avoidance of this topic because they may believe that older adults are not interested in or capable of sexual activities. If the older adult does not have a traditional marital relationship, the stereotype may be further reinforced, and sexual function thus may be viewed as a moot issue.

Adverse Medication and Chemical Effects

Before the 1980s, the role of medication as a cause of disorders of sexual function was largely ignored. In the past decade, however, adverse medication effects have received increased attention, primarily because younger men are experiencing sexual dysfunction from their use of antidepressants, antihypertensives, and cardiac medications. This problem was brought to the public's attention almost 2 decades ago in a *New York Times* article that cited medications as the single largest cause of erectile dysfunction in men and listed more than 50 medications with potentially adverse sexual effects (Brody, 1983). Brody's article referred to a study, published in the *Journal of the American Medical Association* (Slag et al., 1983), of 1180 male patients in a medical clinic. Of these subjects, 401 were impotent, and 25% of the 188 subjects who subsequently underwent further evaluation were found to have medication-induced erectile dysfunction.

Research on medication-related sexual dysfunction is growing because of the increased awareness of adverse medication effects and their impact on quality of life. Most scientific literature on medication-induced sexual dysfunction focuses on men, particularly middle-aged or younger men. The lack of attention to medication-induced sexual dysfunction in women and older adults is not the result of an absence of such problems in these groups. Rather, it is attributable to the fact that investigators usually select younger men as their subjects because of cultural biases and the relative ease with which male sexual response is measured compared to female sexual response. One recent article concluded that more than one third of young patients taking serotonin selective-reuptake inhibitors for depression experienced difficulties with sexual function, and that this figure is likely to be much higher in older patients (Jenike, 1997).

Medications adversely affect sexual function through a variety of mechanisms, including their influence on the release of hormones and their actions on the autonomic and central nervous systems. For example, serotonergic and cholinergic actions of antidepressants can interfere with libido, erection, ejaculation, and orgasm. Specific adverse medication effects that interfere with sexual function in men include a decreased or absent libido, difficulty obtaining or maintaining an erection, and premature or retrograde ejaculation. A less common adverse medication effect is priapism, or prolonged erection, which is associated with some neuroleptics, antidepressants, and medications used for the treatment of erectile dysfunction. Women may experience any of the following medication-induced limitations in sexual function: diminished vaginal lubrication, decreased or absent libido, and inability to achieve orgasm. Table 16-1 lists some of the medications that are commonly associated with sexual dysfunction. These effects usually disappear when the medication is discontinued; occasionally, the effects will disappear with a mere decrease in the dose.

As alcohol is a central nervous system depressant, it can interfere with sexual function. Also, in men, alcohol interferes with sexual function because it interferes with the release of testoster-

one and gonadotropins. In some social settings, alcohol decreases inhibitions and heightens sensual and sexual interest. In excessive amounts, however, the depressant effect of alcohol on the central nervous system usually counteracts any beneficial effects and interferes with sexual performance. Moderate amounts of alcohol normally would not interfere with sexual performance; however, in combination with other risk factors, such as medications or pathologic conditions, even small amounts of alcohol may be detrimental to the sexual performance of older adults.

Although little research has been done on the effects of nicotine on sexual function, smoking is a contributing factor to erectile dysfunction because it accentuates the effects of other risk factors, such as hypertension and vascular disease (National Institutes of Health, 1992). One study of smoking, diabetes, hypertension, and hyperlipidemia as arterial risk factors in 440 impotent men revealed that, although all factors were significantly associated with erectile dysfunction, the factor with the highest association of the four was smoking (Virag et al., 1985). Authors of another study that addressed smoking as a risk factor for penile arterial insufficiency advised that cessation of smoking should be encouraged to promote even marginal improvement in penile arterial flow (Mulligan and Katz, 1988).

Functional Impairment

Any chronic illness that causes serious functional impairment, such as arthritis or respiratory disease, can interfere with sexual interest and performance. People with limited energy, agility, or respiratory capacity may experience difficulties in their sexual activities unless they use compensatory measures. Some functional impairments, such as incontinence, might contribute to sexual dysfunction in people of any age. Problems with a sexual relationship also may arise when a person depends on the sexual partner for assistance in activities of daily living.

TABLE 16-1
Medications/Chemicals That Can Interfere with Sexual Function

Cardiovascular Agents	*Antihistamines*
Antiadrenergic agents	Diphenhydramine
Beta-adrenergic blockers	Chlorpheniramine
Beta-blockers	*Gastrointestinal Agents*
Hydralazine	Anticholinergics
Digoxin	Histamine H_2 antagonists
Diuretics	
Cholesterol-lowering agents	*Antiparkinsonian Agents*
Antidepressants	Benztropine
All antidepressants except trazodone	Trihexyphenidyl
Phenothiazine	*Miscellaneous Agents*
Benzodiazepines	Alcohol
	Decongestants
	Barbiturates
	Amphetamines
	Cytotoxic agents

Some of the tasks that require the highest level of motor coordination, such as cleansing the genitalia and rectal area, are those activities that are also the most personal. When a person depends on a sexual partner for assistance with these daily activities, conflicts may arise because these activities are closely connected with sexual activities.

People with a readily apparent disability often are viewed by society as asexual because of cultural biases that tend to correlate a visible disability with additional invisible disabilities. This perception, along with other effects of disabilities on self-image, may have a negative impact on sexual function. This may be more problematic for men because society tends to associate male sexual performance with physical vigor. Although these effects are not unique to older adults, functional limitations increase with advancing age and are likely to combine with other risk factors to interfere with sexual function. One study of sexual function among chronically ill men revealed that self-reported poor health was a significant risk factor for sexual dysfunction, particularly in older subjects (Mulligan et al., 1988). In the study by Mulligan and co-workers, the likelihood of being sexually dysfunctional was 6 times greater for middle-aged men with subjectively poor health, and 40 times greater for men older than 75 years of age, as compared with subjects of the same age who viewed themselves as healthy.

Because sensory stimulation is an important part of sexual pleasure and intimate communication, sensory impairments can interfere with sexual pleasure. An older adult whose hearing ability is seriously impaired may find it difficult or impossible to carry on the intimate conversations that are often a part of sexual stimulation with a partner. Hearing impairments may also interfere with professional efforts to assess and counsel the older adult on this sensitive topic. Likewise, impairments affecting vision, smell, or touch can interfere with some of the usual sensual stimulation associated with sexual activities.

Environmental Constraints

Privacy is generally considered to be a requisite for sexual activity, and it is usually arranged with ease by adults who live in their own homes. However, older adults who live in institutions, group settings, or family homes may find it difficult or impossible to arrange for privacy, especially if their sexual needs are ignored or considered abnormal by their caregivers or those with whom they live. Even if private time is provided in institutional settings, the inability to lock doors and ensure total privacy may interfere with sexual activities. Another environmental constraint for older adults in long-term care settings is the unavailability of anything larger than a single bed.

Functional Consequences

Sexual function involves reproduction, interest in sexual activity, and response to sexual stimulation. Whereas reproduction is directly affected by age-related changes, the other two aspects of sexual function are affected more directly by risk factors than by age-related changes.

Reproductive Ability

The loss of reproductive ability is the most clear-cut functional consequence for postmenopausal women. With the gradual decrease in the release of ova during the premenopausal years, women lose their ability to conceive, and those ova that are fertilized are more likely to result in a defective fetus. Reproductive ability usually ceases within 1 year of the last menstrual cycle. In contrast to the complete cessation of reproductive ability in women, the reproductive ability of men does not cease, but gradually declines.

Response to Sexual Stimulation

The Kinsey reports (1948, 1953) are recognized as landmark studies of human sexual behaviors, whereas the Masters and Johnson investigation (1966) is recognized as the landmark study of human physiologic response to sexual stimulation. The Masters and Johnson study of 694 adults in a laboratory setting identified four phases of physiologic response to sexual stimulation in men and women. An analysis of data on older subjects led to the conclusion that the ability of older adults to respond to sexual stimulation is maintained, but their response is slower and less intense. Masters and Johnson also concluded that older adults who engage in sexual activity experience fewer changes in their response to sexual stimulation than those who are sexually inactive. Any additional changes in an individual's response to sexual stimulation or ability to be sexually stimulated are thought to be associated with the many risk factors that commonly occur in older adults.

In the Masters and Johnson study (1966), only 31 of the 100 so-called aging subjects were 61 years or older, and only 9 of the subjects were 71 years or older. Subjects were grouped by gender and decade, and women aged 41 years and older and men aged 51 years and older were compared with women and men of ages 20 to 40 or 50 years. Additional information about "geriatric" sexual behaviors was obtained from sociosexual histories provided by 152 women and 212 men aged 51 to 90 years who participated in an interview, but not in the laboratory phase of the study. Despite the underrepresentation of older adults in this study, the findings of Masters and Johnson have been widely accepted as the knowledge base about age-related changes in physiologic response to sexual stimulation. Normal male and female responses to sexual stimulation and the associated age-related changes that were identified by Masters and Johnson are discussed in the following sections and are summarized in Table 16-2.

Response of Women to Sexual Stimulation

During the initial excitement phase of sexual stimulation, the following physiologic changes occur in women: the breasts enlarge and the nipples become erect; the skin over the upper chest becomes flushed; voluntary muscles be-come tense; the heart rate and blood pressure increase; the labia and clitoris enlarge and become vasocongested; the vaginal barrel expands, distends, and becomes lubricated and vasocongested; and the uterus elevates slightly. Older women are likely to experience some changes in the intensity of these responses. For instance, the breasts enlarge to a smaller degree; the sexual flush is absent or less noticeable; the length and width of vaginal expansion are diminished; vaginal lubrication is decreased and takes longer to occur; the elevation of the uterus is delayed and less marked; and the labia are less vasocongested.

During phase two—the plateau phase—the following responses normally occur: the breasts enlarge to a greater degree and the areola become engorged; the sexual flush spreads over the body and becomes more intense; the voluntary muscles become more tense; the rectal sphincter is voluntarily contracted; the blood pressure, heart rate, and respiratory rate increase; the clitoral shaft and glans withdraw; the vaginal barrel increases further in width and depth; the uterus elevates fully and the cervix elevates; the labia become more vasocongested; and Bartholin's glands secrete mucoid material. Because of age-related changes, older women experience these responses to a lesser degree, as summarized in Table 16-2.

The orgasmic phase of female sexual response is characterized by the following: sexual flush increases in intensity, parallel to the intensity of orgasm; muscle groups contract involuntarily; the rectal sphincter contracts involuntarily; pulse, blood pressure, and respirations increase further; the orgasmic platform contracts at intervals, with gradual lengthening of the intervals and weakening of the contractions; and the uterus contracts with an intensity parallel to that of the orgasm. As with other phases of sexual excitement, all the responses of the orgasmic phase are less intense in older females. In addition, the involuntary rectal sphincter contractions occur only with high tension levels, and the number of orgasmic contractions decreases

TABLE 16-2
Age-Related Changes in Response to Sexual Stimulation

Female Response	Male Response
Excitement Phase	
Breasts not as fully engorged	Longer time required to attain erection
Sexual flush absent or diminished	Less firm erection
Delayed or diminished vaginal lubrication	Longer maintenance of erection before ejaculation
Decreased expansion of vaginal wall	
Decreased vasocongestion of labia	Increased difficulty regaining an erection if lost
	Reduced or absent scrotal and testicular vasocongestion
Plateau Phase	
Decreased areolar engorgement	Diminished or absent nipple turgidity and sexual flush
Less intense sexual flush	
Less intense myotonia	Less intense muscle tension
Decreased degree of deepening of labial color	Slower penile erectile response
Decreased vasocongestion of labia	No color change in glans penis
Reduced Bartholin's gland secretions	Delayed and diminished testicular elevation
Slower/less marked uterine elevation	
Orgasmic Phase	
Decreased frequency of rectal sphincter contractions	Decreased frequency of rectal sphincter contractions
Decreased number and intensity of orgasmic contractions	Diminution of ejaculatory expulsion force by about 50%
	Absent or diminished sense of ejaculatory inevitability
	Fewer and less intense ejaculatory contractions
Resolution Phase	
Slower loss of nipple erection	Slower loss of nipple erection
Quicker return to pre-excitement stage	Longer refractory period
	Very rapid penile detumescence
	Very rapid testicular descent

by about 50%. Because postmenopausal women are no longer concerned about the reproductive consequences of sexual intercourse, however, their anxieties might be decreased and their capacity for orgasm may actually be increased. Some women experience orgasm or multiple orgasms for the first time during their postmenopausal years.

The resolution phase involves a gradual return to the pre-excitement state, beginning with a loss of deep vasocongestion. The breasts return to their normal appearance, the sexual flush disappears, muscle tone returns to a normal state within 5 minutes, vital signs return to normal, and all pelvic organs resume their pre-excitement characteristics. With the exception of a slower loss of nipple erection, the resolution phase occurs more rapidly in older women.

Response of Men to Sexual Stimulation

During the excitement phase of sexual stimulation, men experience the following physiologic changes: nipples may become erect; voluntary muscles become more tense; heart rate and blood pressure increase; the penis becomes erect; the scrotal sac flattens and elevates; and the testes become partially elevated. The most noticeable age-related change in this phase is a delay in attaining erection because of the need for longer or more intense stimulation. In addition, the erection may be less firm, but it can be maintained longer before ejaculation. If the erection subsides before ejaculation, however, a refractory period occurs and older men may have greater difficulty than younger men regaining a full erection. Scrotal and testicular vasocongestion is markedly reduced in older men, as is testicular elevation. In general, all responses of the excitement phase are less intense and are influenced more by arousal conditions than by autonomic nervous system responses.

During phase two, or the plateau phase, men experience the following: the nipples become erect and turgid; the skin over the head and trunk becomes flushed; voluntary and involuntary muscle tone increases; the rectal sphincter is voluntarily contracted; the pulse, respirations, and blood pressure are increased; penile circumference increases at the coronal ridge; the testes elevate and enlarge by 50%; and Cowper's glands emit pre-ejaculatory fluid. Age-related changes in these responses include an absence of or great diminution in sexual flush, nipple erection, and muscle tension. Full penile erection often occurs later in this stage, just before ejaculation, and testicular elevation is delayed or diminished because of less intense vasocongestion.

The orgasmic phase, which represents the peak response to sexual stimulation, is characterized by the following changes: the skin flush is well developed and parallels the intensity of excitement; there is a loss of voluntary control of muscles, and the rectal sphincter and some muscle groups involuntarily contract; heart rate, blood pressure, and respirations increase above normal; the penis contracts at intervals and with an expulsive force; and a sensation of ejaculatory inevitability is experienced and the ejaculatory process is initiated. Masters and Johnson (1966) identified the following changes in the orgasmic phase in older men: ejaculation is less powerful; seminal fluid emerges under less pressure; penile contractions are fewer and less intense; rectal sphincter contractions occur less frequently; and intercontractile intervals lengthen rapidly after the second expulsive contraction. Older men also reported a decreased sense of ejaculatory inevitability.

During the resolution phase, the manifestations of sexual excitement gradually disappear, and all physiologic responses return to the pre-excitement state. A refractory period occurs, during which the man is unable to redevelop an erection that is accompanied by ejaculation. With the exception of a slower loss of nipple erection, if present, all other responses to sexual stimulation return to their pre-excitement state more rapidly in older men as compared to younger men. In older men, the refractory period may last for a day or two, but erection without ejaculation may be able to be achieved during this time.

Sexual Interest and Activity

The first large-scale surveys of human sexual behavior, conducted by Kinsey and associates, were published in 1948 (*Sexual Behavior in the Human Male*) and 1953 (*Sexual Behavior in the Human Female*). These surveys of the sexual behaviors of more than 20,000 adults in the United States, collectively referred to as the "Kinsey Report," are widely considered to be landmark studies of the sexual activity of adults in the United States. Although fewer than 300 participants in the Kinsey Report were aged 61 years or older, these surveys provided the first information available regarding the sexual activity of older adults. Just as important, the Kinsey Report was a major step in bringing information about adult sexual behavior to public attention. Because of this report, many of the existing myths about sexual activity were challenged, and further interest in and research on this previously taboo topic were stimulated.

Although the Kinsey Report has been criticized for its biased sampling, many of its conclusions have been confirmed by subsequent studies. With regard to older adults, the Kinsey Report's conclusions about the occurrence of a gradual decline in sexual activity were confirmed by a 1978–1979 Consumers Union survey of more than 4000 people between the ages of 50 and 93 years (Brecher, 1984). As with the Kinsey Report, conclusions from the Consumers Union survey must be interpreted cautiously because of its biased sample. However, most, if not all, surveys on this topic are biased and self-selected because of the nature of the subject. It is interesting to note that 61% of the participants in the Kinsey Report and 73% of those participating in the Consumers Union survey were born between 1905 and 1924 (Brecher, 1984, p. 17). Thus, when considered together, these two surveys provide a historical picture of the sexual activity of a select group of people who currently are between 75 and 94 years of age.

Since the publication of Kinsey's survey in 1948, many smaller studies have been undertaken to investigate various aspects of sexual behavior in older adults. In recent years, studies of sexuality and aging have included an increased number of subjects older than 80 years of age, and they have focused on broader aspects of sexual function. For example, a study of 202 men and women aged 80 to 102 years addressed levels of sexual interest and enjoyment, as well as a variety of sexual activities, including touching and caressing without sexual intercourse (Bretschneider and McCoy, 1988). The results of such studies on sexuality and aging (Matthias et al., 1997; Wiley and Bortz, 1996; Bretsch-

neider and McCoy, 1988; White, 1982) can be summarized as follows:

1. Although the frequency of sexual activity gradually declines with increasing age, the level of sexual interest and the competence of older adults do not decline. In the absence of risk factors, there is no age at which interest in and ability to enjoy sexual activities are curtailed.
2. The decrease in sexual activity with advancing age is not attributable to age-related physiologic changes, but is associated with social circumstances, pathologic conditions, and other risk factors.
3. The social circumstances that most frequently lead to decreased sexual activity are spousal death or illness and lack of an available partner. The sexual activity of older women is more often affected by these conditions than is that of men.
4. Sexual interest, attitudes, activity, and satisfaction are a continuation of lifelong patterns and do not change significantly with advanced age.
5. Throughout life, men are more sexually active than women.

Although much progress has been made in identifying patterns of sexual interest and activity in older adults, very little emphasis has been placed on more complex, and perhaps more important, aspects of sexual function. Affection, friendships, and intimacy in homosexual and heterosexual relationships have been ignored by the Kinsey Report and by researchers, not only with regard to older adults, but also with regard to sexual function at any age. For older adults, these aspects of sexual function may increase in importance in proportion to the decreasing number of acceptable opportunities for direct sexual activities. In one of the few studies addressing sexual behaviors other than intercourse and masturbation, the most common sexual activities in both male and female subjects were touching and caressing without sexual intercourse (Bretschneider and McCoy, 1988). Another recent study revealed that older men and women reported that the sexual activities of kissing, hugging, and hearing loving words were more important than masturbation, oral sex, or sexual conversation (Johnson, 1996). In this same study, older women ascribed greater importance to sexual activities of sitting and talking, making oneself more attractive, and saying loving words than did men. By contrast, older men reported greater interest in sexual activities, such as erotic movies and readings, sexual daydreams, and physically intimate activities. In the light of these findings, conclusions drawn from studies considering only the frequency of masturbation or sexual intercourse as indicators of sexual activity might be quite limited in their applicability to older adults.

Older residents of long-term care facilities are, perhaps, the most overlooked population with regard to studies of sexual interests and activities. Although the sexual needs and interests of institutionalized older adults do not necessarily decrease, their opportunities for sexual expression are severely limited by social, attitudinal, and environmental constraints that do not affect community-living older adults. One of the few studies investigating the sexual interest of institutionalized older adults has revealed that nursing home residents are similar to community-living older adults in that their sexual interest exceeds their sexual activities (White, 1982).

Erectile Dysfunction

Since the mid-1990s, knowledge about erectile dysfunction has been growing at a rapid pace, and much of the information that was thought to be accurate is now being disproven. Even the term "impotence" is considered to be outdated and the term "erectile dysfunction" is now being used to emphasize that this is a very common and reversible condition that should be addressed by health care professionals (Godschalk

et al., 1997; Burnett, 1998). Erectile dysfunction is defined as the inability to achieve or maintain an erection sufficient for satisfactory sexual performance (National Institutes of Health, 1992). Although it is a common problem for older men, it is not an inevitable consequence of aging, nor is it likely to be psychogenic in origin. Recent estimates suggest that psychological disorders contribute to erectile dysfunction in only about 15% of cases (Salcido, 1997; Stern, 1997). Adverse medication effects are one of the most common causes of erectile dysfunction, as discussed in the section entitled Risk Factors. Other physiologic factors that may cause or contribute to erectile dysfunction include trauma, alcohol, nicotine, complications of pelvic surgery, and circulatory, endocrine, and neurologic conditions (e.g., diabetes mellitus and cardiovascular disorders). Other conditions that may cause or contribute to erectile dysfunction include dementia, depression, anxiety, and myths and misunderstandings about age-related changes in sexual function. As Masters and Johnson have reported, "Fears [of failure to perform] were expressed, under interrogation, by every male subject beyond forty years of age, irrespective of reported levels of formal education" (1966, p. 202). They concluded that "the fallacy that secondary impotence is to be expected as the male ages is probably more firmly entrenched in our culture than any other misapprehension" (1966, p. 202).

Additional Physiologic Consequences

Because of age-related changes, older adults are more susceptible to gender-specific pathologic conditions. For example, women are more susceptible to urethritis and vaginitis because of the thinning of the vaginal tissue and the decreased acidity and quantity of vaginal secretions. After intercourse, women may experience urinary urgency and burning that persists for several days. Fibroid cysts also are more likely to develop in older women than in younger women. Prostatic hyperplasia is a pathologic condition that affects 50% of 50-year-old men and 90% of 90-year-old men; it is caused, at least in part, by age-related hormonal changes. Although prostatic hyperplasia is not necessarily accompanied by functional consequences, the following problems often occur when prostatic hyperplasia obstructs the flow of urine: urinary urgency, retention, frequency, and hesitancy; urinary tract infections; and varying degrees of urinary incontinence.

One of the most noticeable effects of estrogen deficiency in menopausal women is the occurrence of hot flashes. Hot flashes affect 65% to 85% of all menopausal women, and 20% to 25% experience them for 5 years or longer. Although hot flashes do not necessarily cause functional consequences, they do cause discomfort, embarrassment, and brief interruptions in activities. For some women, hot flashes may occur frequently throughout the day and night and last for as long as half an hour. When hot flashes are frequent or prolonged, they can interfere with sexual enjoyment and many daily activities.

Most older men are unaware of changes in the frequency and characteristics of nocturnal penile tumescence, which is a reflex erection that occurs during sleep. Nocturnal penile tumescences gradually diminish in frequency and become less rigid in older men. Although this consequence is largely unnoticed, the presence or absence of nocturnal penile tumescence has been viewed as a diagnostic indicator that may be useful in differentiating between organic and psychogenic erectile dysfunction. However, this distinction has been challenged recently because of questions about whether nonsexual and sexual erections have the same physiologic basis (Stern, 1997).

Psychosocial Consequences

Attitudes, stereotypes, and lack of information about age-related changes in sexual function can have serious detrimental psychosocial consequences that are closely related to negative functional consequences. For example, if an older man experiences a delayed or diminished erectile response, he may assume he is impotent. Also, because of the high value placed on sexual performance in our society, any decline in sexual function may have a negative impact on self-esteem. One study of the relationship between sexuality and self-esteem in younger and older subjects identified specific effects of sexuality on self-esteem for male and female subjects and compared the findings for younger and older subjects (Stimson et al., 1981). These researchers concluded that sexuality is as crucial to self-esteem and self-organization in older men as it is in younger men. For younger men, however, the quantity of sexual activity was the important variable, whereas for older men, the quality of performance was the factor that sustained pride and social comfort. With regard to women, the study demonstrated a strong relationship between self-esteem and perceived youthfulness and attractiveness, and this relationship was particularly detrimental for older women. This study concluded that, because older women often feel unattractive, they also feel socially rejected and become less sure of their overall worth.

Summary of Consequences

In summary, older adults do not lose their interest in or capacity for sexual activity because of age-related changes. Any diminution in sexual function is related to social circumstances, pathologic conditions, adverse medication effects, or myths and attitudes. Because of age-related changes, however, the response of older men and women to sexual stimulation is slower, less intense, and of shorter duration. As one 79-year-old man confided to this author, "It's like sparklers, not fireworks."

Figure 16-1 illustrates the age-related

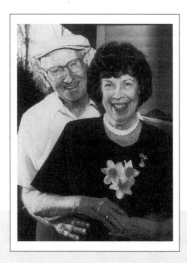

AGE-RELATED CHANGES

- *Female:* Atrophy of reproductive organs, thinning and drying of vaginal wall, diminished vaginal length and width, decreased vaginal lubrication
- *Male:* Degenerative changes in reproductive organs

NEGATIVE FUNCTIONAL CONSEQUENCES

- Less intense response to sexual stimulation owing to age-related factors
- Decreased sexual activity owing to risk factors

RISK FACTORS

- Myths and misunderstandings
- Social circumstances (e.g., loss of partner)
- Medications (e.g., antihypertensives)
- Relationship problems
- Systemic disease (e.g., diabetes, arthritis)
- Illness of partner
- Environmental factors (e.g., lack of privacy)
- Alcohol

FIGURE 16-1. Sexual function in older adults.

changes, risk factors, and negative functional consequences that affect sexual function.

Nursing Assessment

On a conceptual level, sexual function is viewed as an integral part of a functional assessment of any adult. However, on a practical and personal level, sexual function is most often neglected in an assessment. Even on a conceptual level, sexual function is neglected in most writings about the assessment of older adults. Although an assessment of sexual function is not a necessary component of every nursing assessment, it should be included in any comprehensive functional assessment. It is especially important in settings, such as nursing homes, group homes, and private homes, where care is focused not on acute care issues, but on quality-of-life issues that affect the person's day-to-day function on a long-term basis.

When one considers the high degree of privacy associated with sexual function, it is easy to understand why this aspect of function is neglected in the assessment process. When one adds to that the "sexless senior" stereotype that is prevalent in our society, it is even easier to understand why sexual function is neglected in assessment instruments developed for older adults. If there are gender or generational differences between the health professional and the older person, these differences may create additional barriers to an assessment of sexual function. Although all of these factors may explain why sexual function in older adults is so often overlooked, they do not justify the exclusion of this important aspect of function. Rather, when one considers the potential detrimental consequences of ignoring the sexual needs of older adults and the relatively easy educational interventions that can be initiated to address this quality-of-life issue, an assessment of the sexual function of older adults should be viewed as an essential component of gerontological nursing care.

Nurses' Attitudes About Sexual Function in Older Adults

Because of the private nature of sexual function and the intense emotional responses and cultural factors associated with this topic, nurses are often uncomfortable discussing it. Additional discomfort stems from the fact that many nurses do not learn about sexual function and assessment, especially regarding older adults, in their professional education. If older adults are involved in same-sex or other nontraditional relationships, nurses may experience additional discomfort if they have not first examined their own attitudes about nontraditional relationships. Thus, an assessment of personal attitudes about sexuality and aging is a prerequisite for the gerontological nurse who is addressing the sexual function of older adults. Display 16-1 lists some of the questions nurses can use to examine their attitudes toward the sexual function of older adults. The list includes assessment questions specific to attitudes of nursing staff in long-term care facilities because of the importance of addressing sexual function as a quality-of-life issue and because of the dominant role that nurses play in addressing this issue in long-term care facilities. Also included are questions about the nurse's attitudes toward nontraditional sexual activities, as these attitudes can influence the assessment and care of people who do not conform to the nurse's expectations. Recommendations for assessing the sexual issues of older gays and lesbians emphasize the need to be nonjudgmental and to develop an awareness of gay and lesbian culture. Additional recommendations include the need to understand the importance of relationships for older lesbians and of sexual activity for older gays (Pope, 1997). The goal of examining personal attitudes about the sexual function of older adults is to increase the nurse's level of comfort with, openness to, and sensitivity about issues of sexual function. Information included in the accompanying Culture Box should be incorporated in nurses' communica-

---

DISPLAY 16-1
Assessing Personal Attitudes Toward Sexuality and Aging

What Do I Believe About Sexuality and Aging?

- Do I believe that older people, especially unmarried ones, are no longer interested in or capable of sexual activities?
- Do I believe the subtle messages associating sexual activities with youth and attractiveness?
- Do I hold age-specific standards regarding sexual activity and romantic relationships? (For example, do I think it is OK for young adults to kiss or hold hands, but inappropriate or "cute" for older people to do this?)

What Do I Believe About the Nurse's Role with Regard to the Sexual Function of Older Adults?

- Do I believe that sexual function is strictly a private matter that should not be addressed by health professionals?
- Do I view sexual function as an activity of daily living that should be included in a comprehensive assessment of long-term care needs of older adults?
- Do I feel more comfortable discussing sexual function with people who are of the same gender and age range as myself, but very uncomfortable in discussing this matter with people who are old enough to be my parents or grandparents?
- Do I avoid discussion of sexual function with older adults because I believe they are not interested in sexual activity or are uncomfortable discussing this topic?
- Do I avoid discussing sexual function with older adults who are not in traditional marital relationships?

- Do I hold different beliefs about the assessment of sexual function based on the age of the person? For example, do I think sexual function should be assessed in sexually active teenagers who are at risk for unwanted pregnancy, but not older people?

What Is My Attitude About Various Expressions of Sexual Activity?

- How do I view sexual activity and romantic relationships between unmarried people, or between people of the same gender?
- How do I view masturbation?
- Do my views about masturbation or sexual activity between unmarried or same-gender people influence my assessment of and interventions for people who engage in these activities?
- Am I tolerant and nonjudgmental toward people whose views and practices are nontraditional or different from mine?

For Nurses in Settings Where Long-Term Needs Are Addressed:

- How do I feel about the rights of residents to engage in sexual activity in private, either with themselves or people of their own choosing?
- Do I try to ensure privacy for those residents who desire it?
- If I am aware of the sexual activities of a resident, do I think that I should inform the administrator, a family member, or another "responsible adult"?

---

tions with older adults and in their assessments of sexual function.

Sexual Function in Older Adults

The goals of assessment of sexual function in older adults are: (1) to provide an opportunity for the older adult to address any issues related to sexual function that are important or relevant; and (2) to identify risk factors, particularly attitudinal influences and lack of information, that interfere with the older person's sexual function and quality of life. Although the extent of the assessment will vary according to individual circumstances, the assessment should include, at a minimum, questions about the gyne-

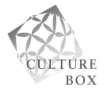

CULTURE
BOX

Cultural Aspects of Sexual Function

Expressions of Sexuality and Intimacy

- In some cultures, direct eye contact, especially between a man and woman, is interpreted as an expression of intimacy.
- In some cultures, it is taboo for a man to be alone with a woman other than his wife.
- Touching another person (particularly of the opposite sex) is considered taboo in many cultures.
- In some cultures, heterosexual men and women commonly hold hands with another person of the same gender.
- Only a few cultures value sexual equality between men and women.
- Homosexuality is accepted in some cultures but is considered taboo or is kept secret among family members in others.

Assessment Considerations

- In some cultures, it is considered taboo for postmenopausal women to have their breasts or vagina examined, even by a health care provider.
- Menopausal manifestations may vary in different cultural groups (e.g., most Japanese women do not experience hot flashes).

cologic aspects of female sexual function and the genitourinary aspects of male sexual function. These questions are easily incorporated into a routine assessment of overall function. If these questions are followed by an open-ended question about sexual interest and activities, the nurse can then respond to the needs of the older adult on an individual basis. If problems or risk factors are identified, the nurse is not expected to conduct an in-depth assessment of all aspects of sexual function, but should obtain enough information to suggest appropriate resources for further evaluation. Display 16-2 summarizes various techniques that may facilitate the assessment interview, and it lists specific assessment questions.

Nursing Diagnosis

When the nursing assessment identifies risks that interfere with sexual function, or when older adults express an interest in discussing their sexual function, the appropriate nursing diagnosis is Altered Sexuality Patterns. This is defined as "the state in which an individual experiences or is at risk of experiencing a change in sexual behaviors or sexual health" (Carpenito, 1997, p. 811). Related factors commonly identified in older adults include medication effects (e.g., from antihypertensive medications); endocrine diseases (e.g., diabetes); cardiovascular diseases (e.g., congestive heart failure); genitourinary conditions (e.g., vaginitis, prostatitis, incontinence); functional impairments secondary to chronic conditions (e.g., limited range of motion as a result of arthritis); psychosocial circumstances (e.g., lack of a partner); and myths and misunderstandings about age-related changes. The case example at the end of this chapter addresses this nursing diagnosis.

Nursing Goals

One nursing goal for older adults with the diagnosis of Altered Sexual Patterns is to address the risk factors that are reversible. Problems with

---

DISPLAY 16-2
Guidelines for Assessing Sexual Function

Interview Atmosphere and Communication Techniques

- Ensure both privacy and comfort.
- Be nonjudgmental and matter-of-fact in verbal and nonverbal communication.
- If feasible, sit face-to-face in chairs, rather than conducting the interview while the person being interviewed is in bed.
- If feasible, allow the person being interviewed to wear usual daytime clothing, rather than a hospital gown.

Initiation and Discussion of the Topic

- Begin by acknowledging feelings of discomfort and by stating the reason for discussing this topic. (For example, "I know that sexuality is a private matter and people are often uncomfortable discussing this topic. However, as a nurse, I consider sexuality to be an aspect of health and well-being, and it may have a significant bearing on your overall care.")
- Include statements that address stereotypes and require a response from the older adult. (For example, "Our society tends to view old people as being uninterested in sex, but for most older people, this is not true. Many older people are less sexually active than when they were younger, but this is not because of age-related changes. "Have you experienced any changes in your sexual activities in the past few years?")
- Initiate the topic near the end of a comprehensive assessment interview, and begin with questions about the physiologic aspects of male or female function, such as those that follow.

Interview Questions to Assess Male Sexual Function

- Have you ever had prostate problems or related surgery? Have you ever been told that you have or had an enlarged prostate?
- How often do you undergo a complete medical examination? When was your last complete physical?

- Do you ever experience dribbling of urine or have problems holding your water?
- Do you have any trouble initiating the stream of urine?
- After you have urinated (passed water), do you still feel like you haven't emptied your bladder completely?
- Do you have to get up during the night to empty your bladder? If so, how many times?
- Have you ever noticed any blood in your urine?
- Do you ever have any discharge from your penis?
- Do you have any sores, lumps, ulcers, irritations, or areas of inflammation on your penis or scrotum?
- Do you have any trouble with erection or ejaculation?

Interview Questions to Assess Female Sexual Function

- How many children, if any, have you had? How many pregnancies?
- At what ages did your menstrual periods begin and end?
- Have you ever had a PAP (Papanicolaou) test? When was your most recent PAP test and gynecologic examination?
- Have you ever had a mammogram? When was the most recent one?
- Have you ever been taught to examine your breasts for lumps?
- Do you examine your breasts for lumps? How often?
- Have you noticed any changes in your breasts? Do you ever have any discharge from your nipples?
- Do you have any burning, itching, or irritation in the vaginal area?
- Do you ever have any vaginal discharge or bleeding?
- Do you have any difficulties with sexual intercourse?

DISPLAY 16-2
Guidelines for Assessing Sexual Function (Continued)

Principles for Assessing Sexual Interest and Activities

- If the older adult makes a clear statement that this topic is irrelevant, do not insist on further questions. If the older adult responds to questions, however, do not discontinue the interview because of your own discomfort.
- Do not assume that an assessment of sexual function is irrelevant to unmarried people.
- For both married and unmarried older adults, use open-ended questions to elicit information about intimate relationships (e.g., "Is there anything you would like to ask or discuss about intimate relationships?").
- For a married person, open-ended questions may be asked about the partner's influence on sexual activities (e.g., "Has your husband experienced any changes in his health that have affected your sexual activities?").
- Listen for statements that reflect myths, a negative self-image, or self-fulfilling prophecies,

such as "Of course, I stopped being interested in sex after menopause," or "I can't have an erection because I have prostate trouble."
- If risk factors, such as certain medications or pathologic conditions, have been identified earlier in the interview, ask additional questions, such as "Have you had any difficulties with sexual activities since your heart attack?" or "Do you have any questions about the possible effects of diabetes on sexual activity?"
- Emphasize the clinical reason for the questions. ("Sometimes certain illnesses or medications interfere with sexual function, and we want to identify any problems you might be having in this area.")
- Use open-ended questions that allow for either closure of the topic or a further discussion of issues. ("Is there anything you would like to discuss with regard to your sexual relationships?")

---

sexual function in older adults often are caused by myths, attitudes, stereotypes, and misinformation. Therefore, the provision of accurate information about sexual function is the primary intervention for achieving this goal. The effects of other risk factors, such as medications and medical conditions, can be diminished or eliminated through the provision of care and counseling by a health professional. An additional goal is to assist older adults in addressing medical or psychogenic causes of problems with sexual function. This is achieved by facilitating referrals to appropriate professional resources (refer to the Educational Resources listed at the end of this chapter).

Maintaining quality of life is another goal that might be addressed, particularly in home care and nursing home settings. This is achieved through staff education and team interventions that address the sexual needs of older adults in

nursing home settings. The following sections discuss health education interventions that can be used by nurses. Also discussed is the role of the nurse in educating older adults about sexual function, because this is not usually considered an essential aspect of nursing care for older adults.

Nursing Interventions

Role of the Nurse in Education About Sexual Function

The role of the nurse in educating older people about sexual function is distinct from that of a primary health care provider or sex therapist; the nurse is not expected to provide direct interventions (other than educational interventions) or sex counseling. Rather, the aim of nursing interventions is to provide information that will debunk myths, clarify misinformation, and change the attitudes of older adults and caregivers. Also, nursing interventions are directed toward facilitating appropriate referrals for further evaluation and treatment of identified problems. Gerontological nurses are not expected to know all the answers about sexual function; however, they are expected to provide accurate information about normal sexual function, age-related changes, risk factors that cause or contribute to problems with sexual function, and resources for dealing with identified problems and risk factors.

Eliminating Risk Factors Through Health Education

Older adults, as well as their caregivers, need to be educated about age-related changes that affect sexual function. This is not always easily accomplished, however, because of strong feelings about this topic being private. Excellent leadership and communication skills are requisites for providing information about sexual function in older adults. Because of the nature of the topic, education may be more effective when delivered in a group setting, rather than on a one-to-one basis. A recent study of the effect of several sex education sessions with older adults showed positive attitudinal changes and improved knowledge, confidence, and sensitivity on the part of group participants (Wiley and Bortz, 1996). A number of articles, including ones by Tunstull and Henry (1996), Boyer and Boyer (1982), Shomaker (1980), and Guarino and Knowlton (1980), provide useful information on nursing models for group education programs on the topic of sexual function in older adults. Recently, the results of a survey sent to men and women aged 50 years or older were published, providing guidelines for discussions between health care providers and older adults with regard to sexual concerns (Johnson, 1997). A major theme of these guidelines is that health care professionals should use open, re-spectful, nonjudgmental, and "plain English" communication to address the sexual concerns of older adults.

Written materials are helpful in providing a basis for education and discussion. Many excellent resources, which can be used by professionals and lay people alike, are available in bookstores and on the Internet. Display 16-3 is a sample of a teaching tool that is written in nontechnical terms so that it can be used for older adults and caregivers as a basis of discussion about sexual function. Table 16-2 also may be used as a basis for a more detailed discussion of age-related changes that affect sexual function in older adults. Displays 16-6 and 16-7, along with the Alternative and Preventive Health Care Practices boxes relating to menopause and loss of libido and erectile dysfunction, can be used as a basis for discussing with older adults the topics of menopause, erectile dysfunction, hormonal replacement therapy, and loss of libido. Gerontological nurses can use these educational materials to encourage older women and men to seek further advice about these conditions from their primary care provider or other appropriate health care professional.

Addressing Risk Factors Related to Medication/Chemical Effects and Pathologic Conditions

In addition to providing education aimed at correcting myths and changing attitudes, the nurse must also provide information that can help to eliminate or minimize the effects of medication/chemical use or pathologic conditions on sexual function. When such risk factors are identified, the nurse must decide whether to inform the older adult about the potential causal relationship between the medication/chemical or pathologic condition and sexual dysfunction. Table 16-1 can be used to identify some of the medications and chemicals that can interface with sexual function. In the absence of any reported sex-

---

DISPLAY 16-3
Fact Sheet on Sexual Function for Older People

- Older people remain fully capable of enjoying orgasm, but their response to sexual stimulation usually is slower, less intense, and of shorter duration. Increasing the amount and diversity of sexual stimulation and experimenting with different positions can compensate for these changes and increase sexual enjoyment.
- The "use it or lose it" principle applies to sexual activity.
- Sexual problems in older people occur for the same reasons they occur in younger people. That is, they may be related to illness or disability, medications or alcohol, or psychological and relationship factors. The only cause of sexual problems that is unique to older people is the self-fulfilling prophecy of the "sexless senior" stereotype.
- The following habits enhance sexual enjoyment: exercising regularly, avoiding or limiting consumption of alcohol, maintaining optimal health and nutrition, using hearing aids and corrective lenses as needed, and engaging in sexual activities when you are relaxed and your energy level is at its peak.
- If you experience problems with sexual function, seek advice from a professional who is skilled in working with older people. Medical help can be obtained from a urologist, gynecologist, or other medical specialist. If there is no medical basis for the problem, a sex therapist or marriage counselor might be helpful.

Facts Specific to Older Men

- Periodic difficulties with erection and ejaculation do not necessarily indicate that you are impotent.

- After you've reached orgasm, it may be 1 or 2 days before you are able to reach full orgasm again.
- Many new treatment options are available for treating erectile dysfunction (impotence). If your health care provider cannot provide up-to-date information about these options, ask for a referral for an appropriate evaluation and discussion of various options.

Facts Specific to Older Women

- Using a water-soluble lubricant will compensate for decreased vaginal lubrication. Do NOT use petroleum jelly, as it is not a very effective lubricant for this purpose and it can predispose you to infection.
- Estrogen is beneficial in preventing some problems with sexual function, but the relative risks and benefits of such therapy should be considered and discussed thoroughly with your primary care provider.
- You may have vaginal irritation or urinary tract infections, especially after sexual intercourse, because of age-related thinning of the vaginal wall. Such problems may be avoided by the following interventions:

1. Drink plenty of fluids.
2. Use an estrogen cream or vaginal lubricant.
3. Maintain good hygiene in the vaginal area.
4. If you have a male partner, have him thrust his penis downward, toward the back of your vagina.
5. Empty your bladder before and after intercourse.

---

ual dysfunction, sharing of this information may prove to be detrimental because introduction of the topic may have the effect of a self-fulfilling prophecy. If, however, the older adult has acknowledged a problem with sexual function and also has a pathologic condition, takes a medication, or uses a chemical substance that might be a contributing factor, the nurse can educate the older adult about the potential relationship between the two, as discussed in the section on Adverse Medication and Chemical Effects. This is especially important when the nurse has identified pertinent risk factors, but the older adult attributes sexual dysfunction to old age.

ALTERNATIVE
AND
PREVENTIVE
HEALTH
CARE
PRACTICES

Preventing or Alleviating Loss of Libido and Erectile Dysfunction

Herbs
- Aphrodisiacs: anise, ginseng, fennel, cardamom, ashwaganda, fava bean, dong quai, yohimbe (use yohimbe only under professional supervision)
- For erectile dysfunction: ginkgo biloba, fava bean

Homeopathic Remedies
- For inhibited sexual desire: ignatia, pulsatilla, natrum muriaticum
- For erectile dysfunction: conium, caladium, lycopodium, agnus castus, argentum nitricum

Nutritional Considerations
- Foods: soy beans, fava beans
- Zinc and vitamins A and E

Preventive Measures and Additional Approaches
- Yoga, massage, imagery, relaxation, meditation, polarity, reflexology
- Aromatherapy: rose, ginger, jasmine, cinnamon, clary sage, ylang ylang

Education about these risk factors requires a high degree of tact, caution, sensitivity, and good judgment. In conjunction with educating the older adult about the potential relationship between risk factors and problems with sexual function, the nurse should assist the older adult in obtaining the appropriate professional consultations for assessment and treatment. A complete medical evaluation by a primary care provider who is knowledgeable about the sexual problems of older adults is usually the best starting point. After any medical problems have been satisfactorily addressed, the older adult may be referred to a mental health professional for counseling if problems with sexual function persist. Also, the alternative and preventive health care practices summarized in the box on this page may be appropriate once interventions have been addressed.

Sexual Function and Arthritis

Arthritis is one of the most common pathologic conditions affecting older adults, and it is often self-managed with little or no medical supervision. Often, the symptoms are not severe enough

to motivate the older adult to seek medical evaluation and treatment, but they may be severe enough to interfere with sexual activities. In such cases, the nurse may be the health professional most likely to address the sexual problems that may be caused by the pain, fatigue, and joint limitations associated with arthritis. Simple interventions may be effective in improving the quality of sexual activities for the older adult with arthritis, and education about these interventions can be provided by the nurse. Pamphlets about arthritis and sexual activity are available from local chapters of the Arthritis Foundation. In addition, Display 16-4 can be used as a teaching tool regarding sexual activity for the older adult who has arthritis.

Sexual Function and Cardiac Disease

One of the pathologic conditions often associated with sexual dysfunction is coronary artery disease, especially in those who have had myocardial infarctions or who have undergone coronary artery bypass surgery. It has become increasingly common for nurses to include information about sexual function in individual

---

DISPLAY 16-4
Tips on Sexual Activity for the Person with Arthritis

The pain, fatigue, and joint limitations of arthritis may interfere with, but do not have to curtail, your enjoyment of sexual activity. In fact, sexual activity can be beneficial to you because it stimulates the release of cortisone, adrenalin, and other chemicals that are natural pain relievers. The following actions may enhance your sexual enjoyment and minimize the effects of arthritis:

- Engage in sexual activity when you feel least fatigued and most relaxed.
- Use analgesic medications and other methods of pain relief before engaging in sexual activity.

- Use relaxation techniques before engaging in sexual activity. Relaxation techniques that may be helpful for arthritis include warm baths or showers and the application of hot packs to the affected joints.
- Maintain optimal health through good nutrition and a proper balance of rest and activity.
- Experiment with different sexual positions and use pillows for comfort and support.
- Increase the time spent in foreplay.
- Use a vibrator if your ability to massage is limited by arthritis.
- Use a water-soluble jelly for vaginal lubrication.

---

and group educational programs designed for patients with cardiac disease. However, this information may not have been provided to older adults who sustained myocardial infarctions before the 1980s. Likewise, even in this decade, information may not have been provided if the nurse believed that it was irrelevant because of old age or if the older adult was reluctant to discuss the topic. It is not unusual, therefore, for a gerontological nurse to care for an older adult who has long-standing problems with sexual function arising from fears related to cardiac illness. Moreover, these older adults may never have discussed their problems with a health professional. In these situations, the nurse can present the general guidelines outlined in Display 16-5 and encourage the older adult to discuss his or her concerns with a primary care provider.

DISPLAY 16-5
Tips on Sexual Activity for the Person with Cardiac Disease

- Participation in a medically supervised exercise program can reduce oxygen requirements during sexual activity and improve the quality of your sex life.
- The typical energy expenditure for sexual intercourse is equivalent to that used for climbing two flights of steps.
- Do not engage in sexual activity in extremely hot and humid environments.
- Wait 3 hours after consuming alcohol or a large meal before initiating sexual activity.
- Engage in sexual activity when your energy is at its peak and you are feeling rested and relaxed.

- Avoid sexual activity during times of intense emotional stress.
- Avoid engaging in sexual activity with a partner with whom you are uncomfortable (e.g., an extramarital partner).
- Experiment with different positions to find one that is least demanding of your energy.
- Consider using nitroglycerin, if ordered by your primary care provider, as needed before sexual activity.
- Consult your primary care provider if you experience chest pain during or after sexual activity, or breathlessness or heart palpitations persisting for 15 minutes after orgasm.

Hormonal Replacement Therapy for Women

For many years, synthetic estrogen has been widely prescribed in the United States for menopausal and postmenopausal women. For decades, hormonal replacement therapy (HRT) was viewed as a safe and effective way of alleviating hot flashes, vaginal atrophy, and other manifestations of menopause that interfered with comfort, sexual function, and quality of life. During the 1970s, however, studies began showing an association between estrogen and breast and uterine cancers, and many questions were raised about the risk-to-benefit ratio of HRT. Around the same time, studies also revealed that estrogen was effective in preventing osteoporosis-related fractures in postmenopausal women. By the 1980s, studies were indicating that HRT had far-reaching benefits and might even reduce mortality, prevent skin aging, and decrease the incidence of depression, memory loss, and cardiovascular disease. At the same time, still other studies raised further questions about the increased incidence of endometrial cancer and hyperplasia; these studies suggested that the cyclic administration of estrogen and progestin could reduce or eliminate such risks.

During the 1990s, there has been increasing consensus about the benefits of HRT with regard to preventing heart disease, osteoporosis, and fractures. There also has been increasing evidence that estrogen may be beneficial in reducing the risk of developing Alzheimer's disease. The controversy about whether the risk of breast cancer is increased with HRT persists, with various studies showing increased risk, decreased risk, or no difference in risk. Much of the controversy about the findings centers around the length of time that HRT is used, and researchers are awaiting results of well-controlled, long-term studies that can address this issue. Consideration is being given to the duration of and time frame for HRT, with some researchers suggesting that women should wait until 60 years of age or older to start HRT, or

that the duration of therapy be limited to 5 to 10 years. These variable recommendations and findings have made decisions about HRT very complex. Research studies are also being developed to answer questions about different doses and combinations of estrogen and progesterone. Adding to the confusion and complexity are recent questions about natural versus synthetic forms of hormones, and about the influence of testosterone, which is already included in some regimens of HRT.

Because of these controversies, and the growing trend toward public awareness about health-related issues, women are taking a more active role in decisions regarding HRT. In making these decisions, women are likely to consult nurses for opinions, information, and clarification of information already obtained. Thus, it is important that nurses be knowledgeable about these issues so that they can provide accurate, complete, and objective information. Women need to understand that decisions about HRT are highly individualized and should be made only after careful consideration by the woman and her health care practitioner. Display 16-6 summarizes considerations regarding HRT. Because HRT is currently being subjected to intense investigation, nurses should keep abreast of the latest knowledge and research results by frequently reviewing reliable sources of information. In addition to considering the use of HRT, menopausal women may also wish to consider the use of various alternative and preventive health care practices, as summarized in the box on page 468.

Addressing Erectile Dysfunction

Before the mid-1990s, erectile dysfunction was viewed as a relatively inevitable and untreatable condition of older adulthood, but the recent development of diverse types of interventions has changed this picture. In 1998, approval by the Food and Drug Administration (FDA) of the first oral medication for erectile dysfunction (sil-

DISPLAY 16-6
Considerations Regarding Hormonal Replacement Therapy (HRT)

Known and Potential Benefits of HRT

- HRT has beneficial effects in preventing fractures, osteoporosis, and heart disease.
- HRT has been found to reduce overall mortality rates.
- HRT may be beneficial in reducing the probability of developing Alzheimer's disease.
- HRT may be beneficial in reducing the risk of tooth loss.
- HRT may be beneficial in preventing and treating depression.
- For most menopausal women, HRT alleviates hot flashes, urethritis and associated infections, and vaginal dryness and associated vaginitis and dyspareunia (painful sexual intercourse).

Known and Potential Adverse Effects of HRT

- Studies have revealed an increased incidence of endometrial hyperplasia and cancer associated with estrogen use. The risk of endometrial hyperplasia and cancer, however, may be eliminated or greatly reduced with the addition of progestin.
- If endometrial cancer develops from HRT, the 5-year survival rate is 95%.
- The potential association between estrogen and breast cancer is under intense scrutiny, and results of various studies are controversial. The evidence thus far is weighing in the direction of little or no increase in the risk of breast cancer.
- Women with known or suspected breast cancer, or a personal or family history of the disease, should not take estrogen.
- Additional contraindications to HRT include endometriosis, thrombophlebitis, liver impairment, migraine headaches, neuro-ophthalmologic disease, estrogen-dependent cancer, heavy cigarette smoking, undiagnosed vaginal bleeding, and a history of endometrial cancer.
- The adverse effects of estrogen or estrogen-progestin combinations include edema, headache, depression, weight gain, withdrawal bleeding, and breast fullness and tenderness.

Duration and Methods of Estrogen Administration

- The dose of hormones should be the lowest possible dose that will produce the desired effect.
- The duration of therapy should be considered in relation to the risks and benefits. For example, if the primary reason for HRT is to alleviate hot flashes, treatment can be discontinued to evaluate the presence or absence of hot flashes, which usually disappear naturally within 5 years. If the primary purpose is for prevention of osteoporosis in a woman who is at high risk for fractures, then lifelong therapy may be required, because bone loss will resume as soon as the estrogen is discontinued.
- A variety of hormonal products are available (including oral, vaginal, transdermal, natural, and synthetic forms). Each product has advantages and disadvantages.
- HRT can be administered cyclically or continuously, with each regimen having both advantages and disadvantages.
- Women should discuss the various options of HRT with their primary care provider to identify the best dosing regimen and form of medication.
- The form, regimen, and duration of therapy should be reviewed at least annually, with consideration of up-to-date information about new products and the risks and benefits of HRT.

denafil) simplified the treatment of this disorder and stimulated much public debate and attention. At the time, additional oral or sublingual medications for erectile dysfunction were expected to be approved by the FDA in 1999, and pharmaceutical companies were exploring the use of oral medications for sexual dysfunctions in both men and women. Erectile dysfunction

ALTERNATIVE
AND
PREVENTIVE
HEALTH
CARE
PRACTICES

Alleviating the Effects of Menopause

Herbs
- Sage, ginseng, fenugreek, motherwort, chaste tree, dong quai, black cohosh

Homeopathic Remedies
- Sepia, sulphur, lachesis, pulsatilla, natrum muriaticum, amyl nitrosum
- Bryonia (to increase vaginal lubrication)

Nutritional Considerations
- High intake of foods high in plant estrogens: beans, nuts, seeds, corn, dates, wheat, apples, carrots, celery, whole grains, soy products
- High intake of foods rich in boron (to increase estrogen retention): beans, peaches, prunes, cabbage, broccoli, tomatoes, strawberries, asparagus
- Avoidance of foods that stimulate the adrenal glands: salt, sugar, caffeine, alcohol, refined carbohydrates
- Vitamins and minerals: zinc, chromium, magnesium, selenium, vitamin B-complex, and vitamins C, D, and E

Preventive Measures and Additional Approaches
- Yoga, music, massage, imagery, relaxation, meditation, reflexology, therapeutic touch
- Aromatherapy: rose, fennel, lavender, chamomile, sandalwood, geranium, clary sage
- Natural progesterone: capsules, skin cream, wild yam
- Acupuncture (to balance the hormonal system)
- Ice water compresses on the neck and chest for 3 minutes (to alleviate hot flash symptoms)

is now viewed as a common but very treatable condition that should be addressed by health care professionals.

The primary responsibility of the gerontological nurse is to keep up-to-date on the types of interventions that are available and to educate older men about the importance of seeking help for erectile dysfunction. Display 16-7 summarizes some of the most commonly used treatment options, which include penile prostheses and medications administered by a variety of methods. Decisions about appropriate treatment options must be based on a comprehensive evaluation by a urologist or a primary care provider who is knowledgeable about erectile dysfunction. Nurses can use the information in Display

16-7 to provide health education about medical options that were available for the treatment of erectile dysfunction as of 1998.

Surgical procedures, which are used less commonly, include penile implants and vascular surgery. Implants, or penile prostheses, are concealed inside the body and require manipulation before and after intercourse to control erection. Although this intervention is the most invasive, it is the only intervention that is permanent. Vascular surgery to restore normal circulation to the penis is appropriate only when the blood flow is blocked. Psychotherapy and behavioral therapy may be used as primary or adjunctive treatment options to address the psychosocial issues that may be contributing to erectile dys-

DISPLAY 16-7
Medical Treatments for Erectile Dysfunction Available in 1998

Type of Intervention	Mode of Action	Comment
Vacuum erection devices	A vacuum is created around the penis, using an airtight plastic cylinder. A constriction band is then placed around the base of the penis to retain the erection, after which the cylinder is removed.	Requires a high degree of manual dexterity; is intrusive and cumbersome; may cause ejaculatory discomfort; very safe.
Intracavernosal injection of vasoactive drugs	Self-injection of a medication into the erectile tissue; causes vasodilation and relaxation of the smooth muscles of the penis.	Use must be limited to twice weekly. Adverse effects include priapism, bruising, and local pain.
Transurethral alprostadil (prostaglandin) administration	A plastic applicator containing a micro-suppository of alprostadil is inserted into the urethra, where the medication is released.	Can be used twice daily; adverse effects include hypotension and a temporary burning sensation in the urethra.
Yohimbine (sometimes combined with trazadone)	A traditional African aphrodisiac that increases sympathetic outflow.	Low success rate; adverse effects include nausea, insomnia, nervousness, dizziness, and hypertension.
Testosterone replacement therapy	Oral, sublingual, or injectable preparations, or scrotal or transdermal patches, may be effective for the small number of men who have testosterone deficiency.	May worsen prostate problems or trigger prostate cancer.
Topical medications (e.g., herbal combinations, vasodilators)	May assist in enhancing erection but not approved by the FDA for this purpose.	Vasodilators should not be used by people with cardiovascular disease.
Oral medications (e.g., sildenafil)	Increases blood flow to the penis.	Cannot be used by men who are taking any nitrate medication. Adverse effects include headache, indigestion, and facial flushing.

function. Pelvic muscle exercises, commonly performed as a treatment for urinary incontinence, may also be useful in the treatment of erectile dysfunction. The technique for performing these exercises is discussed in Chapter 9. If medications are causing or contributing to erectile dysfunction, the primary care provider should consider alternative medications or reduced doses if medically feasible. For example, people with hypertension are less likely to have sexual dysfunction when treated with calcium channel blockers, angiotensin-converting enzyme inhibitors, or peripheral alpha-receptor blockers (Stern, 1997).

Maintaining Quality of Life in Long-Term Care Facilities

In addressing the sexual needs of older adults, the responsibilities of nurses in long-term care facilities differ from those of nurses in acute care or home settings in the following ways:

1. Because of the intense medical needs of patients in acute care settings, sexual needs are often irrelevant or have a very low priority.
2. Because of the short duration of stay in acute care settings, it is not necessary to address the long-term sexual needs of patients.
3. Because people in their own homes have a high degree of privacy and autonomy in meeting their personal needs, a nurse who provides home care does not routinely have to be concerned about sexual needs.

In contrast to these situations, residents of long-term care facilities generally are not acutely ill, are planning to stay in the facility for a long time, and depend on the nursing staff for ensuring the privacy necessary to meet their personal needs. Thus, the nurse in long-term care facilities must address the sexual needs of residents as an integral part of the overall care plan.

Because many of the barriers to meeting the sexual needs of older adults in long-term care facilities are based on myths and attitudes of the staff, education of the staff is the most effective starting point for addressing these issues. Studies of the effects of sex education programs on older adults, nursing home staff, and adult family members of older adults have documented a positive impact of such programs on the sexual attitudes and knowledge of all three groups of subjects (White and Catania, 1982; Hillman and Stricker, 1994; Tunstull and Henry, 1996). Additional benefits for the older adults involved included an increase in the perceived importance of sexual feelings and a reported increase in the frequency of sexual activity.

Education of staff members in long-term care facilities can be accomplished through in-service programs that address issues related to various aspects of sexual function, including the lifelong interest in and need for sexual activity and intimate relationships. Audiovisual materials can be used to stimulate discussion about the unique aspects of meeting sexual needs in institutional settings and about the responsibilities and limitations of staff. When staff express concerns about the ability of a cognitively impaired resident to give informed consent, a model for assessing competence to participate in an intimate relationship may be used. An example of such a model is discussed by Lichtenberg (1997) and can be used by an interdisciplinary team.

Emphasis should be placed on the rights of residents, as defined by the federal government in the Residents' Rights Bill (Health Care Financing Administration, 1980). Specific rights pertaining to the sexual needs of residents of long-term care facilities include: (1) the right to private visits with a spouse and the right to share a room with a spouse unless medically contraindicated; as well as (2) the right to associate, communicate, and meet privately with people of their choice, unless this infringes on the rights of another resident. The effectiveness of in-service programs may be enhanced if social service and administrative staff members are included as planners and participants. Presenters and discussion leaders should be nonjudgmental and matter-of-fact in their approach so as to provide the staff with an appropriate role model for addressing this sensitive topic.

In addition to educating staff members about the sexual needs and rights of residents, direct actions must be taken to ensure privacy for those residents who desire it. If a resident does not have a private room, efforts must be made to provide privacy, while still respecting the rights of any roommates. Sometimes, the role of the nurse will be that of a negotiator, assisting residents in reaching mutually acceptable agreements about privacy and shared space.

Evaluating Nursing Care

Nursing care for older adults with the diagnosis of Altered Sexuality Patterns is evaluated by the degree to which risk factors are eliminated, particularly through the provision of accurate information. For example, older adults may verbalize an improved understanding of the age-related changes that affect response to sexual stimulation. In turn, this information can alleviate anxiety about sexual performance and may improve the older adult's quality of life. Interventions to alleviate risk factors, such as medical conditions or adverse medication/chemical effects, would be judged to be successful if the older adult follows through with a referral to an appropriate resource. One measure of successful intervention in nursing home settings would be that staff members increase their understanding of the sexual needs of older adults and are more comfortable allowing appropriate means of sexual expression by the residents.

Chapter Summary

Age-related changes do not interfere with the ability of older adults to pursue and maintain satisfying sexual activities and relationships. Risk factors commonly interfere with sexual expression, but most of these risk factors can be addressed or alleviated. Myths and lack of knowledge about age-related changes and risk factors that influence sexual function are important risk factors that can be alleviated through educational interventions. Risk factors that cannot be alleviated, such as medical conditions or social circumstances, may be addressed through referrals for further evaluation or counseling.

Nursing assessment is directed toward identi-fying the concerns that older adults have about their sexual function. Nursing assessment also aims to identify any risk factors that interfere with an older adult's sexual function and quality of life. Assessment of sexual function is particularly important in home and long-term care settings, where nursing care is focused on quality-of-life issues that affect the older adult's daily life. Because nurses usually are not well prepared to assess sexual function, it is helpful for them to begin with a self-assessment of their personal attitudes toward sexual function in older adults.

Altered Sexuality Patterns is an appropriate nursing diagnosis for older adults who express concerns about, or who have risk factors that interfere with, their sexual function. Nursing goals are to improve or maintain the older adult's quality of life and to address or alleviate any risk factors. These goals are achieved through educational interventions and referrals for counseling or further evaluation. Nursing care is evaluated according to the degree to which the older adult increases his or her knowledge about age-related changes and risk factors that influence sexual function. Another measure of successful interventions would be that the older adult expresses improved satisfaction with sexual activities and relationships.

Critical Thinking Exercises

1. Describe the attitudinal risk factors, on the parts of society, older adults, and health care providers, that can interfere with healthy sexual function in older adults.
2. Summarize the functional consequences that are likely to affect sexual function in healthy older men and women.
3. What are the responsibilities of nurses in each of the following settings with regard to assessment of sexual function in older adults: community setting, acute care facility, and long-term care facility?

4. Describe the assessment and health education approaches you might use for a 73-year-old married man who confides that he has difficulty making his wife "happy in bed."

5. Spend a few minutes answering all the questions included in Display 16-1, "Assessment of Personal Attitudes Toward Sexuality and Aging." What did you learn about yourself?

Case Example and Nursing Care Plan

Pertinent Case Information

Mr. and Mrs. S. come regularly to your nursing clinic in the assisted living facility where they live. Mr. S. is 73 years old and has a history of hypertension and a history of myocardial infarction. He takes clonidine, 0.3 mg q.d., and digoxin, 0.125 mg q.d. Mrs. S., who is 71 years old, describes herself as generally healthy, but with osteoporosis and some arthritis. She states, "I have to live with old Arthur, who keeps my knees stiff and sometimes is a pain in the hip." She takes ibuprofen, 400 mg q.i.d., premarin, 0.625 mg q.d., and provera, 2.5 mg q.d.

Mr. and Mrs. S. moved to the facility because they needed help with transportation and they wanted to live in a place where they had fewer responsibilities and more time to enjoy life. During one of their appointments, Mrs. S. becomes tearful and says she has been disappointed in their move from their own home. She says, "Now we have the time to enjoy our life together, but we seem to be in each other's way all the time. When we lived in our own home we were so busy with the yard and the housekeeping and all the daily chores, we never had time to think about what we enjoy together. Now I don't have to cook meals and worry about getting to the grocery store, but we aren't enjoying the time we have together."

Nursing Assessment

On further discussion, Mrs. S. acknowledges that she has talked with her husband about having more "intimate time and resuming sexual activities that have petered out in the past few years because we were always so tired and never seemed to have much time." In reply, Mr. S. has stated that "We're probably too old to do those things, and old people shouldn't expect to have the fun we used to have." Mrs. S. says she used to believe that, but recently she's been talking with some of the other women in the assisted living facility who seem to be enjoying sexual activities. Mr. and Mrs. S. relate that they had a good sexual relationship until Mr. S.'s heart attack 5 years ago. After that, he lost interest in sexual activities, even though he was told he could resume all his usual activities except for very strenuous activity, such as shoveling snow. Mrs. S. says she masturbates occasionally, but she doesn't find that very satisfying. She says she has no problems with vaginal dryness or infections because she takes hormones. Mrs. S. expresses concern about being comfortable in the sexual position they used previously because her arthritis has gotten worse in the past few years.

Nursing Diagnosis

You address Altered Sexuality Patterns as your nursing diagnosis for Mr. and Mrs. S. Related factors include myths and lack of information about the age-related changes and risk factors that influence sexual function. Potential risk factors that you identify are Mr. S.'s medications and his lack of information about post–heart attack sexual function.

Goals	Nursing Interventions	Evaluation Criteria
To increase Mr. and Mrs. S.'s knowledge about age-related changes and risk factors that affect sexual function	Use Display 16-3 as a basis for discussion of sexual function in later adulthood.	Mr. and Mrs. S. will verbalize correct information about sexual function in older adulthood.
To address the risk factors associated with Mr. S.'s heart attack and medication regimen	Explain that many medications for heart problems and high blood pressure are associated with problems with sexual function. Use Display 16-5 as a basis for discussing sexual activity as it relates to people with heart problems. Encourage Mr. S. to talk with his primary care provider about his medication regimen and about his heart condition. Suggest that he inquire whether an alternative medication would effectively treat his high blood pressure without interfering with sexual function.	Mr. S. will agree to talk with his primary care provider about the potential relationship between his medications and heart condition and his lack of sexual activity.
To address the risk factors associated with Mrs. S.'s arthritis	Use Display 16-4 to discuss sexual activity as it relates to people with arthritis.	Mrs. S. will identify ways to increase her comfort during sexual activities.

Educational Resources

American Association of Sex Educators, Counselors and Therapists
P.O. Box 238, Mount Vernon, IA 52314–0238
www.aasect.org
• Referral list of certified sex counselors and sex therapists arranged by state (Send a self-addressed stamped envelope.)

American Menopause Foundation, Inc.
350 Fifth Avenue, Suite 2822, New York, NY 10118
(212) 714–2398

North American Menopause Society
P.O. Box 94527, Cleveland, OH 44101
(216) 844–8748
www.menopause.org

Pride Senior Network
1756 Broadway, Suite 11H, New York, NY 10019
(212) 757–3203
www.pridesenior.org

Senior Action in a Gay Environment (SAGE)
305 Seventh Avenue, 16th Floor, New York, NY 10001
(212) 741–2247

Sexuality Information and Education Council of the United States
130 West 42nd Street, Suite 350, New York, NY 10036–7802
(212) 819–9770
www.siecus.org

References

Boyer, G., & Boyer, J. (1982). Sexuality and aging. *Nursing Clinics of North America, 17,* 421–427.

Brecher, E. M. (1984). *Love, sex, and aging: A Consumers Union report.* Boston: Little, Brown & Company.

Bretschneider, J. G., & McCoy, N. L. (1988). Sexual interest and behavior in healthy 80- to 102-year-olds. *Archives of Sexual Behavior, 17,* 109–129.

Brody, J. E. (1983, September 28). Drugs can be bad medicine for lover. *New York Times,* p. III, 1:1.

Burnett, A. L. (1998). Erectile dysfunction: A practical approach for primary care. *Geriatrics, 53*(2), 34–48.

Carpenito, L. J. (1997). *Nursing diagnosis: Application to clinical practice* (7th ed.). Philadelphia: J. B. Lippincott.

Covey, H. C. (1989). Perceptions and attitudes toward sexuality of the elderly during the middle ages. *The Gerontologist, 29*(1), 93–100.

Cutler, S. J. (1985). Ageing and attitudes about sexual morality. *Ageing and Society, 5,* 161–173.

Godschalk, M. F., Sison, A., & Mulligan, T. (1997). Management of erectile dysfunction by the geriatrician. *Journal of the American Geriatrics Society, 45,* 1240–1246.

Guarino, S. C., & Knowlton, C. N. (1980). Planning and implementing a group health program on sexuality for the elderly. *Journal of Gerontological Nursing, 10,* 600–603.

Health Care Financing Administration (1980, July 1). Rule 5101:3-3-08. Residents' rights in long-term care facilities. Washington, DC: U.S. Government Printing Office.

Hillman, J. L., & Stricker, G. (1994). A linkage of knowledge and attitudes toward elderly sexuality: Not necessarily a uniform relationship. *The Gerontologist, 34*(2), 256–260.

Jenike, M. A. (1997). Managing sexual side effects of psychotropic drugs. *Journal of Geriatric Psychiatry and Neurology, 10,* 131–132.

Johnson, B. (1997). Older adults' suggestions for health care providers regarding discussions of sex. *Geriatric Nursing, 18*(2), 65–66.

Johnson, B. K. (1996). Older adults and sexuality: A multidimensional perspective. *Journal of Gerontological Nursing, 22*(2), 6–15.

Keil, J. E., Sutherland, S. E., Knapp, R. G., Waid, L. R., & Gazes, P. C. (1992). Self-reported sexual functioning in elderly Blacks and Whites. *Journal of Aging and Health, 4*(1), 112–125.

Kinsey, A. C., Pomeroy, W. B., & Martin, C. E. (1948). *Sexual behavior in the human male.* Philadelphia: W. B. Saunders.

Kinsey, A. C., Pomeroy, W. B., & Martin, C. E. (1953). *Sexual behavior in the human female.* Philadelphia: W. B. Saunders.

Lichtenberg, P. A. (1997). Clinical perspectives on sexual issues in nursing homes. *Topics in Geriatric Rehabilitation, 12*(4), 1–10.

Masters, W. H., & Johnson, V. E. (1966). *Human sexual response.* Boston: Little, Brown & Company.

Matthias, R. E., Lubben, J. E., Atchison, K. A., & Schweitzer, S. O. (1997). Sexual activity and satisfaction among very old adults: Results from a community-dwelling Medicare population survey. *The Gerontologist, 37*(1), 6–14.

Morley, J. E. (1991). Endocrine factors in geriatric sexuality. *Clinics in Geriatric Medicine, 7*(1), 85–92.

Muller, J. E., Mittleman, M. A., Maclure, M., Sherwood, J. B., & Tofler, G. H. (1996). Triggering myocardial infarction by sexual activity. *Journal of the American Medical Association, 275,* 1405–1409.

Mulligan, T., & Katz, P. G. (1988). Erectile failure in the aged: Evaluation and treatment. *Journal of the American Geriatrics Society, 36,* 54–62.

Mulligan, T., Retchin, S. M., Chinchilli, V. M., & Bettinger, C. B. (1988). The role of aging and chronic disease in sexual dysfunction. *Journal of the American Geriatrics Society, 36,* 520–524.

National Institutes of Health, Consensus Statement (1992, December 7–9). *Impotence, 10*(4). Washington, DC: National Institutes of Health.

Nieschlag, E., Lammers, U., Freischem, C. W., Langer, K., & Wickings, E. J. (1982). Reproductive functions in young fathers and grandfathers. *Journal of Clinical Endocrinology and Metabolism, 55,* 676–681.

Pope, M. (1997). Sexual issues for older lesbians and gays. *Topics in Geriatric Rehabilitation, 12*(4), 53–60.

Quam, J. K., & Whitford, G. S. (1992). Adaptation and age-related expectations of older gay and lesbian adults. *The Gerontologist, 32*(3), 367–374.

Salcido, R. (1997). New remedies for an old problem? *Topics in Geriatric Rehabilitation, 12*(4), 86–89.

Schlesinger, B. (1983). Institutional life: The Canadian experience. In R. B. Weg (Ed.), *Sexuality in the later years: Roles and behavior.* New York: Academic Press.

Shomaker, D. M. (1980). Integration of physiological and sociocultural factors as a basis for sex education to the elderly. *Journal of Gerontological Nursing, 10,* 311–318.

Slag, M., Morley, J. E., Elson, M. K., Trence, D. L., Nelson, C. J., Nelson, A. E., Kinlaw, W. B., Beyer, H. S., Nuttall, F. Q., & Shafer, R. B. (1983). Impotence in medical clinic outpatients. *Journal of the American Medical Association, 249*, 1736–1740.

Slusher, M. P., Mayer, C. J., & Dunkle, R. E. (1996). Gays and lesbians older and wiser (GLOW): A support group for older gay people. *The Gerontologist, 36*(1), 118–123.

Stern, M. F. (1997). Erectile dysfunction in older men. *Topics in Geriatric Rehabilitation, 12*(4), 40–52.

Stimson, A., Wase, J. F., & Stimson, J. (1981). Sexuality and self-esteem among the aged. *Research on Aging, 3*, 228–239.

Tunstull, P., & Henry, M. E. (1996). Approaches to resident sexuality. *Journal of Gerontological Nursing, 22*(6), 37–42.

United States Bureau of the Census. (1996). *Projections of the population of the United States, by age, and sex: 1995 to 2050.* Washington, DC: U.S. Bureau of the Census.

Virag, R., Bouilly, P., & Frydman, D. (1985). Is impotence an arterial disorder? *Lancet, 1*, 181–184.

White, C. B. (1982). Sexual interest, attitudes, knowledge, and sexual history in relation to sexual behavior in the institutionalized aged. *Archives of Sexual Behavior, 11*, 11–21.

White, C. B., & Catania, J. A. (1982). Psychoeducational intervention for sexuality with the aged, family members of the aged, and people who work with the aged. *International Journal of Aging and Human Development, 15*(2), 121–138.

Wiley, D., & Bortz, W. M. (1996). Sexuality and aging—Usual and successful. *Journal of Gerontology: Medical Sciences, 51A*(3), M142–M146.

Winn, R. L., & Newton, N. (1982). Sexuality in aging: A study of 106 cultures. *Archives of Sexual Behavior, 11*, 283–298.

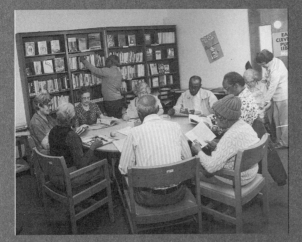

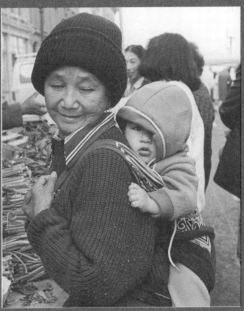

Multidimensional Aspects of Care

Overall Functional Assessment

Chapter

17

The intent of this chapter is to provide guidelines for an assessment of the older adult's ability to perform activities of daily living (ADL) and instrumental activities of daily living (IADL). As such, its format is similar to that of Chapter 5 (Psychosocial Assessment). That is, it does not address the age-related changes, risk factors, functional consequences, or interven-

tions specific to one area of function. Rather, it provides a basis for assessing the physiologic aspects of function in older adults and is meant to be used as a guide for assessing ADL and IADL. This chapter can be used with Chapter 5 as a basis for a comprehensive assessment of all aspects of psychosocial and physiologic function of older adults. The aspects of physiologic function that are discussed in Parts 3 and 4 of this text are outlined in Appendix A, at the end of this book.

Functional Assessment

The concept of functional assessment, which is central to the functional consequences theory of gerontological nursing, is used consistently in this text to address specific aspects of physiologic and psychosocial function. Although the concept is thoroughly discussed throughout this text as it applies to specific aspects of function, the term "functional assessment" is generally used in a more restrictive sense to refer to the measurement of a person's ability to fulfill responsibilities and perform tasks for self-care. In this chapter, the concept is discussed from a historical perspective as it has been used by health care professionals, with particular emphasis on the recent application of functional assessment to older adults. In addition, a model for a nursing functional assessment of ADL and IADL is presented. Several sections of Chapter 2 present a further explanation of the concept of functional assessment as it relates to the functional consequences theory of gerontological nursing.

History of and Current Trends in Functional Assessment

The concept of functional assessment was first used in relation to workers' compensation. In the 1920s, the primary purpose of such an assessment was to measure the loss of function in work activity for the purpose of assigning a cash value to an impairment (Frey, 1984). Initially, there were no standards for a functional assessment, and the determination was based solely on a physician's opinion. In the 1940s, primarily as a result of World War II, the number of people with functional impairments increased dramatically, and with this increase came a new emphasis on rehabilitation. Concomitantly, there was a surge of interest in functional assessment for rehabilitation, and in 1954, the term "activities of daily living" was first coined (Frey, 1984).

Beginning in the late 1950s, a few forward-thinking gerontological practitioners published articles about the interrelationships between ADL, chronic disease, and older people (e.g., Benjamin Rose Institute, 1959; Katz et al., 1963). During the next decade, gerontological research was undertaken to develop functional assessment instruments that would be applicable to older people in a number of situations (Lawton and Brody, 1969). Lawton and Brody's study used a point-system scale to measure six ADL items (toileting, feeding, dressing, grooming, bathing, and ambulation), as well as more complex tasks they identified as IADL, such as shopping and housekeeping. Another development during the 1960s was the broadening of the concept of functional assessment to include person-environment interactions. In this context, the functional assessment was used to identify the impact of environmental modifications and other rehabilitation interventions on the person's level of function.

In the 1970s, gerontologists began recognizing the utility of functional assessment measures, particularly in research and planning. It was not until the 1980s, however, that the clinical value of these assessment tools was recognized by gerontological practitioners. This appreciation of the functional assessment approach was closely related to a growing recognition of the inadequacy of diagnostic labels in describing the health needs of people with chronic illnesses. In 1983, the National Institute on Aging convened a special conference to focus on functional assessment of older people. At this conference, physicians caring for older patients were advised to use a functional assessment tool along with their traditional, disease-oriented, diagnostic evaluations. Moreover, the suggested approach to geriatric medical care was to assist the patient and family in maintaining the greatest degree of functional independence possible (Williams, 1983). In addition, the concept that functional impairments are the best early manifestation of active illness in older people was emphasized (Besdine, 1983).

By the mid-1980s, geriatricians were using functional assessment as an approach to medical rehabilitation, and at least one conceptual framework for functional assessment was developed (Jette, 1986). As part of the nursing home regulations that were included in the 1987 Omnibus Budget Reconciliation Act, all Medicaid- and Medicare-funded nursing homes were required to use a standardized assessment form. This form, known as the Minimum Data Set (MDS) for Resident Assessment and Care Planning, included measures of ADL and other functional parameters. One part of the MDS was the Resident Assessment Instrument (RAI), a structured, multidimensional resident assessment and problem identification system. The purpose of this form was to reinforce a holistic view of residents and to provide nursing home staff with a basis for planning residents' care so as to address both current and potential levels of function (Morris et al., 1990). By October of 1991, the RAI was being used in all Medicaid- and Medicare-funded nursing homes. Its implementation has led to significant improvements in the quality of care provided to nursing home residents (Fries et al., 1997; Hawes et al., 1997; Phillips et al., 1997). In 1995, a second version of the MDS supplanted the initial assessment tool, and subsequent nursing research has supported the reliability and clinical utility of this latest version (Morris et al., 1997b). One evaluation of a home care version (MDS-HC) used in Medicaid- and Medicare-funded home care programs concluded that the core set of items in MDS 2.0 was equally applicable to and reliable in nursing home and community settings (Morris et al., 1997a). A recent study revealed that the benefits of using the comprehensive geriatric assessment in home settings included improved functional status of and decreased nursing home use by the older adults who participated in this program (Alessi et al., 1997). Another recent study underscored the need for functional assessment as part of hospital discharge planning as a tool to identify home care needs of older adults (Rosswurm and Lanham, 1998).

Currently, increasing attention is being paid to the interrelationship between function and environmental factors. Based on this recognition, it is essential to assess the environment as it influences a person's abilities to perform ADL and IADL. Chapters 6, 7, and 12 of this text contain information about environmental factors that should be considered in relation to the functional assessment of older adults. Another trend that has evolved in the late 1990s is the application of functional assessment to hospitalized older adults. Indeed, a nursing standard of practice protocol for assessment of function in acute care settings has recently been published (Kresevic et al., 1997).

There has also been a growing recognition of the strong interrelationship between cognitive abilities and performance of ADL and IADL (Gill et al., 1996). In recent years, a need for functional assessment tools—applicable to people with dementia in a variety of settings and to community-living people who are only slightly or moderately cognitively impaired—has been identified. Assessment tools are currently being developed in an effort to identify the "everyday cognitive competence" of community-living older adults. Cognitive competence is defined as "the ability to perform adequately those cognitively complex tasks of daily living considered essential for living on one's own in this society" (Willis, 1997 p. 595). The assessment tool includes both ADL and IADL, but focuses on the cognitive abilities involved in carrying out these tasks. Some assessment instruments that have been designed for people with dementia divide the ADL items into smaller components that may be affected by the underlying cognitive impairment (Patterson et al., 1992). Examples of these kinds of assessment tools can be found in the geriatric literature (e.g., Loewenstein et al., 1989; Mahurin, 1991; Spector, 1997). Another recent trend is the use of a

		Date	PTA	ADM	DISCH		
Personal Care	Bathing 5 completely dependent 4 dependent with some assist 3 heavy partial 2 light partial 1 independent with devices 0 independent						
	Dressing 5 complete assist 3 partial assist 1 compensated 0 independent						
	Mouth care 5 totally unable to do 3 some assist 1 independent with device 0 independent						
	Hair care 5 completely unable 3 some assist 1 independent with device 0 independent						
	Dietary intake 5 total assist 4 assist with feeding 3 supplements 2 set up/encouragement 1 independent with device 0 independent						
Mobility	Transfer 5 completely unable 4 3-person/portalift 3 2-person 2 1-person 1 independent with device 0 independent						
	Ambulation 5 completely unable 4 3-person assist 3 2-person assist 2 1-person assist 1 independent with device 0 independent						
	Bed 5 unable to move in bed 3 needs assist 1 independent with device 0 independent						
Mental Status	Mental 5 totally impaired 4 assist with simple tasks 3 assist with complex tasks 2 inconsistent 1 compensated 0 no impairment						

FIGURE 17-1. Functional assessment of older adults. *Source:* Fairview General Hospital, Cleveland, Ohio 44111-5659. Used with permission.

		Date	PTA	ADM	DISCH		
Elimination	*Bladder* 5 completely incontinent 3 occasionally incontinent 1 continent with assist/device 0 continent/independent						
	Bowel 5 completely incontinent 3 occasionally incontinent 1 continent with assist/device 0 continent/independent						
	Assist/device codes A bedside commode E ostomy I catheter, intermittent B bathroom F incontinence pads J verbal cuing/supervision C urinal G catheter, external K other _____ D bedpan H catheter, indwelling						
Instrumental Activities of Daily Living	*Meal preparation* 5 unable to do 3 assist/supervise 1 independent with resources 0 independent						
	Shopping 5 unable to do 3 assist/supervise 1 compensated 0 independent						
	Telephone 5 unable to do/doesn't have 3 assist 1 independent with device 0 independent						
	Transportation 5 completely homebound 3 assist 1 arranges own 0 independent						
	Medications 5 unable to take 3 assist 1 independent 0 doesn't use						
	Housekeeping 5 unable to do 3 assist 1 independent with resources 0 independent						
	Laundry 5 unable to do 3 assist 1 independent with resources 0 independent						
	Money management 5 unable to handle 3 assist 1 independent with resources 0 independent						
	Total Points						

ADM, admission; *DISCH,* discharge, *PTA,* prior to admission.

combination ADL/IADL scale to measure disability (Spector and Fleishman, 1998).

Functional Assessment Instruments

Some of the goals of a functional assessment are: (1) to prevent disability through early identification of functional loss; (2) to develop treatment plans that enhance functional performance; (3) to ensure that the care addresses the issues most likely to maximize the patient's quality of life; (4) to improve compliance by focusing on the problems that the patient feels are most limiting; and (5) to determine the efficacy of treatment modes by measuring changes in functional performance over time (Granger et al., 1986). Functional assessment instruments generally include a scale for measuring a person's level of independence in performing specific ADL and IADL. ADL include activities that are essential to personal care, whereas IADL comprise the more complex activities that are essential in community-living situations. The assessment of ADL performance is important in determining the level of assistance needed on a daily basis, and this assessment is particularly helpful in planning long-term care for older adults. Likewise, an evaluation of IADL is important in determining the level of assistance needed by people in independent or semi-independent settings.

In a review of 43 functional assessment indices, Feinstein and co-workers made the following suggestions for more effective use of these indices in clinical settings: (1) indices must be able to measure changes that occur over time; (2) functional assessment must address concomitant psychosocial factors, as well as physiologic factors, that influence functional abilities; and (3) when multiple functional impairments are identified, the relative importance the patient assigns to each must be considered in establishing priorities (Feinstein et al., 1986). A model of functional assessment, illustrated in Figure 17-1, is discussed in the following sections.

Functional Assessment Format

The functional assessment tool illustrated in Figure 17-1 was developed by nurses in a geriatric rehabilitation setting and can be used to measure a person's functional status at different times. An initial assessment can be done at the time of admission, and this information can then be used as a baseline for establishing goals for care. The form also has a column for information about the person's reported level of function before admission. This information is helpful in determining the person's potential level of function. At the time of discharge, the reassessment information enables the staff to determine whether the goals were met. In settings in which postdischarge follow-up is possible, or in settings in which the person is readmitted at different times, the same assessment form is used to measure changes over time. Each category of activity is assigned a numeric value based on the criteria listed in Displays 17-1 and 17-2. The numeric values are used as a guide to measure progress toward goals as the person's level of function changes.

The functional assessment form in Figure 17-1 differs from many others in two ways. First, allowance is made for measurement of changes over time. The three time designations indicated on the form signify the period prior to admission (PTA), the time of admission (ADM), and the day of discharge (DISCH). The unmarked columns may be used at any time after discharge, or upon readmission. In a rehabilitative or long-term care setting, these measurements over time are particularly helpful in evaluating progress and reevaluating goals. The second major difference in this assessment form is that for each activity category, the number 1 rating is used to indicate that the person does not depend on others, but depends on some adaptive device or equipment for independent function in that area. The adaptive device might be as small as a shoehorn or as complex as an electric wheelchair. The importance of this designation

Bathing

5 Unable to assist in any way

4 Able to cooperate but cannot assist

3 Able to wash hands, face, and chest with supervision; needs help with completing the bath

2 Able to wash face, chest, arms, and upper legs; needs help with completing the bath

1 Bathes self but requires devices (e.g., long-handled sponge)

0 Bathes self independently

Dressing

5 Needs total assistance

4 Needs total supervision, but is able to dress self if clothing articles are given one at a time or set out in the order they are needed

3 Needs reminding and encouragement and some assistance with clothing selection, but can dress with little supervision

2 Dresses self, but needs help with activities requiring fine motor skills (e.g., zippers, shoelaces)

1 Dresses self using assistive devices (e.g., zipper pullers, long-handled shoehorn)

0 Dresses independently

Mouth Care

5 Cannot perform oral hygiene, but requires that it be done by others

4 Needs total supervision; needs toothpaste put on brush

3 Needs reminding and some supervision

2 Needs reminding but is otherwise independent

1 Performs oral hygiene using devices (e.g., toothbrush with built-up handle)

0 Performs oral hygiene independently

Hair Care

5 Cannot perform hair care, but requires that it be done by others

4 Needs total supervision

3 Needs some assistance with daily care

2 Performs daily care independently, but needs assistance with washing hair

1 Performs hair care using devices (e.g., hairbrush with built-up handle)

0 Performs all hair care (including washing) independently

Dietary Intake

5 Cannot prepare or obtain food; cannot feed self; nutritional requirements would not be met without total assistance

4 Needs assistance in obtaining and preparing food; needs total supervision with eating, but can feed self; nutritional requirements would not be met adequately without assistance

3 Needs assistance in tasks that involve complex skills (e.g., cutting meat, opening packages, preparing and obtaining food), but feeds self; nutritional needs would be met partially without assistance

2 Requires some assistance with obtaining and preparing food, but eats independently; would maintain adequate nutrition with encouragement or a little assistance

1 Needs assistive devices for food preparation and consumption (e.g., plate rings, rocker knife); adequately maintains nutritional requirements

0 Requires no assistance

Transfer Mobility

5 Cannot transfer, except with extreme difficulty

(continued)

Transfer Mobility (continued)

4 Needs assistance of three people for transfers, or needs two people and a lifting device
3 Needs the assistance of two people
2 Needs the assistance of one person
1 Transfers independently with a device (e.g., sliding board)
0 Transfers independently

Ambulation

5 Completely unable to walk
4 Walks with the assistance of three people
3 Walks with the assistance of two people
2 Walks with the assistance of one person
1 Walks independently with device (e.g., walker, quad cane)
0 Walks independently

Bed Mobility

5 Unable to move in bed
4 Needs the assistance of two people
3 Needs the assistance of one person
2 Needs to be encouraged and supervised
1 Moves independently with device (e.g., uses side rails or trapeze)
0 Moves independently in bed

Mental Status

5 Has extremely poor memory function; cannot follow directions; has minimal ability to identify and express needs; requires a totally structured environment

4 Has obvious memory impairment that interferes with daily life; has poor judgment and may undertake inappropriate actions; may be aware of the deficit and, consequently, may be anxious or depressed; can participate in daily routine but needs supervision; requires a strong orientation and reminder program
3 Fluctuates between levels two and four; unpredictable on a routine basis; requires monitoring and some supervision; may engage in risky behaviors at times
2 Minimal short-term memory loss; able to perform most daily tasks with only minimal reminding or supervision; has good to fair judgment and occasionally needs assistance, but does not engage in any risky behaviors
1 Is dependent on self-initiated reminders and cues for daily activities
0 No observable impairment in memory; no cognitive or psychosocial impairment that interferes with daily activities

Bladder and Bowel Elimination

5 Consistently soils self
4 Needs supervision and assistance on a regular basis
3 Needs reminding on a regular basis
2 Generally controls elimination; has accidents no more than once a week
1 Maintains control of elimination with devices (listed in Fig. 17-1)
0 Fully continent without any assistance

is that the staff is then aware that the person has compensated for a deficit, but that the compensatory mechanism must be available for the person's use.

Nurses obtain assessment information for Figure 17-1 from several sources. When older adults are able to provide reliable information about their level of function before admission, data for the column marked "PTA" are obtained through an interview with the patient/resident within 24 hours of the admission to the care facility. When older adults are not able to provide this information, as is often the case, the nurse interviews a family member or other person who is knowledgeable about the person's level of function before admission. Nurses use direct observation of the person's current level of function in performing ADL to complete the columns marked "ADM" and "DISCH." Much of the information for the sections on IADL must be obtained by questioning the older adult or their caregivers, as many of these activities pertain only to community-based settings.

The source of information is noted on the chart, and any discrepancies between objective and subjective information also are noted. In interviewing the older adult or caregiver, it is important to ask specific details about how tasks are accomplished, rather than asking open-ended questions, such as "Do you have any difficulty with . . . ?" Also, it is important to find out whether the task is meaningful to the person, rather than assuming that the person wants or needs to do the task. For example, in the IADL categories, a person who lives with other people might never have to participate in grocery shopping or money management. Therefore, assessment information, particularly regarding IADL, must be considered in relation to the person's support system and living arrangements.

Activities of Daily Living

The following areas of function are those generally considered in an assessment of ADL: grooming, bathing, dressing, eating, elimination, and mobility. The assessment format illustrated in Figure 17-1 further specifies these activities as follows: bathing, dressing, mouth care, hair care, dietary intake, transfer mobility, ambulation, bed mobility, and bladder and bowel elimination. In addition, a brief mental status assessment is included on the ADL form. This approach is taken, rather than using a separate mental status assessment tool, because it reinforces the fact that cognitive function is an integral component of ADL. In addition, it helps to determine whether ADL impairments are attributable, at least in part, to cognitive impairments, rather than primarily to physical limitations. Display 17-1 lists the functional assessment criteria for each of the ADL, as well as for mental status.

Instrumental Activities of Daily Living

In institutional settings, IADL are less important than in community settings. In institutional settings, however, an assessment of IADL is an important consideration in discharge planning. When older adults cannot perform IADL independently, caregivers often provide the assistance that enables the person to remain in a community setting. When older adults cannot perform IADL and have no caregiver to help with the task, community resources often are available to meet these needs. Home-delivered meals programs, for example, might be appropriate for older adults who have difficulty with shopping or meal preparation. Community resources often can be arranged with one or two phone calls, and they can be effective and efficient ways of improving an older adult's ability to perform IADL. Display 17-2 lists the assessment criteria for the IADL that are included in Figure 17-1.

DISPLAY 17-2
Functional Assessment Criteria for Instrumental Activities of Daily Living

Meal Preparation

5 Unable to prepare even simple meals
4 Can assist with meal preparation
3 Prepares meals, but cannot obtain groceries
2 Prepares meals with reminding or supervision

1 Prepares meals and obtains food using resources (e.g., specialized equipment, Meals on Wheels program, transportation to the grocery store)
0 Independent in obtaining and preparing food

(continued)

DISPLAY 17-2
Functional Assessment Criteria for Instrumental Activities of Daily Living (Continued)

Grocery Shopping

5   Cannot participate in shopping
4   Can accompany someone else and assist with food selection
3   Can shop and select appropriate food with some supervision
2   Can shop, but has difficulty obtaining transportation
1   Is able to arrange for necessary help with shopping
0   Shops independently

Telephone Use

5   Cannot dial or answer the phone, or carry on a routine phone conversation
4   Can talk on the phone, but cannot dial or answer it
3   Can use the phone with assistance (e.g., help in dialing)
2   Can use the phone with supervision
1   Depends on adaptive devices for telephone activities (e.g., automatic dialing system, speaker phone)
0   Independent in phone-related activities

Transportation

5   Does not leave home, even for medical care
4   Leaves home only for medical care or in rare circumstances
3   Needs assistance in arranging for transportation and needs special accommodations (e.g., wheelchair lift)
2   Needs assistance in arranging for transportation, but can get in and out of cars with little or no help
1   Arranges for own transportation, but depends on others for any transportation other than walking
0   Independent in traveling from one place to another (e.g., drives a car)

Medications

5   Unable to obtain or take medications without assistance or complete supervision
4   Cannot obtain medications, but can take them with assistance or supervision

3   Can obtain and take medications with reminders from others or with a system set up by others
2   Can obtain and take medications with a self-initiated reminder or set-up system
1   Safely takes and prepares all medications
0   Does not use medications

Housekeeping

5   Cannot perform any routine household tasks
4   Can assist with household tasks (e.g., bed making, dusting, vacuuming)
3   Can perform household tasks if supervised during the activity
2   Can perform household tasks if encouraged to do so
1   Arranges for housekeeping assistance
0   Is independent in all routine tasks

Laundry

5   Cannot perform any laundry tasks
4   Can assist with folding clothes; cannot wash or iron clothes
3   With assistance, can perform laundry tasks adequately
2   Can perform laundry tasks with supervision and reminding
1   Arranges for laundry to be done
0   Completes all laundry tasks independently

Money Management

5   Unable to manage any aspect of finances
4   Can handle simple cash transactions, but no other financial transactions (e.g., writing checks)
3   Can write checks with supervision or assistance; cannot handle any higher-level transactions (e.g., bank withdrawals)
2   Maintains checkbook, pays bills appropriately, and understands currency exchanges, but needs some assistance or supervision with these tasks
1   Arranges for someone else to handle financial matters
0   Handles all finances independently

References

Alessi, C. A., Stuck, A. E., Aronow, H. U., Yuhas, K. E., Bula, C. J., Madison, R., et al. (1997). The process of care in preventive in-home comprehensive geriatric assessment. *Journal of the American Geriatrics Society, 45,* 1044–1050.

Benjamin Rose Institute. (1959). Multidisciplinary studies of illness in aged persons: II. A new classification of functional status in activities of daily living. *Journal of Chronic Disease, 9,* 55.

Besdine, R. W. (1983). The educational utility of comprehensive functional assessment in the elderly. *Journal of the American Geriatrics Society, 31,* 651–656.

Feinstein, A. R., Josephy, B. R., & Wells, C. K. (1986). Scientific and clinical problems in indexes of functional disability. *Annals of Internal Medicine, 105,* 413–420.

Frey, W. D. (1984). Functional assessment in the '80s: A conceptual enigma, a technical challenge. In A. S. Halpern & J. J. Fuhrer (Eds.), *Functional assessment in rehabilitation* (pp. 11–43). Baltimore: Paul H. Brookes.

Fries, B. E., Hawes, C., Morris, J. N., Phillips, C. D., Mor, V., & Park, P. S. (1997). Effect of the National Resident Assessment Instrument on selected health conditions and problems. *Journal of the American Geriatrics Society, 45,* 994–1001.

Gill, T. M., Williams, C. S., Richardson, E. D., & Tinetti, M. E. (1996). Impairments in physical performance and cognitive status as predisposing factors for functional dependence among nondisabled older persons. *Journal of Gerontology: Medical Sciences, 51A*(6), M283–M288.

Granger, C. V., Hamilton, B. B., Keith, R. A., Zielezny, M., & Sherwin, F. S. (1986). Advances in functional assessment for medical rehabilitation. *Topics in Geriatric Rehabilitation, 1* (3), 59–74.

Hawes, C., Mor, V., Phillips, C. D., Fries, B. E., Morris, J. N., Steele-Friedlob, E., Greene, A. M., & Nennstiel, M. (1997). The OBRA-87 Nursing Home Regulations and implementation of the Resident Assessment Instrument: Effects on process quality. *Journal of the American Geriatrics Society, 45,* 977–985.

Jette, A. M. (1986). Functional disability and rehabilitation of the aged. *Topics in Geriatric Rehabilitation, 1*(3), 1–7.

Katz, S., Ford, A. B., Moskowitz, R. W., Jackson, B. A., & Jaffee M. W. (1963). Studies of illness in the aged: The index of ADL, a standardized measure of biological and psychosocial function. *Journal of the American Medical Association, 185,* 914–919.

Kresevic, D. M., Mezey M., & The NICHE Faculty. (1997). Assessment of function: Critically important to acute care of elders. *Geriatric Nursing, 18,* 216–221.

Lawton, M. P., & Brody, E. M. (1969). Assessment of older people: Self-maintaining and instrumental activities of daily living. *The Gerontologist, 9,* 179–186.

Loewenstein, D. A., Amigo, E., Duara, R., Guterman, A., Hurwitz, D., Berkowitz, N., et al. (1989). A new scale for the assessment of functional status in Alzheimer's disease and related disorders. *Journal of Gerontology: Psychological Sciences, 44*(4), P114–P121.

Mahurin, R. K., DeBettignies, B. H., & Pirozzolo, F. J. (1991). Structured assessment of independent living skills: Preliminary report of a performance measure of functional abilities in dementia. *Journal of Gerontology: Psychological Sciences, 46*(2), P58–P66.

Morris, J. N., Fries, B. E., Steel, K., Ikegami, M., Bernabei, R., Carpenter, G. I., et al. (1997). Comprehensive clinical assessment in community setting: Applicability of the MDS-HC. *Journal of the American Geriatrics Society, 45,* 1017–1024.

Morris, J. N., Hawes, C., Fries, B. E., Phillips, C. D., Mor, V., Katz, S., Murphy, K., Drugovich, M. L., & Friedlob, A. S. (1990). Designing the National Resident Assessment Instrument for Nursing Homes. *The Gerontologist, 30,* 293–307.

Morris, J. N., Nonemaker, S., Murphy, K., Hawes, C., Fries, B. E., Mor, V., & Phillips, C. (1997). A commitment to change: Revision of HCFA's RAI. *Journal of the American Geriatrics Society, 45,* 1011–1016.

Patterson, M. B., Mack, J. L., Neundorfer, M., Martin, R. J., Smyth, K. A., & Whitehouse, P. J. (1992). Assessment of functional ability in Alzheimer's disease: A review and a preliminary report on the Cleveland scale for activities of daily living. *Alzheimer Disease and Related Disorders, 6*(3), 145–163.

Phillips, C. D., Morris, J. N., Hawes, C., Fries, B. E., Mor, V., Nennstiel, M., & Iannacchione, V. (1997). Association of the Resident Assessment Instrument (RAI) with changes in function, cognition, and psychosocial status. *Journal of the American Geriatrics Society, 45,* 986–993.

Rosswurm, M. A., & Lanham, D. M. (1998). Discharge planning for elderly patients. *Journal of Gerontological Nursing, 24*(5), 14–21.

Spector, W. D. (1997). Measuring functioning in daily activities for persons with dementia. *Alzheimer Disease and Associated Disorders, 11* (Suppl. 6), 81–90.

Spector, W. D., & Fleishman, J. A. (1998). Combining activities of daily living with instrumental activities of daily living to measure functional disability. *Journal of Gerontology: Social Sciences, 53B,* S46–S57.

Williams, T. F. (1983). Comprehensive functional assessment: An overview. *Journal of the American Geriatrics Society, 31*(11), 637–641.

Willis, S. L. (1996). Everyday cognitive competence in elderly persons: Conceptual issues and empirical findings. *The Gerontologist, 36,* 595–601.

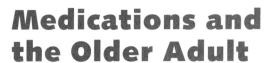

Medications and the Older Adult

Chapter

18

1. *Delineate age-related changes that influence patterns of medication consumption and actions of medications.*

2. *Examine risk factors that affect medication action and consumption in older adults.*

3. *Identify non-Western sources of care and alternative practices that are likely to be used by people of various cultural groups.*

4. *Discuss the functional consequences of age-related changes and risk factors that increase the potential for altered therapeutic action and adverse effects of medications.*

5. *Explain the purposes of medication assessment and the relationship between the medication assessment and the overall assessment of older adults.*

6. *Describe observations and interview questions that are relevant to performing a comprehensive and culturally relevant assessment with regard to medications and other remedies.*

7. *Examine the use of herbs and homeopathic remedies, including potential problems with herb use.*

8. *Identify interventions directed toward enhancing the therapeutic effectiveness of medications, reducing the risks for adverse effects, and minimizing the negative functional consequences of adverse effects.*

The topic of medications and the older adult is not a distinct category of function in the same sense as physiologic and psychosocial aspects of function, such as vision and cognition. Within the functional consequences framework, however, medication use by the older adult is an extremely important consideration, and it can be addressed in the same manner as other aspects of function. This chapter addresses the age-related changes that influence medication effects, as well as those changes that can influence patterns of medication use. Similarly, the risk factors that can influence medication action and those that may affect medication-taking behaviors are discussed. The negative functional consequences for older adults are the effects of the age-related changes and the risk factors that influence medication actions. Nursing care for older adults with actual or potential medication-related problems is also addressed.

Age-Related Changes

Age-related changes influence patterns of medication consumption and actions of medications in the body. Specific age-related changes that affect medication action include alterations in homeostasis, renal function, cardiac output, liver function, serum albumin level, body composition, and receptor sensitivity. The following factors also modify medication action in the body: food; gender; body weight; chemical characteristics of the medication; and medication interactions with caffeine, alcohol, nicotine, and other medications. Although the latter influences are not unique to older adults, they combine with age-related changes to increase the unpredictability of medication effects in older adults.

Appropriate consumption of oral medications depends on the following factors: motivation; some level of understanding about the purpose of the medication; an ability to obtain the correct amounts of medications; an ability to distinguish the correct container and an ability to read directions; an ability to hear and remember verbal instructions; an ability to understand the correct timing for medication administration and to follow the correct dosage regimen; fine motor movement and coordination to remove medications from containers and place them in the mouth; and an ability to swallow the particular form of medication. Additional skills related to coordination, manual dexterity, and visual acuity may be required when medications are administered nasally, transdermally, subcutaneously, or by any other method. Many of these skills are influenced by age-related changes, and all of them can be influenced by risk factors that commonly affect older adults. For example, a hearing or vision impairment can interfere with a person's ability to understand instructions and read directions, especially labels on medicine bottles. Any limitations in fine motor movement of the hands may interfere with the ability to remove lids from medication containers, especially when the lids are tamper-resistant.

Body Composition

An age-related decrease in total body water and an increase in the proportion of body fat to lean body mass can alter medication action in older adults. Between the ages of about 20 and 80 years, the following changes in body composition occur: body fat gradually increases by 15%

to 20%, lean tissue decreases by about 20%, and total body water is reduced by 10% to 15%. With some exceptions, these age-related changes will affect a particular medication according to its degree of fat or water solubility. Thus, drugs that are distributed primarily in body water or lean body mass may reach higher serum concentrations in older adults, and their effects may be more intense. Similarly, the serum concentration of highly fat-soluble medications, which are distributed and stored in fat tissue, may be lowered, and these medications have an increased tendency to accumulate in adipose tissue. The end result is that fat-soluble medications may have a prolonged duration of action, their overall effect may be erratic, and their short-term effects may be less intense. Studies of the impact of age-related changes on the volume of distribution of particular medications have confirmed these effects for many, but not all, medications. Table 18-1 list some of the medications that are known to be affected by changes in body composition.

Serum Albumin Level

As medications are distributed and metabolized in the body, some molecules are bound to proteins, primarily to serum albumin. The bound

TABLE 18-1

Some Medications Affected by Changes in Body Composition

Decreased Volume of Distribution	Increased Volume of Distribution
Antipyrine	Chlordiazepoxide
Cimetidine	Chlormethiazole
Digoxin	Clobazam
Ethanol	Midazolam
Gentamicin	Phenobarbital
Morphine	Prazosin
Quinine	Thiopental
	Tolbutamide

portion thus becomes inactive, whereas the unbound molecules remain active. Because the unbound portion is the amount available for metabolism, tissue perfusion, and renal excretion, the protein-binding capacity of a drug is an important determinant of its potential for both therapeutic and adverse effects. The degree of protein binding of each medication varies, with some medications, such as warfarin, having a protein-binding capacity of 99%. The binding capacity of protein-bound medications can be influenced by diminished serum albumin levels in older adults. Additional determinants of the degree of protein binding for any medication include the strength of the binding and the number of chemicals competing for the binding sites.

Although researchers disagree about the extent and cause of decreased serum albumin levels in older adults, it is generally agreed that the serum albumin level diminishes by as much as 20% in the later decades of life. Diminished serum albumin levels are associated with a combination of factors, including nutrition, disease processes, decreased mobility, and age-related liver changes. A recent study has revealed that laxative use in older adults is independently associated with hypoalbuminemia (Pahor et al., 1994). Regardless of the cause, a decrease in serum albumin level will lead to an increased amount of the active portion of protein-bound medications. Highly protein-bound medications, which are commonly taken by older adults, are especially likely to be affected. A few examples of medications that are likely to be altered by low serum albumin levels and decreased binding opportunities are furosemide, phenylbutazone, phenytoin, salicylic acid, theophylline, thiopental, tolbutamide, and warfarin.

When more than one medication is consumed, the influence of decreased albumin level is intensified. Even in the presence of adequate serum albumin levels, highly protein-bound medications compete for the same sites. Thus, if the serum albumin level is low, the competi-

TABLE 18-2
Some Medications That Compete at Protein-Binding Sites

Salicylates and oral hypoglycemics
Sulfonamides and oral hypoglycemics
Warfarin and chloral hydrate
Warfarin and clofibrate
Warfarin and nalidixic acid
Warfarin and phenylbutazone
Warfarin and sertraline

tion will be increased, as will the potential for altered effects. Table 18-2 identifies a few of the medication combinations that are competitive by virtue of their protein-binding capabilities, and which, therefore, have an increased risk of altered effects in the presence of diminished serum albumin levels.

Renal and Liver Function

An age-related decline in glomerular filtration rate begins in early adulthood and progresses at an annual rate of 1% to 2%. More than any other age-related change, diminished renal function has a profound impact on medication action. As with other aspects of pharmacokinetics, however, the specific chemical characteristics of each medication determine the degree to which age-related changes affect excretion. For example, medications excreted largely unchanged through the kidneys, such as aminoglycoside antibiotics, will be more directly influenced by diminished renal function than those that are metabolized more extensively in the liver before excretion. Likewise, the effect of diminished renal function will be greater on medications that have a narrow therapeutic index, like digoxin, than on medications with a wide therapeutic index.

Hepatic blood flow declines by 45% between the ages of 25 and 65 years. This age-related change may influence the serum concentration and volume of distribution of some medications. For example, the effect of medications that are rapidly metabolized and, therefore, greatly influenced by the speed of delivery to the liver may be affected by diminished hepatic blood flow. The specific impact of these age-related liver changes on medication metabolism is unclear, however. Definitive conclusions about the influence of age-related changes on medication metabolism are thwarted by the simultaneous and stronger influence of other factors, such as diet, disease, and smoking.

Two measures of the efficiency of metabolism and elimination are elimination half-life and clearance rate. Elimination half-life is the time required to decrease the drug concentration by one-half of its original value. It takes five half-lives to reach steady-state concentrations after a drug is initiated. Similarly, it takes five half-lives to eliminate a medication from the body after a drug is discontinued. The clearance rate measures the volume of blood from which the medication is eliminated per unit of time. An increase in half-life or a decrease in clearance rate may result in accumulation of the medication. The end result is that the therapeutic effect is likely to be altered, and the risk of adverse effects is likely to be increased. Table 18-3 lists examples of medications with half-lives that may be increased or with clearance rates that may be decreased in older adults.

Gastrointestinal Changes

A controversy persists in geropharmacology as to the extent to which gastrointestinal changes occur as a result of normal aging, and to what degree, if any, these changes affect medication absorption. Absorption refers to the passage of a medication from its site of introduction, usually the gastrointestinal tract, into the general circulation. Absorption of medications can be affected by diminished gastric acid, increased gastric pH, and delayed gastric emptying. Because most oral medications are absorbed by

TABLE 18-3
Some Medications That Are Likely to Be Altered in Older Adults

Some Medications Whose Half-Lives Are Likely to Be Increased

Ampicillin	Kanamycin
Barbiturates	Penicillin
Cimetidine	Salicylate
Desmethyldiazepam	Tetracycline
Digoxin (not digitoxin)	Thiopental
Gentamicin	

Some Medications Whose Clearance Rates Are Likely to Be Decreased

Ampicillin	Gentamicin
Atenolol	Lithium
Cimetidine	Meperidine
Chlordiazepoxide	Nortriptyline
Desmethyldiazepam	Quinidine
Digoxin	Tetracycline

passive diffusion across the small intestine—a process that is not pH-dependent—they are not usually affected by any alterations in gastric acidity. Recent research also suggests that healthy older adults do not have diminished gastric acidity (Hurwitz et al., 1997). However, the lack of agreement regarding the existence of age-related changes in gastric emptying time or gastrointestinal absorptive surfaces raises further questions about potential age-related effects on medication absorption.

The unique chemical properties of each medication determine the degree to which it is susceptible to any gastrointestinal changes, regardless of age. For example, pH-sensitive medications, such as penicillin and ferrous sulfate, are more likely to be affected by altered gastric acid levels or by prolonged exposure to these acids because of delayed emptying. In addition, product-to-product differences in inert ingredients may be significant determinants of medication absorption. Examples of medications whose effects may be altered by product-to-product differences are digitalis, lithium, phenytoin, and thyroid products (Todd, 1985). Finally, absorption of some medications is likely to be altered by antacids, which often are viewed as harmless products because they are sold over the counter.

Although it may be logical to conclude that absorption of oral medications is influenced by age-related gastric acid changes, these conclusions are not supported by research. A review of 48 studies of the effect of age on medication absorption after oral administration of 35 medications has revealed a wide range of results, from no age-related effects to significant age-related effects (Vestal and Dawson, 1985). Even the results of two or more studies of the same medication often differ. It is now thought that drug absorption is not significantly altered in healthy older adults (Avorn and Gurwitz, 1997). The most accurate conclusion is that some medications may be affected by gastrointestinal factors, but that these factors are probably related to pathologic conditions or medication interactions rather than to age-related changes.

Homeostatic Mechanisms

Thermoregulation, fluid regulation, and baroreceptor control over blood pressure are homeostatic mechanisms that become less efficient with increasing age. Age-related changes in these mechanisms influence medication action; likewise, medication action influences these mechanisms. Thus, interactions between medications and homeostatic mechanisms potentially have the double effect of altering the medication action and impairing the homeostatic mechanism. For example, inefficient fluid regulation may alter the action of medications, such as lithium, that are particularly sensitive to fluid and electrolyte balance. An example of impaired homeostasis from medication action is the increased potential for medication-induced hypothermia or hyperthermia because of altered thermoregulation. Postural hypotension is more common in older adults than in younger populations and

is exacerbated by medications that act on the central and autonomic nervous system, and by medications with other modes of action. Medications affecting thermoregulation are discussed in Chapter 15, and medications affecting postural hypotension are discussed in Chapter 10.

Receptor Sensitivity

Independent of any other changes, age-related changes in receptor sensitivity can influence medication action. Although research on age-related receptor site changes is scarce, these changes are thought to contribute to the increased sensitivity of older adults to some medications, such as warfarin. In addition, an increased sensitivity of the older brain to centrally acting psychotropic medications may potentiate both the therapeutic and adverse effects of these medications. Age-related changes, either in homeostatic mechanisms or receptor sites, also are thought to account for the adverse effects of impaired psychomotor function and increased postural sway associated with some medications. Until further research identifies specific age-related changes, however, the most accurate conclusion is that age-related alterations in receptor sensitivity are likely to influence the therapeutic and adverse effects of some medications.

Table 18-4 summarizes the age-related changes that influence medications. Risk factors are discussed in the following section.

Risk Factors

In addition to being influenced by age-related changes, medication action and consumption are influenced by risk factors that are common in older adults. Pathologic processes usually are present in medicated older adults and may profoundly affect medication action and consumption. The consumption of more than one medication greatly increases the potential for adverse effects and altered therapeutic effect. Because

TABLE 18-4
Age-Related Changes That May Influence
Medication Effects

Age-Related Change	Effect on Some Medications
Decreased body water, decreased lean tissue, increased body fat	Increased or decreased serum concentration, depending on the drug's degree of fat or water solubility
Decreased serum albumin level	Increased amount of the active portion of protein-bound medications
Decreased renal and hepatic function	Increased serum concentration
Decreased gastric acid, increased gastric pH	Altered absorption of medications that are sensitive to stomach pH
Altered homeostatic mechanisms	Increased potential for adverse effects
Altered receptor sensitivity	Increased or decreased therapeutic effect

older adults take a disproportionately greater number of medications than do younger people, they have an increased susceptibility to adverse or altered medication effects. Additional risks arise from myths and misunderstandings that affect the medication consumption patterns of older adults. Finally, certain factors that are unrelated to age, such as gender and smoking habits, combine with age-related changes and risk factors to further increase the risk of adverse and altered effects.

Weight and Gender

Because body size affects volume of distribution, changes in body size influence medication concentration and thus alter medication effects. In an older adult who is particularly small or who has lost or is losing weight, these changes may influence medication concentration. Despite these associations, body weight is not always considered when determining adult medication

doses. A study of almost 1800 older patients revealed that their mean weight declined progressively with age, but that prescribed doses for the three medications reviewed in the study were not adjusted. As a result, there was a marked and statistically significant increase in the mean dose on a milligram-per-kilogram basis (Campion et al., 1987).

Women are at higher risk than men for altered therapeutic effects and increased adverse medication effects. Although little is known about causal relationships, altered medication effects may be associated with any of the following factors that affect women to a greater degree than men: smaller size, hormonal influences, and a higher proportion of body fat to lean body tissue. Also, studies indicate that women take more prescription and nonprescription medications than do men (Chrischilles et al., 1992).

Pathologic Processes

Because the purpose of any medication is to relieve or control symptoms of pathologic conditions, it can be assumed that a medicated older adult has at least one disease-related symptom. Disease processes may influence not only the action of medications in the body, but also the skills related to medication consumption, especially if functional limitations accompany the disease process. Medication-disease interactions may manifest themselves in any of the following ways:

1. Disease processes tend to exacerbate age-related changes that would otherwise have little or no impact on the medication. (For example, malnutrition further decreases serum albumin levels, thereby increasing both the therapeutic and adverse effects of medications with a high binding capacity.)
2. Disease processes potentiate the therapeutic and adverse effects of medications. (For instance, congestive heart failure decreases both the metabolism and the excretion of most medications.)

3. Adverse medication effects alter disease processes. (For example, anticholinergics may exacerbate prostatic hyperplasia, causing acute urinary retention.)

Behaviors Based on Myths and Attitudes

Medication consumption patterns are influenced by myths and attitudes held by older adults, as well as those held by their caregivers. These myths and attitudes promote the use of medicatio... ...edies, for... ...though th... ...adults as... ...mental to... ...symptom... ...medicatio... ...terparts.

A pot... ...by comm... ...able sy... ...harmless... ...such as '... ...age the... ...tra-stren... ...older a... ...remedie... ...function and ... over-the-counter preparations may be relatively safe for healthy younger adults, they often create problems for older adults, particularly in the presence of pathologic conditions and in combination with other medications. Many over-the-counter preparations, like remedies for colds and insomnia, contain anticholinergic ingredients that have adverse effects in older adults.

Attitudes about medications as quick-fix remedies also influence the prescribing patterns of primary care practitioners. When over-the-counter remedies are ineffective, people expect their health care practitioners to provide an otherwise unobtainable remedy, via a prescription, for their discomfort. An extensive national sur- vey of physicians in the United States has revealed that internists and general practice and family practice physicians prescribed medications in more than 80% of the office visits of people aged 65 years and older (National Center for Health Statistics and Cypress, 1982). Moreover, pharmaceutical companies encourage the use of prescription medications through the widespread distribution of free samples.

In addition to the attitudes of patients that foster quick-fix remedies, the attitudes of primary care practitioners also contribute to the proliferation of prescriptions. Health care prac... ...ioners may feel more satisfied after writing a ...ion, even if they have not identified the ...g cause of the presenting problem or ...uld have suggested nonmedication rem... ...though nonmedication remedies can al... ...ome disorders without adverse effects, ...medies usually demand more of the ...ner's time and some degree of patient ...ion. Sleep and anxiety complaints are ...es of conditions that respond to non... ...tion treatments, but that are often ad... ...by prescription medications because of ...es of the patient or primary care prac... ...ause older adults often perceive their pri... ...care practitioners as all-knowing, they ...esitate to challenge or question the use of prescription medications. Although the image of the infallible physician is subsiding, older adults are still inclined to accept advice from prescribing practitioners without question. In a survey of more than 1000 health care consumers, 70% of the older adults polled said they wanted their physicians to make treatment and prescription decisions for them ("Survey," 1987).

Lack of confidence in one's communication skills may further inhibit someone from discussing prescriptions and other treatments with a health care practitioner. Because of the tremendous expansion of medical knowledge since the mid-1950s, older adults and other health care consumers may feel somewhat ignorant about these matters and may be reluctant to discuss medical decisions. Hearing impairments and other sensory impairments that are common in older adults also may interfere with patient-directed discussions of a medication plan. Other communication barriers, such as an attitude of impatience on the part of the health care practitioner, also may thwart discussion. In addition, poor command of the English language, on the part of either the older adult or the health care practitioner, can interfere with a discussion of health issues and lead to misunderstandings.

Lack of Information

Despite the fact that older adults are the primary consumers of prescription and over-the-counter medications, our knowledge about medications and the older adult is in its infancy. Before the mid-1970s, research on the influence of age on the action of specific medications was virtually nonexistent. During the late 1970s and early 1980s, research concentrated on age-related influences on pharmacokinetics. To date, age-related and disease-related influences on medication action have not been addressed adequately. In addition, because these studies have been cross-sectional rather than longitudinal, the conclusions are based on age differences, rather than age changes.

In the past, when pharmaceutical companies determined adult doses, they overlooked age-related changes and based their recommendations on tests done on healthy men in their mid-20s. In 1982, the United States Pharmacopeia, which sets the official standards for medications in the United States, established a geriatrics advisory panel to examine age-related influences on medication action. Although geriatric doses are not always recommended, progress is being made in addressing age-related changes that affect the therapeutic and adverse effects of medication. Geriatricians also are identifying and ad-

dressing medication-related problems that are specific to older adults. For example, in the early 1990s, a panel of noted geriatricians developed and published criteria for identifying inappropriate medication use in nursing home residents (Beers et al., 1991). In 1997, these criteria were updated and expanded to include potentially inappropriate medication use for any person 65 years of age or older (Beers, 1997).

Information about medication-medication interactions also is lacking, especially for newly approved medications. Because the Food and Drug Administration (FDA) does not require the testing of a medication as it interacts with other medications, medication-medication interactions may not be identified until after the medication has been marketed. Thus, unpredictable effects might occur in older adults who consume more than one medication. Cimetidine is an example of a medication that is relatively safe when taken alone, but that is likely to interact with other medications, potentially causing serious adverse effects, such as mental changes, especially in older people. Examples of other medications that are likely to cause serious adverse effects when consumed with another medication include alcohol, phenytoin, digoxin, analgesics, theophylline, anticoagulants, and psychotropic agents. Also, any recently approved medication should be used cautiously in older adults who are taking more than one medication.

In the late 1980s, two trends emerged in the pharmaceutical industry that may benefit older adults. First, some pharmaceutical companies began testing medications on older adults. Second, they began focusing on adverse medication effects, including medication interactions. Consequently, when new medications are released today, pharmaceutical companies recommend dosage adjustments for older adults. They also are likely to provide information about interactions and adverse effects. In addition, because of the emphasis on adverse reactions, new medications are promoted not only for their therapeutic effectiveness but also for their lack of unwanted effects.

Inadequate Monitoring and Polypharmacy

Many factors interfere with adequate medication monitoring from the time of the initial prescription until the termination of treatment, including the following:

1. Patient consultations with multiple health care providers, who usually do not communicate about the patient's care;
2. Health care practitioners' lack of information about medications obtained from a variety of sources (i.e., prescription medications offered by friends and relatives, or nonprescription products, such as herbs, nutritional supplements, and over-the-counter products);
3. Health care practitioners' lack of information about a patient's noncompliance with a treatment regimen;
4. A patient's fear of disclosing information about folk remedies or about medications obtained from sources other than the prescribing health care practitioner;
5. A patient's fear about disclosing information about self-directed changes in the medication regimen;
6. An assumption by the patient or health care practitioner that, once most medications are started, they should be continued indefinitely;
7. An assumption by the patient or health care practitioner that, once an appropriate medication dosage is established, it will not need to be changed;
8. An assumption by the patient or health care practitioner that a lack of adverse effects early in the course of treatment indicates that adverse effects will never occur;
9. Changes in the patient's weight, especially weight loss, which may affect pharmacokinetics;
10. Changes in the patient's daily habits, which may affect pharmacokinetics (e.g., smoking, activity level, or nutrient and fluid intake);
11. Changes in the patient's mental-emotional status, which may affect medication consumption patterns;
12. Changes in the patient's health status, which may affect medication actions, increasing the potential for adverse effects; and
13. Financial limitations that can influence a patient's medication consumption patterns.

Lack of Awareness of Adverse Medication Effects

Manifestations of adverse effects often are overlooked or misinterpreted because of their similarity to age-related changes or common pathologic conditions of older adults. When an older adult experiences an adverse medication reaction, two or three potential causes, other than the medication, usually can be identified. For example, when an older adult becomes depressed, a psychosocial factor, such as widowhood, may be identified as the source of the depression. Even if the person is taking a medication, such as reserpine, which is known to cause depression, the depression may be viewed as a primary problem. This incorrect assumption may lead to treatment with additional medications, rather than the direct and more appropriate approach of dealing with the adverse effect. Although adverse effects are not unique to older adults, they occur more commonly with increasing age and are more likely to be attributed erroneously to pathologic conditions or age-related changes and circumstances. Table 18-5 summarizes adverse medication effects that are likely to remain unrecognized in older adults because of their similarity to age-related changes.

TABLE 18-5
Some Adverse Medication Effects That May Remain Unrecognized in Older Adults

Manifestation	Medication Type	Specific Examples
Cognitive impairment	Antidepressants; antipsychotics; anti-anxiety agents; anticholinergics; hypoglycemics; OTC cold, cough, and sleeping preparations	Perphenazine, amitriptyline, chlorpromazine, diazepam, chlordiazepoxide, benztropine, trihexyphenidyl, cimetidine, digoxin, barbiturates, tolazamide, tolbutamide, chlorpheniramine, pyrilamine
Depression	Antihypertensives, antiarthritics, anti-anxiety agents, antipsychotics	Reserpine, clonidine, propranolol, indomethacin, haloperidol, barbiturates
Urinary incontinence	Diuretics, anticholinergics	Furosemide, doxepin, thioridazine, lorazepam
Constipation	Narcotics, antacids, antipsychotics, antidepressants	Codeine, chlorpromazine, calcium carbonate, aluminum hydroxide, amoxapine
Vision impairment	Digitalis, antiarthritics, phenothiazines	Digoxin, indomethacin, ibuprofen, chlorpromazine
Hearing impairment	Mycin antibiotics, salicylates, loop diuretics	Gentamicin, aspirin, furosemide, bumetanide
Postural hypotension	Antihypertensives, diuretics, antipsychotics, antidepressants	Guanethidine, furosemide, propranolol, chlorpromazine, imipramine, clonidine
Hypothermia	Antipsychotics, alcohol, salicylates	Haloperidol, aspirin, alcohol, fluphenazine
Sexual dysfunction	Antihypertensives, antipsychotics, antidepressants, alcohol, antihypertensives	Timolol, clonidine, thiazides, haloperidol, amitriptyline, alcohol, cimetidine, propranolol, methyldopa
Mobility problems	Sedatives, antianxiety agents, antipsychotics, ototoxic medications	Chloral hydrate, diazepam, furosemide, gentamicin
Dry mouth	Anticholinergics, corticosteroids, bronchodilators, antihypertensives	Chlorpromazine, haloperidol, prednisone, furosemide, sertraline, theophylline
Anorexia	Digitalis, bronchodilators, antihistamines	Digoxin, theophylline, diphenhydramine
Drowsiness	Antidepressants, antipsychotics, OTC cold preparations, alcohol, barbiturates	Amitriptyline, haloperidol, chlorpheniramine, secobarbital
Edema	Antiarthritics, corticosteroids, antihypertensives	Ibuprofen, indomethacin, prednisone, reserpine, methyldopa
Tremors	Antipsychotics	Haloperidol, chlorpromazine, thioridazine

OTC, over-the-counter.

Functional Consequences

An increased potential for both altered therapeutic action and adverse medication effects is a functional consequence of age-related changes. The presence of risk factors further increases the potential for these negative functional consequences. Age-related changes and risk factors also affect medication consumption patterns, increasing the possibility of noncompliance and the potential for adverse and altered therapeutic effects.

Altered Therapeutic Effects

Risk factors and age-related changes can alter the therapeutic action of medication in older adults. Little information on therapeutic effects is available, however, because research has focused primarily on adverse effects. There is agreement, for example, about the increased sensitivity of older adults to the adverse effects of digoxin, but little information is available about any age-related alterations in its therapeutic effect. Other medications that are thought to have increased therapeutic effectiveness in older adults include morphine, lidocaine, halothane, lithium, temazepam, and pentozocine. As research on the therapeutic effects of medications increases, many more medications will likely be identified as having altered therapeutic effects in older adults.

Increased Potential for Adverse Effects

Adverse medication effects are the unintended outcomes of a medication that occur because of its chemical components. These effects usually are undesirable and harmful; however, a few of these secondary effects can be beneficial. Adverse medication effects occur in healthy younger adults, but they are more likely to occur as a result of a combination of age-related changes, disease-related conditions, or medication-chemical interactions. In older adults, the risk of adverse effects is 2 to 3 times higher than in younger adults. One recent study revealed that 35% of older outpatients, who took an average of eight medications, had adverse drug events during a 1-year period (Hanlon et al., 1997). In fact, experts in geropharmacology caution that, "Any symptom in an elderly patient may be a drug side effect until proven otherwise" (Avorn and Gurwitz, 1997, p. 60). Although research has not been able to distinguish between the unique influences of age-related, disease-related, and medication-related factors, studies have identified certain risk factors for adverse medication effects. The risk factors that are generally agreed upon include pathologic processes, the number of medications consumed, the duration of medication consumption, and a history of adverse reactions. Consequences of adverse drug effects include a decline in function, an increased number of visits for health care services, admission to a hospital or prolongation of a hospital stay, and death (Gerety et al., 1993; Hanlon et al., 1997; Gray et al., 1998).

In recent years, it is becoming increasingly important to recognize the use of herbs by older adults in the United States. Although most herbs are safe and may have therapeutic effects, a few herbs can be particularly hazardous for older adults and for people with certain conditions, such as those listed in Display 18-4. Even in healthy people, herbs can affect blood pressure, electrolyte balance, blood clotting mechanisms, and heart rate and rhythm. In older adults, these adverse effects may be more serious than in younger adults. Also, it is likely that older adults are more susceptible to the adverse effects of herbs because of age-related changes. Table 18-6 lists some of the potential adverse effects of certain herbs, which are likely to be more serious in older adults. This table can be used in conjunction with Display 18-4 for health education with regard to herbs.

Medication-Chemical Interactions

Medication-chemical interactions can arise from herbs, caffeine, nutrients, alcohol, nicotine, and other medications. These interactions are not limited to prescription medications, and they can occur between two over-the-counter preparations, or between any chemical and one over-the-counter preparation. Outcomes of medica-

TABLE 18-6
Potential Adverse Effects of Some Herbs

Black cohosh	Bradycardia, hypotension, joint pains
Bloodroot	Bradycardia, arrhythmia, dizziness, impaired vision, intense thirst
Boneset	Liver toxicity, mental changes, respiratory problems
Coltsfoot	Fever, liver toxicity
Dandelion	Interactions with diuretics, increased concentration of lithium or potassium
Ephedra	Anxiety, dizziness, insomnia, tachycardia, hypertension
Feverfew	Interference with blood clotting mechanisms
Garlic	Hypotension, inhibition of blood clotting, potentiation of antidiabetic drugs
Ginseng	Anxiety, insomnia, hypertension, tachycardia, asthma attacks, postmenopausal bleeding
Ginkgo biloba	Increased anticoagulation
Goldenseal	Vasoconstriction
Guar gum	Hypoglycemia
Hawthorn	Hypotension
Hops, skullcap, valerian	Drowsiness, potentiation of antianxiety or sedative medications
Kava	Damage to the eyes, skin, liver, and spinal cord from long-term use
Licorice	Hypokalemia, hypernatremia
Lobelia	Hearing and vision problems
Motherwort	Increased anticoagulation
Nettle	Hypokalemia
Senna	Potentiation of digoxin
Yohimbe	Anxiety, tachycardia, hypertension, mental changes

tion-chemical interactions can include altered or erratic therapeutic effect, increased potential for adverse effects, and, in rare cases, a decreased potential for adverse effects.

Medication-Medication Interactions

The risk of adverse effects from interactions between two or more medications increases exponentially according to the number of medications being consumed. Because older adults are more likely than younger people to take two or more medications concurrently, they are at increased risk for medication-medication interactions. Medication-medication interactions are often caused by the competitive action of chemicals, but they may be caused by any mechanism that influences the absorption, distribution, metabolism, or elimination of any of the medications. Table 18-7 lists medication-medication

TABLE 18-7
Medication-Medication Interactions

Type of Interaction	Example of Interaction Effect
Interacting agents in stomach or small intestine	Digoxin combined with aluminum or magnesium antacids decreases the serum digoxin level.
Competition for albumin-binding sites	Phenylbutazone competes with warfarin, thereby increasing the warfarin effect.
Altered volume of distribution	Quinidine, when combined with digoxin, may double the serum concentration of digoxin.
Altered medication metabolism	Phenobarbital decreases the effect of warfarin.
Receptor site competition	Methyldopa decreases the amount of norepinephrine available at nerve endings.
Diminished elimination	Probenecid interferes with the elimination of ampicillin and prolongs the action of ampicillin.
Competing drug actions	Nonsteroidal anti-inflammatory drugs may diminish the effectiveness of antihypertensives.

interactions that occur commonly in older adults.

Nutrient-Medication Interactions

The interactions between a medication and caffeine, alcohol, or nicotine usually affect only the action of the medication, but nutrient-medication interactions can affect both the nutrient and the medication. In this chapter, the discussion of nutrient-medication interactions is limited to the influence of nutrients on medications, as the influence of medications on nutrients has already been addressed in Chapter 8.

The sources of nutrients include food, enteral formulas, and nutritional supplements. Nutrients, food preparation methods, and the nonnutrient components of food may alter medication action in any of the following ways:

1. The absorption rate of medication may be delayed, with or without affecting the total amount absorbed, thereby increasing the time required to reach peak serum levels.
2. Heavy or fat-containing meals can slow stomach emptying, increasing the amount of medication that is absorbed in the stomach before it passes into the small intestine.
3. Charcoal broiling of food and consumption of certain foods (e.g., cocoa, coffee, fiber, alcohol, protein, cabbage, caffeinated tea, and brussels sprouts) can alter medication metabolism.

Table 18-8 summarizes common nutrient-medication interactions.

Alcohol-Medication Interactions

Alcohol-medication interactions are similar to medication-medication interactions; however, they are more likely to be overlooked or to remain unrecognized. Because of societal attitudes about alcohol consumption, health professionals may not inquire about a patient's use of alcohol. Even when people are asked, they may not accurately acknowledge the amount of alcohol used. Alcohol is consumed not only in beverages, but also in over-the-counter preparations, some of which are composed of up to 40% alcohol. Categories of over-the-counter preparations that are most likely to contain alcohol include mouthwashes, vitamin and mineral tonics, and liquid cough and cold preparations. When taken in combination with medications, alcohol can alter the therapeutic action of the medication and increase the potential for adverse effects. Some of the medications that are most likely to be affected by alcohol, whether consumed in beverages or medications, are listed in Table 18-9, along with the effects of these interactions.

TABLE 18-8
Nutrient-Medication Interactions

Effect on Medication	Example of Interaction Effect
Delayed absorption rate, no effect on amount absorbed	Ingestion of food may delay absorption of cimetidine, digoxin, and ibuprofen.
Reduced rate and amount of absorption	Calcium decreases absorption of tetracycline. A high-protein or high-fiber meal decreases absorption of levodopa.
Reduced absorption because of non-nutrient components	Caffeinated tea and fiber intake interfere with iron absorption.
Increased absorption	High-fat foods increase serum levels of griseofulvin.
Decreased therapeutic effect	Vitamin K decreases the effectiveness of warfarin. Charcoal broiling of foods diminishes the effectiveness of aminophylline or theophylline
Increased rate of metabolism	A high-protein diet increases the metabolism of theophylline.

TABLE 18-9
Alcohol-Medication Interactions

Type of Interaction	Example of Interaction Effect
Altered metabolism of benzodiazepines when combined with alcohol	Increased psychomotor impairment and adverse effects
Altered metabolism of barbiturates and mepro-bamate when combined with alcohol	Central nervous system depression
Competition between alcohol and chloral hydrate at metabolic sites	Increased serum levels of alcohol and chloral hydrate
Altered metabolism of alcohol when combined with chlorpromazine	Increased serum levels of alcohol and acetyl-hyde; increased psychomotor impairment
Enhanced vasodilation as a result of a combination of alcohol and nitrates	Severe hypotension and headache, enhanced absorption of nitroglycerin
Altered hepatic gluconeogenesis, which influences the action of oral hypoglycemics, as a result of alcohol	Potentiation of oral hypoglycemics by alcohol

Interactions with Caffeine, Nicotine, and Herbs

Caffeine-medication, nicotine-medication, and herb-medication interactions have received little attention despite the widespread use of these substances and the fact that these interactions can be as harmful as medication-medication interactions. In addition to food and beverages, many over-the-counter analgesics and cold preparations are sources of caffeine. Most caffeine-medication interactions affect the action of the medication rather than that of the caffeine; however, a few medications alter caffeine metabolism and increase its half-life. Examples of caffeine-medication interactions are summarized in Table 18-10.

Nicotine-medication interactions arise from cigarette smoking and are affected by fluctuations in smoking habits. Nicotine acts as a vasoconstrictor and a central nervous system stimulant. Although little research has been done on the effects of nicotine and other chemical components of cigarettes on medication, studies indicate that the benzopyrenes in cigarettes may alter the metabolism of many medications through their action on liver enzymes. Most often, the nicotine-medication interaction interferes with the therapeutic action of the medication. With benzodiazepines and phenothiazines, however, cigarette smoking may have the beneficial effect of decreasing the adverse effect of drowsiness in some people. In many cases,

TABLE 18-10
Caffeine-Medication Interactions

Type of Interaction	Example of Interaction Effect
Caffeine-induced increase in gastric acid secretion	Decreased absorption of iron
Caffeine-induced gastrointestinal irritation	Decreased effectiveness of cimetidine; increased gastrointestinal irritation from corticosteroids, alcohol, and analgesics
Altered caffeine metabolism	Prolonged effect of caffeine when combined with ciprofloxacin, estrogen, or cimetidine
Caffeine-induced cardiac arrhythmic effect	Decreased effectiveness of antiarrhythmic medications
Caffeine-induced hypokalemia	Exacerbated hypokalemic effect of diuretics
Caffeine-induced stimulation of the central nervous system	Increased stimulation effects from amantadine, decongestants, fluoxetine, and theophylline
Caffeine-induced increase in excretion of lithium	Decreased effectiveness of lithium

smokers may require higher doses of a medication than nonsmokers to achieve the same therapeutic effects. For example, smokers may require increased doses of insulin, anticoagulants, antihypertensives, and pain relievers (Lee and D'Alonzo, 1993). Table 18-11 summarizes common nicotine-medication interactions that have been identified.

With the recent dramatic increase in the use of herbs by people in the United States, it is becoming increasingly important to address potential interactions between herbs and other bioactive agents. Although herbs are relatively safe, many herbs are similar, in terms of their bioactivity, to over-the-counter or prescription medications. Because of this similarity, it is impera-

TABLE 18-11
Nicotine-Medication Interactions

Type of Interaction	Example of Interaction Effect
Nicotine-induced alteration in metabolism	Decreased efficacy of analgesics, lorazepam, theophylline, aminophylline, beta-blockers, and calcium channel blockers
Nicotine-induced vasoconstriction	Increased peripheral ischemic effect of beta-blockers
Nicotine-induced central nervous system stimulation	Decreased drowsiness from benzodiazepines and phenothiazines
Nicotine-induced stimulation of antidiuretic hormone secretion	Fluid retention, decreased effectiveness of diuretics
Nicotine-induced increase in platelet activity	Decreased anticoagulant effectiveness (heparin, warfarin); increased risk of thrombosis with estrogen use
Nicotine-induced increase in gastric acid	Decreased or negated effects of H_2 antagonists (cimetidine, famotidine, nizatidine, ranitidine)

TABLE 18-12
Herbs and Medications with Similar Bioactivity

Medication	Herb
Aspirin	Birch bark
	Willow bark
	Wintergreen
	Meadowsweet
Anticoagulants	Feverfew
	Garlic
	Ginkgo biloba
Caffeine	Guarana
	Kola nut
Ephedrine	Ephedra
Estrogen	Black cohosh
	Fennel
	Red clover
	Stinging nettle
Lithium	Thyme
	Purslane
Monoamine oxidase inhibitors	Ginseng
	St. John's wort
	Yohimbe
Nicotine	Lobelia
Calcium channel blockers	Angelica

tive that health care professionals consider the possibility that herbs might have adverse, as well as therapeutic, effects resembling those of medications. Likewise, herbs can potentiate the effects of medications. Table 18-12 lists some herbs and medications that have similar bioactivity.

Mental Changes as Manifestations of Adverse Effects

Any medicated person may experience delirium, dementia, or depression as adverse medication effects. Older adults, however, are at increased risk for these effects because of the increased likelihood of medication-medication interactions in this population, and because of age-related changes in homeostatic mechanisms and the central nervous system. Even so, mental changes in older adults, especially if they are subtle or superimposed on a dementia, are not usually attributed to adverse medication effects. Nurses need to be alert to the possibility that even a simple over-the-counter product, such as aspirin, may be the underlying, undetected cause of mental changes in older adults (Bailey and Jones, 1989; Courts, 1996). If aspirin is taken with an herb that has a similar action, the potential for toxicity may be increased (refer to Table 18-12).

Delirium is an acute confusional state that can be precipitated by any medication or by medication interactions. Older adults are particularly susceptible to medication-induced delirium because of altered neurochemical activity in the brain. Moreover, their risk of medication-induced delirium is increased by some pathologic conditions, such as dementia, dehydration, malnutrition, head injury, or central nervous system infection. Older adults are particularly susceptible to delirium resulting from the anticholinergic actions of many psychotropic agents and of over-the-counter preparations for coughs, colds, and insomnia. Even at nontoxic serum levels, or at doses considered to be normal, medications can cause mental changes in older adults. Some medications that are likely to cause mental changes in older adults, as well as the mechanisms underlying these adverse actions, are listed in Table 18-13.

Tardive Dyskinesia

Tardive dyskinesia, a potential side effect of most antipsychotic medications, can cause serious and irreversible negative functional consequences, especially in older adults. Signs include involuntary movements of the jaw, lips, mouth, and tongue; rhythmic movements of the trunk or extremities; and, less commonly, respiratory irregularities. The earliest signs are usually fine, wormlike movements of the tongue. Other early signs include chewing, grimacing, lip smacking,

TABLE 18-13

Mechanisms of Action for Mental Changes Caused by Adverse Medication Reactions

Mechanism of Action	Examples
Anticholinergic interactions	Atropine, scopolamine, antihistamines, antipsychotics, antidepressants, antispasmodics, antiparkinsonian agents
Decreased cerebral blood flow	Antihypertensives, antipsychotics
Depression of respiratory center	Central nervous system depressants
Fluid and electrolyte alterations	Diuretics, alcohol, laxatives
Altered thermoregulation	Alcohol, psychotropics, narcotics
Acidosis	Diuretics, alcohol, nicotinic acid
Hypoglycemia	Hypoglycemics, alcohol, propranolol
Hormonal disturbances	Thyroid extract, corticosteroids
Depression-inducing action	Reserpine, methyldopa, indomethacin, barbiturates, fluphenazine, haloperidol, corticosteroids

jaw clenching, eye blinking, and side-to-side jaw movements. The onset of these signs occurs as early as 3 to 6 months after initiation of antipsychotic medications, or even earlier in older people.

Although tardive dyskinesia is relatively rare in comparison to other adverse medication effects, it deserves special attention with regard to older adults for the following reasons:

1. Older adults are 5 to 6 times more likely than younger adults to experience tardive dyskinesia.
2. Advanced age correlates with both an earlier onset and increased severity of tardive dyskinesia.
3. The chance of reversing tardive dyskinesia decreases with increasing age.

4. When combined with age-related changes and risk factors, tardive dyskinesia can seriously impair the ability of the older adult to perform activities of daily living (ADL).
5. When combined with psychosocial influences, the negative impact of tardive dyskinesia on self-esteem can be especially detrimental.
6. Tardive dyskinesia is associated with the long-term use of antipsychotic medications, which are sometimes used inappropriately in older adults for behaviors that could be managed with nonmedication interventions.

The incidence of tardive dyskinesia increases with increased age of the patient and duration of therapy, and it is associated equally with all antipsychotic medications. One study revealed that tardive dyskinesia developed in 35.4% of older patients taking neuroleptic drugs (Yassa et al., 1992). Factors that may increase the risk for development of tardive dyskinesia include dementia, depression, age-related neurochemical changes, and early extrapyramidal reactions to medications. Anticholinergic medications, often prescribed in combination with an antipsychotic to decrease medication-induced tremors, may worsen or precipitate tardive dyskinesia. The reversibility of tardive dyskinesia depends on early detection of the signs and discontinuation of the causative medication(s). In recent years, vitamin E has been used effectively to reverse tardive dyskinesia in some patients.

Noncompliance

Many studies have been conducted on patient compliance with medication regimens. Definitions and conclusions vary, but much emphasis has been placed on the high incidence of noncompliance among older adults. Although advanced age may be a factor that contributes to noncompliance, it is widely agreed that noncompliance occurs in about 50% of all adults for whom long-term medication regimens have been prescribed. Other factors that have been found to contribute to noncompliance include living alone, financial considerations, type of disease, adverse medication effects, complex medication regimens, increased frequency of dosing, cognitive and sensory impairments, poor understanding of the medication regimen, and the relationship between the patient and the primary care practitioner.

Psychosocial Consequences of Adverse Effects

Older adults experience serious psychosocial consequences when adverse medication effects precipitate mental changes, especially if the cause of the mental change is not recognized. Depression, delirium, and dementia interfere with one's functional abilities and quality of life and, if not reversed, may have long-term or permanent detrimental effects. It is important to keep in mind that medication-induced mental changes do not always subside immediately after the offending medication is discontinued. In some cases, it may take several weeks after the medication is decreased or discontinued before mental function returns to the premedication level. Other adverse medication effects can cause serious and long-term detrimental psychosocial consequences through their effects on functional abilities. For example, medication-induced postural hypotension has been identified as a contributing factor in falls and fractured hips. Figure 18-1 summarizes age-related changes, risk factors, and functional consequences as they relate to medications and the older adult.

Nursing Assessment

The purposes of the medication assessment are: (1) to determine the effectiveness of the medication regimen; (2) to identify any factors that interfere with the correct regimen; (3) to ascertain risks for adverse effects or altered therapeutic actions (with particular attention to older adults at increased risk), and (4) to detect ad-

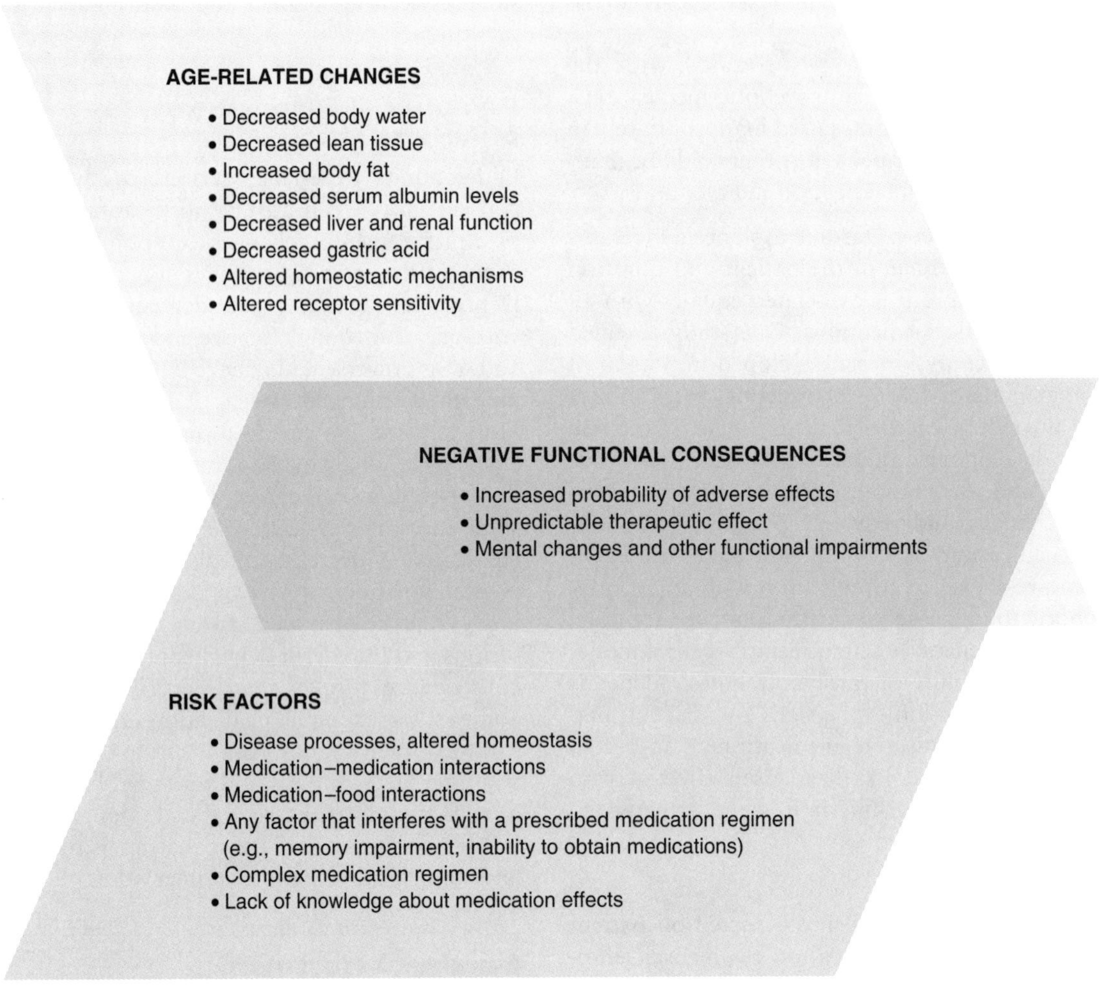

AGE-RELATED CHANGES

- Decreased body water
- Decreased lean tissue
- Increased body fat
- Decreased serum albumin levels
- Decreased liver and renal function
- Decreased gastric acid
- Altered homeostatic mechanisms
- Altered receptor sensitivity

NEGATIVE FUNCTIONAL CONSEQUENCES

- Increased probability of adverse effects
- Unpredictable therapeutic effect
- Mental changes and other functional impairments

RISK FACTORS

- Disease processes, altered homeostasis
- Medication–medication interactions
- Medication–food interactions
- Any factor that interferes with a prescribed medication regimen
  (e.g., memory impairment, inability to obtain medications)
- Complex medication regimen
- Lack of knowledge about medication effects

FIGURE 18-1. Medications and older adults.

verse medication effects. During a medication interview, the nurse clarifies the prescribed medication regimen, as well as the actual medication-taking behavior, which may differ from the prescribed regimen. Interview information and observations about medications are then incorporated into the overall functional assessment to accomplish the goals of the medication assessment.

Techniques for Obtaining Medication Information

Obtaining accurate information about prescribed medications and actual medication-taking behaviors is difficult for a variety of reasons. First, older adults may be reluctant to answer questions about their medications because they perceive this information, along with information about the use of alcohol, as being very private. Many older adults have received care from primary care practitioners who have communicated an attitude of secrecy about prescription medications, blood pressure readings, and other aspects of medical care. Although this attitude of secrecy is no longer common among health care providers, many older adults have learned not to ask questions, and they may believe that they are not entitled to information about medical aspects of their care. Also, they may be unsure of what questions to ask. Many older adults welcome the opportunity to discuss medications with a nurse, but they may initially hesitate to ask questions or share information. Once the nurse has established a trusting relationship and has initiated a medication interview, the assessment often provides an excellent basis for uncovering and discussing many questions about medications.

A second barrier to obtaining accurate medication information is the older adult's fear of judgment, especially if the prescribed regimen is not being followed exactly, or if home remedies, alternative therapies, or over-the-counter medications are being used. Because people are reluc-

tant to admit that they do not follow the health care practitioner's orders exactly as expected, they are likely to recite the prescribed regimen, rather than describe what they actually do. People also may be reluctant to discuss the reasons they do not follow a medication regimen, and this can create additional barriers. For example, older adults who cannot afford medications may be embarrassed to discuss their limited finances.

Therefore, it is essential that the nurse ask open-ended questions and convey a nonjudgmental attitude during the medication interview. For example, if the question "Are you taking anyone else's medications?" is asked in a matter-of-fact way, an honest response may be elicited. However, asking the question "Do you ever miss a dose of medication?" rather than asking "What do you do when you miss a dose of medicine?" may elicit a defensive denial. People are more likely to be honest if they view the nurse as a problem solver, rather than as an authority figure bent on criticizing their health habits. Information about the use of home remedies and over-the-counter preparations is more likely to be elicited by posing open-ended questions than by asking specific questions about medications used for particular problems. For example, the question "What do you do to help you sleep?" is more open-ended than the question "Do you take any medications for sleep?" because the latter may be interpreted only in relation to prescription medications.

Questions about the person's ability to obtain prescribed medications may elicit information about transportation or financial problems that interfere with adherence to the medication regimen. Other barriers can be identified by asking questions such as, "Do you have any trouble swallowing these capsules?" or "Do you have any difficulty getting the caps off your medication bottles?" Someone who cannot remember to take all the medications as prescribed, or who is not motivated to take all of the medications, may be reluctant to acknowledge these factors. Thus, the nurse must assess the cognitive and motivational factors that influence the person's medication-taking behaviors.

Time limitations and lack of a trusting relationship may present additional barriers to obtaining an accurate medication assessment. Medication interviews often are very time-consuming, and so it may be necessary to obtain the information during two or more visits. The older adult may not think of all the information during the first interview or may be reluctant to reveal accurate information. Information obtained from an interview with the older adult can be supplemented by information derived from caregivers and direct observations of the older person. A nonthreatening technique that may elicit more accurate information than direct questions is to ask about the person's method of organizing medications. For example, people taking medications often have a method of organizing their regimen by using divided medication boxes or written charts or schedules. They usually are willing to show this to the nurse and, in fact, may be proud to discuss their method with the nurse during the medication assessment.

If the interview is conducted in the home setting, it is helpful to ask the older person to show the nurse all the medications used. In settings other than the home, the person may be willing to bring medications to the interview if asked to do so ahead of time. In community settings, such as senior meal programs, nurses might sponsor a "brown bag" medication session. Program participants are asked to bring all their medications with them to an educational session, during which the nurse provides group education and individual assessment and counseling regarding medications. Because older people often are very comfortable discussing medications with their peers, this method is both nonthreatening and quite effective.

Direct observation of medication containers can also provide useful information, such as the actual prescription instructions and the dates of prescription refills. Nurses must use this information cautiously, however, because the labels on prescriptions are not always up-to-date, and the medications in the containers may not be the ones that originally were in the containers. Inconsistencies between the labels and the contents of prescription containers may be used as a basis for further questioning. For example, if the label indicates that the original prescription was for 30 pills and the prescription has not been refilled for 1 year, the nurse might inquire about the reason for this. The patient may explain that the prescription is so expensive that the person takes it only occasionally. Often the nurse will find that the original container is not being used because it has a childproof cap that the person cannot manipulate. The pills may then be stored in incorrectly labeled containers, which increases the risk of inaccurate consumption.

Another reason for direct examination of medication containers is to discover information about sources of care and duplication of medications. People who are seeing more than one health care practitioner may not acknowledge multiple sources of prescriptions, but this information can be discovered by reading prescription labels. Nurses also may discover that the same or similar medications are being prescribed by more than one health care practitioner, or under more than one brand name. With the growing popularity of generic medications and the increasing number of brand names and similar medications, the likelihood of duplicate medications is increasing. The person taking the medication often is unaware of duplications, especially if the medications are dispensed with different names on the labels.

Dates on labels also reveal important information that can lead to additional questions. For example, if there are three types of antihypertensive medications, each prescribed at a different time, the nurse can inquire whether the second or third medication was supposed to replace or supplement the original medication. Finally, checking the prescription container can provide valuable clues to compliance. By looking at the date on the label, the amount of the last refill, and the contents of the prescription container, nurses can make a rough estimate of the consumption pattern.

In the 1960s, Doris Schwartz, a nurse-researcher who was among the first to investigate problems of medication use and the elderly, advocated the use of a 24-hour drug history, similar to a nutrition history, to gather information (Schwartz et al., 1962). Such a history may be obtained by asking the older person about a typical day: "When you first get up in the morning, what medicine do you take?" "What medicine is next?" and so on, continuing through the day and night in this way. This approach is more likely to elicit accurate information than simply asking the person to recite the prescribed regimen. Additional examples of tools for assessment of medications can be found in the recent nursing literature (e.g., Hahn and Wietor, 1992).

Components of a Comprehensive Medication Assessment

During the medication interview, the nurse should inquire about prescription and over-the-counter medications, home remedies, vitamins and minerals, and herbal and homeopathic remedies, as well as alcohol, caffeine, and nicotine. Questions should be asked, not only about pills and liquid medications administered orally, but also about remedies and medications administered by any other route (e.g., nasal, aural, topical, optical, injection, or dermal patch medications). Nurses must be alert to the increasing use of alternative products and should include open-ended questions about any products that might be considered nontraditional in Western cultures. It may be advisable to include a question about various sources of health care, particularly when interviewing someone who may be likely to seek health care from non-Western health care practitioners. Herbalists, spiritual healers, naturopathic practitioners, and Ayurvedic doctors may be sources of alternative and complementary remedies. The Culture Box on p. 512 summarizes some culturally specific sources of health care and treatment modalities that might be used by older adults.

Most herbs, home remedies, and alternative products contain relatively safe doses of active ingredients; however, some have the potential for interactions and adverse effects (see Tables 18-6 and 18-12). A discussion of home remedies and alternative health care practices may be valuable in identifying health beliefs and in obtaining information about medication-taking behaviors. Also, it is important to elicit information about medications that are used only sporadically or as needed, because these can contribute to medication interactions, erratic medication effects, and adverse effects when they are taken. Information about doses of vitamins and minerals is important because megavitamins or high doses of some preparations may be harmful. For example, pyridoxine (vitamin B_6) can interfere with coordination or cause peripheral neuropathy at doses greater than the recommended dietary allowance. Moreover, even low doses of iron or calcium carbonate can be constipating.

Information about the brand names of over-the-counter medications is important in identifying additives that may be causing problems or increasing the risk of altered medication action. Examples of additives that may cause difficulties are caffeine in some analgesics, lactose in some antacids, or highly allergenic sulfites in some bronchodilators. Reading the labels on over-the-counter medications is a reliable way of finding out about some additives, such as caffeine, if the nurse is not familiar with ingredients in specific brand names. Keep in mind, however, that the FDA does not require the listing of so-called inert ingredients, such as sulfites, other preservatives, or dissolving agents.

One of the most important aspects of the medication interview is assessing the person's

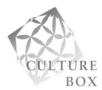

Culturally Specific Health Care Sources and Practices

Cultural Group	Sources of Care*	Common Practices*
African Americans	Home remedies, faith healers, "church nurses"	Folk remedies (e.g., teas, herbs); magic or voodoo (especially in rural areas)
American Indians	Native practitioners	Roots, herbs, physical modalities (e.g., purification rituals)
Cambodians (Khmer)	Vietnamese or Cambodian practitioners	Herbs, medicated strips of adhesive tape, and physical modalities
Chinese Americans	Herbalists, acupuncturists	Herbs, food, beverages, and other remedies to balance yin and yang
Japanese Americans	Herbalists	Herbs, self-care practices
Mexican Americans	Traditional healers, pharmacists	Herbs, teas, soups, rituals, physical modalities (massage, manipulation)
Puerto Ricans	Pharmacists	Tea, herbs, folk remedies
Russians	Folk remedies	Herbal teas, sweet liquor, physical modalities (oils, ointments, enemas, mud baths)
South Asians (Indo-Americans)	Homeopathic or Ayurvedic doctors, spiritual healers	Yoga, diet, fasting, prayer, rituals

Source: J. G. Lipson, S. L. Dibble & P. A. Minarik, (1996), *Culture & nursing care: A pocket guide* (San Francisco: UCSF Nursing Press).

*In the United States, Western practitioners and medicine often are used in conjunction with these sources of care and common practices.

understanding of the purpose of medications. This information reflects not only the person's understanding of the medication regimen, but also the person's understanding of overall health problems. Misinformation or a lack of information can provide clues about the communication patterns between the patient and the primary care practitioner, as well as about the person's interest in and understanding of his or her own health status. As with other parts of the medication assessment, it is essential to phrase questions in as open-ended and nonjudgmental a manner as possible. Asking "What do you take this pill for?" with a tone of curiosity will likely elicit more information than asking questions such as, "What do you take for your heart?" or

"Why do you take digoxin?" Nurses cannot assume that the person has been told the reason for a particular medication, or that the person fully understood the explanation that was provided. The person's explanations for taking or not taking medications can lay the groundwork for many hours of health teaching!

Another aspect of the nursing assessment is obtaining and documenting information about the person's perception of and preferences for various forms of medications (see the Culture Box below). This information may be important in decisions about medication interventions, especially when there are several options that may be equally effective. Similarly, nurses should assess the older adult for any cultural factors that might influence compliance or the person's understanding of the purpose of the medication. For example, Chinese people are likely to perceive illness as an imbalance of hot and cold forces. If the illness makes the body hot, then the remedy should make it cooler. Teaching about medications should be framed accordingly. Practical information about illness and health

beliefs from many cultural perspectives is described in an excellent pocket guide, written by nurses, entitled *Culture and Nursing Care* (Lipson et al., 1996).

Finally, information about allergies and adverse reactions is important because anyone with a history of medication-related problems will need to be closely monitored, especially if the medications being administered are similar to those that caused the reaction. Sometimes people state that they are allergic to a medication, but when they are asked about the symptoms, they describe an adverse effect, rather than an allergic reaction. Therefore, rather than simply documenting that the person is allergic to a certain medication, the nurse should document the specific reaction that occurred if the person can describe it. Nurses can organize the data about medication regimens in a list or chart that is revised and updated as additional information is obtained and changes are made in the regimen. Older adults in community settings can be taught and encouraged to keep their own medication charts. Display 18-1 summarizes the in-

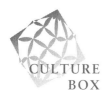

CULTURE BOX

Cultural Considerations with Regard to Medication Assessment and Interventions

- Medications that are not readily available or that are prescription medications in the United States may be available over the counter in other countries, such as Mexico, Canada, and Latin American countries.
- Older Hispanics may view wine and other forms of alcohol as a food staple, not a social drug, because it may be used as a healthy alternative to potentially contaminated water in their home country.
- People of Vietnamese and other cultural groups may view injections as being more effective than pills, and pills as being more effective than drops.
- Some Chinese and other Asian people may have the following preferences:

  - Balms and ointments rather than pills for local pain
  - Teas and soups rather than antacids for indigestion
  - Herbs rather than prescription drugs

- Teaching about medications should be done in the context of culturally based beliefs about health, illness, and remedies.

DISPLAY 18-1
Guidelines for Medication Assessment

Information About the Therapeutic Agents

- Prescription pills, liquids, injections, eye drops, ear drops, nasal sprays, transdermal patches, and topical preparations
- Over-the-counter preparations (identified by brand names) that are used regularly or occasionally
- Vitamins, minerals, and nutritional supplements
- Pattern of alcohol, caffeine, or tobacco use
- Herbs and herbal preparations
- Homeopathic remedies
- Home remedies
- Sources of health care

Interview Questions to Assess Medication-Taking Behaviors

- How would you describe your usual daily routine for taking medications and remedies, beginning when you get up in the morning?
- Is there anything else you do or use to treat illness or to maintain your health, such as using herbs, ointments, home remedies, or nutritional supplements?
- Are you taking anyone else's medications?
- What do you do when you miss a dose of medication?
- What do you take for constipation? What do you do to help you sleep (or to alleviate any other identified problem)?
- How do you get your prescriptions filled? (Where do you get your remedies?)
- Do you have any difficulty taking your pills?
- What method do you use to keep track of your medications and remedies?
- Is there anything you do to help you remember to take your medicines or remedies at the appropriate time?

Interview Questions to Assess the Person's Understanding of the Purpose of Medications and Other Remedies

- What is this medication (or herb, etc.) for?
- For medications (or remedies) that are used

as needed (p.r.n.): How do you decide when to take this pill (or remedy)?
- What did your health care practitioner tell you about this medication (or herb, etc.)?
- What problems were you having when the health care practitioner prescribed this medication (or suggested that you use this remedy)?

Interview Questions to Elicit Additional Information

- Are there any medications or remedies you were taking at one time, but are no longer taking?
- Have you ever had an allergic reaction, or any other bad reaction, to a medication or remedy? (If yes, describe what happened.)
- Where do you store your medications and remedies?

Questions and Observations Based on Reading of Prescription Labels

- Who is the prescribing health care practitioner?
- If there is more than one health care practitioner, does each practitioner know all the medications that are being used?
- Are any medications the same or similar and prescribed by different health care practitioners?
- If the dates on various prescriptions are different, were the later medications supposed to be added to the medication regimen, or were they intended to replace previously prescribed medications?
- Are the date of the last refill and the number of pills in the bottle consistent with the prescribed regimen?

formation that is included in a medication assessment.

Relationship Between the Medication Assessment and the Overall Assessment

The nurse uses information from the medication interview in conjunction with the overall health assessment in several ways. First, information about past and present medication behaviors may provide clues to identified problems or complaints. For example, if the person complains of nervousness or difficulty sleeping, the nurse can inquire about the use of caffeine-containing medications. Information about recent medication-taking behaviors can also shed light on current problems, such as the recurrence of symptoms that once were controlled by medications. For example, if someone stopped taking an antiarrhythmic medication, symptoms of dizziness may be related to this. Recent medication-taking behaviors also may account for health problems that are residual or latent adverse medication effects. Examples of residual adverse effects include arthritic changes after a vaccination, blood dyscrasia after a course of chloramphenicol, diarrhea occurring after a course of antibiotics, and gastrointestinal symptoms arising from the administration of anti-inflammatory medications.

Second, the overall health assessment provides the basis for evaluating the effectiveness of a medication regimen. Nurses are responsible for determining the expected and actual outcomes and usual dosage of medications. The expected outcomes of medications usually are evaluated through subjective and objective assessment information. For example, analgesic effectiveness is measured by the person's report of pain relief, and the effectiveness of antihypertensive medications is judged according to lowered blood pressure readings. Third, the overall health assessment will help answer the question Can the person, or caregivers, safely and effectively administer medications? This is a complex question that addresses all of the following functional areas: cognitive ability to understand the regimen and remember to perform medication-related tasks; motivation to perform the tasks; and physical skills to obtain and administer the medication. Some physical skills that may be required include visual acuity, manual dexterity, and an ability to swallow. The environment also should be assessed in relation to certain conditions, such as accessibility of water and the availability of a refrigerator (if this is necessary for medication storage), that can affect medication-taking behaviors. The overall assessment also might provide information about financial limitations or mobility or transportation problems that interfere with obtaining medications.

Fourth, if the home environment can be observed as part of the overall assessment, important clues to health problems and medication-taking behaviors may be disclosed. For example, observing that nitroglycerin is stored on a window sill may explain why the medication is not effective in relieving angina. An assessment of the home environment also may lead to additional pertinent information, as when the nurse notices over-the-counter preparations and home remedies on a kitchen counter and asks about these items. Finally, the overall health assessment serves as the basis for identifying older adults who are at high risk for adverse effects or altered therapeutic effects. Many physiologic and psychosocial factors can increase the risk for altered medication effects, and many older adults have more than one risk factor. In contrast to the more clearly evident risk factors, such as several concurrent illnesses or multiple medications, some risk factors may be subtle and could be overlooked unless a comprehensive assessment is undertaken. For example, exposure to environmental chemicals is a potential health hazard that may become increasingly significant in those who are taking medications. Environmental chemicals can increase the burden on the liver and renal pathways by raising

DISPLAY 18-2
Characteristics of People Who Are at High Risk for Altered
Medication Effects

- Inclusion of several medications in the drug regimen
- Debilitated or frail state
- Malnourishment or dehydration
- Multiple illnesses
- An illness that interferes with cardiac, renal, or hepatic function
- Cognitive impairment
- Medication allergy

- History of adverse medication effects
- Exposure to certain environmental chemicals
- Fever, which can alter the action of certain medications
- Recent change in health or functional status (e.g., as a result of an accident, surgery, mental changes, or insertion of a nasogastric tube)

the "total body chemical burden." People who may be exposed to environmental chemicals include farmers who work with pesticides, cab drivers who are exposed to automotive exhaust, and painters and other people who work with paints and solvents. Information about occupational activities that increase the risk for exposure to environmental chemicals should be considered in conjunction with the medication assessment. Display 18-2 summarizes some of the factors that increase the risk of altered medication effects. The presence of one or more of these risk factors markedly increases the potential for adverse effects and altered therapeutic effects.

Recognition of Adverse Effects

The first, and sometimes most difficult, step in alleviating adverse medication effects is to recognize their existence. Because many adverse effects are subtle and superimposed on one or more symptoms of illness, they often are attributed to pathologic conditions rather than to the treatment of the condition. Nurses often are the first to recognize adverse medication effects because they generally spend more time with patients than do primary care practitioners. Nurses also are more attentive to long-term monitoring of changes in day-to-day function, in contrast to the focus on acute illnesses of medical practitioners. Especially in long-term care and home

settings, the nurse is the health professional most likely to notice subtle changes in function that may be attributable to adverse medication effects. In community settings, older adults often view the nurse as the health care professional who is most accessible for a discussion of medication regimens.

Primary care practitioners may hesitate to discuss adverse medication effects with patients for any of the following reasons: (1) they may be uncertain about the potential adverse effects of a prescribed drug, especially when newer medications are prescribed; (2) they may assume that the power of suggesting possible adverse effects will become a self-fulfilling prophecy; or (3) they may fear that the patient will choose not to take the medication. The nurse can serve as an interpreter between the prescribing practitioner and the patient by emphasizing the medication's benefits, as well as pointing out the problems that are most likely to arise. The nurse also can educate the patient about ways to avoid adverse effects. For example, if a medication is likely to cause stomach irritation, this adverse effect may be avoided by taking the medication after meals or with milk. The nurse should not automatically initiate a discussion of all the potential adverse effects of a medication, but when a change in the person's health status may be related to adverse medication effects, the nurse can raise that possibility.

Changes in mental status are a potentially devastating adverse medication effect that is often overlooked as such, especially when superimposed on an existing dementia. Any medication-related change in mental status, such as confusion, lethargy, depression, or agitation, can be sudden and obvious or subtle and gradual. Mental status changes, such as delirium or hallucinations, usually are very obvious, but they may be attributed mistakenly to pathologic processes, rather than to medication effects. Whenever an older person experiences changes in mental status, medication intake must be assessed carefully. Over-the-counter medications and alcohol consumption must be considered, especially in relation to medication interactions. Questions that must be asked include the following:

- Can any medications be eliminated?
- Can any doses be lowered?
- Is the mental change interfering with consumption patterns and causing additional problems? (For example, if the person's memory is impaired because of adverse medication effects, is the person taking too much medication and experiencing further mental changes?)

The alleviation of adverse medication effects does not always immediately follow discontinuation of the medication or a dosage adjustment. It may take a few days or several weeks before mental function returns to the premedication level. The resolution time depends on the particular medication(s) involved, the length of time it was consumed, and the person's general health status.

Nursing Diagnosis

When the nursing assessment identifies factors that interfere with the correct medication regimen, the nurse can address these problems with an appropriate nursing diagnosis. The nursing diagnosis of Noncompliance is defined as "the state in which an individual or group desires to comply but factors are present that deter adherence to health-related advice given by health professionals" (Carpenito, 1997, p. 574). Related factors that might be identified include functional impairments, complex medication regimens, inadequate social supports, adverse effects of medication(s), lack of money or transportation, and lack of understanding of instructions. When a functional deficit (e.g., impaired cognition, sensory impairment) is the underlying problem that interferes with safe medication self-administration, the nursing diagnosis of Instrumental Self-Care Deficit could be used. This is defined as "a state in which the individual experiences an impaired ability to perform certain activities or access certain services essential for managing a household" (Carpenito, 1997, p. 752).

If the nursing assessment identifies adverse effects of medications, particularly those that affect one's quality of life, the nurse might address these through a nursing diagnosis that is specific to the adverse effect. Examples of nursing diagnoses that might be related to adverse medication effects include Constipation, Urinary Incontinence, Altered Nutrition, Impaired Cognition, Ineffective Thermoregulation, Sexual Dysfunction, Sleep Pattern Disturbances, Impaired Physical Mobility, and High Risk for Injury because of medication-related falls and postural hypotension. These nursing diagnoses are discussed in other chapters of this text.

Nursing Goals

Nursing care of medicated older adults is directed toward enhancing the therapeutic effectiveness of medications, reducing the risk of adverse effects, and minimizing the negative functional consequences of adverse effects. Two goals for an older adult with the nursing diagnosis of Noncompliance are that the person verbalize correct information about their medication regimen and that they demonstrate the ability to take their medications as directed. A nursing goal for an older adult who is experiencing an adverse medication effect is that the negative consequence be alleviated or controlled. These goals are accomplished by educating older adults and their caregivers and by facilitating communication between older adults and health care providers. Decreasing the number of medications is another intervention designed to achieve these goals.

Another goal is to reduce the risk of adverse medication effects. A well-nourished and adequately hydrated person is less likely to experience adverse medication effects than a person who is undernourished or malnourished, or underhydrated or dehydrated. Therefore, any interventions that improve the person's hydration or nutritional status will decrease the risk of adverse effects. Similarly, a mentally alert person is less likely than a cognitively impaired person to experience adverse medication effects. Thus, any interventions aimed at improving mental alertness, including elimination of unnecessary psychotropic medications, will decrease the risk of adverse medication effects.

Nursing Interventions

Educating Older Adults and Their Caregivers

Medications are most therapeutic and least risky when they are taken as prescribed, and when the medication regimen is periodically reevaluated for maximum effectiveness and minimal risk of adverse reactions. Because most community-living older adults take medications with little advice or supervision from health professionals, education about medications can be an effective intervention to promote responsible medication-taking behaviors.

An easy and nonthreatening way to begin medication education is to have the person write a list of all medications taken, including over-the-counter preparations. This list also should specify any medication allergies. The nurse should explain that the list should be carried with the person at all times because it is a convenient way of helping health professionals keep track of the person's medications. If the person seeks the care of more than one health care practitioner, this list is especially important. The nurse should explain that a medication list facilitates communication and reminds the health care practitioner to reevaluate the medication regimen. The nurse can discuss each medication as it is listed and provide appropriate information based on an assessment of the person's knowledge and understanding. The person might ask additional questions, and the nurse usually will have ample opportunities for medication education while the list is being written.

People often are unsure about what information they are entitled to know about their medications. Older adults, especially, may perceive an aura of secrecy about prescription medications or may be reluctant to question their health care practitioners. Therefore, in any discussion of medications, the nurse should suggest pertinent questions that older persons might ask their primary health care provider. In addition, nurses can educate older adults and their caregivers about obtaining medication-related information from knowledgeable sources, such as pharmacists. People need to understand that prescribing practitioners are skilled in diagnosing illnesses and deciding the most appropriate interventions, and that pharmacists are the health care professionals who are most knowledgeable about the specific actions and interactions of medications. Nurses can explain which medication questions are most appropriate for prescribing practitioners and which are most appropriate for pharmacists. Display 18-3 can serve as a basis of medication education for older adults.

DISPLAY 18-3
Tips for Older Adults to Ensure the Safe and Effective Use of Medications

- Carry an up-to-date list of all your medications, including herbs and over-the-counter preparations, and show the list to your health care practitioner(s).
- When your health care practitioner suggests a medication, ask if there is any way to take care of the problem without medication.
- Ask your health care practitioner the following questions about each new, regularly scheduled medication:
  - What is the reason for taking the medication?
  - How will I know if it's doing what it's meant to do?
  - How soon can I expect to feel the beneficial effects?
  - What will happen if I don't take it?
  - How often am I supposed to take it?
  - How long should I continue taking it?
  - What should I do if I miss a dose?
  - When will you want to see me again, and what will you want me to tell you so that you can determine whether the medication is effective?
- Ask your health care practitioner the following questions at follow-up visits:
  - Do I still need to take this medication?
  - Can the dosage be reduced?
- Ask your health care practitioner the following questions about each medication that is prescribed on an "as-needed" (p.r.n.) basis:
  - What is the reason for taking the medication, and how should I determine whether I need the medication?
  - How often can I take it? Is there a range of frequency?
  - What is the maximum dose I can take within 24 hours?
  - What should I do if the medication does not relieve the symptoms (e.g., if chest pain continues after taking several nitroglycerin tablets)?
- Ask your pharmacist the following questions:
  - What are the generic and brand names for this medication?
  - Is it likely to interact with the other medications I'm taking?
  - Is it likely to interact with herbs, cigarettes, alcohol, or any nutrient?
  - What is the best time of day to take it?
  - Does it matter if I take it before or after meals?
  - Are there any side effects I should watch for?
  - Is there anything I can do to minimize the risk of side effects (e.g., taking the medication with milk or meals to reduce stomach irritation)?
  - Is there anything I should avoid while I'm taking this medication (e.g., milk, certain foods, driving)?
  - Are there any special instructions for storing this medication?

Nurses also can educate older adults and caregivers about using consumer references for information about herbs, homeopathy, medications, and alternative therapies. Particularly in community settings, the nurse might use such a book with the older adult and demonstrate how to obtain pertinent information. People taking medications may be interested in purchasing a reference, obtaining one from the library, or using the Internet for information. The nurse can indicate that some good references have been published in recent years, but that some of the books are biased and some information should be used cautiously. Although older adults may find valuable information in these references, they should be advised that it is best to discuss specific remedies and medications with a health professional who can interpret the information in relation to the person's unique situation.

Finally, education of older adults and caregivers must address economic issues that influence the purchase of medications. For example, nurses may be asked to give advice about the most economical way to purchase medications, or about the use of generic medications or sample medications. Although many generic medications are approved as bioequivalent by the FDA, studies have found variations in the bioavailability of insulin, lithium, phenytoin, prednisone, digitalis, tetracycline, sulfonamides, thyroid preparations, and many other medications (Todd, 1985). Differences between generic and brand name medications, as well as differences between brand names, can be the basis for an altered therapeutic effect or an increased risk for adverse effects. Older adults should be encouraged to purchase their medications from a reputable pharmacy and to ask questions about generic and brand names. If possible, they should avoid changing products; if a change is made, they should watch for possible alterations in medication effects.

When people begin a new medication regimen, they may have the entire prescription filled because this is more economical than purchasing smaller quantities. Nurses can instruct patients to explain to the pharmacist that they have a new prescription and that they want only a few days' supply of the drug so they can determine its effectiveness. Many pharmacists will fill the smaller quantity at the same cost rate as the larger quantity if the customer intends to purchase the entire prescription after the trial doses. This method saves money if the medication is not effective. In addition, this method deters the person from finishing the prescribed medication, even if it is not effective, or from saving the unused portion just because it has been purchased.

Economic issues arise when new medications are prescribed and the person cannot afford the typical cost of a dollar or more per day for medications. Even a person who has an adequate income may decide that a medication is not worth the cost, especially on an ongoing basis. A person taking the generic form of an older medication, especially one that costs only a few cents per pill, may strongly object to switching to a newer medication that costs 50 cents or more per pill. Nurses can encourage older adults to be candid with their health care practitioners in discussing this issue, and to inquire whether a less costly medication might be just as effective as the more expensive one.

Communicating with Health Care Professionals

Because good communication skills are essential to obtaining answers to the questions listed in Display 18-3, it may be necessary for the nurse to suggest ways of communicating effectively with pharmacists and other health care practitioners. For example, before visits for health or medical care, the person can prepare a list of questions to discuss with the health care practitioner. The nurse can help write this list and can suggest which questions are most important for each medication. Regarding communication with pharmacists, nurses can suggest that older adults call the pharmacist at a time of day, such as late morning, that is less likely to be as busy as a peak time. Again, it is helpful to prepare a list of questions that the pharmacist can answer about each medication. In home settings, nurses might call the health care practitioner to discuss medications in the presence of the older adult or caregiver. By demonstrating good communication skills, the nurse will serve as a role model. If older adults or their caregivers can hear the nurse discussing medications using plain English, rather than medical terminology, they may acquire confidence about their own ability to communicate with health professionals.

Decreasing the Number of Medications

Because the chance of adverse medication effects increases in proportion to the number of medications consumed, a key intervention is to decrease the number of medications to as few as possible. This is accomplished by coordinating the efforts of the prescriber(s) to discontinue duplicate medications or medications that are no longer appropriate, and by educating the older person about the judicious use of medications that are not medically necessary. Nurses have many opportunities to raise questions about medication regimens and to communicate with prescribing practitioners about medications. In long-term care facilities, nurses have a great deal of autonomy regarding medications. In home settings, also, nurses have a great deal of autonomy in working with older adults and their caregivers regarding medication regimens, especially those medications prescribed as needed, rather than on a regular schedule.

When older adults are admitted to acute care facilities, they may receive care from a primary care practitioner who has not cared for them before or who has not prescribed many of their medications. The nurse usually is the health professional who obtains the medication history on admission, and the prescribing practitioner may automatically order the medications that are listed on the nursing assessment. Careful questioning of the older adult, or the caregivers of dependent older adults, by the nurse may help identify some medications that are either unnecessary or duplicative. The nurse may even discover that medications or medication interactions contribute to or directly cause the problem for which the patient is hospitalized. The nurse is responsible for raising questions about preadmission medication regimens, rather than assuming that the regimen is safe, effective, and warranted. The hospital admission may be the ideal time to reevaluate the medication regimen, and the medication history obtained by the nurse on admission may provide a basis for this evaluation.

When medications are prescribed for comfort, or for behavioral rather than medical reasons, the nurse is responsible for educating the older adult and his or her caregivers about these medications and potential nonmedication alternatives. Older adults may request antianxiety medications because they perceive medications as a simple and safe solution to "nervousness."

Nursing staff in institutional settings or caregivers of dependent older adults in home settings may request medications for management of undesirable behaviors. After these medications are prescribed, they often are given or taken over long periods of time without reevaluation, even though the situation may have changed. It is especially important, therefore, to educate older adults and their caregivers about medications, such as alcohol, hypnotics, and antianxiety agents, which are used for symptoms that might respond to nonmedication remedies. If the older person has symptoms serious enough to warrant the long-term use of antipsychotic or antidepressant medications, consultation with a mental health professional may be helpful.

In community settings, it is important to educate older adults and caregivers about criteria for using p.r.n. medications, because this is a particularly difficult aspect to assess, and nonmedication interventions may be effective. For example, a person with dementia may become agitated only when the environment is very noisy, but the caregiver might think the agitation is an inherent part of the illness and use medications unnecessarily to decrease the agitation. In contrast to this situation, a caregiver may withhold medications that could improve the quality of life for the older person and the caregiver because of misunderstandings or lack of information about the use of medications. Nurses can educate caregivers about nonmedication interventions, as well as the appropriate use of medications in behavior management.

In institutional settings, nurses must establish clear criteria for administering medications for behavior management. These criteria must be based primarily on the patient's needs, rather than primarily on the staff's needs. In home settings, different criteria for behavioral medication might be justified, and the needs of the caregivers may take precedence over the needs of the dependent older adult. For example, if nighttime wakening of a dependent older person interferes with the caregiver's sleep, medication intervention might be warranted. In an institutional setting, however, the nursing staff who are paid to provide around-the-clock care might try nonmedication interventions or allow the person to be awake at night, rather than immediately turning to the use of medications.

Behavioral problems are one example of the types of symptoms that can be managed medically but might be managed just as well, and with fewer risks, through nonmedication interventions. Other types of problems that can be managed without pharmacologic agents are those that are related to comfort, anxiety, and chronic illnesses. The nurse is the health professional who is best able to encourage the use of nonmedication interventions for certain health problems, such as the ones listed in the displays on Alternative and Preventive Health Care Practices throughout this book.

Providing Information About Alternative Therapies

Homeopathy, herbal medicine, and folk remedies are viewed as nontraditional approaches to preventing and treating illness, despite the fact that these approaches have a long tradition in many non-Western cultures. In recent years, there has been a growing trend in the United States toward the use of alternative healing products that have not traditionally been a part of Western medicine. Thousands of alternative healing products are widely available and are being used increasingly by older adults. Even the National Institutes of Health have established an Office of Alternative Medicine and have funded clinical trials of herbs, such as Ginkgo biloba and St. John's wort. Nurses, primary care providers, and other health care practitioners need to be knowledgeable about a variety of therapies so that health care consumers can be advised about their use and effectiveness and so that some of these therapies can be used judiciously in clinical practice (Dossey, 1997; Eisenberg, 1997). The challenge for health care professionals is to be able to educate health care consumers about these remedies, just as people are educated about prescription medications and standard, over-the-counter products. Throughout this text, information is provided about some of the alternative remedies that are being used more commonly in the United States for particular conditions. This information should be considered in the broader context of the precautions and information discussed in the following sections. This chapter provides information about herbal and homeopathic products in general, and Display 18-4 summarizes information that can be used to teach older adults about the use of herbal and homeopathic remedies. Like Display 18-3, the information is written in plain English so that it can be used as a health education tool with older adults.

Herbs

Herbs were perhaps the original "over-the-counter" products used by people who found the remedies they needed in their natural environment. In fact, prior to the last half of this century, the natural environment was the primary source for all healing agents. Most herbs are safe, but some have side effects and some can cause serious harm (see Table 18-6). Also, herbs can interact with prescription and over-the-counter medications, as discussed in the section on medication-chemical interactions.

Because herbs have been used for centuries in European and non-Western cultures, a wealth of information is available. There is much concern about their increasing popularity in the United States, however, because there has been very little testing that meets the standards established by the FDA for medications. Because herbs are considered to be dietary supplements, they are not required to be tested for safety or efficacy. Also, there is no way of knowing any of the following information about herbal products: the additional ingredients, the potential harmful effects, the exact quantity of active ingredients, and whether the ingredients are in a

---

DISPLAY 18-4
Tips on the Use of Herbs and Homeopathic Remedies

- Before treating any symptom with a nonprescription product, make sure you are not overlooking a condition that requires medical attention.
- Discuss the use of any nonprescription product with your primary health care provider(s).
- Be cautious about substituting herbal or homeopathic products for prescribed medications.
- Seek information from objective sources and check any warnings on the label or package.
- Observe for beneficial and harmful effects.
- Report any possible side effects to your primary health care provider for evaluation.
- Keep in mind that some products are not required to meet FDA standards for safety and efficacy.
- Introduce only one new substance at a time.
- Older adults should start with low doses.
- Doses may need to be lowered when combining two or more herbs or an herb and a medication.
- Some herbs and homeopathic remedies are for short-term use only.
- Some herbs need to be taken for 1 to 3 months before effects are noticed (e.g., ginkgo biloba, St. John's wort).

- Herbs can interact with all of the following: other herbs, food, beverages, caffeine, nutrients, prescription medications, and over-the-counter medications.
- Some herbs are contraindicated in people with the the following conditions: stroke, glaucoma, diabetes, hypertension, heart disease, thyroid disorder, and any bleeding disorder or condition requiring anticoagulation.
- Some herbs are most effective when taken on an empty stomach.
- Many herbs can cause gastrointestinal effects (e.g., anorexia, nausea, diarrhea).
- Some herbs, especially those that are applied externally, can cause skin rashes.
- Herbs can cause allergic reactions.
- Some herbs are extremely toxic, or fatal, if ingested.
- A few herbs, or ingredients in herbs, can be toxic when taken in large doses or for a long time. (For example, Oregon grape, used for prostatitis, may cause heart failure.)
- A few herbs are thought to be carcinogenic.
- Herbs that are used for anxiety or insomnia should not be taken before driving a car.
- Be skeptical about exaggerated claims; if it sounds too good to be true, it probably is!

---

form that can be used by the human body. Health care consumers, therefore, need to obtain herbal products and information from reputable sources that do not have a vested interest in selling a particular product.

Homeopathy

Three concepts are key to understanding homeopathy as it was proposed 2 centuries ago by a German physician, Samuel Hahnemann. First, there is the law of similars, or "like cures like." According to this concept, homeopathy treats an illness by stimulating the body's self-healing abilities through the use of a small amount of a substance similar to the substance that caused the illness. For example, quinine can produce symptoms of malaria in a healthy person, and it can cure malaria when administered in minute doses. The second key concept is that the more a substance is diluted, the more potent it becomes. Based on this concept, homeopathic remedies are diluted repeatedly, and each dilution is vigorously shaken to increase its potency. The third concept is that illnesses are highly individualized and, therefore, the treatment must be individualized. Based on this principle, homeopathic practitioners focus on treating the person, not the disease, and they spend a lot of time interviewing patients. Homeopathy is widely used in India, Russia, Mexico, and European countries, and it is gaining acceptance in the United States as a safe alternative to conventional medicine. Although most homeopathic remedies are now available for self-treatment, a few are available only through health care practitioners. Unlike herbs, homeopathic remedies are regulated by the FDA as over-the-counter products. Remedies come in a variety of single-substance or combination forms, including powders, wafers, small tablets, and alcohol-based liquids. Over-the-counter homeopathic products are too weak to cause adverse effects, and there are very few precautions, interactions, or contraindications that apply to these products. People who are taking homeopathic remedies are advised to limit the amount taken and the length of time they are taken. Other precautions include avoiding food, caffeine, beverages, toothpaste, and mouthwashes for 15 to 60 minutes before and after taking the substance. Also, oils of camphor, eucalyptus, and peppermint should be avoided during homeopathic treatments. Information about homeopathic remedies and homeopathic practitioners can be obtained from the National Center for Homeopathy (see the listing in the Educational Resources section).

Evaluating Nursing Care

Nursing care of older adults with medication-related nursing diagnoses is evaluated according to the degree to which the older adult follows a safe and effective medication regimen. This involves an evaluation of medication-taking behaviors, as well as an evaluation of the therapeutic effects of the medication. Another evaluation criterion is the extent to which negative functional consequences, such as side effects and medication interactions, are avoided, alleviated, or controlled. Nurses in home settings have the ideal opportunity to evaluate the effectiveness of their health education about medication regimens through observations of the medication-taking patterns of the older adult. In any setting, nurses can evaluate the knowledge of the older

adult and his or her caregivers about safe and effective medication management.

Chapter Summary

Age-related changes in many physiologic mechanisms affect medication action, potentially altering the therapeutic effect and increasing the likelihood of adverse effects. The impact of these age-related changes on any particular medication is determined by the chemical characteristics of the medication, the extent of the age-related changes, and the presence of risk factors. The risk factors that can significantly influence medication action in older adults include disease processes, medication interactions, and myths and misunderstandings that influence medication-taking behaviors. The primary functional consequence of these age-related changes and risk factors is that older adults are likely to experience altered therapeutic effects and an increased chance of adverse effects of medications. Additional and serious consequences occur when adverse medication effects are not recognized as such in older adults.

The purpose of the nursing assessment is to determine the effectiveness of the medication regimen and to identify the factors that influence medication-taking behaviors. The assessment also focuses on detecting adverse effects and identifying the factors that increase the risk of adverse effects or altered therapeutic effects. Nurses also assess cultural factors that influence medication-taking behaviors, such as usual sources of health care and common health care practices. Noncompliance and Instrumental Self-Care Deficit are two nursing diagnoses that may be applicable for older adults with medication-related problems. Nursing goals include enhancing the therapeutic effectiveness of medications, reducing the risk of adverse effects, and eliminating or minimizing the negative functional consequences of adverse effects. Nursing interventions include educating older adults and their caregivers, facilitating communication between older adults and health care providers, and decreasing the number of medications. Nursing care is evaluated by the degree to which the older adult adheres to a safe and effective medication regimen and avoids adverse effects.

Critical Thinking Exercises

1. You are asked to give a 1/2 hour presentation on "Medications and Aging" to a local senior citizens group. Describe the following:
   a. What points would you cover about age-related changes?
   b. How would you address the risk factors that affect medication action and medication-taking behaviors?
   c. What tips would you give about taking medications?
   d. What educational materials would you use?
   e. How would you involve the group participants in the discussion?

2. Carefully read the interview questions in Display 18-1 and decide which questions you would use and how you would phrase the questions in your own words for each of the following situations:
   a. You are doing an admission interview for a 78-year-old man who lives alone and has been admitted to the hospital for the third time in 18 months for congestive heart failure.
   b. You are working in a Senior Wellness program in an urban setting with a large number of older adults who were born in Mexico. You are preparing for 15-minute interviews with older adults who have agreed to participate in an educational session to which they must bring all their pills in a bag and ask the nurse about them.

3. Carefully read the information in Displays 18-3 and 18-4 and describe what information you would be likely to use in each of the following situations.
   a. Discharge planning for the 78-year-old man described in Exercise 2a
   b. Health education for the people described in Exercise 2b.

Case Example and Nursing Care Plan

Pertinent Case Information

Mrs. M., who is 76 years old, is being discharged to her home after a stay in a nursing home for rehabilitation following a stroke. Residual problems from the stroke include left-sided weakness and visual-perceptual difficulties. In addition to the stroke, Mrs. M.'s medical problems include glaucoma, depression, and congestive heart failure. Her medications include the following: Centrum Silver, 1 tablet q.d.; furosemide, 20 mg, 2 tablets b.i.d.; Lanoxicaps, 0.1 mg q.d. except Mondays and Thursdays; Ecotrin, 81 mg, 1 tablet q.d.; Transderm-Nitro, 0.2 mg/hr q.d.; Zoloft, 50 mg q.d.; Cardizem, 60 mg t.i.d.; and Timoptic, 0.25% b.i.d. The nursing home regimen for administering the medications is as follows:

7:30 A.M.: Lanoxicaps (except Mondays and Thursdays)
Cardizem, 60 mg

Furosemide, 20 mg, 2 tablets
Timoptic, 0.25% in each eye
9:00 A.M.: Transderm-Nitro, 0.2 mg/hr
1:00 P.M.: Centrum Silver
Ecotrin, 81 mg, 1 tablet
Cardizem, 60 mg
3:30 P.M.: Furosemide, 20 mg, 2 tablets
7:30 P.M.: Timoptic, 0.25% in each eye
Cardizem, 60 mg
9:00 P.M.: Zoloft, 50 mg

Nursing Assessment

Your assessment reveals that, before her hospitalization and nursing home stay, Mrs. M. administered her medications independently, but that the only medications she took were the eye drops, furosemide (20 mg once daily), and Lanoxicaps. The functional assessment indicates that Mrs. M. has weakness and limited use of her left arm and hand, causing difficulty performing tasks that require fine motor movements. She has full use of her right upper extremity, and she is right-hand dominant. She ambulates independently, but slowly, with a walker. A mental status assessment reveals that Mrs. M. is alert, oriented, and has no memory deficits; however, her abstract thinking and time perception have been impaired by the stroke. She has some expressive aphasia, but she seems to understand instructions, especially if ideas are reinforced by using concrete examples and demonstrations.

Mrs. M. expresses motivation to take her medications, but she admits to being overwhelmed by the complexity of the regimen, stating that, at the nursing home, they administered her medications at six different times. She is also concerned about self-administering her eye drops because she used to use her left hand to hold her eyelids open. With regard to the furosemide, she says she does not like taking it twice a day because it makes her go to the bathroom too much. While at the nursing home, she has not had any trouble with incontinence, but she worries about what she'll do at home because there is no bathroom on the first floor. She asks whether she can take the entire dose of furosemide at nighttime so that she will only have to get up during the night to go to the bathroom, which is located near the bedroom.

In response to your questions about medication management routines before her stroke, Mrs. M. reports using a compartmentalized medication container and taking her two medications and the eye drops after breakfast, around 9:30 A.M. She would administer the second dose of eye drops around 9:30 P.M., before getting ready for bed. She had no difficulty remembering the medications because she kept the pill container and one bottle of eye drops near the toaster, and she kept a second bottle of eye drops on her nightstand. Now, though, she expresses concern about the number of times she must take medications if the regimen remains the same as in the nursing home, and she thinks that she will need six pill containers, but is not sure where she should put all of them. She also worries about the cost of all the medications.

Mrs. M. lives with her husband, who is physically healthy but has early-stage Alzheimer's disease. Their daughter lives nearby and visits 2 or 3 times weekly to assist with grocery shopping, laundry, and household chores. She also provides transportation to stores and appointments.

Nursing Diagnosis

You decide on a nursing diagnosis of Noncompliance because Mrs. M. expresses a desire to take her medications, but several factors deter adherence to the current regimen. Related factors include functional impairments, complex medication regimens, negative side effects of furosemide, and concern about the cost of medications.

Goals	Nursing Interventions	Evaluation Criteria
To simplify the medication routine	Work with the pharmacist and the prescribing practitioner to simplify the medication regimen. • Discuss with Mrs. M.'s prescribing practitioner the problem of the complexity of the regimen and the cost of medications. Ask Mrs. M.'s prescribing practitioner if she can take Cardizem CD, 180 mg q.d., rather than Cardizem, 60 mg t.i.d. (This will be less expensive and will eliminate two doses of medication daily.) • Ask the pharmacist about combining medications to allow twice-daily administration. Assist Mrs. M. in establishing a routine for self-administering medications that will fit in with her usual activities. At least 3 days before discharge from the nursing home, arrange for Mrs. M. to assume responsibility for her own medication management, using pill containers that she herself fills.	Mrs. M. will be able to follow a twice-daily medication dosing schedule.

(continued)

Goals	Nursing Interventions	Evaluation Criteria
To address Mrs. M.'s concerns about furosemide	Explain the importance of taking furosemide, as ordered, to control congestive heart failure effectively. Suggest that Mrs. M. obtain a portable commode for use downstairs during the day.	Mrs. M. will take her furosemide as ordered and will not experience difficulty with urinary incontinence.
To address Mrs. M.'s concerns about the cost of medications	Encourage Mrs. M. to talk with her primary care practitioner about her concerns over the cost of the prescribed medications. Suggest that Mrs. M. consider using the pharmacy services provided by the American Association of Retired Persons (AARP) to obtain her prescriptions.	Mrs. M. will be able to afford her prescribed medications.
To identify a system for self-administering eye drops	Ask an occupational therapist to evaluate Mrs. M.'s ability to self-administer her eye drops and to identify any assistive devices that may increase her independence and reliability in performing this task. Have Mrs. M. practice self-administering her eye drops before she is discharged from the nursing home, with staff providing whatever assistance is necessary. Talk with Mrs. M. about the possibility of her husband assisting with the eye drop procedure if she is unable to do this independently. Ask Mrs. M.'s ophthalmologist whether the eye drop regimen can be simplified to once-daily dosing by prescribing an extended-action eye drop formula.	Mrs. M. will self-administer her eye drops or will receive the assistance she needs for eye drop administration from her husband.

Educational Resources

American Association of Retired Persons
601 E Street, NW, Washington, DC 20049
(202) 434–2277
www.aarp.org
• Mail-order pharmacy service for members

Center for the Study of Pharmacy and Therapeutics for the Elderly
University of Maryland, School of Pharmacy, 20 North Pine Street, Baltimore, MD 21201–1180
(410) 706–3011
• Elder Health Program, a nationwide drug education program for community-living older adults
• Health education materials for professionals and consumers

Food and Drug Administration
5600 Fishers Lane, HFE-88, Rockville, MD 20857
www.fda.gov

National Council on Patient Information and Education
666 Eleventh Street, NW, Suite 810, Washington, DC 20001–4542
(202) 347–6711
http://library.nyam.org/keystone
• *Prescription Medicines and You*, educational booklet, available in English, Spanish, Chinese, Korean, Vietnamese, and Cambodian
• Annual "Talk About Prescriptions" program with posters, educational materials, and a planning guide
• Videos, reports, patient handouts, and other educational materials

Office of Alternative Medicine, National Institutes of Health
P. O. Box 8218, Silver Spring, MD 20907–8218
(888) 644–6226
http://altmed.od.nih.gov

References

Avorn, J., & Gurwitz, J. H. (1997). Principles of pharmacology. In C. K. Cassel, H. J. Cohen, E. B. Larson, D. E. Meier, N. M. Resnick, L. Z. Rubenstein, & L. B. Sorenson (Eds.), *Geriatric medicine* (3rd ed., pp. 55–70). New York: Springer.

Bailey, R. B., & Jones, S. R. (1989). Chronic salicylate intoxication: A common cause of morbidity in the elderly. *Journal of the American Geriatrics Society, 37,* 556–561.

Beers, M. H. (1997). Explicit criteria for determining potentially inappropriate medication use by the elderly: An update. *Archives of Internal Medicine, 157,* 1531–1536.

Beers, M. H., Ouslander, J. G., Rollingher, I., Brooks, J., Reuben, D., & Beck, J. C. (1991). Explicit criteria for determining inappropriate medication use in nursing homes. *Archives of Internal Medicine, 151,* 1825–1832.

Campion, E. W., Avorn, J., Reder, V. A., & Olins, N. J. (1987). Overmedication of the low-weight elderly. *Archives of Internal Medicine, 147,* 945–947.

Carpenito, L. J. (1997). *Nursing diagnosis: Application to clinical practice* (7th ed.). Philadelphia: J. B. Lippincott.

Chrischilles, E. A., Foley, D. J., Wallace, R. B., Lemke, J. H., Semla, T. P., Hanlon, J. T., et al. (1992). Use of medications by persons 65 and over: Data from the established populations for epidemiologic studies of the elderly. *Journal of Gerontology: Medical Sciences, 47*(5), M137–M144.

Courts, N. F. (1996). Salicylism in the elderly: "A little aspirin never hurt anybody!" *Geriatric Nursing, 17,* 55–59.

Dossey, B. M. (1997). Complementary and alternative therapies for our aging society. *Journal of Gerontological Nursing, 23*(9), 45–51.

Eisenberg, D. M. (1997). Advising patients who seek alternative medical therapies. *Annals of Internal Medicine, 127*(1), 61–69.

Gerety, M. B., Cornell, J. E., Plichta, D. T., & Eimer, M. (1993). Adverse events related to drugs and drug withdrawal in nursing home residents. *Journal of the American Geriatrics Society, 41,* 1326–1332.

Gray, S. L., Sager, M., Lestico, M. R., & Jalaluddin, M. (1998). Adverse drug events in hospitalized elderly. *Journal of Gerontology: Medical Sciences, 53A,* M59–M63.

Hahn, K., & Wietor, G. (1992). Helpful tools for medication screenings. *Geriatric Nursing, 13,* 160–166.

Hanlon, J. T., Schmader, K. E., Koronkowski, M. J., Weinberger, M., Landsman, P. B., Samsa, G. P., & Lewis, I. K. (1997). Adverse drug events in high risk older outpatients. *Journal of the American Geriatrics Society, 45,* 945–948.

Hurwitz, A., Brady, D. A., Schaal, S. E., Samloff, I. M., Dedon, J., & Ruhl, C. E. (1997). Gastric acidity in older adults. *Journal of the American Medical Association, 278,* 659–662.

Lee, E. W., & D'Alonzo, G. E. (1993). Cigarette smoking, nicotine addiction, and its pharmacological treatment. *Archives of Internal Medicine, 153,* 34–48.

Lipson, J. G., Dibble, S. L., & Minarik, P. A. (1996). *Culture and nursing care: A pocket guide.* San Francisco: UCSF Nursing Press.

National Center for Health Statistics, & Cypress, B. K. (1982). *Drug utilization in office visits to primary care physicians: The national ambulatory care survey, 1980* (Vital and Health Statistics, No. 86). Hyattsville, MD: U.S. Public Health Service. (Publication No. 82–1250).

Pahor, M., Garulnik, J. M., Chrischilles, E. A., & Wallace, R. B. (1994). Use of laxative medication in older persons and associations with low serum albumin. *Journal of the American Geriatrics Society, 42,* 50–56.

Schwartz, D., Wang, M., Zeitz, L., & Goss, M. (1962). Medication errors made by elderly, chronically ill patients. *American Journal of Public Health, 52,* 2018–2029.

Survey: Elderly most health conscious, listen to their physicians more. (1987). *Geriatrics, 42*(10), 16.

Todd, B. (1985). Product-to-product variability. *Geriatric Nursing, 6,* 57–58.

Vestal, R. E., & Dawson, G. W. (1985). Pharmacology and aging. In C. E. Finch & E. L. Schneider (Eds.), *Handbook of the biology of aging* (2nd ed., pp. 744–819). New York: Van Nostrand Reinhold.

Yassa, R., Nastase, C., Dupont D., & Thibeau, M. (1992). Tardive dyskinesia in the elderly psychiatric patient: A 5-year study. *American Journal of Psychiatry, 149,* 1206–1211.

Impaired Cognitive Function: Dementia

Chapter

19

Most older adults have no cognitive impairment, but for those who do, the loss of intellectual abilities may be the most devastating loss that they and their caregivers must confront. Indeed, older adults and their caregivers have described this loss as a "loss of self." Because nurses focus on people's response to actual or potential health problems, gerontological nurses working with cognitively impaired older adults are challenged to assist them and their caregivers to maintain as great a degree of dignity and quality of life as possible, despite the serious and progressive losses associated with dementia.

Overview of Impaired Cognitive Function

An understanding of impaired cognitive function is complicated by the many terms that have been used interchangeably to describe cognitive impairments. More than any other terms used in reference to older adults, those associated with cognitive impairments are the most misunderstood and emotionally charged. Some of the terms, such as Alzheimer's disease (AD), may

be associated with social stigma or images of bizarre behaviors. Other terms, such as senility, may be associated with a false belief that the symptoms are a normal part of aging, rather than a pathologic process. Different terms are more or less acceptable to different people in the same way that various terms associated with cancer are more or less acceptable to different people. Even different health professionals perceive various terms as more or less acceptable. The following are some of the terms that are used in reference to cognitive impairment in older adults: confusion, dementia, senility, AD, small strokes, memory problems, organic brain syndrome, and hardening of the arteries.

Sometimes, the selection of a term is based on emotional preferences; other times, it is based on a lack of understanding. Because cognitive impairment is an emotionally charged aspect of care, nurses must understand the correct terminology and then choose the most appropriate term for the circumstances. The choice of a defining term is based on an understanding of the underlying causes for the impairment and an assessment of what is most acceptable to older adults and their caregivers. Therefore, before any discussion of theories about dementia, the terminology relating to dementia must first be reviewed.

Confusion about the classification of dementia is an issue that is closely related to the terms used to refer to impaired cognitive function. As gerontologists have become more knowledgeable about dementia, they have become increasingly aware of the complexity of this syndrome. It is now widely recognized that multiple, interacting causes are associated with AD, and that there are interacting factors between AD and vascular dementia. Recently, many questions have been raised about interacting causative factors and overlapping pathologic and clinical manifestations among the various types of dementia. Indeed, the more that is learned about dementia, the more questions are raised about the interrelating factors that contribute to this syndrome. Information about current systems of classification for dementia is presented in the sections discussing theories about dementia.

Evolution of "Senility" Terminology

To understand the correct use of terms relating to dementia, one must begin by looking at the way they have been used to describe older people with cognitive impairments. "Senility" was the first term applied to cognitive impairment in older adults. By definition, senility means old age, or pertaining to old age, and originally, it was a neutral term. Only in the past 2 centuries has the term referred to a state of being mentally and physically infirm as a result of old age, and only in the last century has it consistently been associated with disease conditions and feeble-mindedness. Unfortunately, the use of this term to describe cognitively impaired older adults implies that the impairments are a necessary consequence of being old. As recently as the 1970s, senility was applied to age-related conditions that required no explanation, no investigation, and no treatment. In reality, significant and progressive cognitive impairments are a conse-

quence of diseases, which affect fewer than 5% of people aged 65 to 74 years and at least 30% of people older than 85 years of age.

Hardening of the Arteries and Organic Brain Syndrome

In the early 1900s, the phrase "hardening of the arteries" became a popular diagnostic label for cognitive impairment in older adults. This label was an improvement over the senility label because it referred to a causative factor; however, the causative factor still was viewed as an inevitable, albeit pathologic, consequence of aging. This new label, therefore, did nothing to challenge the myth that cognitive impairments were part and parcel of aging.

By the 1950s, the phrase "organic brain syndrome" (OBS) had become the popular medical label for cognitive impairment in older adults. This label described a constellation of manifestations that could be attributed to the neurologic effects of underlying pathologic conditions. Along with the use of the term OBS, there also came a distinction between acute and chronic conditions. Acute organic brain syndrome, also called delirium, was viewed as a manifestation of a pathologic process that would resolve after the underlying cause was treated. By contrast, chronic organic brain syndrome (COBS) was viewed as the manifestation of irreversible brain damage, and it was thought to be closely associated with underlying vascular pathology. The use of the terms OBS and COBS was a step in the right direction, in that cognitive impairments no longer were considered to be an inevitable result of old age per se. The step was not a very big step, however, as the cause of cognitive impairments in older adults still was attributed to untreatable vascular disease.

In the 1960s, autopsy examination of brain specimens provided the first scientific evidence about the underlying causes of cognitive impairments. Based on this research, knowledgeable practitioners began to realize that many of the changes previously attributed to COBS or untreatable vascular diseases actually were manifestations of treatable conditions. By the early 1980s, much of the geriatric literature was reporting that 15% to 25% of older adults had been misdiagnosed as senile or having COBS when they actually had treatable conditions. Since the early 1990s, very few cognitively impaired older adults who undergo a comprehensive geriatric assessment have been misdiagnosed as having an untreatable condition.

Dementia

Dementia is currently the term that is accepted as most accurate when referring to progressive impairments in cognitive function. Dementia is characterized as a persistent decline in several acquired intellectual functions in the presence of a stable level of consciousness. In addition, noncognitive manifestations, such as changes in personality and behavior, are associated with dementia.

Unfortunately, this medical term is also associated with the lay term "demented," which has a long history of pejorative use in popular language. Indeed, the derogatory use of the word demented has been traced as far back as Cicero, who sarcastically applied it to one of his political opponents (Veterans Administration, 1985, p. III-1). The term demented reinforces the notion of being "out of one's mind," and it may be viewed as even more derogatory than the word "senile." Because of these connotations, nurses should avoid referring to people as demented. Rather, phrases such as "a person with dementia" or "a person with a dementing illness" accurately refer to the medical syndrome of impaired cognitive function while avoiding pejorative connotations.

An additional point must be emphasized with regard to the term dementia. Because dementia is not a single disease but a syndrome, the term refers to a unique combination of symptoms that indicate the need to look for an underlying cause. In every country except Japan, AD is thought to be the most common type of progressive dementing condition, accounting for one half to two thirds of the cases of dementia. In Japan, vascular dementia is more common than dementia of the Alzheimer's type. Because AD accounts for most cases of dementia, health care professionals and lay people in the United States frequently use the terms AD and dementia interchangeably, even though this may not be entirely accurate in all situations.

Health professionals today are less apt than their predecessors to use outdated and inaccurate terms, and they are more likely to understand that significant cognitive impairments are not inevitable markers of old age, but are manifestations of underlying disease conditions, some of which are treatable. Despite our current understanding of dementia, however, health care practitioners who are not knowledgeable about the latest research may still use inaccurate or detrimental labels. In a commentary on terms that should never be used in reference to older adults, a leader in gerontological nursing made the following statement:

> The word senile is an archaic, negative, prejudicial term which usually refers to general mental decline in the elderly. . . . But the word senile is not a professional term and should never be used to describe an older person (Hogstel, 1988).

Pseudodementia

As knowledge about dementia increased, one of the discoveries was that some progressive cognitive impairments may be totally or partially reversed when the underlying causes are treated. Based on this knowledge, the term "pseudodementia" was applied to those conditions that resembled dementia, but did not cause irreversible cognitive impairments. The first systematic study of pseudodementia was published by Kiloh (1961), who used the term to refer to conditions that were not true dementias, but which "very closely mimicked" dementia. The psychiatric literature also has applied the term to various mental illnesses, including schizophrenia and malingering, in prisoners as well as other younger populations (McAllister, 1983).

In the geriatric literature, the term "pseudodementia" was used initially to refer exclusively to psychiatric disorders that caused cognitive impairments. In recent years, however, it has been applied by Libow (1973) and other geriatricians to dementias that are associated with physiologic conditions. The term is now applied primarily to depression, but it may also refer to physiologic conditions masquerading as a dementing disorder. This term has been challenged recently, and British and American journals periodically publish articles arguing for or against the continued use of this term. The current trend is to avoid the use of this term because of an increasing capability of identifying specific underlying causes of dementia.

Delirium

Delirium is an acute confusional state that is characterized by a disturbance of consciousness, a change in cognition (e.g., deficits in thinking, memory, perception), and an alteration in sleep-wake cycle. Although this disorder can occur in people of any age, it is 4 times more common among people aged 40 years and older, and it is most common in people aged 70 years and older (Cummings et al., 1997). Studies have demonstrated that up to 24% of older adults in general medical hospital settings have delirium on admission, and that delirium develops in up to 35% of older adults during hospitalization (Levkoff et al., 1992). A recent study of community-living people with AD revealed that 22% had had episodes of delirium during the course of their dementia (Lerner et al., 1997). Dementia may increase the risk of delirium by two- to threefold (Francis, 1997). In addition to impaired cognitive function, factors that are likely to increase the risk of delirium include infection, dehydration, fracture, multiple diseases, surgical procedures, adverse medication effects, and advanced age (80 years of age or older).

Particular problems arise when delirium occurs in older adults because the manifestations are likely to be subtle. Studies have found that nurses are more likely than physicians to identify the symptoms of delirium in hospital settings (Francis, 1992). Also, when delirium occurs in older adults with dementia, the acute changes are likely to be superimposed on already existing cognitive deficits, and the recent changes may be attributed to dementia. Another complicating factor is that the manifestations of delirium may persist for months or years, even after the underlying causes are detected and treated (Levkoff et al., 1992; Goldstein and Fogel, 1993; Rockwood, 1993). Also, delirium in older adults often causes a severe and long-term decline in and loss of physical function (Murray et al., 1993). Some of the physiologic causes of delirium in older adults are listed in Table 19-1, in the section on risk factors for impaired cognitive function. Simon and colleagues (1997) have presented a nurse-physician collaboration model that has been used effectively in hospital settings to detect, assess, and treat patients with delirium.

Theories and Types of Dementia

Medical scientists have speculated about impaired cognitive function for the past 2 centuries, and the review of terminology just discussed reflects a growing understanding of this syndrome. Despite this long history of interest in impaired cognitive function, theories to explain dementia are still evolving. In particular, theories to explain AD, the most common type of dementia, are developing rapidly. Knowledge about other types of dementia, such as vascular and frontotemporal dementias, also is growing rapidly. This section reviews past and current theories about the dementias and reviews current knowledge about the various types of dementia.

Early Theories

In the 1800s, European physicians discovered senile (neuritic) plaques in the brains of older adults and identified these changes as the cause of senility, or senile dementia. In 1906, Alois Alzheimer, a German physician, discovered similar changes during autopsy examination of brain specimens from a woman who was 55 years old at the time of her death and had initially manifested cognitive and behavior changes around the age of 50 years. Alzheimer concluded that these pathologic brain changes caused a relatively rare disease called presenile dementia, and his findings were published in a psychiatric journal (Alzheimer, 1907). By 1920, AD was accepted as a disease entity distinguishable from senile dementia by virtue of the age at onset, and this theory remained intact until the last third of this century (Holstein, 1997).

Around the same time that these changes were identified, medical scientists discovered that, in older adulthood, arteries throughout the body lose their elasticity and become hardened. They theorized that the cause of mental changes in older adults, then, was hardening of the arteries and diminished blood to the brain. Combining this deduction with the available information about neurofibrillary changes, Alzheimer and other medical scientists concluded that presenile dementia was caused by neuropathologic conditions, and that senile dementia was caused by vascular conditions. Simply stated, if the onset of the cognitive impairment occurred before the age of 65 years, it was called AD, whereas if the onset took place after the age of 65 years, it was called hardening of the arteries.

Recent Theories and Advances in the Diagnosis of Dementia

The chronologic distinction between senile and presenile dementia was not challenged until the 1960s. Questions were first raised on the basis of autopsy studies in which no association was found between the degree of arteriosclerotic brain changes and the clinical manifestations of dementia during the person's lifetime (Corsellis and Evans, 1966; Worm-Petersen and Pakkenberg, 1968). In addition, landmark studies by Tomlinson and colleagues (1968, 1970) led to the current theory that the neuropathologic changes of AD represent a single disease process, regardless of the age at onset. Furthermore, studies of autopsy brain specimens from subjects with and without dementia revealed that AD was the underlying cause of progressive dementia in most cases. Based on these and other studies, the underlying causes of irreversible dementia were delineated as follows: 50% of the cases were attributable to AD; 15% were the result of multi-infarct dementia (MID); an additional 25% were attributable to a combination of AD and MID; and the remaining 10% were the result of less common causes, such as frontotemporal dementias.

In 1974, a landmark paper asserted that cerebral atherosclerosis as the cause of cognitive impairments in older adults was the "most common medical misdiagnosis" (Hachinski et al., 1974). Furthermore, these scientists denounced the use of the phrase "hardening of the arteries" and suggested that MID be used to describe dementias of cerebrovascular origin. Their rationale was that dementia was not caused by atherosclerosis or chronic ischemia, but by the occurrence of multiple cerebral infarcts. Another major contribution of this publication was that Hachinski and colleagues supported the findings of Tomlinson and associates, emphasizing that AD was the most common cause of progressive dementia. Since 1975, the Hachinski ischemia score has been used as a guide to the clinical diagnosis of MID. In the early 1990s, questions about the narrow scope of the term MID led to the use of the broader term "vascular dementia," and criteria were proposed for the diagnosis of ischemic vascular dementia (Chui et al., 1992). Current theories about vascular dementia are discussed later in this section.

It was not until 1984 that the National Institute of Neurologic and Communicative Disorders and Stroke/Alzheimer's Disease and Related Disorders Association (NINCDS/ADRDA) developed criteria for the clinical diagnosis of probable and possible AD (McKhann et al., 1984). Criteria such as these have resulted in an improvement in diagnostic accuracy from 73% in 1986 to about 90% in recent years. During the early 1990s, questions were raised about the usefulness of the NINCDS/ADRDA criteria in diagnosing AD in its earliest stages and about the application of these criteria to diverse ethnic and cultural groups (Loewenstein and Rupert, 1992). These criteria are now considered to be outdated because of the new information that has recently become available. Late in 1996, the Agency for Health Care Policy and Research (Costa et al., 1996) published guidelines for assessing dementia and a quick reference for clinicians, which is available to health care professionals without charge (see the list of Educational Resources at the end of this chapter). One very recent development is the current view that AD is no longer a diagnosis of exclusion. Although there is still no single diagnostic test that can be used to determine the underlying cause of dementia, there are many combinations of diagnostic tools that can be used to support the diagnosis (Reisberg et al., 1997). Because of the complexity of dementia, it is imperative that the diagnostic approach be multidisciplinary. Also, it is essential that all gerontological health care practitioners keep abreast of rapidly evolving developments relating to the diagnosis of dementia.

Current Theories About Alzheimer's Disease

As of the late 1990s, no one theory has emerged to explain AD, but knowledge of dementia is progressing at such a rapid pace that major breakthroughs are likely to occur soon. Nurses, therefore, are advised to update their knowledge of developments regarding dementia continually. The Alzheimer's Disease and Related Disorders Association (Alzheimer's Association) and numerous Internet sites, some of which are listed in the Educational Resources list at the end of this chapter, provide lay and professional information about the most recent scientific developments. Some of the pathologic brain changes that have been identified in people with AD are reviewed in the following section. In addition, some of the theories about the causes of AD are summarized in the subsequent sections.

Brain Changes

Neuritic plaques and neurofibrillary tangles are the specific pathologic changes that Alzheimer discovered in the early 1900s. Beginning in the 1960s, when autopsy studies of brain tissue were first done, the pathologic criteria for AD were based on the presence of moderate or severe concentrations of neuritic plaques and neurofibrillary tangles, particularly in the neocortex. The discovery of deposits of beta-amyloid protein in the plaques and blood vessels of people with AD became another pathologic hallmark of AD in the early 1990s (Joachim and Selkoe, 1992). This finding laid the groundwork for much of the current research on the role of beta-amyloid and its precursor protein, as discussed later in this section. Loss or degeneration of neurons and synapses, particularly in the neocortex and hippocampus, is another central feature of the brain changes associated with AD. Also, AD is associated with a marked reduction in brain weight.

Beginning in the mid-1990s, much more information about brain changes became available, particularly through Alzheimer's research centers in the United States and other countries. Of particular interest are some of the longitudinal studies that include extensive background information about younger adulthood and lifestyle patterns, longitudinal information about cognitive function during later life, and autopsy information about brain changes (e.g., "The

Nun Study," Snowden, 1997). Information from recent and ongoing studies such as these has raised questions about some previous conclusions. For example, some of the studies do not show a consistent relationship between Alzheimer-type brain changes and cognitive impairments.

Recent studies also are raising questions related to differences between normal aging and pathologic changes associated with dementia. For example, by the early 1990s, it was clear that most of the brain changes associated with dementia could be found to some degree in older people who did not have dementia. It was widely believed that the difference between people with dementia and those without dementia was the density and distribution of the tangles and plaques. Questions about this assumption were first raised in 1993 when it was speculated that AD may have a long preclinical phase during which the pathologic lesions accumulate in the brain, but do not affect the person's function (Kazee et al., 1993). Now, in the late 1990s, gerontologists are addressing questions about whether AD and normal aging are part of a continuum, or whether they are distinct entities. Some gerontologists are now proposing that there are three distinct groups of people that can be classified according to the degree of brain changes and level of cognitive function (Leon et al., 1997; Morrison and Hof, 1997; Petersen et al., 1997; Reifler, 1997). One group is composed of people who do not have degenerative brain changes but who do have age-associated memory impairment or benign senescent forgetfulness (as discussed in Chapter 4). The second group is composed of people who are in a predementia stage and might be diagnosed as having mild cognitive impairment (also called minimally cognitively impaired). People with mild cognitive impairment do not meet the criteria for dementia, but have some cognitive impairment beyond that which is considered to be normal for their age. This second group is very likely to progress to dementia, which constitutes the third group in this categorization. As gerontologists learn more about brain changes and cognitive function, further conclusions will be drawn about the relationship, if any, between normal aging and pathologic conditions. Currently, there is intense interest in this issue, as well as in the relationship between brain changes and cognitive function. One prevailing consensus is that accurate conclusions about any individual can only be made when information about brain changes is addressed in relation to the person's functional abilities.

Several factors need to be kept in mind with regard to brain changes. First, although gerontologists have identified brain changes that are closely associated with AD, as of 1998, they had not yet identified a cause-and-effect relationship. Much additional research is needed to answer questions about brain changes and to make a practical contribution to the prevention and treatment of dementia. Second, before the 1990s, most of the information on brain changes was based on autopsy studies. During the 1990s, however, brain imaging techniques became more widely available; as a result, much of the current research incorporates information from these scans. Computed tomography (CT) and magnetic resonance imaging (MRI) provide information about structural brain changes and about brain lesions that may cause cognitive impairment. Single photon emission computed tomography (SPECT) and positron emission tomography (PET) scans provide specific information about brain function, such as metabolism rates for glucose and oxygen. Although the diagnostic and therapeutic value of these scans, as well as their cost effectiveness, is a topic of much heated debate, these techniques do provide a wealth of information for dementia research programs.

Neurotransmitters

Many theories have been proposed to address the neurophysiologic changes that occur in AD, and these theories are being used to develop drugs that might cure or reverse AD and other neurodegenerative disorders. These theories also are being used to develop drugs that are effective in treating dementia-related behaviors. Cholinergic, dopamine, serotoninergic, and noradrenergic neurotransmitter systems have been implicated as causative factors in AD. Changes in neurotransmitter mechanisms that have been associated with AD include: (1) a loss of serotonin receptors and reduced serotonin uptake into platelets; (2) a 50% or greater reduction in the production of acetylcholine in the areas of the brain that contain plaques and tangles; (3) a reduction in the amount of acetylcholinesterase, which serves to break down acetylcholine after it has been secreted; and (4) a reduction in the amount of choline acetyltransferase, with the greatest reduction in the areas most affected by plaques and tangles. Some of these changes, particularly diminished choline acetyltransferase in the hippocampus and cerebral cortex, are thought to be associated with impaired memory and other cognitive functions. These changes also are directly associated with dementia-related behaviors, such as psychoses and depression (Sunderland et al., 1997).

Based on these findings, potential medical interventions initially were directed toward increasing the brain's supply of choline and choline precursors by the use of such substances as choline and lecithin. Because this approach was not successful, the focus shifted to finding ways of preventing or slowing the breakdown of acetylcholine (e.g., through cholinesterase inhibitors). Tacrine (Cognex) and donepezil (Aricept) were the first two cholinesterase inhibitors approved by the FDA for the treatment of AD. Other drugs in this category are likely to be approved before the end of the 1990s (see Table 19-4). Another approach that addresses the cholinergic system is to increase the amount of acetylcholine through the use of drugs that enhance its synthesis and release (e.g., nicotinic agonists). A third approach is to replace choline selectively by using muscarinic agonists. One such drug—

xanomeline—has been shown in clinical trials to improve behavior and cognitive function in people with AD, but its use is limited by significant adverse effects. A transdermal form of this drug was being tested in clinical trials in 1998 (Bodick et al., 1997). Current efforts also are directed toward finding drugs that affect serotonin and other neurotransmitters. Table 19-4 lists some of the neurotransmitter-affecting drugs that have been approved or that were being investigated, as of 1998, for the treatment of AD. The use of these drugs, as well as other noncholinergic drugs, in people with AD is discussed in more detail in the section on Medication Interventions.

Beta-Amyloid and Amyloid Precursor Protein

Beta-amyloid was first described as a "peculiar substance" by Alzheimer in 1907, but it was not named or defined until 1984. It is now understood that beta-amyloid is a tiny, insoluble, protein fragment of a much larger protein called the amyloid precursor protein (APP). The exact functions of APP have not been identified, but researchers recognize that this protein has multiple essential roles in cells throughout the body. In late 1992, it was discovered that beta-amyloid was not an abnormal substance, but that it was produced by many cells in the body and released by APP. It is not known how beta-amyloid is released from APP. In some cases, a genetic mutation is thought to be an underlying factor, as discussed in the next section. What is known is that excessive amounts of beta-amyloid are found in the neuritic plaques and the walls of the blood vessels in the brains of people with AD and Down syndrome. These deposits cause damage by destroying nerve cells and triggering a low-grade inflammation in the brain.

Much of the focus of research is on whether this abnormal accumulation results from excessive production or insufficient removal of beta-amyloid. Researchers also are addressing questions about whether the accumulation of beta-amyloid is the cause or the effect of pathologic processes. In addition, researchers are trying to find enzymes to reduce beta-amyloid, perhaps through drugs that stop its production. They also are trying to find ways of reducing the toxicity of beta-amyloid and reducing the associated inflammation of the brain. This theory may help explain the recent discovery that anti-inflammatory agents may have a role in preventing and treating dementia.

Genetic Factors

Questions about genetic factors as a cause of AD were first raised in the mid-1930s, but it was not until the late 1970s that the phrase "familial Alzheimer's disease" first appeared in the literature (Cook et al., 1979). Recent studies in twins indicate that genetic factors significantly increase the risk for AD, but that environmental factors also influence this risk (Gatz et al., 1997). Studies conducted over the past 2 decades have identified subtypes of AD with strong genetic links. In these types of AD, the children of an affected parent have a 25% to 50% chance of having AD if they live to be old enough for the disease to manifest itself.

Recent discoveries related to beta-amyloid, chromosomal mutations, and APP are the bases for much genetics research. For example, it is known that people with Down syndrome have an extra chromosome 21, where the APP gene is located. It is also known that people with Down syndrome inevitably show AD-like brain changes at around the age of 40 years. In addition, there is an increased risk of Down syndrome in the families of individuals with AD. These clues are the bases for studies designed to identify a causative relationship between AD, chromosome 21, and APP. Another finding of recent studies is that the average age at onset of AD may be associated with various genetic mutations. For example, early-onset AD is associated with abnormalities in chromosomes 1, 14, and 21, whereas late-onset AD is associated with abnormalities of the genotypes of apolipoprotein E (apo E) on chromosome 19.

Intensive research efforts are being directed toward elucidating the role of apo E in the development of late-onset AD, which is the most common form of AD, accounting for up to 98% of cases. A relationship between apo E and AD was discovered by Allen Roses in the 1990s in conjunction with research on triglyceride metabolism and cholesterol levels in cardiovascular disease. What is known is that there are three variants of the APOE gene, designated as APOE-ε2, APOE-ε3, and APOE-ε4. Each person inherits one APOE gene from each parent, so there are six possible combinations (2/2, 2/3, 2/4, 3/3, 3/4, and 4/4). The inherited combination may be at least partially predictive of the age at onset, as well as the risk for AD. An increased risk of developing AD and a younger age at onset of AD is associated with APOE-ε4. By contrast, APOE-ε2 is associated with both a decreased risk for AD and a later age at onset if the disease does develop. As of 1997, the apo E genotype was thought to be the single most common genetic determinant of susceptibility to AD, accounting for as much as 50% of the risk (Goate, 1997). Current research is focusing on the practical implications of the role of apo E in causing or preventing AD. For example, Roses proposes that, if a safe medication could be developed to mimic the function of APOE-ε2 in the brain, then people who lack the APOE-ε2 allele might benefit from the use of this drug to delay the onset of AD (Roses, 1995).

Theories About Aluminum, Calcium, and Other Trace Elements

One of the earliest and most widely publicized findings regarding AD was that the brains of people with AD contained higher-than-normal levels of aluminum. Subsequent studies have confirmed this finding, which suggests a possible association between AD and aluminum. One study found prominent aluminum accumulation, as well as abnormally high levels of iron, in the neurofibrillary tangles of the brains of people who died of AD (Good et al., 1992). As of 1998, however, studies had not determined whether increased aluminum levels were a cause or an effect of AD. Studies are attempting to answer questions about the link between AD and aluminum, but there is no reason to believe that increased aluminum levels are related to the amount of aluminum ingested through the diet. Nor is there adequate evidence that high levels of aluminum are a causative factor in AD. Although some scientists continue to examine the link between aluminum and AD, this question is not a major focus of research in the late 1990s in the United States.

Scientists are also studying other minerals as potential contributing factors in AD, either alone or in combination with aluminum. For example, some studies have suggested that high fluoride levels in drinking water may have a preventive role in AD, perhaps because fluoride can block absorption of aluminum in the intestinal tract. Another factor that is being investigated is the relationship between calcium and aluminum in the brain. Finally, zinc levels are known to be relatively low in people with AD, but, as with aluminum and AD, a cause-effect relationship has not yet been established.

Additional Theories

Theories about a viral cause for AD were first generated by the discovery of a viral origin for some dementias, such as Creutzfeldt-Jakob disease. To date, the possibility of a viral origin, at least for some subtypes of AD, has been neither ruled out nor confirmed. Among the additional factors currently being investigated in the United States and other countries as possible causes for AD are head trauma, environmental toxins, nutrient deficiencies, food-borne agents, the flow of calcium in and out of brain cells, and the possibility that AD is a systemic metabolic disorder with some specificity for brain tissue. Also, recent and current research is focusing on the possibility that AD is an inflammatory process. As stated earlier, no one theory can explain the causes of AD, and studies are pointing toward

multiple, perhaps interactive, causative factors. Scientists are now suggesting that AD, like dementia in general, is actually a syndrome of different diseases and factors that interact and share the same clinical pathologic endpoint (Shua-Haim and Ross, 1998). Perhaps in the near future, gerontologists will be able to identify several subtypes of AD, as well as several preventive and treatment modalities.

Current Theories About Vascular Dementia

The role of vascular disease as a cause of dementia is increasingly being recognized, and much progress has been made in our understanding of MID and other vascular dementias. Since the 1970s, it has been known that symptoms of dementia are not caused by arteriosclerosis or atherosclerosis per se. Rather, dementia is caused by cerebral infarcts, or the death of nerve cells in the regions nourished by the diseased vessels. It also is known that dementia occurs when cerebral infarcts are extensive enough to destroy a certain amount of brain tissue. The three types of cerebral infarcts involved include the following: (1) one or more strokes caused by blockage of the large cerebral blood vessels; (2) lacunar strokes affecting the small arteries; and (3) microinfarcts affecting the smallest blood vessels in the brain. Any of these processes can cause MID.

In the late 1980s, a number of questions arose concerning the diagnosis of MID. The term was viewed as too narrow because it referred only to completed infarcts. Hence, during the early 1990s, the term "vascular dementia" replaced the term MID. Vascular dementia includes, but is not limited to, dementia arising from the following causes: single or multiple infarcts; diffuse lesions involving the white matter; small- or large-vessel disease; thrombotic, hemorrhagic, or hypoxic-ischemic cerebral lesions; and hypoperfusion secondary to global brain ischemia following cardiac arrest or profound hypotension. In the late 1990s, gerontologists began to question whether vascular dementia was being too closely linked with the concept of MID, as they believed that vascular dementia was a much broader diagnostic category. Vascular cognitive impairment is now being viewed as a syndrome—like AD and dementia—with diverse causes and multiple manifestations (Erkinjuntti, 1997).

The main features distinguishing vascular dementia from AD are its tendency to have an abrupt onset and its stepwise progression. Also, its manifestations usually can be traced, through diagnostic procedures, to damage incurred by particular areas of the brain. Early manifestations of vascular dementia include gait disturbances, psychomotor slowing, urinary incontinence, falls and unsteadiness, and personality and mood changes. Another important characteristic of vascular dementia is that it is likely to be associated with identifiable risk factors, such as smoking, hypertension, hyperlipidemia, previous strokes, cardiovascular pathology, and a sedentary lifestyle, all of which can be addressed through preventive and treatment measures. By contrast, preventive measures for AD have not yet been identified.

Other Types of Dementia

In addition to AD and vascular dementia, researchers are also investigating frontotemporal dementias (FTD). In the early 1990s, gerontologists began to recognize FTD as a group of dementias affecting primarily the frontal lobes of the brain and being characterized by neuronal atrophy rather than plaques and tangles (Kumar and Gottlieb, 1993). By the late 1990s, an attempt was being made to distinguish between the behavioral manifestations and other characteristics of FTD and those of AD, vascular dementia, and late-life depression (Lund and Manchester Groups, 1995; Cherrier et al., 1997; Swartz et al., 1997). A characteristic that is

unique to FTD in its early stage, in contrast to other types of dementia, is the predominance of behavioral disturbances, rather than cognitive disturbances. Additional, common, early-stage manifestations include apathy, disinhibition, personal neglect, emotional lability, urinary incontinence, and personality changes. Also, early-stage cognitive changes tend to involve speech-language skills and abstract thinking rather than memory skills. As FTD progresses, cognitive and behavioral characteristics become more similar to those of other dementias. Other distinguishing features include a family history of a similar disorder and an onset before the age of 65 years. Pick's disease is one of the most common types of FTD, and some gerontologists consider Pick's disease and FTD to be synonymous.

Another type of dementia that currently is under intense investigation is dementia with Lewy bodies (DLB), also known as cortical Lewy-body disease. Some gerontologists consider this condition to be a subtype of AD because many of the brains studied show Alzheimer-type pathology as well as Lewy bodies in the neocortex and brain stem. Others consider DLB to be a form of Parkinson's disease because it is always accompanied by pathologic changes characteristic of Parkinson's disease. Still others consider it a separate type of dementia. Lewy bodies are spherical, intraneuronal inclusions that are formed by a protein in the neuron. Early-stage clinical features of DLB include parkinsonism, prominent visual hallucinations, and fluctuating cognition with variations in attention and alertness. Additional manifestations are neuroleptic sensitivity, systematized delusions, hallucinations (other than visual), and transient loss of consciousness (McKeith et al., 1996). Neuroleptic sensitivity has important clinical implications because people with DLB are likely to have extreme, sometimes fatal, reactions to cholinergic-type medications, such as antipsychotics, even in very small doses. Other clinical implications include a rapid progression of disease and heightened responsiveness to cholinesterase inhibitors (e.g., tacrine and donepezil) (McKeith et al., 1996).

Current Knowledge About Dementia

What should be clear from this discussion is that the more that is learned about dementia, the more questions are rasied. Although there is much disagreement about dementia, there is consensus that this is a most complex syndrome that probably involves several syndromes within the broad category of dementia. There is also consensus that AD is a heterogeneous disorder with multiple causes, and that several factors interact to cause dementia. There is also increasing agreement that AD, vascular dementia, and other types of dementia may have common pathologic features, as well as some distinct features.

The diagnosis of dementia is currently viewed as a two-step process. The first step is to determine that the person has dementia; the second step is to determine the type of dementia. Despite many recent advances in diagnostic modalities, the specific type of dementia still cannot be determined definitively until autopsy findings are considered in conjunction with information about the person's functional level during the course of the illness. This may change before the end of the 1990s, however. Comprehensive geriatric assessment programs and research settings have a high rate of accuracy in determining the causes of dementia. It is important to keep in mind that the accuracy of a diagnosis of a specific type of dementia generally improves as the disease condition evolves over time, although some of the distinguishing features of various dementias are most obvious during the early stages. Also, it is important to understand that some, or even many, people with dementia will have more than one disease condition that might be contributing to the dementia.

Studies in the United States and other countries have led to important clues about the causes of AD and other dementias, but research is still in its infancy stage. Of course, the primary goal of research is to find ways of preventing and treating various forms of dementia. In 1993, tacrine became the first drug approved in the United States for the treatment of AD, but 5 years later, drug treatments for AD offered only modest benefits for people in the mid stages of AD. Before the end of the 1990s, however, at least 10 more drugs will likely become available for the treatment of dementia, and some drug interventions may be available for the prevention of dementia in people who are at risk for AD.

It is clear that advances in our knowledge of dementia are bringing us closer to the day when we will be able to diagnose accurately, treat successfully, and perhaps prevent the cognitive impairments associated with dementia. As emphasized previously, it is imperative that health care professionals keep apace with ongoing developments in dementia research by using the resources listed in the Educational Resources section.

Risk Factors

Epidemiologic studies of cognitively impaired older people have flourished in the past decade, with emphasis placed on identifying those people who have underlying conditions that are reversible or treatable. As discussed earlier, dementia is, by definition, a condition of progressive decline. Although dementia is a common underlying cause of impaired cognitive function in older adults, it is not the only causative factor. Many, if not most, cognitively impaired older adults have at least one treatable underlying or concurrent condition. An accurate assessment is essential to ensure that treatable conditions are identified, as serious and unnecessary functional consequences can develop when underlying factors are not treated. Also, it is important to distinguish between primary conditions and secondary manifestations before initiating treatment. For example, if a cognitively impaired person has delusions, it is important to determine whether the delusions are associated with a dementia, a depression, or a delirium, rather than simply treating the delusions with an antipsychotic medication.

In addition to being one of the most important aspects of the care of older adults, the identification of risk factors for cognitive impairments is one of the most complex aspects of their care because it is not always possible to attribute the cognitive changes to one risk factor, to the exclusion of others. For example, depression is likely to coexist with dementia and contribute to functional impairment. When the depression is treated, the person's level of function may improve, despite continued cognitive impairment. Therefore, it is essential to identify any treatable risk factor, such as depression or physiologic disturbance, to avoid attributing all the manifestations to an untreatable dementia.

Rather than discussing the many specific risk factors, this section contains a review of the physiologic disorders that are most likely to cause cognitive impairments in older adults. Many of these factors are associated with delirium, as discussed in the section on theories. Two other risk factors—adverse medication effects and depression—are discussed at length in Chapters 18 and 20, respectively, and must be considered in any assessment of dementia. Finally, risk factors arising from attitudes and misunderstandings are discussed because these are significant aspects of gerontological nursing. The two risk factors that have been consistently associated with AD are age and family history of dementia (Hendrie, 1998). Risk factors specific only to AD are not discussed at length because the focus of this chapter is on the broader aspects of impaired cognitive function.

Physiologic Causes of Impaired Cognitive Function

Categorically, the most common risk factors for cognitive impairments are physiologic disturbances. The most common treatable physiologic disturbances in older adults with dementia are adverse medication or chemical effects and metabolic diseases (Larson et al., 1985). Based on this and other studies, many references state that there are more than 100 possible physiologic causes of impaired cognitive function. Some of the causes that are most commonly found in older adults are summarized in Table 19-1.

Attitudes, Misunderstandings, and Cultural Perspectives

Although overlooking reversible causes of impaired cognitive function is becoming an issue of the past, there is still much progress to be made in understanding and identifying treatable underlying causes. Because knowledge of dementia is evolving at a rapid pace, any practitioner who does not keep up with the newest developments in this area is likely to be ill-prepared to work with cognitively impaired older adults. The most devastating effect of a lack of knowledge on the part of health care practitioners is the tendency to attribute cognitive impairments to normal aging. When this happens, treatable conditions are likely to be overlooked and allowed to progress to the point at which the cognitive impairments are no longer reversible. Although nurses do not have primary responsibility for diagnosing dementia, they do have primary responsibility for raising questions about whether the older adult's level of function can be improved. Therefore, nurses must question any attitudes on the part of other professionals or lay people that reflect the "what-do-you-expect-you're-old" syndrome. When these attitudes are not challenged, they become risk factors for progressive cognitive impairments.

TABLE 19-1
Some Physiologic Causes of Impaired Cognitive Function

Fluid and Electrolyte Disturbances
Dehydration
Volume depletion
Acidosis/alkalosis
Hypercalcemia
Hypokalemia
Hyponatremia/hypernatremia
Hypoglycemia/hyperglycemia

Nutritional Deficiencies
Folate or vitamin B_{12} deficiency
Anemia
Niacin deficiency
Magnesium deficiency

Cardiovascular Disturbances
Myocardial infarction
Congestive heart failure
Arrhythmias
Heart block

Respiratory Disorders
Chronic obstructive pulmonary disease
Pulmonary embolism
Tuberculosis
Pneumonia

Miscellaneous
General anesthesia
Surgery
Pain, trauma
Bowel impaction
Acute abdominal disorder
Malignant disease
Heavy metal or carbon monoxide intoxication

Infections
Septicemia
Meningitis, encephalitis
Urinary tract infection

Metabolic and Endocrine Disorders
Hypothyroidism/hyperthyroidism
Hypopituitarism/hyperpituitarism
Parathyroid disorders
Hypoadrenocorticism/hyperadrenocorticism
Postural hypotension
Hypothermia/hyperthermia
Hepatic or renal failure

Central Nervous System Disorders
Alzheimer's disease
Vascular dementia
Head trauma
Tumors
Neurosyphilis
Seizures and postconvulsive states
Normal-pressure hydrocephalus

Collagen and Rheumatoid Disease
Polymyalgia rheumatica
Temporal arteritis
Periarteritis nodosa
Lupus erythematosus

Chemicals and Medications
Alcoholism
Medications (see Chapter 18)

Attitudes about dementia are highly influenced by cultural factors, such as perceptions of aging and illness. For example, some cultural groups accept dementia as a normal process in old age, whereas other cultural groups view dementia-related behaviors as shameful. The Culture Box on page 546 presents a summary of some cultural differences in attitudes toward dementia. It is imperative that all health care providers demonstrate sensitivity toward various cultural interpretations of aging, illness, and dementia-related behaviors. Many such cultural interpretations create barriers to treatment and support services. As more treatment options be-

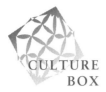

CULTURE
BOX

Cultural Differences in Attitudes Toward Dementia

African Americans
- Old age is more of a survival process than an adaptive process.
- Less attention is directed toward cognitive abilities than affective function.
- Self-worth is maintained when the elder with dementia can perform some role (Lewis and Ausberry, 1996).

American Indians
- Dementia is part of normal aging.
- There is no stigma from or embarrassment about dementia because elders are respected and accepted.
- Dementia-related behaviors provide the elder with a way of communicating with an afterlife during a period of transition to the next world (John et al., 1996).

Chinese Americans
- Dementia is part of normal aging.
- People with dementia may be referred to in terms that translate into English as "stupid and silly" or "less smart."
- Dementia-related behaviors may be viewed as signs of a mental illness and, therefore, as extremely shameful.
- Dementia may be interpreted as fate, an imbalance of energy, or as retribution for the sins of one's ancestors (Elliott et al., 1996).

Cubans and Puerto Ricans Living in the United States
- Caregivers may believe they are being punished for some sin.
- Social stigma and embarrassment are common when dementia-related behaviors are noticed by others.
- Family members may be mortified by an elder who wanders or is not dressed appropriately, or by any incontinence-related odors (Henderson, 1996).

Japanese Americans
- Dementia is a mental illness and, therefore, is shameful.
- Family members should conceal the dementia or they, too, will be considered impaired and thus undesirable (Tempo and Saito, 1996).

Mexican Americans
- Dementia is viewed as a part of normal aging.
- The brain "dries up" and causes child-like behaviors.
- Memory impairment may be caused by "nerves" or "the evil eye" and, therefore, can be cured by the *curandero* (folk healer) (Gallagher-Thompson et al., 1996).

come available, it will become increasingly important to facilitate acceptance of appropriate diagnostic and treatment programs. Some suggestions for developing and implementing culturally sensitive interventions are summarized in a Culture Box that appears later in this chapter (p. 571).

Functional Consequences

The functional consequences of impaired cognition are discussed primarily in relation to AD. This approach is taken for the following reasons:

1. Although not all dementias are attributable to AD, it is an underlying factor for most chronic dementing processes.
2. Because AD has been the focus of most clinical studies of dementia, the functional consequences that are likely to occur can be described relatively accurately.
3. The functional consequences of AD often are present in other dementias, and the major distinguishing characteristic is the course of the illness. As any of the dementias progress, the manifestations become increasingly similar.

Specifically, the following aspects are discussed: the incidence and prevalence of dementia, the functional consequences of each stage of AD, the emotional responses, the behavioral manifestations, and the impact on caregivers.

Incidence and Prevalence of Alzheimer's Disease

Various figures on the prevalence of AD have been quoted, with some estimates suggesting that 50% of individuals aged 85 years and older will have AD. Although this figure is controversial, it is widely agreed that between 70% and 80% of nursing home residents—the population having the most impaired older people—have

dementia. It is also widely agreed that the chance of having AD is highly associated with advancing age. For example, one recent study found that 10% of cognitively intact people between the ages of 85 and 88 years developed dementia each year (Aevarsson and Skoog, 1996). Other studies cite an annual incidence rate of 12% for people aged 80 years and older (Howieson et al., 1997) and 16% for people aged 85 years (Brayne et al., 1995). Current consensus on prevalence rates—that is, the number of people who have AD at a particular age—indicates the following rates: 1% to 3% of people aged 65 to 74 years, 6% to 11% of people aged 75 to 84 years, and 30% of people aged 85 years and older. Recently, attention has been focused on variations in the rates of AD and vascular dementia among different ethnic groups, both worldwide and in the United States. The Culture Box on page 548 summarizes some of the information that is known about variations in dementia by ethnic categories.

Stages of Alzheimer's Disease

The first reference to stages of AD was published in 1952 by Sjögren in a Scandinavian psychiatry journal (Office of Technology Assessment Task Force, 1988). According to Sjögren, the stages of AD are: (1) memory loss; (2) impairment of language, motor ability, and object recognition; and (3) the terminal stage, which is marked by loss of continence, ambulation, and all language skills. In 1982, a more detailed approach to the stages of AD was proposed by an American psychiatrist, Barry Reisberg, and his colleagues. This staging scheme has since been updated and refined, and has been found to be valid and reliable for staging AD in diverse settings. It is now referred to as the Global Deterioration Scale/Functional Assessment Staging, or GDS/FAST (Auer and Reisberg, 1997). Table 19-2 summarizes the functional aspects of each of the seven stages identified in the GDS/FAST. It is

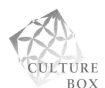

Cultural Differences in the Prevalence of Dementia in the United States

- Prevalence rates for vascular dementia, arranged in order from highest to lowest, are as follows: African Americans, Asian/Pacific Islanders, Whites, Hispanics (Yeo et al., 1996).
- Whites have the highest rate of AD, compared with Blacks, Hispanics, and Asian/Pacific Islanders (Yeo et al., 1996).
- Although data are very limited and there are wide intracultural variations, Native Americans are thought to have a low rate of dementia (John et al., 1996).
- The APOE-ε4 allele is a strong risk factor for AD in Whites, an intermediate risk factor for Hispanic Americans, and not a risk for African Americans (Mayeux, 1993).
- Genes other than the APOE genotype may contribute to the increased risk of AD in Hispanic Americans and African Americans (Tang et al., 1998).

TABLE 19-2
Stages of Alzheimer's Disease (AD) According to Functional Consequences

Stage	Functional Manifestations	Diagnosis
1	No deficits or complaints	Normal adult
2	Forgets names and location of objects; decreased ability to recall appointments; no objective findings	Normal older adult
3	Deficit in complex tasks, especially in demanding social and employment settings; deficits noted by others for the first time; denial may be strong	Compatible with early AD or other disease state
4	Deficits in memory, calculation, fund of knowledge; assistance required for complex tasks, such as shopping and money management; can perform ADL; may be depressed and may withdraw from challenging situations; strong denial	Mild AD
5	Obvious cognitive deficits; may be disoriented to time or place; assistance required for complex ADL, such as clothing selection; no longer able to live independently or drive a car	Moderate AD
6	Increasingly obvious disorientation and other cognitive deficits; personality and emotional changes; may be anxious, agitated, or delusional; assistance required in personal care; urinary and fecal incontinence occur later	Moderately severe AD
7	Progressive loss of all verbal and psychomotor abilities; eventually needs total assistance in all activities	Severe AD

Source: B. Reisberg, (1986), Dementia: A systematic approach to identifying reversible causes, *Geriatrics, 41*(4), 30–46.

important to keep in mind that a diagnosis of AD is based on a progression of manifestations, and that the subtle manifestations of the early stages are attributed to AD only retrospectively.

Reisberg subdivides the last two stages, but he acknowledges that these substages may be less distinct than those marking the major functional stages (1986). Stage 6 is subdivided to reflect a progressive loss of ability to put clothing on properly, to bathe independently, to toilet independently, to maintain urinary continence, and to maintain fecal continence. Reisberg believes that these five functional abilities are lost in sequential order, but that two functions may be lost simultaneously. Reisberg points out that this sequence applies only to uncomplicated AD, and that the sequence may not apply to AD when concomitant conditions affect functional abilities.

Reisberg subdivides stage 7 to reflect the sequential loss of six additional functional abilities: (1) a diminution in speech ability to six or fewer intelligible words; (2) a further reduction in intelligible vocabulary to one word; (3) loss of the ability to ambulate; (4) loss of the ability to sit; (5) loss of the ability to smile; and (6) loss of the ability to hold up the head. In discussing these functional consequences, Reisberg points out that the cognitive changes of AD seem to occur in reverse order to the gains in these areas that occur during normal human development (1986). Similarly, it has been suggested that there is an inverse relationship between the stages of early childhood development and the loss of abilities in the later stages of AD. This concept has been used to develop intervention guidelines to address the stage-specific psychosocial changes that occur during the later stages of AD (Holthaus, 1997).

Although the seven stages of the GDS/FAST scheme are widely accepted, some questions have been raised about the consistency and predictability of these changes. In particular, emphasis has been placed on the fact that cognitive skills and competence in life deteriorate at differ-ent rates in different people. There is unanimous agreement that cognitive declines are progressive through the remaining lifetime of the person with AD. There also is much agreement that many emotional responses and behavioral changes occur as the cognitive deficits increase. Finally, there is agreement that, as the cognitive deficits progress, the behaviors of the person with AD are increasingly influenced by the environment and other variables.

Of major interest to researchers, clinicians, and caregivers of people with AD is information about predictors of the disease course. There is wide individual variability in the rate of progression, and no patient characteristics have been found to relate consistently to the rate of decline. Some of this variability is associated with the fact that AD is a very heterogeneous disease that may, in fact, represent multiple entities with a common pathologic basis. Some of the variability also is associated with the presence of additional chronic illnesses and pathologic conditions that affect levels of function. Although some factors have been identified as precipitants of rapid decline, there is currently no consensus on this issue.

The ultimate functional consequence of AD is death. Compared to the life expectancy of healthy people of the same age, the life expectancy of people with AD is reduced by one half to one third. A conclusion of one study of causes of death in people with AD was that illnesses that are potentially amenable to treatment, such as pneumonia, cause death at all levels of disease, but are more likely to do so in the early stages of AD (Kukull et al., 1994). Another study, which identified factors associated with excess mortality in nursing home residents with dementia, concluded that dementia should be viewed as an independent risk factor for increased mortality (Dijk et al., 1992). The following average lengths of time for the progression of AD have been suggested: 2.5 to 3 years between onset of symptoms and diagnosis, about 2 years between diagnosis and placement in a long-term care facility, and 3.5 to 4 years between placement in a facility and death. Using these figures, the average length of time between onset of symptoms and death is 8 to 9 years.

Emotional Responses to Alzheimer's Disease

Early in the course of AD, common emotions and behaviors of the person with the disease include fear, anxiety, depression, diminished affect, and withdrawal from challenging activities. People with AD describe feelings of frustration, inadequacy, being overwhelmed, or as one person stated "feeling tired and in a fog for no good reason" (Gwyther, 1997). Only the people who live, work, or have close contact with a person with AD will notice the initial change(s) in behavior. When the behaviors are noticed, numerous explanations may be applicable, and the behaviors may be attributed to such factors as depression or retirement. Affected individuals may withdraw from complex tasks as a way of protecting themselves from the effects of diminishing cognitive abilities. For example, employed people may retire without acknowledging cognitive impairments as the reason. If the person does not have to cope with intellectual challenges or complex psychomotor tasks, cognitive impairments may not be noticed at all in the early stages of AD. People with AD may be able to conceal or compensate for the cognitive losses until the deficits seriously interfere with activities of daily living (ADL). As the disease progresses, the person with AD will be less able to ignore or cover up the deficits, and people with less intimate contact will begin to question the underlying cause of the deficits.

One of the myths associated with AD is that people with AD deny their symptoms or have no awareness of their deficits. Unfortunately, this fallacy has led to an attitude on the part of some health care professionals of, "If they can ask if they have Alzheimer's disease, then they

don't have it." In recent years, this perception of a high prevalence of denial in people with AD has been challenged by geriatric practitioners who have come to recognize that some people with dementia have full awareness of their deficits, and many people with dementia have at least some awareness. Sometimes, this awareness is accompanied by feelings of fear, shame, loneliness, depression, uselessness, and self-blame. Many people with early-stage AD become distressed when they are challenged to meet unrealistic demands or when their concerns are dismissed with false reassurance (Gwyther, 1997). People in the early and middle stages of AD who do have some awareness of their deficits usually are relieved when they are told that they have an identifiable disease process that can be addressed through interventions.

During the 1990s, gerontologists began researching "anosognosia," or "unawareness of cognitive deficit" in relation to people with dementia. Recent studies have emphasized that there is a great deal of individual variability in awareness of cognitive deficits. Controversy persists about whether there is a relationship between unawareness and severity of dementia, and about whether unawareness varies according to the type of dementia. One recent study concluded that unawareness is more common with AD than with vascular dementia, and that unawareness increases with increased severity of the disease (Wagner et al., 1997). There is some agreement that unawareness is related to specific areas of the brain, with damage to the frontal lobes and right hemisphere being more likely to be associated with anosognosia. A recent article discusses assessment and intervention issues, with emphasis on clinical implications of unawareness (Cotrell, 1997). Cotrell distinguishes between the psychologic defense of denial and neurologically based denial, or anosognosia. When confronted with their deficits, people who are using the defense mechanism of denial tend to become agitated, whereas people with anosognosia tend to be perplexed and less emotionally reactive. Moreover, denial is likely to be present in the early stages when awareness is most threatening, whereas anosognosia may first develop in the middle or later stages of AD (Cotrell, 1997).

Cohen and associates (1984) described six phases of emotional response to AD. According to their model, phase 1 occurs before diagnosis and is characterized by a recognition and concern that something is seriously wrong. Phase 2, which begins when the diagnosis of AD is made, is characterized by denial. After the diagnosis, during phase 3, people with AD and their family members experience and must resolve the following feelings: shock, guilt, anger, depression, confusion, and questioning. Phase 4 is the coping stage, during which the person and family plan for present and future problems. Phases 5 and 6 occur if the person lives long enough after the onset of the disease. Phase 5, called maturation, is characterized both by an acceptance of the necessary losses and a striving to maintain functional abilities. Phase 6, a stage that "no patient has ever been able to express," is the point at which people can react to certain environmental stimuli but do not have the ability to respond actively (Cohen et al., 1984, p. 14).

Nurses must keep in mind that there is significant individual variation in the emotional responses of people with dementia, but there is always some emotional response. Even in the later stages of dementia, when cognitive abilities are severely impaired, emotional response may be blunted or altered, but it is never absent. As dementia progresses, the person is likely to express emotions nonverbally and behaviorally. As emotional expressions become less verbal and more indirect, it is easy to overlook or misinterpret the feelings of the person with AD. Feelings of fear, shame, anger, and anxiety may begin in the early stage and last throughout the course of the disease, but they will vary in their manifestations. One recent study found that people in later stages of AD express a wide range of emotions, including fear, anger, sadness, interest, and happiness (Magai et al., 1996).

Behavioral Manifestations

In addition to their emotional responses to the disease, people with AD exhibit a wide range of behaviors that are associated with their cognitive impairments and declining functional abilities. Recent evidence suggests that these neuropsychiatric manifestations are caused by the cholinergic deficits that characterize some of the dementia-related brain changes (Cummings, 1997). Not all behavioral changes are problematic for caregivers, but the geriatric literature tends to focus on those behaviors that cause management problems. This is unfortunate because it reinforces fears and anxieties about the functional consequences of AD that may never occur. This author has heard such remarks as, "I know he doesn't have Alzheimer's disease because he doesn't hallucinate," or "I know she doesn't have Alzheimer's disease because she's not violent." These comments reflect a false belief that certain difficult behaviors are an inevitable consequence of dementia. Another caregiver recently asked, "Can you tell me if my mother will be the 'nice kind' or the 'mean kind' as her Alzheimer's gets worse?" This question at least acknowledges that not all people with AD are difficult, but it reflects another negative and false belief about categorical types of behaviors in people with AD. A recent consensus statement recommended that the term "behavioral disturbances" be replaced by the phrase "behavioral and psychological symptoms" to emphasize the importance of preventing and treating these behavioral manifestations (Finkel et al., 1998).

Although difficult behaviors are not necessarily a part of AD, almost all people with AD will manifest some troublesome behaviors during the course of the disease. Disruptive behaviors usually are transient, and they may resolve or give way to different behaviors as the disease progresses. One recent longitudinal study comparing different types of aggressive behavior in an adult day care population found that verbally aggressive, physically aggressive, and physically nonaggressive behaviors increased significantly with progression of the disease, but that verbally nonaggressive behaviors did not change (Cohen-Mansfield and Werner, 1998a). Common behavioral changes include:

- anxiety,
- forgetfulness,
- repetition,
- inappropriate social and sexual actions,
- impaired judgment and reasoning,
- personality alterations (apathy),
- psychosis (delusions, hallucination),
- agitation (physical or verbal),
- mood changes (depression, euphoria, emotional lability),
- aberrant motor movements (pacing, rummaging, wandering), and
- neurovegetative changes (appetite changes, sleep disturbances).

The degree of difficulty of behaviors is measured according to the perceptions of caregivers, and these vary depending on the caregiver. Caregivers reportedly are more distressed by depression-related behaviors, such as withdrawal and passivity, than by other dementia-related behaviors (Teri, 1997). The degree of perceived difficulty also is highly associated with the environment. In a locked institutional unit, for example, wandering behaviors might not be problematic, whereas in a home setting, wandering may be both unsafe and otherwise problematic. Likewise, nighttime restlessness creates more problems for a spouse who is the sole caregiver than for nursing staff who are paid to provide 24-hour care.

The term "agitation" is applied to a wide variety of dementia-related behaviors: anxiety, wandering, irritability, sleep disturbances, rest-

less walking, repetitive motor activity, nonaggressive or repetitive vocalizations, or verbally and physically aggressive behavior. In addition to being a dementia-related behavior, agitation can be a manifestation of certain types of depression, or it can arise from physiologic disturbances or adverse medication effects. Like other behaviors, therefore, agitation cannot automatically be attributed to a dementing illness just because it occurs in someone with dementia. In fact, agitation in a person with dementia often is an early and prominent sign of a change in physical condition, such as an infection.

Aggressive behaviors also are strongly associated with dementia, and gerontologists are attempting to identify factors that are associated with these behaviors. Psychotic symptoms, particularly delusions, have been found to be associated with aggressive behaviors (Gilley et al., 1997). One recent study suggested that lifelong personality traits of anger, anxiety, depression, impulsiveness, hostility, and vulnerability may be associated with aggression (Kolanowski et al., 1997). Kolanowski and colleagues found that aggressive nursing home residents were reported to have been more active, assertive, and disagreeable before the onset of dementia than their nonaggressive counterparts.

The phrase "catastrophic reaction" has been applied to a wide range of behaviors exhibited by people who have brain damage. Any action that is threatening to the person may precipitate this type of reaction. The phrase has become popular among lay and professional caregivers of people with AD, largely because of the frequent reference to catastrophic reactions in *The 36-Hour Day* (Mace and Rabins, 1991), one of the most widely used guides to the care of people with AD. A catastrophic reaction is a sudden and exaggerated response that occurs when a person suffering from dementia overreacts to a situation. The onset of a catastrophic reaction may be signaled by a sudden change in mood, increased restlessness, stubbornness, or wandering. In addition, any of the following behaviors may be a component of the catastrophic reaction: anger, crying, shouting, anxiety, irritability, combativeness, and physical or verbal aggression. Caregivers sometimes may be able to identify specific precipitants of these episodes. For example, a catastrophic reaction may be precipitated by the performance of essential ADL that may be perceived as embarrassing or threatening, such as during bathing or incontinence care. At other times, caregivers may be unable to identify any precipitating factor. Catastrophic reactions resolve when the perceived threat is removed, or when the person with dementia again feels safe and secure.

The Impact on Caregivers

"Caregiver" is a term that was absent in the health care literature before the 1980s. Now, many books about caregiving are available in bookstores throughout the United States, and gerontologists and federal policy makers have increasingly addressed caregiving issues. This attention is warranted, because 80% to 90% of the care given to dependent older adults in the community is provided by family and friends, despite the proliferation and availability of formal services for older adults in the United States. Thus, the impact and responsibility of caregiving affect primarily family members, particularly women.

The term "caregiver burden," coined in 1980 by Zarit and colleagues (1980), continues to be used in reference to the "physical, psychological or emotional, social, and financial problems that can be experienced by family members caring for impaired older adults" (George and Gwyther, 1986). Studies have identified the following functional consequences for caregivers (Office of Technology Assessment Task Force, 1988; Cohen et al., 1990; Schulz et al., 1990; Dhooper, 1991):

- infringement of privacy;
- diminished social contact;
- loss of income and assets;
- increased levels of family conflict and distress;
- little or no time for personal or recreational activities;
- increased use of alcohol and psychotropic drugs as compared with control groups;
- changes in family living arrangements, with an increased likelihood of sharing a household;
- increased likelihood of decreasing or giving up job responsibilities because of caregiver responsibilities;
- increased risk of clinical depression;
- increased feelings of anger, guilt, grief, anxiety, depression, helplessness, chronic fatigue, and emotional exhaustion; and
- poorer physical health as compared with that of people without caregiving responsibilities, with a greater frequency of stress-related illnesses and injuries secondary to caregiving.

In recent years, some studies have tried to identify cultural differences in various aspects of caregiving for people with dementia. Reviews of studies comparing African Americans to Whites have concluded that most studies reveal no differences in caregiver burden, although a few have determined that non-White caregivers report lower levels of caregiver stress (Lewis and Ausberry, 1996; Connell and Gibson, 1997). Many studies have found that Americans of non-Anglo heritage are less likely than Whites to use services or seek information. Additional cultural differences with regard to caregivers is discussed in Chapter 3.

Although most attention has been focused on the burdens of caregiving, some of the literature has addressed the positive functional consequences of caregiving. As one article stated, "Several positive aspects have been identified, including the drawing of families closer together through the expression of familial love and fulfillment of familial obligations. Additionally, families often feel that their caregiving services make a difference in guaranteeing appropriate and high-quality care" (Ory et al., 1985, p. 631).

A congressional report discussed the following positive functional consequences: (1) companionship, (2) financial assistance, (3) a broader perspective on other stresses, (4) an increased understanding of the care recipient, (5) increased feelings of usefulness and self-worth, and (6) an improved relationship between the caregiver and the care recipient (U.S. House Select Committee on Aging, 1987). Brody (1985) identified both positive and negative consequences of caregiving in her theory about parent care. She stated that "having an elderly parent is gratifying and helpful. Older people are a resource to their children, providing many forms of assistance. Most people help their parents willingly and they derive satisfaction from doing so. Some adult children negotiate this stage of life without undue strain and experience personal growth during the process" (Brody, 1985, p. 21). Brody further concluded that when the parent's dependency needs disrupt the family homeostasis, the potential for stress occurs (1985, p. 22).

Nursing Assessment

Assessment of cognitively impaired older adults must be based on a multidisciplinary approach, and the nursing assessment provides a basis for planning the nursing care. As in other aspects of assessment, the role of the nurse is to determine the person's level of function, to identify the factors that affect their level of function, and to identify their response to their illness. The nursing assessment of cognitive abilities can serve as the basis for implementing individualized interventions that will help impaired older adults function at their highest level. The assessment of all psychosocial aspects of older adulthood, including cognitive function, has been discussed in one chapter because all aspects are related. Readers, therefore, are referred to Chapter 5 for assessment information regarding cognitive function. In this chapter, the discussion is limited to a summary of guidelines for assessing older adults with dementing conditions (Display 19-1).

With regard to the assessment of specific aspects of function in people already diagnosed with dementia, there is much current emphasis on the importance of individualized assessments based on the unique needs of each person with dementia (e.g., Burgener et al., 1993). One recent article described a functional assessment model for assessing specific behavioral problems in Alzheimer's disease (Bakke, 1997). Moreover, increased emphasis is being placed on assessing not just the disabilities, but also the remaining abilities, of the person with dementia (e.g., Heacock et al., 1997). Recent nursing articles also have addressed the need to assess the behavioral aspects of dementia, such as differentiating between aggressive and resistive behaviors in long-term care residents (Gibson, 1997). Because nursing guidelines for individualized assessment are rapidly evolving, nurses should keep up-to-date with these developments by reading current nursing and gerontological journals and by obtaining information from the Alzheimer's Association.

Nursing Diagnosis

Altered Thought Processes, related to the effects of dementia, is the nursing diagnosis that is most often applied to older adults who have dementia. Carpenito defines Altered Thought Processes as "a state in which an individual experiences a disruption in such mental activities as conscious thought, reality orientation, problem solving, judgment, and comprehension related to coping, personality, and/or mental disorder" (1997, p. 873). Other common related factors for Altered Thought Processes may be delirium or an adverse medication effect. These are particularly likely to occur in hospital settings.

DISPLAY 19-1
Guidelines for Assessing Cognitive Impairment in Older Adults

General Principles

- A thorough assessment will necessitate several visits, and it might include a home assessment.
- The person's rights must be respected, and permission must be sought to obtain information from others.
- Do not assume that the family has drawn accurate conclusions about events of the past. (For example, family members may state that the person retired and then showed cognitive deficits when, in reality, the person retired because of an inability to cope with job demands.)

Focus of the Assessment

- The assessment must be multidisciplinary and must include the following components: complete medical history and physical examination (including a neurologic evaluation and a review of all medications); a functional assessment; a comprehensive psychosocial and formal mental status assessment; and an assessment of environmental and caregiver influences, with particular emphasis on those factors that affect functional abilities.
- The primary purpose of the comprehensive geriatric assessment is to identify treatable causes of the cognitive impairment.
- The assessment must include an interview with caregivers, family members, and other people who can describe the progression of the manifestations of impairment.
- Information about lifelong patterns of personality, coping, and performance characteristics must be obtained and considered in relation to the person's current functional level.
- It may be necessary to ask probing questions to help family members recognize clues to cognitive deficits retrospectively.

Considerations in Assessing Risk Factors

- Never assume that all cognitive impairments and behavioral manifestations stem from a dementing illness.

- Because risk factors can either cause the initial cognitive impairments or develop later, causing additional impairments, they must be reassessed periodically.
- The following categories of risk factors must be assessed, both initially and on an ongoing basis: depression, physiologic alterations, functional impairments, adverse medication effects, and environmental and psychosocial influences.
- Early in the assessment, the assessors must ensure that vision and hearing impairments are compensated for as much as possible, and that the environment does not interfere with the person's performance.
- Assessors must identify and treat those factors that are or might be reversible before deciding on a long-term management plan.
- In planning interventions, the assessment team should begin with those factors that are most acceptable and least threatening to the person, especially when the person denies the deficits.

Multidisciplinary Team Approach to Assessment

- Members of the multidisciplinary team must discuss their assessment findings together; if an in-person discussion is not possible, a phone conference may be arranged.
- In settings in which multidisciplinary teams are not the norm, nurses must be innovative in creating a team. This often involves the cooperation of more than one agency or institution.
- Members of the assessment team must work with the family and other caregivers to determine the appropriate level of involvement of the person with dementia with regard to discussing assessment results and planning care.

Many additional nursing diagnoses may be used to address specific problems that often are associated with the progression of dementia from the early to later stages. In the early stages, nurses may address the person's responses to the diagnosis and the implications of this diagnosis. Nursing diagnoses that might apply include Fear, Anxiety, Hopelessness, Impaired Adjustment, Self-Esteem Disturbance, and Ineffective Individual Coping. In the later stages of dementia, nursing care addresses the many problems associated with functional impairments and declining abilities of the person with dementia. Nursing diagnoses that might be applicable include Constipation, Social Isolation, Altered Nutrition, Urinary Incontinence, Self-Care Deficits, Impaired Physical Mobility, Altered Sexuality Patterns, Impaired Verbal Communication, Sensory-Perceptual Alterations, Diversional Activity Deficit, and High Risk for Injury. At any stage, if the person is taking medications and cannot remember to take the medications correctly, the nurse might apply the diagnosis of Ineffective Management of Therapeutic Regimen.

Nursing diagnoses also may be used to address the needs of caregivers because much of the care of people with dementia focuses on helping the family and other caregivers address the day-to-day needs and issues of the person with dementia. Nursing diagnoses that might be used to address caregiver needs include Altered Family Processes, Ineffective Family Coping, and Caregiver Role Strain (or High Risk for Caregiver Role Strain). During the later stages of dementia, the nursing diagnoses of Social Isolation and Anticipatory Grieving may be appropriate, particularly for spousal caregivers.

Nursing Goals

The primary nursing goal for older adults in any stage of dementia is to promote function at the highest level of independence possible, while providing the supports that are necessary for the highest quality of life. Additional goals related to the care of people with dementia might be to alleviate anxiety, to maintain reality orientation, to promote memory function, and to facilitate maximum communication. These goals are achieved through communication techniques and environmental modifications that address the needs of each person with dementia. In addition, nursing goals address the specific problems associated with dementia, such as those identified in the section on Nursing Diagnosis.

In recent years, gerontologists and ethicists have raised questions about how to assess and address quality of life for people with dementia. This is an essential aspect of establishing goals for care, particularly in situations in which the person with dementia is not able to articulate his or her preferences for care approaches and interventions. One noted gerontologist recently suggested that the essential aspects of quality of life for people with dementia include the following components: environmental quality, social interaction, clinical depression, basic affective states, discretional time use, ADL, and disturbed or agitated behaviors (Lawton, 1997). Using these parameters as a framework, nursing goals for people with dementia would include preventing and alleviating agitation; meeting the individual's needs for all ADL; and providing the most supportive physical and emotional environment possible, including opportunities for meaningful social interaction. Gerontological practitioners also are addressing quality of life issues and goals of care in end-stage dementia. In later-stage dementia care, emphasis is placed on comfort, dignity, psychological well-being, and needs of the caregivers (Teno et al., 1997; Volicer, 1997).

Nursing goals and interventions vary according to the specific setting. What works in one setting may not work or may not be able to be implemented in another. In hospitals, for example, a goal might be to alleviate the confusion and agitation associated with an acute medical condition and a strange environment, and the interventions may include the use of behavior-modifying medications. In homes and residential settings, a goal might be to promote the highest and most independent level of function, and interventions would likely emphasize environmental modifications and communication techniques.

When the person with dementia is cared for by friends, family members, or paid caregivers, nursing goals also will address the needs of the caregivers. In the early stages of dementia, the caregiver's foremost need might be for information about the disease and about resources that address the changing needs of the person with dementia and the caregiver's own needs. Additional caregiver needs are for emotional support and practical assistance, particularly when the person with dementia requires increased care and supervision. Interventions that address caregiver needs include counseling, caregiver support groups, direct assistance with care, and individual or group education. Local chapters of the Alzheimer's Association can provide information about resources that address caregiver needs.

Nursing Interventions

As anyone who has cared for a person with dementia knows, interventions must be highly individualized and frequently modified. An intervention that works for one person may not work for others, and interventions that are effective one day will not necessarily be effective the next day. Currently, there is much emphasis on care plans that incorporate individualized interventions based on the assessment of the person's unique expressions and behaviors. Thus, caring for people with dementia is a creative process, and is, perhaps, the most challenging of all aspects of gerontological nursing.

Interventions for specific behaviors are not discussed in detail in this text for several reasons.

First, the manifestations of AD are very complex, and so the interventions must be highly individualized. Second, there are many practical and comprehensive references available on the management of dementia-related behaviors. Third, nursing roles and interventions vary according to the setting. The approach of this text, therefore, is to provide guidelines for nursing interventions and information about additional references. Nurses are strongly urged to take advantage of the excellent written materials available from the Alzheimer's Association and from other resources listed at the end of this chapter. Nurses also are encouraged to keep up-to-date with gerontological and nursing articles that reflect the increasing knowledge about various interventions for different dementia-associated behaviors and care needs. Table 19-3 lists many of the journal articles that were published in 1997 describing interventions for dementia-associated nursing problems.

Two additional issues are discussed that often are not addressed from a nursing perspective. First, medical treatment of people with AD is addressed, with emphasis on the role of the nurse in decisions about these interventions. Current information is reviewed with regard to medications for dementia and dementia-related behaviors. Also, alternative and preventive health care practices are discussed. Second, a model is presented for decision making about the care of older adults with dementia. This issue is covered in detail because although nurses often are the professional caregivers who are most involved with these decisions, they usually are not prepared for this role and have very few references to use as guides.

Environmental Modifications and Communication Techniques

Environmental modifications and communication techniques are two types of interventions that are most important in caring for people with dementia. One discussion of studies of the

TABLE 19-3
Journal Articles, Published in 1997, on Interventions for Dementia-Related Problems

Authors	Target Problem	Interventions
Cohen-Mansfield & Werner	Verbally disruptive behaviors	Music, social interaction
Cohen-Mansfield et al.	Wandering	Interventions to accommodate the behavior
Denney	Mealtime agitation	Quiet music
Hepburn et al.	Diminished sense of meaning	Family stories
Hoeffer et al.	Aggressive behavior during bathing	Individualized, person-focused approach
Holmberg	Wandering	Volunteer-facilitated walking program
Kayser-Jones & Schell	Problematic mealtime behaviors	Individualized care approaches
Kovach & Meyer-Arnold	Agitated behaviors during bathing	Environmental modifications
Lantz et al.	Disruptive behaviors	Group therapy focused on wellness
Miller	Aggressive behavior during hygienic care	Individualized care approaches
Mistretta & Kee	Diminished quality of life	Specific caregiving strategies
Sloane et al.	Disruptive vocalizations	Individualized care approaches
Taft et al.	Agitation	Individualized, targeted interventions
Teri et al.	Depression	Pleasant events and caregiver problem solving
Whall et al.	Agitation and aggression during bathing	Environmental modification

effects of the environment on people with dementia concluded that there was an inverse relationship between environmental stimuli and functional behaviors. That is, a decrease in environmental stimuli led to improved function, whereas an increase in environmental stimuli led to diminished function (Hall and Buckwalter, 1987). There is also a growing recognition that the influence of the environment may vary, depending on the stage of cognitive impairment. The more cognitively impaired a person is, the more the environment will influence his or her behavior and function. Thus, modifications of the environment are essential aspects of nursing interventions that must be adapted as the person's level of function changes. Environmental interventions may be especially effective in ad-

dressing behavioral problems, such as wandering, incontinence, and agitation (Cohen-Mansfield and Werner, 1998b). Also, environmental modifications are important interventions for fostering independence in ADL, such as dressing and eating. For example, a recent study found that recorded music was effective in decreasing aggressive behaviors of nursing home residents during bathing routines (Clark et al., 1998).

Initially, the approach to environmental modifications was simply to provide stimulation, with emphasis on orientation cues. It was thought that sensory stimulation and orientation cues would benefit any cognitively impaired person. Based on this rationale, reality orientation has been implemented widely, particularly in nursing homes and other residential care settings. Reality orientation involves the repeated use of verbal and nonverbal indicators of time, place, and person in the context of the individual, group, and environment. The goals are to improve the person's awareness of himself or herself and the immediate environment, and to reduce the person's confusion, anxiety, and disorientation. In recent years, questions have been raised about the effectiveness and appropriateness of reality orientation. Although it may be effective for some people with dementia, especially when it is combined with other strategies, reality orientation should not necessarily be applied to all people with dementia, and it must be tailored to individual needs.

Along with environmental modifications, communication techniques are extremely important interventions for people with dementia. It is well known that nonverbal communication, such as facial expressions, can significantly affect the behavior of people with dementia. Validation therapy is a communication strategy that has been promoted since the late 1960s as an alternative to the approach of reality therapy. A recent review of studies on the use of Validation techniques in long-term care facilities emphasized the need for further research into its effectiveness before adopting this approach as a standard intervention for people with dementia (Day, 1997). Currently, emphasis is being placed on individualizing communication to the specific needs of each person with dementia. Techniques discussed in Chapter 5 can be applied to the care of people with dementia. Guidelines for communicating with cognitively impaired people also are presented in Display 19-2.

Long-Term Care Settings

In recent years, nurses and other health care professionals in nursing homes have planned and implemented special care units (SCUs) for older adults with dementia. Essential features of these units for cognitively impaired residents include environmental modifications, family involvement, individualized care plans, dementia-specific activity programs, and specially trained and selected staff. Many positive outcomes of SCUs have been identified for the staff, the residents with dementia, and the families of these residents; however, many of these same outcomes can be achieved in nursing care units that address the individualized needs of the residents even though they are not specifically designated as an SCU. The development of SCUs is another rapidly evolving aspect of dementia-related care, and nurses need to keep pace with these developments by reading pertinent journal articles (e.g., Buettner, 1998; Grant et al., 1998; McAiney, 1998; Teresi et al., 1998).

A theoretical framework for nursing interventions for people with dementia, called the progressively lowered stress threshold model, has been proposed by two nurses (Hall and Buckwalter, 1987) and has been widely implemented in the past decade. Briefly stated, this theory contends that dysfunctional behaviors indicate a progressive lowering of the stress threshold, which, in turn, interferes with the person's function and ability to interact with the environment. The goal of nursing care, then, is to maximize the person's function by relieving stressors that cause excess disability (Hall, 1988). The choice of interventions is based on an ongoing assessment of anxiety "as a barometer to determine how much activity and stimuli the anxious person can tolerate at any point during their illness. As anxious behaviors occur, activities and environmental stimuli are modified and simplified until the anxiety disappears" (Hall and Buckwalter, 1987, p. 403). This approach is highly individualized, and from a nursing perspective, it is analogous to adjusting insulin doses for diabetics according to serum glucose levels. Some of the interventions and underlying principles of this approach are included in Display 19-2, along with additional guidelines for modifying the environment in long-term care settings.

DISPLAY 19-2
Guidelines for Care of People with Dementia

Verbal Communication

- Adapt your level of communication to the abilities of the person with AD.
- Avoid indicators of infantilization (e.g., do not talk "baby talk" or use a demeaning or condescending tone of voice).
- For people in the middle to later stages of AD, use very simple sentences and present only one idea at a time.
- If the person does not understand a statement, repeat the statement using the same words, or simplify the wording.
- In general, do not argue with the person, unless it is a matter of safety.
- Use positive statements (i.e., avoid using statements containing the word "don't" or other negative commands).
- If the person is able to make decisions, offer simple and concrete choices (e.g., "Do you want chicken or steak?" rather than "What do you want to eat?").
- Listen to the feelings the person is trying to express and respond to the feelings, rather than the statement.
- Do not ask questions that you know the person cannot answer correctly.

Nonverbal Communication

- Reinforce verbal communication with appropriate nonverbal communication (e.g., demonstrate what you are asking the person to do).
- Use appropriate touch to gain the person's attention and to reinforce feelings of concern (unless the person responds negatively to touch).
- Maintain good eye contact and pleasant facial expressions.
- Use a relaxed and smiling approach.
- Be aware of your own nonverbal communication. Keep in mind that your nonverbal cues will probably communicate more than your spoken words and will not necessarily be interpreted correctly.
- Closely observe all nonverbal cues exhibited by the person, especially those that express feelings.
- Assume that all nonverbal expressions of the person with dementia are attempts to communicate needs or feelings.

Environmental Modifications

- Modify the environment to compensate as much as possible for sensory deficits and other functional impairments. (Refer to the information presented in Chapters 6 through 9 and 12.)
- Use clocks, calendars, daily newspapers, and simple written cues for orientation (e.g., day, date, names, place, and events).
- Use simple pictures, written cues, or color codes for identifying items and places (e.g., toilet, bedroom).
- Use simple written cues to clarify directions for operating radios, televisions, appliances, and thermostats (e.g., on, off, directional arrows).
- If verbal comprehension is impaired, use pictures rather than written cues.
- Place pictures of familiar people in highly visible places, but use nonglossy pictures and nonglare glass in picture frames.
- Turn lights on as soon as or before it begins to get dark.
- Use night-lights, or leave dim lights on during the night.
- Simplify the environment to avoid overstimulation.

Techniques to Ensure Safety

- Make sure the person carries some form of identification, along with the phone number of someone to call.
- Adapt the environment for safety (e.g., use alarm devices for doors to prevent wandering).
- Keep the environment uncluttered.
- Keep medications, cleaning solutions, and any poisonous chemicals in inaccessible places.
- Enroll the person in a protective program, such as the "Safe Return" program sponsored by the Alzheimer's Association.

Techniques to Facilitate Independent Performance of ADL

- Keep all activities as simple and routine as possible.

DISPLAY 19-2
Guidelines for Care of People with Dementia (Continued)

- For ADL, establish routines that allow for maximum independence and the least amount of frustration.
- While keeping the routines as consistent as possible, recognize that they will have to be changed as the person's level of function changes.
- Lay out one set of clothing in the order in which the items are to be donned.
- If the person needs assistance with hygiene, use matter-of-fact statements, such as "It's time for your bath." Avoid statements such as, "You need a bath now," which may be interpreted as judgmental.
- Arrange personal care items, such as grooming and hygiene aids, in a visible and uncluttered place, in the order in which the items are to be used.
- Leave a toothbrush on the bathroom sink with toothpaste already on it.
- Establish an individualized toileting plan that allows for maximum independence but minimal risk of incontinence episodes.
- Use finger foods and nutritious snacks if the person will not sit at the table to eat a meal.

Principles Based on the Progressively Lowered Stress Threshold Model (Hall & Buckwalter, 1987)

- Maximize safety by modifying the environment to compensate for cognitive losses.
- Control any factors that increase stress, such as fatigue; physical stressors; competing or overwhelming stimuli; changes in routine, caregiver, or environment; and activities or demands that exceed the person's functional ability.
- Plan and maintain a consistent routine.
- Implement regular rest periods to compensate for fatigue and loss of reserve energy.
- Provide unconditional positive regard.
- Remain nonjudgmental about the appropriateness of all behaviors except those that present threats to safety.
- Recognize individual expressions of fatigue, anxiety, and increasing stress, and intervene to reduce stressors as soon as possible.
- Modify reality orientation and other therapeutic interventions to incorporate only that information needed for safe function.
- Use reassuring forms of therapy, such as music and reminiscence.

Acute Care Settings

In some circumstances, an older adult may be hospitalized for an initial evaluation of dementia, especially if there are primary or secondary physiologic causes. In most cases, however, the reason for hospitalizing a person with a dementing illness is to provide care for an acute medical problem, in which case, management of dementia-related behaviors is a secondary but major nursing problem. Therefore, nurses in hospital settings deal not only with the acute illness, but also with the dementia-related behaviors, which often are exacerbated by the medical problem. Problematic dementia-related behaviors often are exacerbated or precipitated by the hospital environment, the unfamiliar caregivers, and the change in routines. Further difficulties stem from

the fact that nurses have little or no control over many of the environmental influences, such as paging systems and other noises, that contribute to management problems in hospitals. Thus, nurses in acute care settings face a tremendous challenge in caring for people with dementia.

One of the most important initial interventions is to involve at least one of the older adult's usual caregivers in planning and implementing nursing care for the cognitively impaired person. Although the person with dementia is likely to exhibit different behaviors in the hospital than at home, nurses must begin by identifying any interventions that were effective in the home environment. During the admission process, nurses may save a lot of time and frustration if they interview the caregivers about specific methods that help or hinder care. For example, knowing that the person eats only sandwiches or needs to be assisted to the toilet at specific times may facilitate the planning of effective interventions. It is important to remember that people with dementia may not express their needs directly or verbally. Usually, family caregivers have a good understanding of the needs of the person and the expressions of those needs, but if this information is not obtained at the time of admission, the person's needs may not be addressed.

In addition to obtaining information from one of the usual caregivers, nurses may consider involving them in the person's care during hospitalization. Although family members and other caregivers certainly deserve a respite from caregiving responsibilities, they may be willing to assist at some level with the care of the patient. This may be particularly helpful during the first few days of hospitalization, and with patients who are especially difficult to manage. Often, the family will be relieved to be able to participate in the care, especially if they have never had any outside assistance. Booklets and other materials with helpful information for nurses in any institutional setting can be obtained from the Alzheimer's Association.

Community Settings

In community settings, professional nurses usually work with family or agency caregivers, rather than directly implementing the interventions for the person with dementia. Thus, their primary responsibilities are to serve as role models and to educate primary caregivers about interventions that will promote the highest level of function for the person with dementia and the least burden for the caregivers. An intervention that might be most effective, as well as efficient, is to encourage caregivers to participate in educational or support groups. The number of groups addressing the needs of caregivers is increasing rapidly, and information about these

groups is available from the Alzheimer's Association or local hospitals. Nurses also can encourage caregivers to purchase one of the many caregiver guides that are available in bookstores or through the Internet and to contact the Alzheimer's Association and other resources for information. The suggestions outlined in Display 19-2 can be used as a guide for developing individualized interventions in community settings.

In addition to educating caregivers about specific management problems, nurses in community settings must be ready to discuss resources for medical care, home services, and other community-based services for people with dementia and their caregivers. As the number and range of services increase, it is becoming more and more difficult to keep up-to-date on the resources in one's own community. Although nurses cannot be expected to know all the details about all available community services, they should know about the general types of services available. In addition, they must be able to suggest at least one information and referral resource from which caregivers can obtain specific information. A good rule of thumb is to suggest that caregivers call the local area agency on aging, because every part of the United States is served by this type of organization. Additionally, local chapters of the Alzheimer's Association provide information about resources for care, and many chapters provide direct services. Information about these services can be obtained from the national Alzheimer's Association, listed in the Educational Resources section at the end of this chapter. Various types of services that may be helpful to people with dementia and their caregivers are discussed in Chapter 21.

Medication Interventions

Three aspects of medication use must be considered when caring for people with dementia: (1) adverse medication effects; (2) medications as a primary intervention for AD; and (3) medications for dementia-related behaviors, including depression. With regard to the first aspect, the most important consideration is to be vigilant about the possibility that cognitive impairment and dementia-like behaviors may be caused by any medication, as discussed in detail in Chapter 18. The discussion in this section is limited to the second and third aspects; however, the information presented in Chapter 18 must be kept in mind when caring for cognitively impaired older adults.

Medications for the Treatment of AD in the United States

Many medications are being investigated for the treatment of AD, as discussed in the section on Neurotransmitters and as summarized in Table 19-4. In addition to drugs that act on neurotransmitters, other types of drugs that are under intense investigation in the late 1990s for the prevention or treatment of dementia include estrogen, ampakines, antioxidants, neurotrophic agents, anti-inflammatory agents,

TABLE 19-4
Drugs for Alzheimer's Disease

Drug Type	Examples	Availability/Status
Cholinesterase inhibitors	Tacrine	Approved (1993)
	Donepezil	Approved (1996)
	ENA-713	Approval pending (1998)
	Metrifonate	Approval pending (1998)
	Eptastigmine	In trials (1998)
	Galantamine	In trials (1998)
	Physostigmine	In trials (1998)
Nicotinic, cholinergic, and muscarinic agonists	Arecoline	Clinical trials in process (1998)
	Nicotine	
	ABT-418	
	AF-102B	
	Milameline	
	Xanomeline	
Calcium channel blockers	Nimodipine	In trials (1998)
	Sabeluzole	
Ampakines	CX-516	In trials (1998)
Neurotrophins, growth factors, and neuroprotective agents	Nerve growth factor	Various research phases
	GM1	
	Acetyl-L-carnitine	
	MAO-A inhibitors	
	MAO-B inhibitors	
Antioxidants	Vitamins C and E	OTC
	Selegiline	Prescription (for other conditions)
Anti-inflammatory agents	Aspirin, ibuprofen, indomethacin, prednisone	OTC and prescription (for other conditions); clinical trials in process (1998)
Estrogen	Estradiol	Prescription (for other conditions); clinical trials in process (1998)

MAO, monoamine oxidase; *OTC*, over-the-counter.

and calcium channel blockers. Since 1993, when the first drug was approved for the treatment of AD, much progress has been made in our knowledge about treatment and prevention strategies. Despite these advances in knowledge, however, as of 1998, no medication had been determined to be effective in reversing or permanently improving the cognitive impairments caused by AD. The next sections summarize what was known in 1998 about some of the most widely discussed and readily available agents under investigation for prevention or treatment of dementia: estrogen, ibuprofen, and vitamin E.

Estrogen is thought to have a neuroprotective effect on brain cells. Several studies have confirmed that hormonal replacement therapy in menopausal women is associated with a reduced risk of developing AD or with a delayed onset of symptoms for those women who do develop AD. Other studies have found that estrogen may improve mental function and delay the progression of the disease in women who already have developed AD. Studies are currently being conducted to determine the appropriate dose and duration of estrogen therapy and to further address risk-to-benefit ratios.

People enrolled in the Baltimore Longitudinal Study of Aging who were taking ibuprofen and other nonsteroidal anti-inflammatory drugs (NSAIDs) for 2 years or longer were found to have a 60% lower risk of developing AD, whereas study participants who were taking aspirin or acetaminophen were not found to have any lower risk of developing AD. It is thought that NSAIDs protect the brain from the inflammatory response associated with the amyloid protein that builds up in the brains of people with AD. As of 1998, however, the association between NSAIDs and a reduced risk of AD was an incidental finding that had not been confirmed through clinical trials.

Results of studies of vitamin E, taken alone or in combination with selegiline (a drug prescribed for the management of Parkinson's disease), indicate that either of these drugs can delay the progression of AD. The effects of the drugs are thought to be attributable to their antioxidant properties, which may improve overall health and function. Current recommendations are that either vitamin E or selegiline be administered to slow disease progression in older adults with moderate AD. However, it must be noted that vitamin E is contraindicated for those who are taking anticoagulants.

Behavior-Modifying Medications

Behavior-modifying medications may be an effective and essential intervention for the safety and comfort of people with dementia, as well as their caregivers. Decisions about the use of these medications must be made carefully, however, because there is always a risk that medications will further interfere with function and perhaps even cause serious harm. Nurses must keep in mind that a dementing illness is not necessarily the basis of difficult behaviors. Another consideration is whether the behaviors justify the risks associated with medications. Bothersome or socially inappropriate behaviors might better be ignored or tolerated than treated with medications. However, if the behavior is unsafe, uncomfortable, or interferes with the function of the person with dementia, then medication intervention is probably justified if nonmedication interventions are not successful. Moreover, if the behavior interferes with the rights of the caregivers or other people in the environment, then consideration might be given to medication management. When medications are used in combination with other interventions, the dose of medication may be able to be lowered, and the effectiveness of the other interventions may be enhanced. Display 19-3 summarizes general principles and specific considerations relating to medications for people with dementia.

Guidelines for Use of Behavior-Modifying Medications for People with Dementia

Considerations Regarding Behavior-Modifying Medications

- Assess whether any of the following factors cause or contribute to the difficult behaviors: environmental conditions; psychosocial factors, such as anxiety or depression; or physiologic factors, such as pain, discomfort, or physical disorders. If any of these factors are implicated, interventions should be directed at the causative factor.
- Are the behaviors caused by adverse medication effects? In this case, the appropriate intervention might be to reduce the dose of or discontinue a medication, rather than begin a new medication.
- Treatment with medication should be implemented for behavior problems only after a trial of nonmedication interventions.
- Do the behaviors truly justify the use of medications, or are the caregivers requesting medications for their own comfort and convenience?

Considerations Regarding the Choice and Dose of Medications

- The specific goals of and expectations for the medication interventions should be clear to all caregivers.
- If the person is depressed, antidepressants may be effective in treating the depression, and some functional improvement may occur as the depression is alleviated.
- Caregivers should not assume that, just because medications are necessary and appro-

priate during one stage of AD, they will be necessary and appropriate on an ongoing basis.
- Medication regimens should be reevaluated as AD progresses or as other conditions, such as medical disorders, affect the person's functional level.
- People with dementia exhibit a wide range of responses to various medications, and the selection of a particular medication should be based on current manifestations, as well as prior experiences with medications.
- Some people with dementia, especially those with DLB, are highly sensitive to even minute doses of psychotropic medications.
- Any behavior-modifying medication is likely to interfere with cognitive function.
- The type of behavior-modifying medication should be appropriate for the type of behavioral manifestations (e.g., antipsychotics for delusions and hallucination, antianxiety agents for anxiety).
- The initial dose should be one half to one third the normal adult dose.
- Dosage should be increased gradually until therapeutic effects are achieved, all the while observing the person for adverse effects.
- Medications with long half-lives (e.g., flurazepam, diazepam, chlordiazepoxide) should be avoided.
- The half-life of a medication should be considered in determining the frequency of doses.

Alternative and Preventive Health Care Practices

Nutrition, exercise, and general mental, physical, and spiritual health practices have long been considered essential components of maintaining optimal cognitive function in people with and without dementia. Recently, however, attention has been focused on a quest for remedies, such as "brain boosters," that can enhance cognitive performance for people of all ages. This quest is particularly applicable to older adults, whether or not they have cognitive impairments. In the late 1990s, information about ginkgo biloba, St. John's wort, and other remedies designed to increase cognitive function or alleviate possible depression could be found daily in the media and on the Internet. Even the National Institutes of Health, many medical institutions, and Alzheimer's research centers in the United States are studying these herbs and other alternative care practices that are widely used in other countries. It is interesting to note that many of the herbs used to enhance cognition contain ingredients that are similar to those in the medications being used or investigated. For example, willow bark has anti-inflammatory effects, stinging nettle is similar to estrogen, and sage and rosemary affect acetylcholine levels and have antioxidant effects. Not only do health care professionals need to keep up-to-date on developments in this area, but they need to maintain a nonjudgmental attitude while sorting out the facts from the myths. In meeting this challenge, nurses must obtain information from many sources, including their own clinical experiences and observations, and then draw conclusions than can be used to educate older adults and their caregivers. Some of the alternative and preventive health care practices that were under investigation or were commonly used or available in the United States in 1998 are summarized in the box on page 567. The next section discusses the responsibilities of nurses with regard to health education about medical and alternative interventions for impaired cognitive function.

Responsibilities of Nurses in Educating People with Dementia and Their Caregivers

People with dementia and their families and caregivers often seek information from nurses about medications and alternative health care practices. Any "breakthroughs" reported in the media generally precipitate a flood of inquiries from families, and nurses must be prepared to answer these questions, just as they answer questions about other medical conditions. For example, it is not unusual nowadays for the family of a long-term care resident to ask if the resident can be treated with Ginkgo biloba or St. John's

wort as part of the usual medication regimen. In dealing with questions such as this, nurses may have to address gaps in the policy of the facility with regard to over-the-counter products that may be unfamiliar to the prescribing health care practitioner. The wide array of possible medication interventions and alternative health care practices presents a dilemma to nurses who are in a position to educate older adults and their caregivers about potential treatment and prevention options for AD. This dilemma is compounded by the fact that many of the interventions are available without prescription, and some products (e.g., herbs) are unregulated in the United States. Nurses need to keep informed about current scientific knowledge with regard to both the prevention of and treatment for AD. Clinical trials are being conducted on agents that are being developed specifically for AD, as well as for agents, such as NSAIDs and estrogen, that are already commonly used. Nurses can suggest that people with AD and their families contact their local Alzheimer's Association for information about clinical trials in their geographic region. The Alzheimer's Association also is an excellent source of information about the prevention and treatment of AD. Nurses can also encourage people with AD and their families to ask their primary care provider(s) about the drugs that have been approved by the FDA for the treatment of AD. Lastly, nurses can keep abreast of the latest developments in the prevention and treatment of AD by adding their name to the free mailing list of the Alzheimer's Association and the Alzheimer's Disease Education and Referral Center at the National Institute on Aging (see the Educational Resources section). Also, numerous Internet sites provide up-to-date information about all aspects of AD.

Decisions About the Care of People with Dementia

Caregivers of people with dementia face complex decisions and often assume uncomfortable levels of responsibility for people who once were

ALTERNATIVE
AND
PREVENTIVE
HEALTH
CARE
PRACTICES

Promoting Cognitive Function

Herbs
- Ginkgo biloba (60 to 240 mg/day)
- Sage, rosemary, horsebalm, club moss, stinging nettle, willow bark, gotu kola

Homeopathic Remedies
- Sulfur, Lachesis, alumina, Anacardium, calcarea, argentum nitricum, baryta carbonica

Nutritional Considerations
- Important nutrients: zinc, choline, lecithin, selenium, magnesium, beta-carotene, folic acid, vitamins C and E

Preventive Measures and Additional Approaches
- Aerobic exercise, 1/2 hour 3 times/week
- Art, dance, yoga, music, quigong, t'ai chi, massage, imagery, meditation, relaxation, acupressure
- Aromatherapy: balm, sage, basil, fennel, lemon, comfrey, rosemary, forget-me-not
- Assessment for food allergies and food intolerance
- Aspirin (81 mg/d) for prevention of vascular dementia
- Chelation therapy for removal of heavy metals from the system (*Note:* questions have been raised about the safety and efficacy of this mode of therapy.)

Special Precautions
- Minor side effects of ginkgo biloba include headache, restlessness, and gastrointestinal symptoms. It may take several months to notice effects. Prolonged use of ginkgo biloba has been associated with intraocular hemorrhage and subdural hematoma. The risk of these adverse effects increases when taken for long periods of time, or when combined with anticoagulants, such as aspirin.
- Willow bark should not be taken by people who are allergic to aspirin.
- High doses of lecithin may cause anorexia, nausea, diarrhea, abdominal bloating, and gastrointestinal pain.
- Chelation may interfere with anticoagulants.

able to make their own decisions. Although some families assume too much decision-making power, most are reluctant to make decisions about dependent older adults. Decision making is especially difficult when the older adult is physically healthy but mentally impaired, or when the person voices strong opinions about unwise or unsafe actions. For example, families of people with dementia often deal with decisions about the person driving a car. Decisions about specific behaviors, like driving, may be relatively easy compared with decisions about long-term care, which most families of people with progressively declining conditions must confront. In addition to basic safety and medical concerns, these decisions involve complex emotional and financial issues. Because several people are involved in these decisions, differing opinions and interests may complicate the process.

Caregivers facing these decisions often turn to nurses and other health care professionals for advice and assistance. If decisions about long-term care are made during a hospitalization, much of the decision-making responsibility may be assumed by or relegated to the primary care provider. When the person is being cared for at home, however, the locus of decision making is usually more nebulous. When the dependent person primarily needs social activities or supervision of daily care, the decision is more psychosocial than medical. In many situations, especially in home or residential settings, nurses are the only health care professionals who maintain close and ongoing relationships with dependent older adults and their caregivers. Thus, the nurse often becomes a support person or a care manager. The following decision-making model, summarized in Display 19-4, may be used by nurses in these situations. It is important to keep in mind that the identification of caregivers and decision makers should be done with a high degree of cultural sensitivity. As discussed in Chapters 3 and 22, decision-making and caregiver patterns are strongly influenced by cultural factors. Practical information about decision making and caregiving roles from many cultural perspectives is described in an excellent, nurse-authored pocket guide entitled *Culture and Nursing Care* (Lipson et al., 1996).

Step I: Assessing the Decision-Making Situation

To facilitate decisions about long-term care for cognitively impaired older adults, nurses should begin by assessing all of the following: (1) physical and psychosocial function of the dependent person, (2) resources that can be used to meet identified needs, and (3) factors that influence the decision on the part of the caregivers and the dependent person. This assessment usually is very complex and time-consuming. If this step is done well, however, the nurse will save time in the long run, and the plan is increasingly likely to succeed. Questions to be considered are outlined in Display 19-4.

Step II: Obtaining Consensus About Problems and Needs

After obtaining as much assessment information as possible, it usually is effective and efficient to gather all the decision makers together. Exceptions may be made if serious conflicts have arisen between the decision makers. In these situations, it may be best to begin with those who are in the greatest agreement, and to plan a strategy to involve or minimize the impact of those who do not agree with the plan. Once the decision makers are gathered together, the nurse leads the conference according to the guidelines presented in Display 19-4. When caregivers do not have a broad perspective on the dependent person's needs, the nurse may provide additional input about the person's needs. For example, the nurse might point out that social activities and interactions with others are important ways of meeting psychosocial needs and helping cognitively impaired people maintain the highest level of function. Although group activities cannot be provided in home settings, they are available in residential facilities or community-based programs, like adult day care centers.

Step III: Discussing Potential Resources

After summarizing the older person's needs, the nurse then initiates and guides a discussion about potential resources for addressing the problems. Attention must be focused on the needs of the caregivers, as well as the needs of the dependent older person. Often, the needs of caregivers may be addressed through support groups or individual counseling. Many families are not aware of the range of housing options and community-based services that are available. Nurses who are not familiar with these resources should arrange for a social worker to participate in the conference.

As resources are identified, advantages and

DISPLAY 19-4
Model for Decision Making About People with Dementia

Step I: Assess the Decision-Making Situation

- What are the typical decision-making patterns in the family?
- Who influences the decision making, either directly or indirectly?
- How do family relationships help or hinder the decision-making process?
- Are there patterns of passive nondecisions, as well as active decisions?
- What is each person's perception of the situation?
- How objective are the perceptions of the various decision makers?
- What does each person in the decision-making process have to gain or lose based on various decisions?

Step II: Obtain Consensus About Problems and Needs

- Have the most involved caregivers describe the problems first.
- After those who are most involved voice their opinions, those who are less involved can be asked to describe the problems.
- Provide objective information to ensure that the various needs of the dependent person are recognized.
- Address the needs of the caregivers, as well as the needs of the person with dementia.
- Summarize the identified needs of the older adult and the caregivers.

Step III: Discuss the Potential Resources

- Ask caregivers to suggest potential solutions and resources.
- Identify resources for the caregivers' needs, as well as for those of the person with dementia.
- Supplement the family's knowledge about resources and potential solutions.
- Discuss the positive and negative consequences of each option for the person with dementia and for the caregivers.

- As the family members discuss solutions, assess their attitudes about using various services and spending family resources to purchase services.
- Provide information about the long-range benefits that the caregivers might not perceive.
- Summarize important points on paper or a blackboard for all participants to review.

Step IV: Agree on a Plan of Action

- Eliminate the least acceptable options.
- Agree on the two or three most acceptable alternatives.
- Emphasize the fact that any plan of action will be given a trial period and should not be viewed as a permanent decision.
- Suggest a time frame and criteria for evaluating the plan of action.
- Identify one or two people who will evaluate the plan and make appropriate changes.

Step V: Involve the Person with Dementia

- Discuss the ability of the person with dementia to understand the decision.
- Identify the most realistic level of involvement for the person with dementia.
- Identify the best approach to take in involving the person with dementia.
- Identify the roles of caregivers and professionals in assisting the person with dementia to understand the decision.

Step VI: Summarize the Plan and Clarify Roles

- Review and summarize the plan of action.
- Have the caregivers state their roles in very specific terms.
- Clarify the role of the nurse and other professionals.
- Assure caregivers that you will be available for further discussion and problem solving, or provide the name of someone who can assume this role.

disadvantages are discussed from various perspectives. The nurse can begin with a statement, such as "As we identify different options, let's look at the good points and bad points of each. We need to look at the financial costs and emotional costs that affect each of you, as well as the person for whom we are planning the care." Because the financial aspects are the most objective, they often are a good starting point. Financial decisions, however, can involve many repercussions for spouses and for anyone who might inherit money from the dependent older adult. Sometimes, some of the decision makers may be more concerned about protecting their own financial interests than implementing a plan that is in the best interests of the dependent elder. Another pertinent question that may be asked regarding the advantages and disadvantages of various options is "What is the cost of not providing this service?" This approach is especially effective in broadening the caregivers' perspective when their viewpoint is very narrow. For example, the nurse may be able to use professional knowledge and experience to convince a family that the long-term benefits of a particular plan may far outweigh the immediate cost of services.

Step IV: Agreeing on a Plan of Action

After reviewing the options, the nurse then summarizes the information and eliminates those options that are least acceptable. The nurse then tries to identify two options that are the best (or only) alternatives. There are always at least two final choices: to do nothing or to make a change. If caregivers are reluctant to accept any of the options identified, the nurse might review the consequences associated with doing nothing, as well as the consequences of implementing one or two of the possible action steps. When neither alternative is deemed acceptable initially, it may be helpful to say, "I realize that neither of these choices may seem desirable, but there are no other options." Families sometimes need to hear this kind of conclusion, and they may accept it

more readily when it is based on professional experience and knowledge. Once the choices are defined, the decision makers must agree on what action to take. At this point it is helpful to emphasize that no decision is permanent, and to set a specific time frame for evaluating the decision after a trial period. If the caregivers understand that the decision can be altered after a fair trial period, they usually are more comfortable with a particular action. Because this decision-making process can be very time-consuming, it is important to identify ways of streamlining the process as much as possible. Therefore, when many people are involved in the conference, one or two key people should be designated as the ones responsible for follow-up. Unless there is a major change in the situation, effective communication networks can eliminate the need for additional conferences with all the decision makers. The evaluation plan may even be carried out through phone contact, rather than in-person contact.

Step V: Involving the Person with Dementia

When the older adult cannot participate in the decision-making conference, the participants must determine the best way of involving that person in the decision. It should be emphasized that the decision-making process just described applies primarily to situations in which the dependent older person is not able to make decisions on his or her own behalf. In any situation, it is crucial to address the rights and wishes of the dependent older person at every step. In situations in which the person has serious cognitive impairments, the decision makers may simply need to identify the best way to gain acceptance and cooperation. In situations in which the person has some problem-solving abilities, the caregivers may identify the person who is best able to discuss the decision. When spouses are involved in the decision making, they usually assume the role of communicating the decision to the dependent older person. At times, the nurse, physician, or other professional person may assume the role of an authority figure to assist in explaining the decision to the dependent older adult.

Step VI: Summarizing the Plan and Clarifying Roles

The final step is to clarify the roles of various people. The nurse and other professionals who are part of the decision-making process should inform the caregivers about their ongoing roles. If several caregivers are involved with the plan, each person should state their understanding of their role. Display 19-4 summarizes the entire decision-making model.

Culturally Sensitive Interventions

As discussed in Chapters 3 and 5, there are many barriers to the use of services by non-Anglo older adults and their caregivers in the United States. Gerontologists, health care practitioners, and other service providers are attempting to remove some of these barriers by developing and implementing culturally sensitive services, particularly in the area of dementia-related services, as summarized in the Culture Box on this page. Educational materials written in other languages and developed for various cultural groups are available from some of the Educational Resources listed at the end of this chapter, including the Internet.

References on Interventions

Many books are devoted to interventions designed to address the needs of cognitively impaired older adults. Although these books may not be viewed as professional nursing references, they are written by highly qualified and experienced caregivers, and they are excellent references for any nurse caring for people with dementing conditions. Numerous caregiver guides are widely available in bookstores, through the

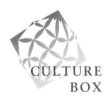

CULTURE BOX

Guidelines for Developing and Implementing Culturally Sensitive Services

- Base all interventions on a knowledge of the ethnocultural values of the community.
- Adapt the services to the needs of the recipients.
- Identify and address the cultural factors that influence the relationship between the service provider and the service recipient.
- In planning, implementing, and evaluating interventions, involve staff and caregivers who share the same cultural background as the person for whom care is being planned.
- Use language and cultural interpreters when necessary.
- Use terminology, in both written and verbal communication, that is educationally appropriate and culturally relevant (e.g., some languages do not have a word for caregiver or respite care).
- Use graphics that are culturally relevant.
- Emphasize the benefits for the person with dementia, rather than for the caregiver.
- Plan on repeated personal contacts with the people who need the services.
- Provide the services in a culturally neutral location, or one that is widely accepted by the people who need the services.

Related references: Henderson et al., 1993; Gallagher-Thompson et al., 1996.

Internet, and through the Alzheimer's Association. This association is continually developing and publishing references for professionals, as well as lay people, and many of their publications are excellent "how-to" references with regard to caring for people with dementia. Some of these references are free, and all of them may be obtained from the national Alzheimer's Association or a local chapter (see the Educational Resources section). Nurses can call the toll-free number to request an up-to-date bibliography and order form, and to obtain information about any of the references available from the Alzheimer's Association. Health care professionals who are interested in modifying or creating environments to meet the needs of people with dementia might obtain the recently published reference entitled *Designing for Alzheimer's Disease: Strategies for Creating Better Care Environments* by Elizabeth C. Brawley (John Wiley & Sons, New York).

Evaluating Nursing Care

Nursing care of people with dementia is evaluated by determining the extent to which these individuals maintain as much dignity as possible and receive the supports they need to maintain the best possible quality of life. Because a decline in function is an inherent part of dementia, evaluation of nursing care must be based on changing expectations as the person's condition worsens. In the final stages of dementia, evaluation criteria may be based on goals that are similar to those applied to someone with a terminal illness—that is, the focus is on comfort.

The degree to which someone's quality of life is maintained is evaluated by receiving feedback from the person about his or her perceived life satisfaction. In the early stages of dementia, the person may be able to express directly his or her degree of life satisfaction. However, as the dementia progresses, it will become more difficult to obtain this kind of information. As the person with dementia loses the ability to communicate his or her feelings and perceptions, the nurse will depend more on feedback from caregivers and the nurse's own judgment about the person's quality of life. One evaluation criterion is the observation that the person enjoys activities in the present, despite their inability to remember the events. Another is that the person participates in activities and interactions that seem to be meaningful to them. As the person's condition declines, measures of quality of life will focus more narrowly on comfort, dignity, and basic physical needs. Also, throughout the course of dementia, the person should be free from fear and anxiety, to the extent that this is possible.

Another important consideration is the extent to which the needs of the caregiver are being addressed. One evaluation criterion is whether caregivers express satisfaction with their own quality of life, despite the demands of the situation. Other evaluation criteria may be a caregiver's attendance at support groups and the use of resources to assist with or guide care.

Chapter Summary

Dementia is a syndrome characterized by a progressive loss of intellectual abilities. AD and vascular dementia are the first and second most common types of dementia, respectively, in the United States. Besides dementia, depression and physiologic disorders can cause cognitive impairments in older adults. These treatable factors should not be overlooked, and cognitive impairments must not erroneously be attributed to "normal aging."

Numerous theories are under intense investigation to identify the causes of AD and other dementias, but as of the late 1990s, no one theory had emerged to explain these diseases. AD is now viewed as a heterogeneous disorder, and many underlying, probably interacting, factors are being studied. Research on drug treatments and alternative approaches also is progressing at a rapid pace. Nurses and lay people can keep up-to-date about any breakthroughs in prevention, diagnosis, and treatment of AD and other dementias by obtaining information from the Alzheimer's Association and from Internet sites.

The functional consequences of dementia can be divided into stages that describe the changes associated with progressive cognitive impairments. Functional impairments, as well as behavioral and emotional manifestations, such as depression, agitation, wandering, and delusions, may be problematic for caregivers. Consideration also should be given to the tremendous emotional impact of dementia, on both the person with dementia and on their caregivers. Assessment must be multidisciplinary and must consider a number of factors. Altered Thought Processes related to the effects of dementia is the nursing diagnosis that is applied most often to older adults with dementia. Additional nursing diagnoses address problems associated with functional impairments, the emotional needs of the person with dementia, and the needs of caregivers.

Nursing goals are directed toward assisting the person with dementia to function at the highest possible level of independence and to maintain the highest possible dignity and quality of life. Nursing goals for caregivers address their needs for information, emotional support, and direct services. Nursing interventions, which include communication techniques and environmental modifications, must be highly individualized and frequently evaluated and modified. Nursing care is evaluated by the extent to which quality of life is maintained for both older adults with dementia and their caregivers.

Critical Thinking Exercises

1. Define each of the following terms and describe the importance and relevance of each term according to our current understanding of impaired cognitive function: senility, organic brain syndrome, hardening of the arteries, pseudodementia, delirium, dementia, Alzheimer's disease, vascular dementia.

2. Describe how you would explain Alzheimer's disease to the following families and what approach you would take to interventions for the person with AD in each of the following situations:
   a. A white person and his family
   b. A Hispanic person and her family
   c. An African American person and his family
   d. A Chinese person and her family
   e. An American Indian and his family

3. You are working in a nursing clinic at a senior center. How would you respond to the following questions, posed by a 74-year-old woman: "I've been having memory problems lately, but I know it's not Alzheimer's because I haven't done anything really stupid. What do you think I should do? My friend says ginkgo helps her a lot, and I was thinking of trying that. Do you know how much of it I should take?"

4. You are asked to present an inservice program to nursing home staff about medications used in the treatment of AD and dementia-related behaviors. What information would you present?

Case Example and Nursing Care Plan

Pertinent Case Information

Mrs. D. is 85 years old and lives with her 86-year-old husband in a high rise apartment for the elderly. Two years ago, Mrs. D. was diagnosed as having AD, but she was able to participate in her usual activities until the past year. Now she is neglecting her personal care and is unsafe in meal preparation.

When she wakes up several times nightly to go to the bathroom, she sometimes goes to the apartment door rather than returning to the bedroom. Mr. D. worries that she will leave in the middle of the night, and his sleep is disrupted because he maintains a state of constant vigilance. Mr. D. has called a home care agency requesting home health aide assistance, and you are the nurse responsible for the initial assessment and for working with the home health aides.

Nursing Assessment

During your initial assessment, you find that Mrs. D. is pleasant and receptive, but has little insight into her need for help. She acknowledges that her doctor has told her she has "a memory problem." Mrs. D. reports that this problem doesn't affect her daily life, except that her husband has to remind her about things like turning the stove off after cooking meals. She acknowledges being lonely and says she misses being able to read books and talk to people. Mrs. D. takes Aricept and vitamin E, and is otherwise physically healthy.

With regard to her ADL, Mrs. D. has not taken a bath or shower in several months, and she gets very angry if Mr. D. suggests that she take one. She gets confused about her clothing and sometimes wears her underwear over her regular clothes, or wears a skirt and slacks at the same time. She insists on doing the meal preparation, but she is unsafe using the stove and gets confused about ingredients in recipes (e.g., she may use salt instead of sugar). Mrs. D. always has done the laundry and housekeeping, but in the past months, she has "made a lot of mistakes," such as using powdered milk for laundry detergent.

Mr. D. reports feeling very stressed about the full-time responsibilities of caring for his wife, and this stress has escalated in the past month because he no longer feels he can leave her alone. Mrs. D. "shadows" him and feels very insecure if he is out of her sight for more than a few minutes. Mr. D. has taken her everywhere with him for the past year, but in the last few months, this has become increasingly more difficult. For example, when they are in the grocery store, Mrs. D. gets very impatient and pushes the cart into other people. Also, while they are waiting in the checkout line, she insists on taking one of each of the tabloids and magazines near the counter, and she creates a big scene if he doesn't buy them for her.

Mr. D. confides that he expected to be able to care for his wife at home "until the end," but now he has doubts about his ability to keep her at home. He perceives her as being "senile" and feels he should be able to meet her needs. There are no nearby family members who can help with her care, but his son and daughter have offered to help pay for some services. Mr. D. is aware of support groups offered by the Alzheimer's Association, but he has not attended any because he cannot leave his wife alone. When asked about his health, Mr. D. says, "I see the doctor for my arthritis and heart problems, but I get along OK, except that I'm supposed to have cataract surgery and I don't know how I'll manage to get that done."

Nursing Diagnosis

Your nursing diagnosis for Mrs. D. is Altered Thought Processes related to the effects of dementia. You use the nursing diagnosis of Caregiver Role Strain for Mr. D. because you recognize the need to address Mr. D.'s problems. Your immediate goal is to arrange for supportive services and assistance with Mrs. D.'s care, as this will improve the quality of life for both Mr. and Mrs. D., and it will alleviate some of the caregiver stress for Mr. D. A long-term goal is to arrange for respite services so Mr. D. can undergo cataract surgery. You also recognize the need for educational and support services for Mr. D.

Goals	Nursing Interventions	Evaluation Criteria
To assist Mrs. D. in functioning at her highest level of independence	Work with Mr. D. to identify ways to improve Mrs. D.'s ability to function safely and independently in performing her ADL. (For instance, Mr. D. can involve Mrs. D. in selecting an outfit to wear and can set out the clothing in the order in which it should be donned.)	Mrs. D. will perform ADL and IADL with minimal assistance.
	Arrange for a home health aide (HHA) to work with Mrs. D. and assist her with complex tasks, such as laundry, housekeeping, and meal preparation.	
	Teach the HHA to assume an "assistant" and "friend" role by providing only subtle supervision and minimal direct help with activities such as laundry.	
To maintain Mrs. D.'s quality of life	Work with Mr. D. and the HHA to identify activities that are interesting, satisfying, and intellectually stimulating (e.g., "word find" games).	Mrs. D. will continue to engage in activities that are satisfying.
	Explore the possibility of Mrs. D.'s attending an adult day care program for group activities.	
	Support Mrs. D. in carrying out familiar roles and meaningful activities.	
Mr. D. will utilize sources of support to alleviate caregiver-related stress	Arrange the HHA's schedule to enable Mr. D. to attend caregiver support groups and educational programs.	Mr. D. will verbalize feelings of being able to cope effectively with caregiver responsibilities.
	Help Mr. D. in identifying one activity per week that he could do to promote his own well-be-	Mr. D. will participate in one activity per week that is focused on his own needs and interests.

(continued)

Goals	Nursing Interventions	Evaluation Criteria
	ing (e.g., going to lunch with a friend).	
	Provide HHA assistance for 4-hour periods to allow Mr. D. time for grocery shopping and pursuing his own interests.	
	Provide Mr. D. with information about the "Caregiver Connection Hot Line" at the Alzheimer's Association, and suggest that he join this telephone support network.	

Educational Resources

Alzheimer's Association
919 North Michigan Avenue, Suite 1000, Chicago, IL 60611
(800) 272-3900
www.alz.org
•24-hour hotline providing information about Alzheimer's disease
•Free publications and newsletter
•Information about local chapters of the Alzheimer's Association

Alzheimer's Disease Education and Referral (ADEAR) Center
P.O. Box 8250, Silver Spring, MD 20907-8250
(800) 438-4380
www.alzheimers.org/adear
•A service of the National Institute on Aging, distributing information about Alzheimer's disease to health professionals, patients, families, and the general public
•Spanish language materials and bibliography
•Progress report on Alzheimer's disease

National Institute of Neurological Disorders and Stroke
Building 31, Room 8A06, 9000 Rockville Pike, Bethesda, MD 20892
(301) 496-5751
www.ninds.nih.gov

National Stroke Association
96 Inverness Drive East, Suite I, Englewood, CO 80112-5112
(800) 787-6537
www.stroke.org

U.S. Department of Health and Human Services Agency for Health Care Policy and Research
AHCPR Publications Clearinghouse, P.O. Box 8547, Silver Spring, MD 20907
(800) 358-9295
www.ahcpr.gov
•Clinical practice guide, clinician's guide, and consumer's guide (written in English and Spanish) on early identification of Alzheimer's disease and related dementias

References

Aevarsson, O., & Skoog, I. (1996). A population-based study on the incidence of dementia disorders between 85 and 88 years of age. *Journal of the American Geriatric Society, 44*, 1455–1460.

Alzheimer, A. (1907). Uber eine eigenartige Erkrankung der Hirnrinde. *Allgemeine Zeitschrift Fur Psychiatrie und Psychisch-Gerichtliche Medicin, 64*, 146–148.

Auer, S., & Reisberg, B. (1997). The GDS/FAST Staging System. *International Psychogeriatrics, 9* (Suppl. 1), 167–171.

Bakke, B. L. (1997). Applied behavior analysis for behavior problems in Alzheimer's disease. *Geriatrics, 52* (Suppl. 2), S40–S43.

Bodick, N. C., Offen, W. W., Shannon, H. E., Satterwhite, J., Lucas, R., Lier, R. van, & Paul, S. M. (1997). The selective muscarinic agonist xanomeline improves both the cognitive deficits and behavioral symptoms of Alzheimer disease. *Alzheimer Disease and Associated Disorders, 11* (Suppl. 4), S16–S22.

Brayne, C., Gill, C., & Huppert, F. (1995). Incidence of clinically diagnosed subtypes of dementia in an elderly population. *British Journal of Psychiatry, 67*, 255–262.

Brody, E. (1985). Parent care as a normative family stress. *The Gerontologist, 25*, 19–29.

Buettner, L. L. (1998). A team approach to dynamic programming on the special care unit. *Journal of Gerontological Nursing, 24*(1), 23–30.

Burgener, S. C., Shimer, R., & Murrell, L. (1993). Expressions of individuality in cognitively impaired elders. *Journal of Gerontological Nursing, 19*(4), 13–22.

Carpenito, L. J. (1997). *Nursing diagnosis: Application to clinical practice* (7th ed.). Philadelphia: J. B. Lippincott.

Cherrier, M. M., Mendez, M. F., Perryman, K. M., Pachana, N. A., Miller, B. L., & Cummings, J. L. (1997). Frontotemporal dementia versus vascular dementia: Differential features on mental status examination. *Journal of the American Geriatrics Society, 45*, 579–583.

Chui, H. C., Victoroff, J. I., Margolin, D., Jagust, W., Shankle, R., & Katzman, R. (1992). Criteria for the diagnosis of ischemic vascular dementia proposed by the State of California Alzheimer's Disease Diagnostic and Treatment Centers. *Neurology, 42*, 473–480.

Clark, M. E., Lipe, A. W., & Bilbrey, M. (1998). Use of music to decrease aggressive behaviors in people with dementia. *Journal of Gerontological Nursing, 24*(7), 10–17.

Cohen, D., Kennedy, G., & Eisdorfer, C. (1984). Phases of change in the patient with Alzheimer's dementia. *Journal of the American Geriatrics Society, 32*(1), 11–15.

Cohen, D., Luchins, D., Eisdorfer, C., Paveza, G., Ashford, J. W., Gorelick, P., Hirschman, R., Freels, S., Levy, P., Semla, T., & Shaw, H. (1990). Caring for relatives with Alzheimer's disease: The mental health risks to spouses, adult children, and other family caregivers. *Behavior, Health, and Aging, 1*, 171–182.

Cohen-Mansfield, J., & Werner, P. (1997). Management of verbally disruptive behaviors in nursing home residents. *Journal of Gerontology: Medical Sciences, 52A*, M369–M377.

Cohen-Mansfield, J., & Werner, P. (1998a). Longitudinal changes in behavioral problems in old age: A study in an adult day care population. *Journal of Gerontology: Medical Sciences, 53A*, M65–M71.

Cohen-Mansfield, J., & Werner, P. (1998b). The effects of an enhanced environment on nursing home residents who pace. *The Gerontologist, 38*, 199–208.

Cohen-Mansfield, J., Werner, P., Culpepper, W. J., & Barkley, D. (1997). Evaluation of an inservice training program on dementia and wandering. *Journal of Gerontological Nursing, 23*(10), 40–47.

Connell, C. M., & Gibson, G. D. (1997). Racial, ethnic, and cultural differences in dementia caregiving: Review and analysis. *The Gerontologist, 37*, 355–364.

Cook, R. H., Ward, B. E., & Austin, J. H. (1979). Studies in aging of the brain. IV. Familial Alzheimer disease: Relation to transmissible dementia, aneuploidy, and microtubular defects. *Neurology, 29,* 1402–1412.

Corsellis, J. A. N., & Evans, P. H. (1966). The relation of stenosis of the extracranial cerebral arteries to mental disorders and cerebral degeneration in old age. In *Proceedings of the Fifth International Congress on Neuropathology* (p. 546). New York: Excerpta Medica.

Costa, P. T. Jr., Williams, T. F., Somerfield, M., Albert, M. S., Butters, N. M., Folstein, M. F., et al. (1996). *Recognition and initial assessment of Alzheimer's disease and related dementias: Clinical practice guideline* (AHCPR Publication No. 97-0702). Rockville, MD: Agency for Health Care Policy and Research, Public Health Service, U.S. Department of Health and Human Services.

Cotrell, V. C. (1997). Awareness deficits in Alzheimer's disease: Issues in assessment and intervention. *Journal of Applied Gerontology, 16*(1), 71–90.

Cummings, J. L. (1997). Changes in neuropsychiatric symptoms as outcome measures in clinical trials with cholinergic therapies for Alzheimer disease. *Alzheimer Disease and Associated Disorders, 11* (Suppl. 4), S1–S9.

Cummings, J. L., Årsland, D., & Jarvik, L. (1997). Dementia. In C. K. Cassel, H. J. Cohen, E. B. Larson, D. E. Meier, N. M. Resnick, L. Z. Rubenstein, & L. B. Sorenson (Eds.), *Geriatric medicine* (3rd ed., pp. 897–916). New York: Springer.

Day, C. R. (1997). Validation therapy: A review of the literature. *Journal of Gerontological Nursing, 23*(4), 29–34.

Denney, A. (1997). Quiet music: An intervention for mealtime agitation? *Journal of Gerontological Nursing, 23*(7), 16–23.

Dhooper, S. S. (1991). Caregivers of Alzheimer's disease patients: A review of the literature. *Journal of Gerontological Social Work, 18*(1/2), 19–37.

Dijk, P. T. M. van, Sande, H. J. van de, Dippel, D. W. J., & Habbema, J. D. F. (1992). The nature of excess mortality in nursing home patients with dementia. *Journal of Gerontology: Medical Sciences, 47*(2), M28–M34.

Elliott, K. S., Minno, M. D., Lam, D., & Tu, A. M. (1996). Working with Chinese families in the context of dementia. In G. Yeo & D. Gallagher-Thompson (Eds.), *Ethnicity and the dementias* (pp. 89–108). Washington, DC: Taylor & Francis.

Erkinjuntti, T. (1997). Vascular dementia: Challenge of clinical diagnosis. *International Psychogeriatrics, 9* (Suppl. 1), 51–58.

Finkel, S. I., Silva, J. C., Cohen, G. D., Miller, S., & Sartorius, N. (1998). Behavioral and psychological symptoms of dementia. *The American Journal of Geriatric Psychiatry, 6*(2), 97–100.

Francis, J. (1992). Delirium in older patients. *Journal of the American Geriatrics Society, 40,* 829–838.

Francis, J. (1997). Delirium. In C. K. Cassel, H. J. Cohen, E. B. Larson, D. E. Meier, N. M. Resnick, L. Z. Rubenstein, & L. B. Sorenson (Eds.), *Geriatric medicine* (3rd ed., pp. 917–922). New York: Springer.

Gallagher-Thompson, D., Talamantes, M., Ramirez, R., & Valverde, I. (1996). Service delivery issues and recommendations for working with Mexican American family caregivers. In G. Yeo & D. Gallagher-Thompson (Eds.), *Ethnicity and the dementias* (pp. 137–152). Washington, DC: Taylor & Francis.

Gatz, M., Pedersen, N. L., Berg, S., Johansson, B., Johansson, K., Mortimer, J. A., et al. (1997). Heritability for Alzheimer's disease: The study of dementia in Swedish twins. *Journal of Gerontology: Medical Sciences, 52A*(2), M117–M125.

George, L. K., & Gwyther, L. P. (1986). Caregiver well-being: A multidimensional examination of family caregivers of demented adults. *The Gerontologist, 26,* 253–259.

Gibson, M. C. (1997). Differentiating aggressive and resistive behaviors in long-term care. *Journal of Gerontological Nursing, 23*(4), 21–28.

Gilley, D. W., Wilson, R. S., Beckett, L. A., & Evans, D. A. (1997). Psychotic symptoms and physically aggressive behavior in Alzheimer's disease. *Journal of the American Geriatrics Society, 45,* 1074–1079.

Goate, A. M. (1997). Molecular genetics of Alzheimer's disease. *Geriatrics, 52* (Suppl. 2), S9–S12.

Goldstein, M. Z., & Fogel, B. S. (1993). Cognitive change after elective surgery in nondemented older adults. *American Journal of Geriatric Psychiatry, 1,* 118–125.

Good, P. F., Perl, D. P., Bierer, L. M., & Schmeidler, J. (1992). Selective accumulation of aluminum and iron in the neurofibrillary tangles of Alzheimer's disease: A laser microprobe (LAMMA) study. *Annals of Neurology, 31,* 286–292.

Grant, L. A., Potthoff, S. J., Ryden, M., & Kane, R. A. (1998). Staff ratios, training, and assignment in Alzheimer's Special Care Units. *Journal of Gerontological Nursing, 24*(1), 9–16.

Gwyther, L. P. (1997). The perspective of the person with Alzheimer disease: Which outcomes matter in early to middle stages of dementia? *Alzheimer Disease and Associated Disorders, 11* (Suppl. 6), 18–24.

Hachinski, V. C., Lassen, N. A., & Marshall, J. (1974). Multi-infarct dementia: A cause of mental deterioration in the elderly. *Lancet, 2,* 207–209.

Hall, G. R. (1988). Alterations in thought process. *Journal of Gerontological Nursing, 14*(3), 30–37.

Hall, G. R., & Buckwalter, K. C. (1987). Progressively lowered stress threshold: A conceptual model for care of adults with Alzheimer's disease. *Archives of Psychiatric Nursing, 1,* 399–406.

Heacock, P. R., Beck, C., M., Souder, E., & Mercer, S. (1997). Assessing dressing ability in dementia. *Geriatric Nursing, 18,* 107–111.

Henderson, J. N. (1996). Cultural dynamics of dementia in a Cuban and Puerto Rican population in the United States. In G. Yeo & D. Gallagher-Thompson (Eds.), *Ethnicity and the dementias* (pp. 153–166). Washington, DC: Taylor & Francis.

Henderson, J. N., Gutierrez-Mayka, M., Garcia, J., & Boyd, S. (1993). A model for Alzheimer's disease support group development in African-American and Hispanic populations. *The Gerontologist, 33,* 409–414.

Hendrie, H. C. (1998). Epidemiology of dementia and Alzheimer's disease. *The American Journal of Geriatric Psychiatry, 6*(2), S3–S18.

Hepburn, K. W., Caron, W., Luptak, M., Ostwald, S., Grant, L., & Keenan, J. M. (1997). The family stories workshop: Stories for those who cannot remember. *The Gerontologist, 37,* 827–832.

Hoeffer, B., Rader, J., McKenzie, D., Lavelle, M., & Stewart, B. (1997). Reducing aggressive behavior during bathing cognitively impaired nursing home residents. *Journal of Gerontological Nursing, 23*(5), 16–23.

Hogstel, M. O. (1988). Forget these three words. *Journal of Gerontological Nursing, 14*(12), 7.

Holmberg, S. K. (1997). A walking program for wanderers: Volunteer training and development of an evening walker's group. *Geriatric Nursing, 18,* 160–165.

Holstein, M. (1997). Alzheimer's disease and senile dementia, 1885–1920: An interpretive history of disease negotiation. *Journal of Aging Studies, 11*(1), 1–13.

Holthaus, J. (1997). I-FAAD (Instrument for Affirming Alzheimer's Disease): Understanding & affirming stage specific cognitive decline as it correlates to early childhood development. *American Journal of Alzheimer's Disease, 12,* 167–170.

Howieson, D. B., Dame, A., Camicioli, R., Sexton, G., Payami, H., & Kaye, J. A. (1997). Cognitive markers preceding Alzheimer's dementia in the healthy oldest old. *Journal of the American Geriatrics Society, 45,* 584–589.

Joachim, C. L., & Selkoe, D. J. (1992). The seminal role of beta-amyloid in the pathogenesis of Alzheimer disease. *Alzheimer Disease and Associated Disorders, 6,* 7–34.

John, R., Hennessy, C. H., Roy, L. C., & Salvini, M. L. (1996). Caring for cognitively impaired American Indian elders: Difficult situations, few options. In G. Yeo & D. Gallagher-Thompson (Eds.), *Ethnicity and the dementias* (pp. 187–203). Washington, DC: Taylor & Francis.

Kayser-Jones, J., & Schell, E. (1997). The mealtime experience of a cognitively impaired elder: Ineffective and effective strategies. *Journal of Gerontological Nursing, 23*(7), 33–39.

Kazee, A. M., Eskin, T. A., Gabriel, K. R., McDaniel, K. D., & Hamill, R. W. (1993). Clinicopathologic correlates in Alzheimer disease: Assessment of clinical and pathologic diagnostic criteria. *Alzheimer Disease and Associated Disorders, 7,* 152–164.

Kiloh, L. G. (1961). Pseudo-dementia. *Acta Psychiatrica Scandinavica, 37,* 336–361.

Kolanowski, A. M., Strand, G., Whall, A. (1997). A pilot study of the relation of premorbid characteristics to behavior in dementia. *Journal of Gerontological Nursing, 23*(2), 21–30.

Kovach, C. R., & Meyer-Arnold, E. A. (1997). Preventing agitated behaviors during bath time. *Geriatric Nursing, 18,* 112–114.

Kukull, W. A., Brenner, D. E., Speck, C. E., Nocklin, D., Bowen, J., McCormick, W., et al. (1994). Causes of death associated with Alzheimer's disease: Variation by level of cognitive impairment before death. *Journal of the American Geriatrics Society, 42,* 723–726.

Kumar, A., & Gottlieb, G. (1993). Frontotemporal dementias: A new clinical syndrome? *The American Journal of Geriatric Psychiatry, 1*(2), 95–108.

Lantz, M. S., Buchalter, E. N., & McBee, L. (1997). The wellness group: A novel intervention for coping with disruptive behavior in elderly nursing home residents. *The Gerontologist, 37*(4), 551–556.

Larson, E. B., Reifler, B. V., Sumi, S. M., Canfield, C. G., & China, N. M. (1985). Diagnostic evaluation of 200 elderly outpatients with suspected dementia. *Journal of Gerontology, 40,* 536–543.

Lawton, M. P. (1997). Assessing quality of life in Alzheimer disease research. *Alzheimer Disease and Associated Disorders, 11* (Suppl. 6), 91–99.

Leon, M. J. de, Convit, A., Santi, S. de, Bobinski, M., George, A. E., Wisniewski, H. M., et al. (1997). Neuroimaging and electrophysiology: Contribution of structural neuroimaging to the early diagnosis of Alzheimer's disease. *International Psychogeriatrics, 9* (Suppl. 1), 183–190.

Lerner, A. J., Hedera, P., Koss, E., Stuckey, J., & Friedland, R. P. (1997). Delirium in Alzheimer disease. *Alzheimer Disease and Associated Disorders, 11*(1), 16–20.

Levkoff, S. E., Evans, D. A., Liptzin, B., Cleary, P. D., Lipsitz, L. A., Wetle, T. T., Reilly, C. H., Pilgrim, D. M., Schor, J., & Rowe, J. (1992). Delirium: The occurrence and persistence of symptoms among elderly hospitalized patients. *Archives of Internal Medicine, 152,* 334–340.

Lewis, I. D., & Ausberry, M. S. C. (1996). African American families: Management of demented elders. In G. Yeo & D. Gallagher-Thompson (Eds.), *Ethnicity and the dementias* (pp. 167–174). Washington, DC: Taylor & Francis.

Libow, L. E. (1973). Pseudo-senility: Acute and reversible organic brain syndromes. *Journal of the American Geriatrics Society, 21,* 112–120.

Lipson, J. G., Dibble, S. L., & Minarik, P. A. (1996). *Culture and Nursing Care: A Pocket Guide.* San Francisco: UCSF Nursing Press.

Loewenstein, D. A., & Rubert, M. P. (1992). The NINCDS-ADRDA neuropsychological criteria for the assessment of dementia: Limitations of current diagnostic guidelines. *Behavior, Health, and Aging, 2*(2), 113–121.

Lund & Manchester Groups. (1995). Clinical and neuropathological criteria for frontotemporal dementia. *Journal of Neurology, Neurosurgery and Psychiatry, 57,* 416–418.

Mace, N. L., & Rabins, P. V. (1991). *The 36-hour day* (2nd ed.). New York: Warner.

Magai, C., Cohen, J., Gomberg, D., Malatesta, C., & Culver, C. (1996). Emotional expression during mid- to late-stage dementia. *International Psychogeriatrics, 8,* 383–395.

Mayeux, R., Stern, Y., Ottman, R., Tatemichi, T. K., Tang, M. X., Maestre, G., et al. (1993). The apolipoprotein epsilon 4 alle in patients with Alzheimer's disease. *Annals of Neurology, 34,* 752–754.

McAiney, C. A. (1998). The development of the empowered aide model: An intervention for long-term care staff who care for Alzheimer's residents. *Journal of Gerontological Nursing, 24*(1), 17–22.

McAllister, T. W. (1983). Overview: Pseudodementia. *American Journal of Psychiatry, 140,* 528–533.

McKeith, I. G., Galasko, D., Kosaka, K., Perry, E. B., Dickson, D. W., Hansen, L. A., et al. (1996). Consensus guidelines for the clinical and pathologic diagnosis of dementia with Lewy bodies (DLB): Report of the consortium on DLB international workshop. *Neurology, 47,* 1113–1124.

McKhann, G., Drachman, D., Folstein, M., Katzman, R., Price, D., & Stadlan, E. M. (1984). Clinical diagnosis of Alzheimer's disease: Report of the NINCDS-ADRDA work group under the auspices of the Department of Health and Human Services task force on Alzheimer's disease. *Neurology, 34,* 939–944.

Miller, M. F. (1997). Physically aggressive resident behavior during hygienic care. *Journal of Gerontological Nursing, 23*(5), 24–39.

Mistretta, E. F., & Kee, C. C. (1997). Caring for Alzheimer's residents in dedicated units. *Journal of Gerontological Nursing, 23*(2), 41–46.

Morrison, J. H., & Hof, P. R. (1997). Life and death of neurons in the aging brain. *Science, 278,* 412–418.

Murray, A. M., Levkoff, S. E., Wetle, T. T., Beckett, L., Cleary, P. D., Schor, J. D., Lipsitz, L. A., Rowe, J. W., & Evans, D. A. (1993). Acute delirium and functional decline in the hospitalized elderly patient. *Journal of Gerontology: Medical Sciences, 48*(5), M181–M186.

Office of Technology Assessment Task Force. (1988). *Confronting Alzheimer's disease and other dementias.* Philadelphia: J. B. Lippincott.

Ory, M. G., Williams, T. F., Emr, M., Lebowitz, B., Rabins, P., Salloway, J., et al. (1985). Families, informal supports, and Alzheimer's disease. *Research on Aging, 7*(4), 623–644.

Petersen, R. C., Smith, G. E., Waring, S. C., Ivnik, R. J., Kokmen, E., & Tangelos, E. G. (1997). Aging, memory, and mild cognitive impairment. *International Psychogeriatrics, 9* (Suppl. 1), 65–69.

Reifler, B. V. (1997). Pre-dementia. *Journal of the American Geriatrics Society, 45,* 776–777.

Reisberg, B. (1986). Dementia: A systematic approach to identifying reversible causes. *Geriatrics, 41*(4), 30–46.

Reisberg, B., Burns, A., Brodaty, H., Eastwood, R., Rossor, M., Sartorius, N., & Winblad, B. (1997). Diagnosis of Alzheimer's disease: Report of an International Psychogeriatric Association special meeting work group. *International Psychogeriatrics, 9* (Suppl. 1), 11–38.

Rockwood, K. (1993). The occurrence and duration of symptoms in elderly patients with delirium. *Journal of Gerontology: Medical Sciences, 48*(4), M162–M166.

Roses, A. D. (1995). Apolipoprotein E and Alzheimer's disease. *Science and Medicine, 2*(5), 16–25.

Schulz, R., Visintainer, P., & Williamson, G. M. (1990). Psychiatric and physical morbidity effects of caregiving. *Journal of Gerontology: Psychological Sciences, 45*(5), P181–P191.

Shua-Haim, J. R., & Ross, J. S. (1998). Alzheimer's syndrome and not Alzheimer's disease: The historical struggle to define the disease. *American Journal of Alzheimer's Disease, 13*(2), 92–95.

Simon, L., Jewell, N., & Brokel, J. (1997). Management of acute delirium in hospitalized elderly: A process improvement project. *Geriatric Nursing, 18,* 150–154.

Sloane, P. D., Davidson, S., Buckwalter, K., Lindsey, B. A., Ayers, S., Lenker, V., & Burgio, L. D. (1997). Management of the patient with disruptive vocalization. *The Gerontologist, 37*(5), 675–682.

Snowden, D. A. (1997). Aging and Alzheimer's disease: Lessons from the Nun Study. *The Gerontologist, 37*, 150–156.

Sunderland, T., Molchan, S. E., Little, J. T., Bahro, M., Putnam, K. T., & Weingartner, H. (1997). Pharmacologic challenges in Alzheimer disease and normal controls: Cognitive modeling in humans. *Alzheimer Disease and Associated Disorders, 11* (Suppl. 4), S23–S26.

Swartz, J. R., Miller, B. L., Lesser, I. M., Booth, R., Darby, A., Wohl, M., & Benson, D. F. (1997). Behavioral phenomenology in Alzheimer's disease, frontotemporal dementia, and late-life depression: A retrospective analysis. *Journal of Geriatric Psychiatry and Neurology, 10*, 67–74.

Tang, M-X., Stern, Y., Marder, K., Bell, K., Gurland, B., Lantigua, R., et al. (1998). The APOE-ε4 allele and the risk of Alzheimer disease among African Americans, Whites, and Hispanics. *Journal of the American Medical Association, 279*(10), 751–755.

Taft, L. B., Matthiesen, V., Farran, C. J., McCann, J. J., & Knafl, K. A. (1997). Supporting strengths and responding to agitation in dementia care: An exploratory study. *American Journal of Alzheimer's Disease, 12*(5), 198–208.

Tempo, P. M., & Saito, A. (1996). Techniques of working with Japanese American families. In G. Yeo & D. Gallagher-Thompson (Eds.), *Ethnicity and the dementias* (pp. 109–122). Washington, DC: Taylor & Francis.

Teno, J. M., Landrun, K., & Lynn, J. (1997). Defining and measuring outcomes in end-stage dementia. *Alzheimer Disease and Associated Disorders, 11* (Suppl. 6), 25–29.

Teresi, J. A., Grant, L. A., Holmes, D., & Ory, M. G. (1998). Staffing in traditional and special dementia care units: Preliminary findings from the National Institute on Aging collaborative studies. *Journal of Gerontological Nursing, 24*(1), 49–53.

Teri, L. (1997). Behavior and caregiver burden: Behavioral problems in patients with Alzheimer disease and its association with caregiver distress. *Alzheimer Disease and Associated Disorders, 11* (Suppl. 4), S35–S38.

Teri, L., Logsdon, R. G., Uomoto, J., & McCurry, S. M. (1997). Behavioral treatment of depression in dementia patients: A controlled clinical trial. *Journal of Gerontology: Psychological Sciences, 52B*(4), P159–P166.

Tomlinson, B. E., Blessed, G., & Roth, M. (1968). Observations on the brains of non-demented old people. *Journal of Neurological Science, 7*, 331–356.

Tomlinson, B. E., Blessed, G., & Roth, M. (1970). Observations on the brains of demented old people. *Journal of Neurological Science, 11*, 205–242.

U.S. House Select Committee on Aging. (1987). *Exploding the myths: Caregiving in America* (Committee Publication No. 99-611). Washington, DC: U.S. Government Printing Office.

Veterans Administration. (1985). *Dementia: Guidelines for diagnosis and treatment* (Information bulletin from the Office of Geriatrics and Extended Care). Washington, DC: Veterans Administration Central Office.

Volicer, L. (1997). Goals of care in advanced dementia: Comfort, dignity, and psychological well-being. *American Journal of Alzheimer's Disease, 12*(5), 196–197.

Wagner, M. T., Spangenberg, K. B., Bachman, D. L., & O'Connell, P. (1997). Unawareness of cognitive deficit in Alzheimer disease & related dementias. *Alzheimer Disease and Related Disorders, 11*(3), 125–131.

Whall, A. L., Black, M. E., Groh, C. J., Yankou, D. J., Kupferschmid, B. J., & Foster, N. L. (1997). The effect of natural environments upon agitation and aggression in late stage dementia patients. *American Journal of Alzheimer's Disease, 12*(5), 216–220.

Worm-Peterson, J., & Pakkenberg, H. (1968). Atherosclerosis of cerebral arteries: Pathological and clinical correlations. *Journal of Gerontology, 23*, 445.

Yeo, G., Gallagher-Thompson, D., & Lieberman, M. (1996). Variations in dementia characteristics by ethnic category. In G. Yeo & D. Gallagher-Thompson (Eds.), *Ethnicity and the dementias* (pp. 21–30). Washington, DC: Taylor & Francis.

Zarit, S. H., Reever, K. E., & Bach-Peterson, J. (1980). Relatives of the impaired elderly: Correlates of feelings of burden. *Gerontologist, 20*, 649–655.

Impaired Affective Function: Depression

Chapter

20

1. *Delineate theories to explain late-life depression.*
2. *Examine risk factors and cultural differences in risk factors that cause or contribute to depression in older adults.*
3. *Discuss the functional consequences of late-life depression.*
4. *Describe the following aspects of assessment of late-life depression: manifestations of depression that differ in younger and older adults, cultural variations in the expression of depression, distinguishing features of dementia and depressive pseudodementia, and potential for suicide.*
5. *Identify interventions for alleviating risk factors for late-life depression, treating depression in older adults, and preventing suicide.*

*D*epression is the most common impairment of psychosocial function in older adulthood, yet it has the unfortunate distinction of being the most undetected and untreated of the treatable mental disorders in older adults. One recent study found that community-residing White men between the ages 65 and 74 years and those 85 years and older are at the greatest risk for underdetection of depression (Garrard et al., 1998). Because depression is viewed as a complaint, a syndrome, and a disease, it is difficult to determine prevalence rates. One approach is to distinguish between the psychiatric diagnosis of major depression and the depression-related affective symptoms of daily life. Using these categories, the prevalence rates for major depression in community-living older adults in most studies is between 1% and 5%, but some studies have reported rates of 12% and 13% (Valvanne et al., 1996; Roberts et al., 1997; Blazer, 1998). Estimates of depressive symptoms in community-living older adults range between 10% and 25%, with an average of 15% (Blazer, 1993). Residents of institutional facilities and people with medical conditions have much higher rates (12% to 16%) for clinical depression and an additional 20% to 30% for depressive symptoms (Blazer, 1998).

Theories About Late-Life Depression

During the 19th century, physicians viewed depression, or melancholia, as the first stage of a progressive psychotic process that eventually ended in dementia (Blazer, 1982). During the 20th century, many classifications have been proposed, and each has become both a source of confusion and a target of debate. Table 20-1 identifies some of the categories of depression that have been identified in the past few decades. The diagnostic guide of the American Psychiatric Association includes major depressive episode and dysthymic disorder as categories of depressive disorders. In addition, the *Diagnostic and Statistical Manual of Mental Disorders* (DSM-IV; American Psychiatric Association, 1994) lists criteria for bereavement and adjustment disorder with depressed mood, which

TABLE 20-1
Terms Used to Categorize Depression

Categories	Rationale for Distinction
Psychotic or neurotic	Severity of symptoms
Agitated or retarded	Type of symptoms
Exogenous or endog-enous	Causative factor
Reactive or autonomous	Causative factor
Reactive or endogenous	Causative factor
Unipolar or bipolar	With or without periods of mania
Situational or chronic	Causative factor and du-ration
Primary or secondary	With or without preex-isting psychiatric illness
Postpartum, premen-strual, or involutional	Specific precipitant event

might be considered to be common types of late-life depression. Display 20-1 summarizes some of the characteristics of major depression and dysthymic disorder, as listed in the *DSM-IV*.

Psychosocial Theories

Psychosocial theories view depression as a re-sponse to the loss of an external love object, and some emphasize that depression results from the failure to replace the lost object. Some theories identify special features of late-life depression, such as having less time and fewer opportunities to replace love objects. A study of community-living adults in the United States found that de-pression "reaches its highest level in adults 80 years old or older, because physical dysfunction and low personal control add to personal and status losses" (Mirowsky and Ross, 1992). Many theories address the unique significance of losses in older adulthood and the personal meaning of life events for the older person. One study found that the impact of an event was determined more by the role changes it caused rather than by the event itself (Lieberman, 1983). Lieberman concluded that "what our data most strongly point to is that it is not the large blockbuster events that create havoc, but rather the insidious alterations of day-to-day

---

DISPLAY 20-1
Characteristics of Various Late-Life Depressions

Dysthymic Disorder
- Chronic depressed mood for at least 2 years
- Presence of at least two of the following: low energy, low self-esteem, sleeping disturbance, feelings of hopelessness, appetite and eating disturbance, poor concentration or difficulty making decisions
- No loss of contact with reality

Major Depressive Episode
- Depressed mood on subjective report (sad or empty) or observed by others (tearful)
- Loss of interest or pleasure in usually pleasur-able activities

- Significant weight loss, or persistent loss of appetite
- Fatigue and loss of energy
- Indecisiveness, difficulty thinking or concen-trating
- Hypersomnia or insomnia
- Psychomotor retardation or agitation
- Feelings of worthlessness, self-reproach, or ex-cessive or inappropriate guilt
- Suicidal thoughts or preoccupation with death or serious illness
- Loss of contact with reality (e.g., delusions, hallucinations)

Source: American Psychiatric Association, (1994), *Diagnostic and statistical manual of mental disorders (DSM-IV) (4th ed)* (Washington, DC: American Psychiatric Association).

life—we are done in more by the drips than the floods" (1983, p. 133).

The learned helplessness theory also has been used to explain late-life depression. A cognitively oriented formulation of this theory describes depression as a deficit in the following four areas: cognitive, motivational, self-esteem, and affective-somatic (Seligman, 1981). According to this theory, depression occurs when people expect bad things to occur, believe they can do nothing to prevent the occurrence, and perceive that the events result from internal, stable, and global factors (Seligman, 1981). The learned helplessness theory has frequently been used to explain why older adults, particularly dependent older adults, become depressed. A recent study of predictors of depression in community-living and institutionalized older adults found that choice, optimism, and personal meaning protected against depression. Specifically, for community-living older adults, the freedom to choose and be responsible for those choices is a predictor of the absence of depression. For institutionalized older adults, the predictors of absence of depression were having a purpose, a sense of order, a reason for existence, and an optimistic outlook (Reker, 1997).

Cognitive Triad Theory

Beck proposed the cognitive triad theory as a way of explaining depression in general, and late-life depression in particular (Beck, 1967; Beck et al., 1979). According to this theory, people appraise themselves by the "cognitive triad" of their self-image, their environment or experiences, and their future. Depressed people appraise these three realms as lacking some features that are necessary for happiness. Examples of negative appraisals are feelings of worthlessness, interpretations of neutral events as bad, and unrealistic feelings of hopelessness. Beck postulates that depression is caused not by adverse events, but by one's distorted perceptions,

which impair one's ability to appraise oneself and the event in a constructive manner.

The second element of Beck's theory involves schemas, or consistent cognitive patterns. Schemas are assumptions, or unarticulated rules, that influence thoughts, feelings, and behaviors. Depressed people typically hold negative assumptions that lead to faulty conclusions. For instance, a depressed person might believe, "I must not be important because the nurse didn't stop to see me." The third component of Beck's theory is the existence of certain logical errors, such as personalization, minimization, magnification, and overgeneralization. Cognitive-behavioral therapy has evolved from this theory, and there is some indication that this interventional approach is effective for and appealing to older adults (DeVries, 1996).

Neuroendocrine and Other Biologic Theories

Theories about disturbed neurotransmitter function as a cause of depression have been discussed for 3 decades, but conclusions have not been drawn about a cause-and-effect relationship. Several theories have addressed the role of neurotransmitters in depression, with particular emphasis on serotonin, dopamine, acetylcholine, and norepinephrine. In addition, the following biochemical changes in the neuroendocrine system are associated with depression: thyroid dysfunction, elevated plasma cortisol levels, and altered growth hormone secretion. Other biologic theories address genetic disorders, decreased cerebral blood flow, and disruption of circadian rhythms, such as sleep.

Theories about relationships between age-related changes in the brain and late-life depression are under intense investigation. Many of the changes associated with depression are similar to age-related changes. Thus, older adults are at increased risk for development of a depressive disorder that is associated with biologic changes and the interactions between these changes and psychosocial factors (Blazer, 1993). Recent attention has also being directed toward the possible relationship between late-life depression and atrophy of brain cells. One study speculated that, like Alzheimer's disease, clinical depression in older adults may be one endpoint in the progressive compromise of neuronal function beyond a critical point (Kumar et al., 1997). In recent years, the potential link between both age-related and pathologic neuroendocrine changes and suicide has been the subject of investigation. One review of such studies concluded that neurochemical alterations increase the risk of suicide, and that aging may further increase the risk through neurobiologic mechanisms (Conwell et al., 1996).

Multiple Causation Theory

Most discussions of late-life depression emphasize the complex interactions between several causative influences. The concept of the "web of causation" refers to all epidemiologic factors and the complex relations between these factors and disease outcome (MacMahon and Pugh, 1970). Using this concept, Blazer (1993) has illustrated some components in the etiology of late-life depression (Figure 20-1). Blazer emphasizes that health care professionals should not be discouraged by the complexity of late-life depression. Rather, they should be encouraged, because interventions can be effective at various points in the web, and "multiple interventions, if orchestrated effectively, are even more likely to be successful" (Blazer, 1993, p. 14).

Risk Factors

Risk factors that are likely to cause or contribute to depression include physiologic disorders, medication and chemical effects, impaired cognitive function, and other functional impair-

ments. Also, there is much current research on the effects of socioeconomic, psychosocial, and cultural factors that are contributory or protective with regard to late-life depression. Although these risk factors increase the vulnerability of people of any age to depression, older adults are more likely than younger people to have one or more of these variables. In the following sections, each category of risk is discussed in relation to older adults.

Physiologic Disorders

At any age, there is a high correlation between depression and medical illnesses. In old age, however, this association is especially significant because older adults have more interacting conditions that complicate the assessment. One study revealed that medical illness was the most common risk factor associated with major depression in older adults and was the best predictor of poor outcome (Caine et al., 1993). Not only are medical conditions themselves risk factors for depression, but somatic complaints, functional impairments, and perceived health have been found to be highly associated with depressive symptoms (Coulehan et al., 1990; Kennedy et al., 1990; Lyness et al., 1993; Callahan et al., 1994). A study of rehabilitation patients aged 54 to 94 years revealed that depression after a catastrophic illness was not related to the person's degree of physical incapacity but to their failure to regain prior abilities (Harris et al., 1988).

Like many other processes in older adults, the relationship between depression and medical illness is cyclical; that is, medical illnesses contribute to depression, and depression contributes to medical illnesses and functional decline. In addition, manifestations of depression may be mistaken for medical conditions, and medical illnesses may be mistaken for depression. In many situations, an older adult has concomitant depression and medical illnesses. Among the ex-

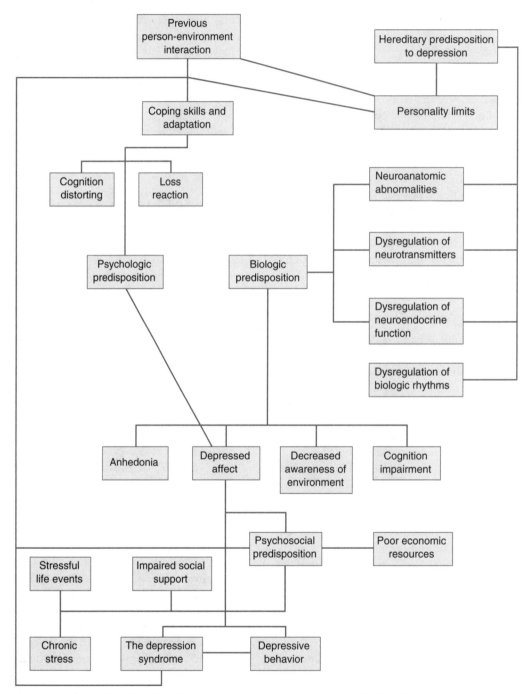

FIGURE 20-1. Possible etiologic factors contributing to depression in late life.
Source: D. G. Blazer, (1993), *Depression in Late Life*, 2d ed. (St. Louis: Mosby). Used with permission.

planat..ons for medical illness as a risk for depression are the following:

1. Chronic illnesses weaken the person by continually or frequently placing demands on coping energy.
2. Physical disease may be a major life event or create daily hassles.
3. Physical illnesses threaten survival, independence, self-concept, role functions, economic resources, and sense of well-being.

Many medical conditions are either mistakenly diagnosed as depression or are underlying causes of depression. Some of these conditions, such as certain vitamin deficiencies, are the same conditions as those that can be diagnosed erroneously as dementia, or that can be underlying causes of dementia. Thus, both depression and subtle medical conditions are likely to be overlooked in older adults, and the manifestations are likely to be attributed falsely to irreversible conditions or inevitable changes of old age. In some of these conditions, the risk for depression is reduced or eliminated once the medical illness has been treated. In other situations, however, the depression is a concomitant condition and must be treated directly. Recent studies emphasize the importance of addressing both depression and medical conditions as distinct entities because patients receiving depression-specific interventions (e.g., antidepressant medications and interpersonal psychotherapy) show greater improvement in more domains of function than do similar patients who receive physicians' usual care (Coulehan et al., 1997). Another study of hospitalized older adults found a strong association between depression at the time of admission and subsequent declines in health status (Covinsky et al., 1997). Covinsky and colleagues stress that symptoms of depression in hospitalized patients deserve medical attention, even in the presence of serious and competing medical conditions. Display 20-2 identifies some of the medical illnesses that are associated with depression.

Effects of Alcohol and Medications

People of any age may experience depression as an adverse medication effect, but older adults are more likely than younger adults to experience medication-related psychiatric problems. One literature review cited 24 studies in which late-life depression was caused by adverse medication effects (Wood et al., 1988). Medications as risk factors for depression can be described as follows:

1. Adverse medication effects can cause a depressive syndrome that improves or disappears when the medication is stopped.
2. Adverse medication effects can induce a depression that does not remit when the medications are stopped.
3. Adverse medication effects can simulate a depressive syndrome by causing lethargy, insomnia, and irritability.
4. A depressive syndrome can result from the withdrawal of certain medications, such as psychostimulants.

One recent review of 12 case reports of depression associated with the use of metoclopramide for gastrointestinal symptoms revealed that the onset of depressive symptoms varied from within 1/2 hour of the initial dose to several months after the initiation of chronic administration (Friend and Young, 1997). This same review found that the older patients included in the study required treatment for depression, and their depressive symptoms took longer to resolve than those affecting younger subjects. Table 20-2 lists some medications that may cause depression as an adverse effect.

Although many medications can cause depression, alcohol continues to be the central nervous system drug that is most commonly used by older people (Blazer, 1993). Moreover, although people of any age may experience adverse effects from alcohol, older people are more sensitive to these adverse effects because of age-related changes. Alcohol and depression have a "vicious cycle" relationship: alcohol causes

---

DISPLAY 20-2
Medical Conditions That Are Highly Correlated with Depression

Central Nervous System Disorders

Parkinson's disease
Dementias
Strokes
Hemorrhage or hematoma
Tumors
Neurosyphilis
Normal-pressure hydrocephalus

Nutritional Deficiencies

Folate or vitamin B_{12} deficiency
Pernicious anemia
Iron deficiency

Cardiovascular Disturbances

Congestive heart failure
Subacute bacterial endocarditis

Miscellaneous

Rheumatoid arthritis
Cancer, particularly of the pancreas or intestinal tract
Tuberculosis
Tertiary syphilis

Metabolic and Endocrine Disorders

Diabetes
Hypothyroidism/hyperthyroidism
Hypoglycemia/hyperglycemia
Parathyroid disorders
Adrenal diseases
Hepatic or renal disease

Fluid and Electrolyte Disturbances

Hypercalcemia
Hypokalemia
Hyponatremia
Hypoglycemia/hyperglycemia

Infections

Meningitis
Viral pneumonia
Hepatitis
Urinary tract infections

---

depression, and depression leads to alcohol abuse. One theory about alcoholism and late-life depression is based on Seligman's learned helplessness theory. According to this perspective, older people view themselves as helpless in the face of inevitable losses, and they use alcohol to reduce their anxiety and restore a sense of control (Hochhauser, 1981). In addition to being a risk factor for depression, alcohol is a significant risk factor for suicide, particularly in older adults (Blazer, 1993).

Impaired Cognitive Function and Other Functional Impairments

There is much agreement about the high correlation between dementia and depression, but there is little agreement about the cause-and-effect re-lationship, or about which condition precedes the other. Depressive pseudodementia refers to a condition that appears to be a cognitive impairment but whose underlying cause is a treatable depression. Such an illness is really a depression, but it is often labeled as a dementia because it is manifested as a cognitive deficit. In many other situations, rather than an underlying depression being the cause of cognitive impairments, the older adult actually has a dementing condition as well as a depression. Recent studies have raised questions about depression being a prodrome or a risk factor for dementia, even suggesting that the term "predementia" be considered in reference to this syndrome (Katz and Parmelee, 1996; Reifler, 1997).

Severe vision and hearing deficits and other functional impairments often lead to social iso-

TABLE 20-2
Adverse Medication Effects as a Cause
of Depression

Types of Medications	Examples
Histamine blockers	Cimetidine, ranitidine
Gastrointestinal stimulants	Metoclopramide
Cardiac medications and antihypertensives	Digoxin, procainamide, reserpine, hydralazine, propranolol, methyldopa, guanethidine, clonidine
Central nervous system depressants, antianxiety agents, antipsychotics	Alcohol, haloperidol, benzodiazepines, meprobamate, flurazepam, barbiturates, fluphenazine
Antiparkinson agents	Levodopa, amantadine
Steroids	Corticosteroids, estrogen, progesterone
Analgesics, nonsteroidal anti-inflammatory drugs	Narcotics, ibuprofen, sulindac, indomethacin
Antineoplastic agents	Asparaginase, tamoxifen

lation, which, in turn, can contribute to depression. Older adults who are most functionally impaired have the highest risk for depressive symptoms and depressive disorders (Blazer, 1993). Studies of the interrelationships between physical disease, functional impairment, and depression have found that functional impairment is a risk factor for depression, even in the absence of disease (Zeiss et al., 1996). A recent study found that increased disability was associated with depression in subjects with dementia and in cognitively intact subjects (Forsell and Winblad, 1998). The risk of depression increases when the functional impairment interferes with the person's ability to participate in enjoyable and meaningful activities. As a corollary, the presence of social supports may offset some of the negative consequences of functional impairment and, therefore, decrease the risk of depression.

Social, Cultural, and Demographic Factors

Demographic factors and personal characteristics that are associated with depression include female gender; low income; low educational level; personal or family history of depression; divorced, widowed, or separated marital status; and early experiences, such as trauma and separation. Other factors, such as cultural background and the effects of the larger society, also may influence the risk for development of depression. For example, longitudinal data suggest that the rate of depression varies according to cohorts, with the current cohort of older people being relatively protected from depression and the cohort of baby boomers having the highest prevalence of depression (Blazer, 1998). A recent focus of research is on cultural differences in the development and expression of depression. The Culture Box on page 590 summarizes some of the studies that have addressed this issue.

The influence of social factors on mental health and psychological well-being is one of the most researched issues in social gerontology. Social factors (i.e., social stressors and social supports) that may trigger or increase the risk of late-life depression include chronic stress, recent social stressors, a stressful social environment, a loss of meaningful social interaction, and the lack of social supports, particularly regarding significant roles and intimate relationships. Studies suggest that having a confidant(e) relationship may protect older adults from depression (Hays et al., 1998). Because social supports are especially effective buffers in stressful situations, only a combination of the presence of stressors and the absence of social supports has been found to increase the risk for depression. Gerontologists emphasize that there are very complex relationships between the social ex-

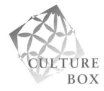

CULTURE BOX

Cultural Differences in Risk Factors for and Functional Consequences of Depression

Risk Factors

- Social supports and chronic illness are significant risk factors for depression in urban and rural older African Americans (Okwumabua et al., 1997).
- Poor health is a more significant risk factor for African American men compared with African American women and White men and women; and low income is a more significant risk factor for African Americans, particularly for African American women, compared with White men and women (Fernandez et al., 1998).
- Different constellations of chronic medical conditions have been found to increase the risk for depression in older Mexican Americans, African Americans, and non-Hispanic Whites (Black et al., 1998).
- Loss of a significant other is a greater risk factor for Blacks than Whites; and decreased social contacts and lack of a sense of control in life are greater risk factors for Whites than for Blacks (Turnball & Mui, 1995).
- A short length of time in the United States and minimal command of the English language are associated with high rates of depression in Chinese Americans (Lam et al., 1997).

Functional Consequences

- Depression is a significant predictor of disability in older Great Lakes American Indians (Lichtenberg et al., 1997).

changes that might contribute to depression and those that might buffer against depression (Okun and Keith, 1998).

Functional Consequences

Depression has serious functional consequences for people of any age. For older adults, especially those who are physically frail, the effects can be life-threatening. This point is evidenced by the fact that older adults, particularly White males, have the highest rate of suicide. Even for older adults who are only mildly depressed, functional consequences can significantly interfere with their well-being and quality of life. This section describes the impact of late-life depression on physical and psychosocial aspects of function. Suicide, the most serious consequence of late-life depression, also is discussed.

Impact of Depression on Physical Function

A distinguishing feature of depression in older adults, as opposed to that which occurs in younger people, is an increased number of physical complaints. Not all physical complaints in depressed older adults are caused by the depression, and the high correlation between medical illness and depression makes it difficult to determine the extent to which physical complaints are risk factors for, or consequences of, depression. One study of the influence of depression, physical health, and other variables on somatic complaints in older adults revealed that depression was the most important factor (Rozzini et al., 1988). The twofold conclusion of this study was that depressed older subjects had significantly more somatic complaints than did those who were not depressed, and that these complaints did not simply result from poorer health status. Another, more recent, study concluded that depressed mood was a strong predictor of health declines over time (Parmelee et al., 1998).

Appetite disturbances, especially anorexia, are among the most common physical complaints of depressed older adults. Sometimes, the depressed person does not complain of anorexia and may even deny the problem, but a caregiver or family member may note that the person is not interested in food and is losing weight. Other gastrointestinal complaints that may be functional consequences of depression include flatulence, constipation, early satiety, and attention to bowels. Any of these disturbances may be attributed to or actually caused by other factors, such as medical conditions or adverse medication effects, but depression must be considered as a possible underlying factor.

Like weight loss and diminished appetite, sleep changes commonly occur in older adults, and they may or may not be caused by depression. One study that addressed this issue revealed a positive correlation between feelings of depression and increased sleep disturbances in general, and early-morning awakening in particular (Rodin et al., 1988). This study concluded that "even when older people have depressed feelings rather than clinical depression, they have greater difficulty than their nondepressed contemporaries in maintaining sleep into the morning hours" (p. P51).

Chronic fatigue and diminished energy are additional functional consequences of late-life depression that are likely to be attributed to or caused by other conditions. Older adults, like seriously depressed people of any age, are likely to experience psychomotor agitation or retardation. Psychomotor retardation is manifested as slowed body movements and slowed verbal responses, sometimes to the point of muteness. A monotonous or whispering tone of voice might also be an indicator of psychomotor retardation.

Affected people often complain of feeling extremely fatigued and having little or no energy. In contrast to people with psychomotor retardation, people with psychomotor agitation present an atypical picture of depression. These people manifest high levels of activity, such as pacing and hand-wringing. They may be unable to sit still and may have verbal outbursts, such as shouting. Another activity associated with psychomotor agitation is compulsive behavior, such as frequent toileting or hand washing. Display 20-3 identifies some additional ways in which depression affects physical function.

Impact of Depression on Psychosocial Function

Depression is inherently characterized by a depressed mood or sad affect, but older adults may not perceive or acknowledge these mood disturbances in themselves. Rather than acknowledging that they are depressed, older adults are more likely to talk about being "blue" or "down in the dumps." Cultural factors may influence the expression of depression, and nurses must consider these in assessing depression. The Culture Box on page 593 identifies some of the cultural variations that are characteristic of depressed older adults.

Depressed older people may feel like crying but may not be able actually to cry or to identify an underlying reason. Depressed older adults also frequently express feelings of diminished life satisfaction, and these feelings may be caused by depression. Anxiety, irritability, diminished self-esteem, and negative feelings about self are some of the more generalized affective consequences of depression. The absence of feelings, or a feeling of emptiness, also can be a functional consequence of depression. A loss of interest in social activities may be the depression-related psychosocial change that is most obvious to others. Similarly, other people are likely to observe that the depressed older person has little or no concern about personal appearance. In addition,

DISPLAY 20-3
Functional Consequences of Late-Life Depression

Impact on Physical Function

- Loss of appetite
- Weight loss
- Digestive system complaints, especially dysphagia, flatulence, constipation, stomach distress, or early satiety
- Insomnia, hypersomnia, frequent awakening, early-morning awakening, and other sleep disturbances
- Fatigue, loss of energy
- Pain, discomfort, dyspnea, general malaise
- Slowed or increased psychomotor activities
- Loss of libido and/or other problems with sexual function

Impact on Psychosocial Function

- Affect: sad, low, "blue," worried, unhappy, "down in the dumps"
- Absence of feelings; feeling numb or empty
- Diminished life satisfaction
- Low self-esteem
- Loss of interest or pleasure
- Passivity, lack of motivation to do things
- Inattention to personal appearance
- Feelings of guilt, hopelessness, self-blame, unworthiness, uselessness, helplessness
- Anxiety, worry, irritability
- Slowed thinking, poor memory, inability to concentrate, poor attention span, inability to make decisions, exaggeration of any mental deficits
- Rumination about past and present problems and failures

the depressed person may be overly or unrealistically worried about illnesses, financial affairs, and family issues.

Cognitive impairments can occur because of depression, and in older adults, these deficits are likely to be viewed as a primary problem rather than as a consequence of another problem. Depressed older adults may, in fact, exaggerate cognitive deficits and make statements about global deficits, such as "I can't remember anything at all." In particular, they may emphasize memory deficits and attribute these to normal aging, when the underlying problem is actually a depression-related difficulty in concentrating. Additional consequences that affect psychosocial function are listed in Display 20-3.

Suicide

Despite the fact that suicide is the most serious functional consequence of late-life depression, nurses and other health care workers tend to overlook this risk. This tendency is partially at-

tributable to the fact that being old is associated with passivity and nonviolence, whereas suicide is associated with aggressiveness and violence. People aged 60 years and older constitute only 18.5% of the population in the United States, but they commit 23% of all suicides in the United States (Blazer, 1982). Suicide rates among older adults in the United States vary significantly by gender and ethnicity, as illustrated in the Culture Box on page 594. Elderly Black and Hispanic men have suicide rates 8 to 10 times higher, respectively, than their female counterparts (National Center for Health Statistics, 1994). Across cultures, there is a general trend for a higher rate of suicide among elderly as compared to young people, and among elderly men as compared to elderly women (Corin, 1996). Recent studies have addressed cross-cultural differences in suicide among elderly persons and are attempting to identify the potential impact of culture on suicide rates (Corin, 1996). This is important because studies of suicide rates among various immigrant groups indicate that the factors that influence

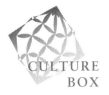

Cultural Variations in Expressions of Depression

Cultural Group	Expressions of Depression
African Americans	Fatigue and somatic complaints. "I sure have a lot of troubles;" "I know God won't give me more than I can handle."
American Indians	Heart problems, being out of harmony
Chinese Americans	Shameful to discuss; may be called "neurasthenia" (i.e., symptoms produced by social stressors)
Cubans	Attribute symptoms to "nerves," anxiety, or extreme stress
Filipinos	Shameful to discuss; may refer to *Lungknot* (i.e., sadness)
Japanese Americans	Shameful to discuss
Koreans	Nonverbal expressions; *Chim-ool haumnida*
Mexican Americans	Sign of weakness, shameful to discuss, common response to stress
Puerto Ricans	References to *Ataque de nervios*
South Asians	References to *Dil uddas hona,* associated with spiritual unhappiness
People from countries with a recent history of war, violence, or political upheaval	May be associated with posttraumatic stress disorder; feelings of helplessness; memories of war-related brutalities

Sources: J. G. Lipson, S. L. Dibble, & P. A. Minarik, (1996), *Culture & nursing care: A pocket guide* (San Francisco: UCSF Nursing Press); and M. M. Andrews & J. S. Boyle, (1995), *Transcultural concepts in nursing care* (2nd ed.) (Philadelphia, J. B. Lippincott).

suicide rates in a country of origin continue to influence suicide rates among immigrants in their new country (Burvill, 1996). In addition to having the highest rate of suicide, older people have the highest rate of completed suicides in proportion to unsuccessful attempts. In contrast to younger adults, older adults are more likely to be successful in committing suicide rather than unsuccessful in a suicide attempt. Also, older adults may indirectly take their own lives through acts such as starvation, not taking medically necessary medications, and other means of self-neglect. Discussions of elderly suicide rates also point out that, if suicide is viewed in the larger context of violent death, then it is important to consider that the lower suicide rates among ethnic minorities living in very harsh conditions in the United States may be offset by the higher rates of homicides and car accidents (Corin, 1996).

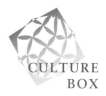

Cultural Differences in Suicide Rates Among the Elderly in the United States According to Race and Gender (1989–1991)

Race and Gender	Deaths per 100,000
White men	43.7
Hispanic men	25.9
Asian and Pacific Islander men	18.5
Black men	16.0
American Indian, Eskimo, Aleut men	11.4
Asian and Pacific Islander women	8.9
White women	6.5
American Indian, Eskimo, Aleut women	3.4
Hispanic women	2.5
Black women	1.9

Source: National Center for Health Statistics, (1994), *Health United States, 1993* (Table 37) (Hyattsville, MD: U.S. Public Health Service).

Nursing Assessment

Chapter 5 of this text addresses all aspects of psychosocial assessment, including depression. Therefore, this section is limited to the following specific aspects of late-life depression: identifying the unique manifestations of depression in older adults, differentiating between dementia and depressive pseudodementia, and assessing suicide risk. The assessment information in Chapter 5, particularly Display 5-6, can be used with the information in the following sections as a guide for assessing depression in older adults. Also, two screening scales—the Geriatric Depression Scale (GDS) and the Center for Epidemiologic Studies-Depression Scale (CES-D)— have been found to be reliable and sensitive for identifying depression in older primary care patients (Lyness et al., 1997). An excellent nursing model for assessing depression in newly admitted nursing home residents can be found in the reference article by Ryden and colleagues (1998).

Unique Manifestations of Depression in Older Adults

Assessment of late-life depression is complicated by a wide array of possible manifestations. The terms "masked" and "atypical" are often used in reference to depression that is not manifested by the expected characteristics. Moreover, manifestations of depression in older adults differ from those in younger adults. Although it is difficult to generalize about manifestations of depression according to age categories, some conclusions about the differences in younger and older adults are summarized in Table 20-3.

Manifestations of Depressive Pseudodementia

In assessing depression in any cognitively impaired older adult, the most problematic area is distinguishing between manifestations of depression and dementia. Although this assessment aspect has been discussed in Chapters 5 and 19, specific features that are most likely to

TABLE 20-3

A Comparison of Various Manifestations of Depression in Young and Old People

Depressed Younger Adults	Depressed Older Adults
More likely to report emotional symptoms	Report more cognitive and physical symptoms
Sense of hopelessness, uselessness, and helplessness	Apathy; exaggeration of personal helplessness
Negative feelings toward self	Sense of emptiness, loss of interest, withdrawal from social activities
Insomnia	Hypersomnia; early morning awakening
Eating disorders	Anorexia, weight loss
More verbal expressions of suicidal ideation than successful attempts; more passive means of suicide	Less talk about suicide, but more successful attempts and more violent means of suicide

be associated with either dementia or depression are summarized in Table 20-4.

Potential for Suicide

Nursing assessment of suicide risk is especially important because older people almost always give clues, sometimes to many people, about potential suicide. These clues, however, may be very subtle, and the person who hears them may not associate them with potential suicide, particularly in older adults. Studies have found that depression, hopelessness, and perceived health status all were predictive of suicidal ideation in older adults (Hill et al., 1988; Rifai et al., 1993; Uncapher et al., 1998). In addition to assessing for clues to suicidal intent, nurses must assess the risk factors that are associated with suicide in older adulthood. Display 20-4 summarizes some of these risk factors, as well as some verbal and nonverbal clues for suicide in older adults.

When risk factors or clues to potential suicide have been identified, an assessment of the imme-diate potential for a suicide attempt must be done. This assessment is multilevel, with each level of questions depending on the response to the prior level. The assessment begins with questions to determine the presence or absence of suicidal thoughts. Health care professionals may be reluctant to initiate questions about suicide because they fear that this line of questioning may "put ideas in the person's head." This fear is unfounded. People who do not have suicidal thoughts usually respect the necessity of the questions but do not begin thinking about suicide just because the topic was broached. Rather than asking a person "Do you ever think about committing suicide?", the nurse can phrase the question in such a way that the person will give clues to his or her intent if it exists, but will not be offended by the question if it does not. Examples of level 1 questions are listed in Display 20-4.

If suicidal thoughts are suspected or identified at level 1, additional questions must be asked. Although level 1 questions can be somewhat indirect, level 2 questions must be more direct, and they are aimed at determining the presence or absence of thoughts about self-harm. If the answer to any of these questions is positive, level 3 questions are asked to determine whether the person has a realistic suicide plan. Questions at this level must be very direct and specific, because this information is crucial to assessing the immediate risk for suicide. If the person describes a detailed plan and has access to all the necessary implements, the potential for suicide is close to 100%. By contrast, if the person has a plan that is vague or that cannot possibly be carried out, the immediate potential for suicide is lower. For example, if the plan involves a gun, but the person does not have a gun and cannot get out of the house, then the chance of a successful suicide is low. By contrast, if the person threatens to consume the bottle of barbiturates that is readily available in the medicine cabinet, then the chance of a successful suicide is quite high. Level 4 questions are asked to further as-

TABLE 20-4
Differentiating Between Dementia and Depression

Parameter	Dementia	Depression
Onset of symptoms	Gradual onset, recognized only by hindsight	Abrupt onset, possibly involving a triggering event
Presentation of symptoms	Unawareness of symptoms, or attribution to nonpathologic causes	Exaggeration of memory problems and other cognitive deficits
Memory and attention	Impaired memory, especially for recent events; poor attention; strong attempts to perform well	Memory and attention deficits attributable to lack of motivation and inability to concentrate
Emotions	Labile affect which changes in response to suggestions; possible apathy owing to cognitive impairments	Consistent feelings of sadness and being "down in the dumps"; unresponsive to suggestions
Response to questions	Evasive, angry, sarcastic; use of humor, confabulation, or social skills to cover up deficits	Slowed, apathetic, frequent response of "I don't know," with no effort expended
Personal appearance	Inappropriate dress and actions owing to impaired perceptions and thought processes	Little or no concern about appearance because of lack of motivation or diminished self-esteem
Physical complaints	Vague fatigue and weakness; complaints are inconsistent and easily forgotten	Anorexia, weight loss, constipation, insomnia, decreased energy
Neurologic features	Aphasia, agnosia, agraphia, apraxia, perseveration	Complaints of dysphagia without any physical basis
Contact with reality	Denial of reality; illusions more predominant than hallucinations; if present, delusions are aimed at explaining deficits	Exaggerated sense of gloom; possible auditory hallucinations or self-derogatory delusions

sess the immediacy of the risk when the person has described a plan. When answers to levels 3 or 4 are positive, the nurse must plan immediate interventions to deal with the suicide risk.

Nursing Diagnosis

If the nursing assessment identifies manifestations of depression, an appropriate nursing diagnosis would be Ineffective Individual Coping. This is defined as "a state in which the individual experiences, or is at risk to experience, an inability to manage internal or environmental stressors adequately due to inadequate resources (physical, psychological, behavioral and/or cog-

nitive)" (Carpenito, 1997, p. 258). Related factors commonly found in older adults are relocation, ageist attitudes, financial concerns, social isolation, caregiving responsibilities, multiple social stressors, loss of significant roles or relationships, functional impairments (including cognitive deficits), and increased dependence (e.g., owing to the loss of the ability to drive).

The nursing diagnosis of Impaired Adjustment would be applicable for an older adult who needs to adjust to a change in his or her abilities. This is defined as "the state in which the individual is unwilling to modify his or her lifestyle/behavior in a manner consistent with a change in health status" (Carpenito, 1997, p. 124). For example, an older adult in the early

DISPLAY 20-4
Guidelines for Assessing Suicide Risk

Risk Factors for Suicide in Older Adults

- Demographic factors: White race, male gender, divorced or widowed, low socioeconomic status
- Depression, especially when accompanied by insomnia, agitation, and self-neglect
- Chronic illness with increasing dependence and helplessness; diagnosis of cancer or a terminal illness
- Poor social supports; social isolation, especially recent isolation
- History of psychiatric illness, especially major depression
- Onset of major depression within the past year
- Family history of suicide; personal or family history of suicide attempts
- Patterns of impulsive behavior
- Alcohol abuse
- Poor communication skills

Verbal Clues to Suicide Intent

- "Pretty soon you won't have to worry about me."
- "I would be better off dead."
- "I don't want to be a burden to others."
- Expressions of hopelessness
- Remarks about life being unbearable
- Reflections on the worthlessness of life

Nonverbal Clues to Suicide Intent

- Making a will; giving belongings away; preparing for own funeral

- Serious self-neglect, especially in people who have no cognitive impairments
- Frequent visits to primary care provider(s)
- Excessive use of medications or alcohol
- Accumulation of prescription medications
- Unusual preoccupation with self and withdrawal from others

Interview Questions to Assess the Immediate Risk of Suicide

Level 1
- "Do you ever think life is not worth living?"
- "Do you ever think about escaping from your problems?"

Level 2
- "Do you ever think about harming yourself?"
- "Do you ever think of taking your own life?"

Level 3
- "Do you have a plan?"
- "What would you do to take your life?"

Level 4
- "Have you ever started to act on a plan to harm yourself?"
- "Under what circumstances would you act on that plan?"

---

stages of Alzheimer's disease may continue to drive, even against medical advice, because the loss of the ability to drive is so threatening to independence.

If the nursing assessment identifies risk factors for suicide, the nursing diagnosis of High Risk for Self-Harm would be applicable. Risk factors and verbal and nonverbal clues to suicide would be identified as related factors. An example is an 85-year-old widower who says his life is no longer worthwhile and who makes frequent

visits to his doctor for complaints of weight loss and sleep disturbance.

Nursing Goals

One nursing goal for older adults with a nursing diagnosis of Impaired Adjustment or Ineffective Individual Coping would be to alleviate the contributing factors. This is accomplished through interventions that improve the person's physical and psychosocial function. Additional goals would be to alleviate the depressive symptoms and to improve the older adult's coping skills. Individual and group therapies can be used to accomplish this goal. Additional interventions include exercise, nutrition, and medical-psychiatric treatments. The following sections discuss the role of the nurse in implementing interventions to address these goals. An overall goal would be to maintain the older adult's quality of life, and this would be achieved through interventions that alleviate the depression and improve the person's coping skills.

For older adults with a nursing diagnosis of High Risk for Self-Harm, the immediate goal would be to protect the person from harm. To achieve this goal, nurses would use communication and counseling skills, as described in Display 20-6 on page 606. Nurses also would use community resources for crisis intervention and psychiatric care. After the immediate risk for self-harm is alleviated, the nurse might address additional nursing diagnoses, such as Ineffective Individual Coping.

Nursing Interventions

Gerontological nurses in any setting are responsible for addressing depression in older adults. Particularly in long-term care settings, nurses are the health care providers most likely to identify manifestations of depression and to request further evaluation and treatment. In recent years, primary care physicians and nurse practitioners have been the health care professionals who are evaluating and managing depression, and referrals to psychiatrists and other mental health professionals for depression have become less common. This trend is due to the emphasis on cost-effectiveness and the availability of safer and more effective antidepressant medications. A recently developed nursing standard of practice protocol for depression in elderly patients emphasizes the important responsibility of

nurses in reducing the negative consequences of depression through early recognition, intervention, and referral of patients with depression (Kurlowicz and NICHE Faculty, 1997). The next sections review the role of the gerontological nurse in planning and implementing interventions for late-life depression.

Alleviating Contributing Factors

When depression is associated with a chronic illness, the related functional impairments often are the risk factors for depression. Any interventions, therefore, that improve physical or psychosocial function also may be interventions for depression. Urinary incontinence, mobility impairments, and sensory impairments are examples of physical problems that might contribute to depression and be amenable to nursing interventions. Dementia is an example of a chronic illness that affects psychosocial function and is highly associated with depression.

As discussed throughout this text, many functional impairments are unnecessary consequences of myths, misinformation, or lack of information. In these situations, the nurse is the professional person most able to provide information and facilitate referrals for a thorough assessment and appropriate interventions. When chronic illnesses and functional impairments challenge the person's coping abilities, individual counseling can be helpful in alleviating feelings of depression. Group interventions, such as support groups, also may be effective in addressing issues that are risk factors for depression.

If adverse medication effects cause or contribute to depression, nurses can educate the person about this potential relationship. Nurses also can discuss problem-solving strategies regarding adverse effects of medications. Most people are not accustomed to questioning their primary care provider about medications. Nurses, therefore, might educate the person about ways of communicating with the prescribing health care provider. For example, if the older person understands that there is a wide array of antihypertensive medications, and that not all of them will cause depression, the person can use this information in discussing the problem with their primary care provider. Nurses also can assure the person that it is acceptable to initiate this kind of problem-solving discussion with health care practitioners. When the nurse, rather than the patient, is the one who communicates with the primary care provider, appropriate questions can be raised about depression as an adverse medication effect. This problem-solving approach is especially important when the primary care provider is considering adding an antidepressant medication to a regimen that includes a depression-inducing medication. In these situations, the solution may be to change medications, rather than to add another medication and increase the risk for adverse effects.

When alcohol consumption is a risk factor for depression, individual and group interventions can be effective, particularly when the alcohol abuse is a reaction to recent losses. Alcoholics Anonymous (AA) is the most widely used group program for alcoholics of any age, and in some areas, age-homogeneous groups have been established, including some for older adults. Nurses can encourage older adults to initiate contact with AA, or they might directly facilitate the referral if the person agrees to this. Individual and family counseling also may be effective, and nurses can suggest or facilitate referrals for these mental health services.

Psychosocial Therapies

In recent years, group therapies have been recognized as an effective and efficient intervention for depressed older adults. Nurses generally do not lead psychotherapy groups as a routine responsibility, but they are increasingly assuming group leadership roles, particularly in community and long-term care settings. Examples of successful nurse-led groups for depressed or be-

reaved older adults have been discussed in the nursing literature (e.g., Utley and Rasie, 1984; Waller and Griffin, 1984; Maynard, 1993; Clark and Vorst, 1994; Phoenix et al., 1997). In addition to groups specifically targeted for depression, groups such as the Healthy Aging Class (described in Chapter 3), which are directed toward developing coping skills, may be effective in alleviating depression. Other group models used as interventions for late-life depression include reminiscence, relaxation, art therapy, focused imagery, creative movement, and cognitive-behavioral strategies. Group interventions for depressed older people are most beneficial when they are active, structured, time-limited, problem-oriented, based on a cognitive or behavioral approach, and not stigmatizing (i.e., emphasizing coping skills rather than psychopathology) (DeVries, 1996).

Individual counseling also can be an effective intervention for depression. In recent years, cognitive-behavioral counseling models, based largely on Beck's cognitive triad theory, have been used effectively for depressed people. Nursing models of this approach are being published in books and journals (e.g., Manderino and Bzdek, 1986; Stuart and Wells-Federman, 1997), and articles have described the application of this approach to depressed older adults in community settings (Hughes, 1991) and in acute care settings (Dreyfus, 1988). One nurse who has researched the use of cognitive-behavioral models for depressed older adults emphasized the effectiveness of this approach and the potential for nurses to become skilled in this approach (Chaisson-Stewart, 1985).

Because social supports significantly affect the mental health of older adults, any intervention that strengthens social supports may prevent or alleviate depression. Nurses can encourage older adults to participate in group meal or social programs. Most communities in the United States have some social programs for older adults, and many provide transportation. Many churches and religious organizations also have programs designed to meet the social needs of isolated older adults. Volunteer visitor or phone call programs, for example, can be used by people who have difficulty getting out of the house. Other programs, such as pet therapy or "Adopt a Grandparent," are available in some home, community-based, and long-term care settings, and they can be helpful in alleviating loneliness and depression.

For older adults who are not seriously depressed, involvement in volunteer activities may enhance their self-esteem and provide them with a meaningful role. The Retired Senior Volunteer Program is one of the many programs in the United States that assists older adults in becoming involved in volunteer activities. Support and self-help groups are available for people coping with life events, such as widowhood or grief reactions. For seriously depressed community-living older people, adult day care programs may be helpful in providing structured social and therapeutic activities. Information about the availability of such programs can be obtained from local offices on aging, and nurses can encourage older adults or their caregivers to seek out such information and take advantage of these programs.

Older adults who are seriously depressed must be referred to appropriate mental health professionals and psychiatric services. Hospital-based geropsychiatric programs, which are becoming increasingly available, can provide assessment and treatment of the unique aspects of late-life depression. Some community mental health centers also are beginning to address the mental health needs of older adults, and they may provide special programs for depressed older adults. Nurses can either suggest or directly facilitate referrals to these programs. Older adults or their caregivers may perceive depression as an untreatable problem, but they may follow through on suggestions for help if they understand that the problem is amenable to interventions. Often, the primary role of the nurse is to convince the older person that depression is not a necessary consequence of old age, and that help is available.

Exercise and Nutrition

The beneficial effects of exercise with regard to anxiety, depression, self-esteem, and other components of mental health are widely acknowledged. Older adults, however, may not view exercise as important, or they may be reluctant to participate in exercise programs because of chronic illnesses, such as arthritis. If older adults understand the benefits of exercise for both their physical and mental health, and an individually tailored program is developed for them, they may be willing to become involved in exercise programs. In community and long-term care settings, nurses can facilitate the establishment of group exercise programs and encourage depressed older adults to participate in them.

Nutrition is an important consideration for three reasons. First, nutritional status often is negatively affected by depression, and this can cause additional negative consequences. Second, good nutrition has a positive effect on mental health and cognitive function. Third, constipation is both a consequence of depression and an adverse effect of some antidepressant medications, and it can be addressed, at least in part, through nutritional interventions. During phases of serious depression, malnutrition can lead to medical problems, which may progress to the point of being life-threatening. Nutritional supplements, hyperalimentation, or tube feedings may be necessary interventions when depression seriously interferes with eating. When depression is severe enough to lead to malnutrition, the older person must be evaluated for psychiatric care. Interventions for less severely depressed older people are aimed at maintaining adequate hydration and nutrition and preventing or managing constipation. The interventions discussed in Chapter 8 can be applied to the care of the depressed older adult.

Medical-Psychiatric Therapies

The two medical-psychiatric modes of treatment for depressed older adults are antidepressant medications and electroconvulsive therapy (ECT). Although nurses in any setting will be involved with decisions regarding antidepressants, only nurses in psychiatric settings will be involved with decisions relating to ECT. Electroconvulsive therapy is discussed in this chapter as an intervention because its use in geropsychiatry is increasing, and most people are misinformed or uninformed about ECT.

Antidepressant Medications

Various types of antidepressants are available for the treatment of depression. The development of antidepressant medications is based on the biochemical theories of depression, with emphasis on alterations in the neurotransmitters serotonin and norepinephrine. For example, the monoamine theory of depression was derived, at least in part, from observations that depression was a common adverse effect of drugs, such as reserpine, which deplete the brain of catecholamine. Pharmaceutical companies have used this theory to develop tricyclic and other cyclic antidepressants, which block the reuptake of chemical messengers at neuronal synapses in the brain.

Monoamine oxidase inhibitors (MAOIs) were the first medications used as antidepressants. After their use became widespread in the 1960s, it was discovered that this category of medication could cause dangerous and even fatal interactions with many other medications and with some types of food. Because of these side effects, these agents have largely been replaced with newer types of antidepressants in the past few decades. Because one contraindication for the use of MAOIs is cerebral vascular disease, they should not be used in older adults. Another contraindication is that they should not be used within 2 weeks of any other antidepressant therapy.

Cyclic antidepressants, used widely since the late 1950s, are thought to be particularly effec-
tive in alleviating the following depression-related symptoms: loss of libido, sleep and appetite disturbances, and loss of interest and pleasure in activities. Newer cyclic antidepressants, called second-generation agents, have been developed in recent years. These differ more in their potential for adverse effects than in their therapeutic effects. Because cyclic antidepressants affect several neurotransmitters, they are associated with a variety of anticholinergic and other detrimental effects. Two particular areas of concern in geriatric care are the potential for adverse anticholinergic and cardiovascular effects. The most likely cardiovascular effects are orthostatic hypotension and altered cardiac rate and rhythm. The most serious anticholinergic effects are blurred vision, urinary retention, and cognitive impairments. Additional common side effects are sedation, constipation, dry mouth, and weight gain. Because of these side effects, people with glaucoma, prostatic hyperplasia, or cardiac conduction abnormalities should not take cyclic antidepressants. Also, cyclic antidepressants should be avoided in people with dementia or Parkinson's disease because of the potential adverse effect of cognitive impairment. Anticholinergic potency varies among the tricyclic antidepressants, with amitriptyline having the strongest anticholinergic effects and desipramine having the weakest. The strength of anticholinergic effects should be considered when cyclic antidepressants are prescribed for older adults.

During the late 1980s, pharmaceutical companies developed a class of antidepressant drugs that were more selective in their action than the cyclic antidepressants. Called selective serotonin reuptake inhibitors (SSRIs), these drugs are chemically unrelated to cyclic or other available antidepressants. They have minimal cholinergic, histaminic, dopaminergic, or noradrenergic effects, and they are now considered to be the first-line drugs for depression because they are effective for most people and have more tolerable and less dangerous adverse effects. An important consideration for older adults is that SSRIs are less likely than cyclics to cause orthostatic hypotension and anticholinergic effects. This is particularly important for mentally frail elderly who are susceptible to confusion and for physically frail elderly who are at high risk for falls. Another consideration in the use of SSRIs is their potential for drug interactions because of their effects on hepatic metabolizing enzymes and because some of them are highly bound to plasma protein. When an SSRI is prescribed, special attention should be paid to potential interactions with nicotine, alcohol, and other medications (including some over-the-counter products). Drug interactions may occur even after an SSRI with a long half-life (e.g., fluoxetine) has been discontinued. Common adverse effects of SSRIs include nausea, vomiting, diarrhea, headache, nervousness, insomnia, tremor, dry mouth, and sexual dysfunction. Withdrawal effects of SSRIs include nausea, tremor, anxiety, dizziness, palpitations, and paresthesias. Fluoxetine, the first available drug in this category, may cause agitation in as many as 20% to 30% of the patients taking it. Also, because of its long half-life, it may take 2 to 4 weeks to reach a steady state in older adults, and side effects may not resolve until 7 to 10 days after the drug is discontinued. Sertraline and paroxetine differ from fluoxetine in that they have shorter half-lives and no anticholinergic effects. Fluvoxamine, like fluoxetine, may have mild anticholinergic effects.

Several other antidepressants, each with a unique type of action on neurotransmitters, are available. These are listed in Table 20-5. With the exception of lithium and trazodone, these unique types were approved during the 1990s. Special considerations in the use of these unique types of antidepressants are as follows: venlafaxine may cause an increase in blood pressure; lithium may be used as a second drug to augment the effects of another antidepressant; trazodone and nefazodone are very sedating and may be useful in the treatment of depression with sleep

disturbances; and buproprion has a stimulating effect, which sometimes can be therapeutic, but is contraindicated in people with a seizure disorder. Psychomotor stimulants (e.g., methylphenidate) have been used for decades for certain types of depression, but these drugs are not antidepressants, and they are not widely used, especially in older adults. In recent years, there has been some evidence that estrogen may have antidepressive effects or may boost the antidepressant effects of SSRIs in postmenopausal women, but this is still under investigation. Table 20-5 lists categories and examples of some of the commonly used antidepressants.

TABLE 20-5
Commonly Used Antidepressants

Category	Examples	Trade Name
Cyclics	Imipramine	Tofranil
	Desipramine	Norpramin, Pertofrane
	Amitriptyline*	Elavil
	Nortriptyline	Aventyl, Pamelor
	Doxepin*	Sinequan, Adapin
	Trimipramine	Surmontil
	Amoxapine	Asendin
	Maprotiline	Ludiomil
	Protriptyline	Vivactil
SSRIs	Fluoxetine	Prozac
	Sertraline	Zoloft
	Paroxetine	Paxil
	Fluvoxamine	Luvox
Unique types	Lithium	Eskalith
	Bupropion	Wellbutrin
	Trazodone	Desyrel
	Nefazodone	Serzone
	Venlafaxine	Effexor
	Mirtazapine	Remeron
MAOIs	Tranylcy-promine*	Parnate
	Phenelzine*	Nardil

*Not recommended for older adults.
SSRIs, selective serotonin reuptake inhibitors; *MAOIs,* monoamine oxidase inhibitors.

Regardless of the type of medication used, the primary purpose of an antidepressant medication is to alleviate depressive symptoms so that the person is able to respond to additional interventions, such as psychosocial therapy. For older adults who have both a depression and a dementia, antidepressant medications may improve the affective symptoms so that overall abilities are improved and the person is able to function more effectively and independently. Nursing responsibilities regarding antidepressant medication therapy include observing for both adverse and therapeutic effects and educating the older adult about the unique aspects of these medication therapies. Guidelines for these nursing responsibilities are listed in Display 20-5.

Electroconvulsive Therapy

For seriously depressed older adults, ECT can be life saving, and it may be safer than antidepressant medications. About 50% of the people

---

DISPLAY 20-5
Guidelines for Antidepressant Medications

Information to Be Shared with the Older Adult

- Immediate improvement will not be evident, but a fair trial must be given to the medication as long as serious adverse effects are not noticed.
- The fair trial may take as long as 12 weeks, but some positive effects should be noticed within 2 to 4 weeks.
- If one type of antidepressant is not effective, another type may be effective.
- Antidepressants cannot be used on an "as needed" basis.
- Antidepressants should be viewed as part of a comprehensive approach to treating depression, and psychosocial therapies should be considered along with antidepressants.
- Antidepressants can interact with alcohol, nicotine, and other medications, including over-the-counter medications, possibly altering the effects of the medication or increasing the potential for adverse effects.
- The prescribing health care practitioner should be asked about potential adverse effects and drug or food-drug interactions.
- The prescribing health care practitioner should be consulted before discontinuing an antidepressant.
- If postural hypotension occurs, the effects can be minimized through such interventions as changing position slowly and maintaining adequate fluid intake.

- If MAOIs are prescribed, certain medications must be avoided, and a low-tyramine diet must be followed (i.e., avoidance of beer, yogurt, red wine, fermented cheese, and pickled foods, as well as excessive amounts of caffeine and chocolate).

Principles Regarding Dosage and Length of Treatment

- Older adults should be started at one half to one third the normal adult dose.
- Dosages can be increased gradually until maximal therapeutic levels are reached, while observing for adverse effects.
- Age-related changes may increase the time needed for medication to reach maximal effectiveness.
- A once-daily regimen usually is effective.
- Bedtime administration of an antidepressant may facilitate sleep as a result of the drug's hypnotic effects, but some antidepressants (e.g., fluoxetine) may be better taken in the morning because of side effects, such as agitation.
- The length of treatment is usually 6 months for a first-time depression, 1 to 2 years for people with a history of a prior depressive episode, and lifetime maintenance for people with a history of three or more depressive episodes.

receiving ECT are older than 60 years of age, and ECT is thought to be safer than many antidepressants for older adults. Some evidence suggests that although older adults are less responsive than younger adults to antidepressants, they are equally responsive as younger adults to ECT (Blazer, 1998). The effectiveness of ECT may be related to its effects on the receptors of chemical messengers. One recent study of ECT in patients older than 85 years of age concluded that it was a safe and effective treatment for extremely elderly patients suffering from an affective or psychotic illness (Tomac et al., 1997). Tomac and colleagues further found that the ECT-related adverse effects were treated successfully and that all psychiatric rating scales showed significant improvements after ECT.

Prevalent negative attitudes about ECT are attributable, in part, to the alleged inhumane use of this procedure when it was first developed a half-century ago. In recent years, however, the technique for administering ECT has been refined, and the risks, discomfort, and side effects are now quite minimal. Except in psychiatric settings, nurses will not be involved with the care of people who are undergoing ECT. Nurses caring for depressed people in any setting, however, need to maintain an open mind about this therapy. In addition, gerontological nurses may be in the position of encouraging older adults or their caregivers to seek advice about ECT from knowledgeable professionals.

Alternative Health Care Practices

In recent years, there has been increasing interest in herbs and other natural remedies for depression. St. John's wort has been widely used in Europe as an alternative to prescription antidepressants, and it has been found to be equally effective for many people. In 1998, the National Institutes of Health Office of Alternative Medicine sponsored double-blind studies in the United States to compare placebo effect, St.

John's wort, and prescription antidepressants. Results of these studies should be available by the end of the 1990s. St. John's wort is widely available, relatively inexpensive, and not likely to cause any serious adverse reactions. As with other herbal preparations, the precautions discussed in Chapter 18 should be heeded. Information about St. John's wort and other alternative and preventive health care practices for depression are summarized in the box on page 605. Keep in mind that many of these remedies have not been subjected to the scientific criteria that are applied to medications approved by the Food and Drug Administration (FDA). These remedies, however, are unlikely to be detrimental, as long as the person seeks appropriate health care for any symptoms that may be associated with a serious condition.

Suicide Prevention

Gerontological nurses do not usually deal with suicidal older adults in the course of their routine duties, but they may have to plan immediate interventions when they identify risk factors. The most important intervention is to seek out psychiatric resources and activate protective service agencies, rather than attempting to deal with potentially suicidal people without the help of specialized resources. All communities have some emergency psychiatric services, and nurses can either make referrals directly or discuss these resources with older adults and their caregivers. Some guidelines for working with people who are potentially suicidal are listed in Display 20-6.

Evaluating Nursing Care

Nursing care of depressed older adults is evaluated by documenting improved coping skills and diminished manifestations of depression. An example of a measure of improved coping skills

ALTERNATIVE
AND
PREVENTIVE
HEALTH
CARE
PRACTICES

Preventing or Alleviating Depression

Herbs
- St. John's wort (300 mg t.i.d.)
- Ginkgo biloba (80 mg t.i.d.)
- Ginger, ginseng, thorowax, dong quai, licorice

Homeopathic Remedies
- Sulfur, sepia, Lachesis, ignatia, Gelsemium, arsenicum, pulsatilla, natrum mur, aurum met, nux vomica

Nutritional Considerations
- Important nutrients: vitamins B-complex and C, magnesium, potassium, selenium, tyrosine
- Tryptophan (eggs, milk, fish, nuts, turkey, bananas, soybeans, pumpkin seeds)
- Phenylalanine (meat, fish, poultry, sunflower seeds, black beans, watercress, soybeans, chocolate)
- Avoidance of excess caffeine and aspartame (artificial sweetener)

Preventive Measures and Additional Approaches
- Aerobic exercise, 1/2 hour 3 times/week
- Avoidance of nicotine
- Art, dance, music, drama, yoga, t'ai chi, qigong, massage, imagery, meditation, relaxation, stress management, spiritual healing
- Psychotherapy, hypnotherapy, autogenic training, cognitive behavioral therapy, individual and group counseling
- Acupuncture, acupressure, reflexology
- Aromatherapy: rose, basil, jasmine, bergamot, lavender, clary sage, chamomile
- Light therapy for seasonal affective disorder

Special Precautions
- People taking antidepressants should talk with their health care practitioner before taking St. John's wort. It may take several months to notice therapeutic effects.
- Minor side effects of ginkgo biloba include headache, restlessness, and gastrointestinal symptoms. It may take several months to notice therapeutic effects. Prolonged use of ginkgo biloba has been associated with intraocular hemorrhage and subdural hematoma. The risk of these adverse effects increases when taken for long periods of time or with anticoagulants, such as aspirin.
- Prolonged use or large dosages (more than 5 g/d) of licorice may cause headache, lethargy, and sodium or water retention. Licorice should not be used by people who have hypertension or who are taking digitalis preparations. Licorice increases one's susceptibility to hypokalemia when taken with diuretics.
- Tyrosine supplements should not be taken by people who have hypertension or migraine headaches.
- Tryptophan supplements should be avoided because of possible side effects.
- Phenylalanine should not be used by people with hypertension.

DISPLAY 20-6
Working with People Who Are Potentially Suicidal

Communicating with Someone Who Is Potentially Suicidal

- Be direct and honest; do not be afraid to ask direct questions, such as "Are you thinking of hurting yourself?"
- Express feelings of concern and confidence.
- Acknowledge the person's feelings of helplessness and hopelessness.
- Encourage the person to talk about the precipitating event, if there is one.
- Emphasize that suicide is only one of several options; then explore other options.
- Emphasize positive relationships; talk about the negative impact of suicide on survivors.
- Maintain a nonjudgmental attitude.

- Make a contract: ask the person to agree to do certain things for limited amounts of time and to call for help if he or she cannot keep the agreement.
- Discuss the problems openly with the family and caregivers.

Crisis Intervention

- Focus on the immediate precipitating event.
- Reduce the immediate danger by removing the implements, interfering with the plan, and providing constant supervision.
- Obtain psychiatric help; call a suicide hot line or activate emergency psychiatric services if necessary.

---

would be that the older person expresses less anxiety about his or her future. Another measure that would reflect improved quality of life would be that the older adult expresses interest in and participates in meaningful activities. Other measures might include improvements in physical manifestations, such as eating and sleeping patterns. Nursing care also could be evaluated by the older adult's participation in individual or group therapies.

Nursing care of older adults who are at high risk for self-harm would be evaluated by the prevention of harm. Another measure would be the degree to which the older adult develops coping skills to deal with the issues that underlie their suicidal thoughts. Nursing care also could be evaluated by whether the older adult obtains mental health services to address underlying problems.

Chapter Summary

Late-life depression occurs because of a combination of factors, including biologic and psychosocial influences. Age-related nervous system changes may increase the risk of depression for older adults. Common risk factors that contribute to depression include physical illness, psychosocial factors, medication and chemical effects, impaired cognitive function, and sensory deficits and other functional impairments. Functional consequences of late-life depression include prominent physical manifestations (e.g., eating and sleep disturbances), emotional manifestations (e.g., sad affect, low self-esteem), and cognitive components (e.g., memory and attention deficits). The most serious functional consequence is a high risk for suicide.

Nursing assessment must address the unique manifestations of depression in older adults and the differences between dementia and depression. Nurses also must assess the risk for suicide and cultural factors in the expression of depression and the risk for suicide. Applicable nursing diagnoses are Impaired Adjustment, Ineffective Individual Coping, and High Risk for Self-Harm. Nursing goals include improving the older adult's coping skills, alleviating contributing factors and depressive symptoms, and maintaining quality of life. For suicidal older adults, the goal is to prevent harm and improve coping skills. Nursing interventions address contributing factors, such as functional impairments. Individual and group psychosocial therapies can be initiated by nurses using models described in this text and in other suggested references. Nurses also have responsibilities for knowing about medical-psychiatric treatment with ECT and antidepressants. Nursing care is evaluated by how well the older adult develops improved coping skills and life satisfaction.

Critical Thinking Exercises

1. Explain why older adults are likely to become depressed.
2. Think of an older adult in your personal life or professional practice who is or has been depressed. What are (were) the risk factors in that person's situation that might play (have played) a part in the depression?
3. Describe at least four cultural variations in the way depression might be expressed.
4. What assessment observations would you make and what questions would you ask to differentiate between dementia and depression in older adults?
5. Make up a case example of someone who is potentially suicidal and who would require all four levels of suicide assessment. Describe how you would phrase the questions for each of the levels.
6. Describe a teaching plan for an 84-year-old woman for whom Paxil 10 mg daily, has been prescribed.

Case Example and Nursing Care Plan

Pertinent Case Information

Mrs. D. is 81 years old and recently has been diagnosed as having vascular dementia. She lives with her husband, who has diabetes, macular degeneration, and severe arthritis. Mrs. D. had managed all household and financial responsibilities until about 1 year ago, when she began having trouble with her memory. Mrs. D. was evaluated at the geriatric assessment program where you work, and she was advised to stop driving and to arrange for some help with complex tasks, such as bill paying and grocery shopping. Two months after the initial evaluation, Mrs. D. returns for follow-up and informs you that she limits her driving to short, daytime trips in familiar areas. When asked about getting help with complex tasks, she states, "I just don't have any energy to make all those calls you suggested. Besides, I don't want anyone else looking at my finances or going to the store for me."

Nursing Assessment

A mental status assessment indicates that Mrs. D.'s level of cognitive impairment is unchanged since her initial evaluation. She has prominent deficits in calculation, short-term memory, abstract thinking, problem solving, and language skills. Your psychosocial assessment reveals that Mrs. D. has a very sad affect and low self-esteem, and she expresses feelings of hopelessness and helplessness. She admits to being overwhelmed with feelings of responsibility for herself and her husband, and she says she feels "paralyzed because there's no light at the end of the tunnel."

When you ask about her daily life, Mrs. D. says she spends most of her time at home because she hasn't had the energy to go out. She admits that she doesn't sleep well and that she has difficulty falling asleep at night. She naps for a couple of hours in the morning and in the afternoon because "I feel tired all the time and I can't go out and do things anyway." Her appetite is poor, and in the past 2 months, her weight has declined from 140 pounds to 126 pounds (her height is 5'6"). She complains of constipation and "heartburn."

When you ask about meaningful activities, she tells you she no longer goes to her weekly bowling club because it meets in the evening and she doesn't want to drive at night. She also has given up her church activities (Thursday discussion club and Sunday service) because she does not want to inconvenience anyone by having them drive her. She feels it's "demeaning to have to tell my friends that I need a ride." She used to enjoy reading, but she hasn't felt like going to the library, and she's not interested in any of the books she has at home.

Nursing Diagnosis

You use the nursing diagnosis of Ineffective Individual Coping, related to depression and declining cognitive abilities. Evidence comes from Mrs. D.'s sad affect, low self-esteem, loss of interest in activities, feelings of hopelessness and helplessness, and inability to address her problems effectively. Physical manifestations are her poor appetite, weight loss, sleep disturbances, and complaints about constipation and heartburn.

Goals	Nursing Interventions	Evaluation Criteria
To help Mrs. D. to identify her coping patterns	Ask Mrs. D. to describe her prior experiences in dealing with her husband's illness.	Mrs. D. will recognize and acknowledge the coping strategies that have been helpful in the past.
	Help Mrs. D. to identify coping strategies that have been helpful in the past.	
To educate Mrs. D. about depression and encourage her to obtain further evaluation of her depression	Talk with Mrs. D. about her signs and symptoms of depression, emphasizing the fact that depression is a treatable condition.	Mrs. D. will follow through with an appointment with a geropsychiatrist.
	Discuss the relationship between depression and the inability to cope effectively with stressful situations.	
	Ask Mrs. D. if she is willing to see a geropsychiatrist for further evaluation and treatment.	
	Explain that antidepressant medications can be very effective when used in conjunction with counseling.	

(continued)

Goals	Nursing Interventions	Evaluation Criteria
To identify and promote effective coping strategies for addressing Mrs. D.'s declining abilities	Discuss with Mrs. D. several options for ongoing support and counseling to assist her in coping with her declining abilities (e.g., the "Something for You" support group for people with memory loss; or individual counseling sessions with the social worker who is affiliated with the geriatric assessment program). Emphasize the importance of developing short-term goals that can be addressed through problem solving (for example, suggest that Mrs. D. begin to address her lack of meaningful activities by going to the library for reading material).	Mrs. D. will attend one support group on a trial basis and talk with you about the experience at her next appointment in 1 month. Mrs. D. will make an appointment for counseling with the social worker. Mrs. D. will participate in one meaningful activity each week for the next month.

Educational Resources

National Senior Service Corps
(formerly the ACTION: Older American Volunteer Program)
1100 Vermont Avenue, NW, Washington, DC 20525
(800) 424–8867

National Mental Health Association
1021 Prince Street, Alexandria, VA 22314–2971
(800) 969–6642
www.nmha.org
• Clearinghouse for information and referrals about depression and other mental illnesses

National Institute of Mental Health
DEPRESSION Awareness, Recognition, and Treatment Program (D/ART)
5600 Fishers Lane, Room 10-85, Rockville, MD 20857
(800) 421–4211
www.nimh.nih.gov

National Depressive and Manic-Depressive Association
730 North Franklin, Suite 501, Chicago, IL 60610–3526
(800) 826–3632
www.ndmda.org

U.S. Department of Health and Human Services Agency for Health Care Policy and Research
AHCPR Publications Clearinghouse, P.O. Box 8547, Silver Spring, MD 20907
(800) 358–9295
www.ahcpr.gov
• Clinical practice guide and consumer's guide on depression (written in English and Spanish)

References

American Psychiatric Association. (1994). *Diagnostic and statistical manual of mental disorders (DSM-IV)* (4th ed.). Washington, DC: American Psychiatric Association.

Beck, A. T. (1967). *Depression: Clinical, experimental and theoretical aspects.* New York: Harper and Row.

Beck, A. T., Rush, A. J., Shaw, B., & Emery, G. (1979). *Cognitive therapy of depression.* New York: Guilford Press.

Black, S. A., Goodwin, J. S., & Markides, K. S. (1998). The association between chronic diseases and depressive symptomatology in older Mexican Americans. *Journal of Gerontology: Medical Sciences, 53A,* M188–M194.

Blazer, D. G. (1982). *Depression in late life.* St. Louis: C. V. Mosby.

Blazer, D. G. (1993). *Depression in late life* (2nd ed.). St. Louis: C. V. Mosby.

Blazer, D. G. (1998). *Emotional problems in later life: Intervention Strategies for professional caregivers* (2nd ed.). New York: Springer.

Burvill, P. W. (1996). Suicide in the multiethnic elderly population of Australia, 1979–1990. In J. L. Pearson & Y. Conwell (Eds.), *Suicide and aging: International perspectives* (pp. 187–201). New York: Springer.

Caine, E. D., Lyness, J. M., & King, D. A. (1993). Reconsidering depression in the elderly. *American Journal of Geriatric Psychiatry, 1,* 4–20.

Callahan, C. M., Hendrie, H. C., Dittus, R. S., Brater, D. C., Hui, S. L., & Tierney, W. M. (1994). Depression in late life: The use of clinical characteristics to focus screening efforts. *Journal of Gerontology: Medical Sciences, 49,* M9–M14.

Carpenito, L. J. (1997). *Nursing diagnosis: Application to clinical practice* (7th ed.). Philadelphia: J. B. Lippincott.

Chaisson-Stewart, G. M. (1985). Psychotherapy. In G. M. Chaisson-Stewart (Ed.), *Depression in the elderly* (pp. 263–287). New York: John Wiley & Sons.

Clark, W. G., & Vorst, V. R. (1994). Group therapy with chronically depressed geriatric patients. *Journal of Psychosocial Nursing and Mental Health Services, 32*(5), 9–13, 44–45.

Conwell, Y., Raby, W. N., & Caine, E. D. (1996). Suicide and aging II: The psychobiological interface. In J. L. Pearson & Y. Conwell (Eds.), *Suicide and aging: International perspectives* (pp. 31–47). New York: Springer.

Corin, E. (1996). From a cultural stance: Suicide and aging in a changing world. In J. L. Pearson & Y. Conwell (Eds.), *Suicide and aging: International perspectives* (pp. 205–224). New York: Springer.

Coulehan, J. L., Schulberg, H. C., Block, M. R., Janosky, J. E., & Arena, V. C. (1990). Medical comorbidity of major depressive disorder in a primary medical practice. *Archives of Internal Medicine, 150,* 2363–2367.

Coulehan, J. L., Schulberg, H. C., Block, M. R., Madonia, M. J., & Rodriguez, E. (1997). Treating depressed primary care patients improves their physical, mental, and social functioning. *Archives of Internal Medicine, 157,* 1113–1120.

Covinsky, K. E., Fortinsky, R. H., Palmer, R. M., Kresevic, D. M., & Landefeld, C. S. (1997). Relation between symptoms of depression and health status outcomes in acutely ill hospitalized older persons. *Annals of Internal Medicine, 426,* 417–425.

DeVries, H. M. (1996). Cognitive-behavioral interventions. In J. E. Birren (Ed.), *Encyclopedia of gerontology: Age, aging, and the aged* (Vol. 1, pp. 289–297). San Diego: Academic Press.

Dreyfus, J. K. (1988). Depression assessment and interventions in the medically ill frail elderly. *Journal of Gerontological Nursing, 14*(9), 27–36.

Fernandez, M. E., Mutran, E. J., Reitzes, D. C., & Sudha, S. (1998). Ethnicity, gender, and depressive symptoms in older workers. *The Gerontologist, 38,* 71–79.

Forsell, Y., & Winblad, B. (1998). Major depression in a population of demented and nondemented older people: Prevalence and correlates. *Journal of the American Geriatrics Society, 46,* 27–30.

Friend, K. D., & Young, R. C. (1997). Late-onset major depression with delusions after metoclopramide treatment. *The American Journal of Geriatric Psychiatry, 5*(1), 79–82.

Garrard, J., Rolnick, S. J., Nitz, N. M., Luepke, L., Jackson, J., Fischer, L. R., et al. (1998). Clinical detection of depression among community-based elderly people with self-reported symptoms of depression. *Journal of Gerontology: Medical Sciences, 53A,* M92–M101.

Harris, R. E., Mion, L. C., Patterson, M. B., & Frengley, J. D. (1988). Severe illness in older patients: The association between depressive disorders and functional dependency during the recovery phase. *Journal of the American Geriatrics Society, 36,* 890–896.

Hays, J. C., Landerman, L. R., George, L. K., Flint, E. P., Koenig, H. G., Land, K. C., & Blazer, D. G. (1998). Social correlates of the dimensions of depression in the elderly. *Journal of Gerontology: Psychological Sciences, 53B,* P31–P39.

Hill, R. D., Gallagher, D., Thompson, L. W., & Ishida, T. (1988). Hopelessness as a measure of suicidal intent in depressed elderly. *Psychology and Aging, 3,* 230–232.

Hochhauser, M. (1981). Learned helplessness and substance abuse in the elderly. *Journal of Psychoactive Drugs, 13,* 127–133.

Hughes, C. P. (1991). Community psychiatric nursing and the depressed elderly: A case for using cognitive therapy. *Journal of Advanced Nursing, 16,* 565–572.

Katz, I. R., & Parmelee, P. (1996). Assessment of depression in patients with dementia. *Journal of Mental Health and Aging, 2,* 243–257.

Kennedy, G. J., Kelman, H. R., & Thomas, C. J. (1990). The emergence of depressive symptoms in late life: The importance of declining health and increasing disability. *Journal of Community Health, 15,* 93–103.

Kumar, A., Miller, D., Ewbank, D., Yousem, D., Newberg, A., Samuels, S., et al. (1997). Quantitative anatomic measures and comorbid medical illness in late-life major depression. *American Journal of Geriatric Psychiatry, 5*(1), 15–25.

Kurlowicz, L. H., & NICHE Faculty. (1997). Nursing standards of practice protocol: Depression in elderly patients. *Geriatric Nursing, 18,* 192–199.

Lam, R. E., Pacala, J. T., & Smith, S. L. (1997). Factors related to depressive symptoms in an elderly Chinese American sample. *Clinical Gerontologist, 17*(4), 57–70.

Lichtenberg, P. A., Chapleski, E. E., & Youngblade, L. M. (1997). The effect of depression on functional abilities among Great Lakes American Indians. *Journal of Applied Gerontology, 16*(2), 235–248.

Lieberman, M. A. (1983). Social contexts of depression. In L. D. Breslau & M. R. Haug (Eds.), *Depression and aging: Causes, care, and consequences* (pp. 121–137). New York: Springer.

Lyness, J. M., King, D. A., Conwell, Y., Cox, C., & Caine, E. D. (1993). "Somatic worry" and medical illness in depressed inpatients. *American Journal of Geriatric Psychiatry, 1*(4), 288–295.

Lyness, J. M., Noel, T. K., Cox, C., King, D. A., Conwell, Y., & Caine, E. D. (1997). Screening for depression in elderly primary care patients. *Archives of Internal Medicine, 157,* 449–454.

MacMahon, B., & Pugh, T. F. (1970). *Epidemiology: principles and methods.* Boston: Little, Brown & Company.

Manderino, M. A., & Bzdek, V. M. (1986). Mobilizing depressed clients. *Journal of Psychosocial Nursing, 24*(5), 23–28.

Maynard, C. (1993). A psychoeducational approach to depression in women. *Journal of Psychosocial Nursing, 31*(2), 9–14.

Mirowsky, J., & Ross, C. E. (1992). Age and depression. *Journal of Health and Social Behavior, 33*(3), 187–205.

National Center for Health Statistics. (1994). *Health United States, 1993* (Table 36). Hyattsville, MD: U.S. Public Health Service.

Okun, M. A., & Keith, V. M. (1998). Effects of positive and negative social exchanges with various sources on depressive symptoms in younger and older adults. *Journal of Gerontology: Psychological Sciences, 53B,* P4–P20.

Okwumabua, J. O., Baker, F. M., Wong, S. P., & Pilgram, B. O. (1997). Characteristics of depressive symptoms in elderly urban and rural African Americans. *Journal of Gerontology: Medical Sciences, 52A,* M241–M246.

Parmelee, P. A., Lawton, M. P., & Katz, I. R. (1998). The structure of depression among elderly institution residents: Affective and somatic correlates of physical frailty. *Journal of Gerontology: Medical Sciences, 53A,* M155–M162.

Phoenix, E., Irvine, Y., & Kohr, R. (1997). Sharing stories: Group therapy with elderly depressed women. *Journal of Gerontological Nursing, 23*(4), 10–15.

Reifler, B. V. (1997). Diagnosing Alzheimer's Disease in the presence of mixed cognitive and affective symptoms. *International Psychogeriatrics, 9* (Suppl. 1), 59–64.

Reker, G. T. (1997). Personal meaning, optimism, and choice: Existential predictors of depression in community and institutional elderly. *The Gerontologist, 37,* 709–716.

Rifai, A. H., Mulsant, B. H., Sweet, R. A., Pasternak, R. E., Rosen, J., & Zubenko, G. S. (1993). A study of elderly suicide attempters admitted to an inpatient psychiatric unit. *American Journal of Geriatric Psychiatry, 1*(2), 126–135.

Roberts, R. E., Kaplan, G. A., Shema, S. J., & Strawbridge, W. J. (1997). Prevalence and correlates of depression in an aging cohort: The Alameda County study. *Journal of Gerontology: Social Sciences, 52B,* S252–S258.

Rodin, J., McAvay, G., & Timko, C. (1988). A longitudinal study of depressed mood and sleep disturbances in elderly adults. *Journal of Gerontology: Psychological Sciences, 43,* P45–53.

Rozzini, R., Bianchetti, A., Carabellese, C., Inzoli, M., & Trabucci, M. (1988). Depression, life events and somatic symptoms. *The Gerontologist, 28,* 229–232.

Ryden, J. B., Pearson, V., Kaas, M. J., Snyder, M., Krichbaum, K., Lee, H., et al. (1998). Assessment of depression in a population at risk: Newly admitted nursing home residents. *Journal of Gerontological Nursing, 24*(2), 21–29.

Seligman, M. E. P. (1981). A learned helplessness point of view. In L. P. Rehm (Ed.), *Behavior therapy for depression* (pp. 123–141). New York: Academic Press.

Stuart, E. M., & Wells-Federman, C. L. (1997). Cognitive Therapy. In B. M. Dossey (Ed.), *Core curriculum for holistic nursing* (pp. 143–152). Gaithersburg, MD: Aspen.

Tomac, T. A., Rummans, T. A., Pileggi, T. S., & Hongzhe, L. (1997). Safety and efficacy of electroconvulsive therapy in patients over age 85. *The American Journal of Geriatric Psychiatry, 5*(2), 126–130.

Turnbull, J. E., & Mui, A. C. (1995). Mental health status and needs of Black and White elderly: Differences in depression. In D. K. Padgett, *Handbook on ethnicity, aging, and mental health* (pp. 73–98). Westport, CT: Greenwood Press.

Uncapher, H., Gallagher-Thompson, D., Osgood, N. J., & Bongar, B. (1998). Hopelessness and suicidal ideation in older adults. *The Gerontologist, 38,* 62–70.

Utley, Q. E., & Rasie, S. (1984). Coping with loss: A group experience with elderly survivors. *Journal of Gerontological Nursing, 10*(8), 8–14.

Valvanne, J., Juva, K., Erkinjuntti, T., & Tilvis, R. (1996). Major depression in the elderly: A population study in Helsinki. *International Psychogeriatrics, 8,* 437–443.

Waller, M., & Griffin, M. (1984). Group therapy for depressed elders. *Geriatric Nursing, 5,* 309–311.

Wood, K. A., Harris, M. J., Morreale, A., & Rizos, A. L. (1988). Drug-induced psychosis and depression in the elderly. *Psychiatric Clinics of North America, 11,* 167–913.

Zeiss, A. M., Lewinsohn, P. M., Rohde, P., & Seeley, J. R. (1996). Relationship of physical disease and functional impairment to depression in older people. *Psychology and Aging, 11,* 572–581.

Impaired Psychosocial Function: Elder Abuse and Neglect

Chapter

21

Learning Objectives

1. Discuss theories regarding elder abuse and neglect.

2. Examine risk factors that increase the potential for elder abuse and neglect.

3. Define elder abuse and neglect and delineate the types of elder abuse.

4. Describe the various aspects involved in detecting and assessing common types of elder abuse.

5. Describe the role and responsibilities of the nurse in interventions for elder abuse.

6. Explain the range of interventions, including legal interventions, directed toward preventing and alleviating elder abuse.

*I*n the context of the functional consequences theory, elder abuse is the most complex and serious negative functional consequence that affects vulnerable older adults. Thus, elder abuse demands the highest level of nursing skill and is the most challenging aspect of gerontological nursing. In this chapter, elder abuse is viewed as a serious impairment of overall function, and it is discussed from the perspective of the functional consequences theory. That is, theories about elder abuse are reviewed, risk factors are discussed, the functional consequences are identified, and guidelines for nursing assessment and intervention are presented. In addition, because legal and ethical concerns are an aspect of elder abuse with which nurses must be familiar, these issues also are discussed.

Overview and Theories

Certain members of any population are vulnerable to abuse and neglect by virtue of being physically or psychosocially impaired or subjugated. In industrialized societies, these groups are protected and cared for through legislative mandates and social programs. For many decades, children and mentally retarded people have been protected in the United States, and in recent decades, two additional groups have been recognized as being in need of protection: victims of domestic violence, and abused or neglected older people. Although the problem of abused or neglected older adults is not new, recognition of elder abuse as a social problem is new. This awareness began in the 1950s and 1960s as the writings of Geneva Mathiasen and Gertrude Hall introduced the concept of protecting vulnerable adults. Centers like the Benjamin Rose Institute in Cleveland, Ohio, developed the concept in the early 1970s through initial demonstration projects, usually specifically related to self-neglect. Awareness of physical abuse, however, did not surface until the late 1970s, and awareness of other types of elder abuse arose during the 1980s.

Elder Abuse as a Social Problem

Recognition by public officials of the problem of domestic elder abuse can be traced to 1977, when congressional hearings on child abuse suggested that the entire scope of family violence be considered (Oakar and Miller, 1983). In 1978, the term "battered parent" was first used by Suzanne Steinmetz at a congressional hearing on domestic violence, and in that same year, two research grants for elder abuse were awarded through the Department of Health and Human Services. In 1979, the first congressional hearing dealing exclusively with elder abuse was held by the U.S. House Select Committee on Aging, and further hearings were held during the 1980s. Several bills were introduced in Congress, and attention was called to the need for federal legislation to address the issue of elder abuse. Although federal legislation was not passed until later, much public interest was stimulated, and state legislatures began to address the issue. By the mid-1990s, all states had passed some form of adult protective services or abuse-reporting laws. On the federal level, a major step was taken in 1989 with the establishment of what is now called the National Center on Elder Abuse, which operates under the auspices of the American Public Welfare Association.

During the late 1980s, a decade after the first research on the subject, elder abuse emerged from the shadows of child and spousal abuse to receive public recognition as a major social problem on its own. Evidence of this comes from newspaper and magazine headlines, such as: "Old and Beaten;" "Hospital Teams Fight 'Adult Abuse;'" "Woman Gets Four-Year Term for Torturing Her Father;" "Love Gone Awry— Some Elderly Suffer Abuse at Hand of Their Own Kin;" and "A Shed of Shame—Woman, 85, Rescued; Court-Appointed Guardian Arrested." Evidence also comes from discussion of the subject on popular television talk shows and news programs. Finally, elder abuse and neglect are topics of concern considered at every major aging-related conference and in public policy agendas.

Elder Abuse as an Issue for Gerontological Care Providers

There are several reasons why elder abuse has emerged as a major social problem and a significant aspect of family violence. First, re-

ports of elder abuse have increased in recent years (Tatara, 1996). This increase is attributable, at least in part, to the fact that those older people who are most likely to experience maltreatment and self-neglect are the same group of older people whose numbers are increasing at the fastest rate. Specifically, the group includes women, the very old, and the frail and impaired. In addition, adult children increasingly are called upon to care for their elderly parents. Some children, however, simply do not have the skills or resources to undertake this responsibility successfully, and abuse and neglect may be the unfortunate outcomes in such situations. Also, elder abuse may be increasing because there are fewer adult children available to share caregiving responsibilities as a result of population mobility and other factors. Therefore, the stress and burden of caregiving accelerates for those who are available, and the perceived stress and burden on caregivers is thought to exacerbate some forms of elder abuse (Steinmetz, 1988). Finally, reports of elder abuse have increased as reporting systems have become more developed and as professionals and the public have become more aware of adult protective services and abuse-reporting laws (Wolf, 1996).

Second, because of the growing number of older people, increased attention is being directed toward all matters affecting this population. In a climate of scarce resources for human concerns, however, special attention has been given to elder abuse and other problems that affect the most vulnerable of the aged. Last, problem recognition has been facilitated by the mushrooming of studies on elder abuse and the subsequent promulgation of experts to champion interest in the subject. Scholars like Rosalie Wolf, Suzanne Steinmetz, Karl Pillemer, and Mark Lachs have kept elder abuse in the forefront through research and publications. In addition, congressional hearings and educational programs have stimulated public and professional interest in the issue.

Elder abuse was first formally brought to the

attention of gerontological practitioners in 1975 through a letter to the editor of the *British Medical Journal,* referring to "Granny-battering" (Burston, 1975). In the same year, Butler discussed the "battered older person syndrome" in his Pulitzer Prize-winning book *Why Survive?: Being Old in America* (Butler, 1975). By the late 1970s, articles began appearing in the gerontological literature in both England and the United States. During the same period, research on elder abuse began with a study at the Chronic Illness Center in Cleveland, Ohio. The study, which reviewed 404 cases handled by nurses, social workers, and other staff, revealed that nearly 10% of the agency's elderly clients had suffered abuse or neglect during the previous year (Lau and Kosberg, 1979). Furthermore, this study identified specific types of elder abuse, including physical and psychological abuse, misuse of property, and violation of rights.

Gerontological nurses have been in the forefront of research and publications on elder abuse. In the late 1970s, articles on the subject began appearing in nursing journals, such as *Nursing Research, Geriatric Nursing, Emergency Nursing, Journal of Gerontological Nursing,* and *Journal of Advanced Nursing.* In 1986, the first clinically oriented text on elder abuse was coauthored by a nurse (Quinn and Tomita, 1986), and in 1987, another important reference was coauthored by a nurse (Fulmer and O'Malley, 1987). Currently, nursing is represented in the field of elder abuse through the continuing research of Hudson (1991, 1994) with the aim of defining elder abuse, and through the work of Fulmer on developing sound clinical interventions (Fulmer and Anetzberger, 1995; Fulmer and Gould, 1996).

Incidence of Elder Abuse

Elder abuse is neither a rare nor an isolated phenomenon in the United States and other industrialized countries. Rather, all indicators suggest that it is widespread, and that it occurs among all subgroups of the aged population.

The prevalence of elder abuse is estimated to be 1% to 10%, with 5% of the nation's elderly being affected by this problem, to a moderate to severe degree, annually (U.S. House Select Committee on Aging, 1990). Although selected studies support these incidence rates (e.g., Block and Sinnott, 1979; Lau and Kosberg, 1979; Steinmetz, 1981; Crouse et al., 1981; Poertner, 1986), only a few prevalence studies of the problem have been conducted. An early study, which examined four types of abuse in a random sample of older New Jersey residents, revealed that 15 of 1000 subjects were subjected to some form of maltreatment (Gioglio and Blakemore, 1983). A more recent study, which surveyed a stratified sample of older Bostonians with regard to three types of abuse, found that 32 of 1000 were maltreated (Pillemer and Finkelhor, 1988). It is reasonable to conjecture that, if these two prevalence studies had considered all forms of abuse, the reported incidence would have been greater. It is also interesting to note that the estimated incidence of elder abuse in the United States is comparable to that found in some other industrialized countries, including Canada, Finland, and Great Britain (Podnieks, 1992; Ogg and Bennett, 1992; Kivela, 1995).

Research further suggests that most maltreatment is repeated, is seldom reported to authorities, and represents more than one form of abuse (Block and Sinnott, 1979; Lau and Kosberg, 1979; O'Malley et al., 1979; Wolf et al., 1984; U.S. House Select Committee on Aging, 1990; Tatara, 1996). Moreover, although the problem can affect any older person, it is most likely to occur among those with certain characteristics. The typical abuse victim is a woman of advanced age who has few social contacts and at least one physical or mental impairment that limits her activities of daily living (ADL). In addition, the typical victim either lives alone or with the abuser, and depends on the abuser for care (Block and Sinnott, 1979; Lau and Kosberg, 1979; O'Malley et al., 1979; Douglass and Hickey, 1983; Wolf et al., 1984; Anetzberger, 1987). In a recent summary of research on elder abuse dynamics, Kosberg and Nahmiash (1996) suggest that, along with characteristics of victims and perpetrators, the social context and cultural norms must be considered in understanding elder abuse. Financial difficulties, a legacy of violence, sharing a household, and intrafamily conflict may contribute to abuse occurrence. Likewise, cultural norms, like ageism, sexism, and stereotyping people with disabilities, provide a climate that can foster elder abuse. To a great extent, the profile of the typical abused elder varies by type of abuse. Victims of physical abuse, for example, are more likely to be younger and married, whereas victims of neglect are more likely to be older and single (Wolf et al., 1986). By comparison, victims of self-neglect are more likely to be male, older, living alone, and isolated from family, and to have dementia, mental illness, or substance abuse (Longres, 1995).

The most commonly reported form of elder abuse is self-neglect (Tatara, 1996). The actual prevalence of different forms of abuse varies, however, in different studies. For instance, early research in Massachusetts and Ohio revealed physical abuse to be the most prevalent form of abuse, whereas studies in Maryland and Michigan documented psychological abuse to be the most prevalent (Block and Sinnott, 1979; Lau and Kosberg, 1979; O'Malley et al., 1979; Sengstock and Liang, 1982). A study of three models of elder abuse investigation and treatment in Massachusetts, New York, and New Jersey revealed psychological abuse to be the most prevalent form in all three locations. The forms that were next in prevalence, however, varied among the geographic sites (Wolf et al., 1984). In a survey of Illinois service providers, neglect was the form of elder abuse most commonly seen, followed in prevalence by verbal or emotional abuse (Poertner, 1986). The Boston random sample survey of three abuse forms revealed considerable incidence of spousal abuse (Pillemer and Finkelhor, 1988). Finally, using similar methods and measures as the Boston survey, studies in Canada and Great Britain revealed

that verbal abuse, followed by exploitation and physical abuse, were the most common forms of elder abuse (Podnieks, 1992; Ogg and Bennett, 1992).

Causes of Elder Abuse

Research on the causes of elder abuse is still in its infancy. Although several recent studies have provided some insight, much of what is known is derived from speculation or analogy with other abused populations. Early theorizing on the subject contrasts with the findings of recent research. Publications before the early 1980s offered lengthy lists of likely explanations, with much emphasis placed on caregiver stress. After holding multiple hearings on elder abuse, the U.S. House Select Committee on Aging (1981) identified more than a dozen major causes, including ageism, retaliation, caregiver stress, caregiver unemployment, environmental conditions, increased life expectancy, resentment of dependence, lack of community resources, lack of financial resources, lack of close family ties, violence as a way of life, a history of personal and mental problems, and a history of alcohol and drug abuse. Likewise, many early theorists suggested that elder abuse was a complex problem with multiple explanations (Block and Sinnott, 1979; Douglass et al., 1980). Most, however, emphasized stress as an underlying cause (O'Malley et al., 1979; McLaughlin et al., 1980; Boydston and McNairn, 1981; Chen et al., 1981; Sengstock and Liang, 1982).

In contrast to the early studies of elder abuse, recent studies have addressed specific types of maltreatment using methods such as comparison groups and interviews of victims or perpetrators. Findings from these investigations indicate that, when elder abuse occurs, it results from multiple, interrelated variables. Etiologies for elder abuse can be divided between those associated with the perpetrator and those associated with the victim. In terms of the former, Pillemer (1986) and Anetzberger (1987), in investigations of physical abuse, found that the dominant underlying factors were social isolation and a pathologic condition on the part of the perpetrator. Both researchers also identified a number of instances in which the abuser was emotionally or financially dependent on the victim, and both came to reject external stress and a history of family violence as salient explanations of the problem. Similarly, in studies comparing forms of abuse, Bristowe (1987) found alcoholism and depression on the part of the perpetrator to be major factors. Likewise, alcohol use and abuse have been identified as significant correlates for elder abuse by adult children (Greenberg et al., 1990; Anetzberger et al., 1994). Phillips (1986) discovered that, although abusing caregivers lacked distinguishing external stressors, they did have fewer contacts in times of trouble than did nonabusing caregivers. By contrast, Steinmetz's study (1988), which involved interviews with caregivers, concluded that caregivers' perceptions of stress and feelings of burden were stronger predictors of elder abuse than were demographic variables or the caregiving tasks performed. In addition, in situations in which the older person used physical violence, the caregiver was found to have experienced increased stress, and was more likely to inflict abuse on the older person.

Characteristics of older people that appear to increase the risk of elder abuse include dementia, poor health, and coresidence with the perpetrator. Health declines involving functional impairment of the older adult may lead to self-neglect or diminished ability for self-defense or escape from maltreatment (Lachs and Pillemer, 1995). Moreover, a number of recent studies have identified dementia, including the onset of new cognitive impairment, as a major correlate of abuse occurrence (Coyne et al., 1993; Lachs et al., 1997). Elder abuse is also likely to occur when cognitive impairment leads to violence or threats of violence by the older adult toward the caregiver (Homer and Gilleard, 1990). Last, there is strong empirical support for shared living arrangements with the perpetrator being an abuse correlate (Pillemer, 1986; Anetzberger, 1987).

The dynamics of living together can reactivate old family conflict and create new conflicts as well, especially when relationship expectations are not met.

Research indicates that there is some association between the type of abuse and the sex of the perpetrator (Sengstock and Liang, 1982). Men are more likely to exploit or physically abuse elders. In part, this reflects a socialization process that encourages men to be more aggressive in their behavior and to control legal and financial decisions in households. By contrast, women are more likely to neglect elders physically or to abuse them psychologically. Female perpetrators may have been socialized to express anger and frustration through words or inactions, rather than actions. Moreover, as the primary caregivers for elderly persons, women are in a critical position to provide either adequate or neglectful care to impaired older people. Finally, women are more likely than men to neglect themselves (Texas Department of Human Services, 1985; Vinton, 1991). This tendency may result from a variety of characteristics of women in old age, including low income, an increased frequency of chronic illnesses, an increased chance of living alone, and an increased likelihood of living into advanced old age.

Questions about cultural variations with regard to elder abuse are currently under investigation. For example, a recent article emphasized that the strong family ties and respect for others that are an inherent value in the Hispanic culture may minimize the incidence of elder abuse, whereas the strong family ties and male/female roles may reduce the incidence of reporting in the Hispanic community (Montoya, 1997). Although there was early speculation that the prevalence and perception of elder abuse may vary by ethnic group, little research was conducted on the subject before the 1990s (Galbraith and Zdorkowski, 1986; Anetzberger, 1987; Stein, 1991). Recently, a number of studies have suggested that the meaning of, incidence of, and response to elder abuse show either cultural variation or commonality. Studies published

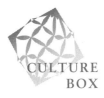

Studies of Cultural Variation and Commonality with Regard to Elder Abuse

- Korean-American elderly women were more likely to judge situations as abusive than either Caucasians or African Americans (Moon and Williams, 1993).
- A study of four ethnic groups in two urban areas found comparability among European Americans, African Americans, Puerto Ricans, and Japanese Americans in the importance placed on psychological abuse and neglect as forms of mistreatment (Anetzberger et al., 1996).
- Asian Indians consider ignoring and not visiting the worst things that family members can do to elderly members (Nagpaul, 1997).
- An investigation of two geographically distinct Plains Indian reservations revealed that elder abuse was more common in the reservation that had the higher unemployment and substance abuse rates and little potential income from the land (Krassen Maxwell and Maxwell, 1992).
- Financial abuse was the most prevalent form of mistreatment among African Americans in rural North Carolina (Griffin, 1994).
- Research that is currently being conducted under the auspices of the National Center on Elder Abuse indicates that Korean Americans hold the most divergent perspectives and attitudes about elder abuse among the six ethnic groups studied (Tatara, 1997).

through 1997 that address this issue are summarized in the accompanying Culture Box. In summary, research on the causes of elder abuse is pointing in the following directions:

1. Causation varies by form of abuse.
2. The etiology of any form of abuse is a composite of several interrelated variables.
3. The origins of elder abuse are found in both the victim and the perpetrator, as well as the relationship between the two.
4. The etiology of elder abuse differs from that suggested for other abused populations in important ways.

Risk Factors

As is clear from the discussion of theories about elder abuse, gerontologists are just beginning to identify specific risk factors. Perhaps the most accurate conclusion that can be drawn at this time is that several serious risk factors must be present for elder abuse to occur. Because these risk factors generally develop over a long period of time, it is difficult to identify a specific point in time at which elder abuse begins. Moreover, risk factors often originate from several sources; that is, they usually are present in the older adult, the caregiver(s) or perpetrator(s), and the environment. Two characteristics, however, tend to be common to all elder abuse situations, regardless of the type of abuse: the invisibility of the problem and the vulnerability of the older person. These risk factors are discussed in the following sections. In addition, some general characteristics of abused older adults and their caregivers have been reviewed in the section on theories, and are briefly discussed as risk factors in the following sections.

Invisibility

Elder abuse is unlike most problems affecting older adults in that one of the major risk factors is its invisibility. Certainly, elder abuse existed in the past. Even in colonial times, tensions between adult children and their parents over property sometimes produced hostility when parents became enfeebled and would not relinquish control. Moreover, the witch-burnings of the 16th and 17th centuries targeted old women in particular, possibly because of the burdens they placed on family resources and their access to property desired by younger relatives (Stearns, 1986).

The authors of one survey on the prevalence of elder abuse underscored the invisibility of abused/neglected elders (Pillemer and Finkelhor, 1988). These researchers found that only 1 of 14 cases of elder abuse came to public attention in Massachusetts, a state with one of the best models of reporting and intervention. There are several reasons that elder abuse has remained hidden so long and continues to be as invisible as it is. First, older people usually have less contact with the community than do other segments of the population, and their circumstances thus remain hidden for longer periods of time. By comparison, children are required to attend school, and thus can be observed by teachers and counselors. Because retired older people are not required or expected to be anywhere, the potential exists for them to remain at home, unobserved, for some time.

The second reason for the invisibility of elder abuse involves the reticence of older people to admit to being abused or neglected. Self-reports are unusual. Sometimes, this reflects the elder's desire to protect the abuser, who typically is a family member. At other times, there is fear of reprisal or a belief that the alternatives, such as nursing home admission, may be worse than the present situation. The last reason for the invisibility of elder abuse reflects society's negative feelings about aging. The myths and stereotypes associated with old age provide a negative image of the last stage of life. One consequence of this image has been a tendency to avoid older people and to ignore their circumstances. As a society, we maintain a strong denial of our own aging, but we hold an even stronger denial of

the social problems associated with vulnerable old people. Another consequence of the negative image associated with old age has been the subjection of older adults to ridicule and even attack. Examples of the vehicles for such ridicule and attack include messages on greeting cards, and portrayals in the media.

Vulnerability

The one characteristic that abused or neglected older people have in common is that they are vulnerable. In sociologic terms, they might be described as needing "protective services," which means they are functionally impaired to the degree that they need formal support services. People who need protective services typically are unable to maintain minimal social standards of care; are unable to meet their own needs for food, shelter, or warmth; are unable to manage their own financial affairs; and represent a danger to themselves or others as a consequence of mental impairment. Moreover, people in need of protective services do not have relatives or others able and willing to provide adequate and appropriate assistance, and they rarely seek services for themselves (Luppens and Lau, 1983; Byers and Lammana, 1993). The degree of psychosocial impairment can range from a lifelong dependent or vulnerable personality to global impairment of cognitive functions.

Anetzberger (1990) has identified four sets of characteristics that can render individual older people vulnerable to elder abuse: (1) personal characteristics, such as impairment and isolation; (2) situational characteristics, such as poverty and pathologic caregivers; (3) environmental factors, including deteriorated housing and crime-ridden neighborhoods; and (4) social factors, such as learned helplessness and growing up in a violent subculture. These individual characteristics tend to increase vulnerability for elder abuse, especially for repeated or chronic maltreatment and self-neglect.

Psychosocial Factors

As indicated before, many abused older adults become vulnerable as a result of impaired cognitive function. Impaired judgment, inability to make safe decisions, and loss of contact with reality are specific impairments that can lead to abuse and neglect. Cognitive impairment may be caused by an underlying dementia, delirium, or depression, or by a combination of pathologic processes. Therefore, anything that can cause cognitive impairments, such as dementia, physiologic disturbances, or adverse medication effects, must be considered a risk factor for impaired psychosocial function. When the older adult denies the cognitive impairment or refuses help or evaluation, the risk increases. Older people who live alone and are aware of their impairments may be afraid of acknowledging them because they fear that they have an untreatable problem that will require nursing home care. Sometimes, this fear leads to social isolation, the overlooking of treatable or reversible causes of impairment, and a progressive but unnecessary decline in function.

Much recent research has revealed a correlation between physical abuse and dementia. Pillemer and Suitor (1992), for example, identified predictors of both violent feelings and violence based on interviews with 236 family caregivers caring for people with dementia. Predictors of violent feelings included physical aggression and disruptive behaviors by the care recipient, along with a shared living situation. Predictors of violence included being a spouse and being very old. In a similar study of 184 patients with Alzheimer's disease and their primary caregivers, Paveza and colleagues (1992) found that important correlates to physical abuse included caregiver depression and a living arrangement in which the older person is residing with immediate family, but without a spouse.

Long-term mental illness predisposes the older adult to abuse or neglect, especially in combination with other factors, such as dementia or the loss of a significant social support. Families who describe an older adult as "always somewhat eccentric" may be masking their own denial of a long-term, progressive problem. Depression can also be an underlying cause of self-neglect because one of its symptoms is a lack of interest in caring for oneself (Rathbone-McCuan and Bricker-Jenkins, 1992; Lustbader, 1996). Moreover, depressed people often refuse or discourage any social contact and then become progressively more isolated. Even if they do not discourage social contact, depressed people may have such a negative outlook that other people choose to avoid them. Thus, any condition that is a risk factor for depression also must be considered to be a risk factor for elder abuse. Additional risk factors arise from social and environmental sources. The lack of a support system is one of the most common contributing factors to self-neglect, especially in old-old people who may have outlived most of the people who once provided support and tangible services. This is especially problematic for people who have been lifelong recluses or who have no children or extended family. More often than not, a combination of risk factors will be present in the older adult, the caregiver(s), and the environment.

Caregiver Factors

Some psychosocial impairment usually can be identified in the caregiver who perpetrates abuse. Any of the psychosocial risk factors for abuse or neglect in older adults can also apply to their caregivers, particularly if the caregivers themselves are old. Caregivers who are physically abusive are more likely to have a psychopathologic condition than nonabusive caregivers. Some of the psychosocial factors that have been identified for abusive and potentially abusive caregivers include a perception of social isolation, a recent decline in health, dependence and coresidence, an external locus of control, and poor interpersonal relations with the dependent elder (Wolf et al., 1986; Anetzberger, 1987; Bendik, 1992). It is not unusual to have a mutually neglectful or abusive situation when an older married couple has several of the psychosocial risk factors just identified and is, in addition, socially isolated.

Functional Consequences

The existence of one or more of the risk factors just discussed predisposes the older person to become the knowing or unknowing victim of elder abuse, which can be defined as the maltreatment of older people. This maltreatment can be intentional or unintentional, and it can result from the actions or inactions of other people, usually caregivers. Self-neglect is a type of elder abuse that occurs when older people fail to provide themselves with adequate food, shelter, medical care, and other life essentials.

Elder abuse is illustrated by the following situations, which have come to the attention of health and social service professionals in both rural and urban communities:

1. A middle-aged alcoholic man hit his aged father during an argument. In turn, both were beaten by their sons/grandsons, who wanted money for drugs.
2. An elderly woman never left home because she feared her memory lapses would prevent her from finding the way back. When she did venture out, she fell on the porch and the local office on aging was called. Outreach workers found she had no food in the house and was malnourished.
3. An unemployed couple kept their impaired grandparents confined to the house, refusing them visitors, abandoning them for days without adequate food, and denying them help for fear of losing access to their Social Security checks.
4. A son visited his mother in the nursing home and sexually assaulted her when staff members were not present.

5. A depressed elderly woman refused to take a needed medication with the result that her legs became so swollen she could not leave her chair.
6. A woman in her 80s—who was weak, incontinent, and had hypertension—was abandoned in an emergency room with a note and the message "Totally dependent! Handle with care."

These situations were selected because they reflect the variety of forms of elder abuse. Most researchers and practitioners agree on the following forms of elder abuse: (1) physical abuse, including hitting and shoving; (2) psychological abuse, including threats and name-calling; (3) physical neglect, including denying adequate food or medication; (4) psychological neglect, including failure to provide proper supervision or social interaction; (5) exploitation, including forcing the elder to change a will or a deed; and (6) violation of rights, including denying privacy or visitors.

More recently recognized forms of elder abuse are abandonment and sexual assault. Early interest in rape and other sexual violence perpetrated against older people emerged during the 1970s when the topic of crime and the elderly was much discussed and researched (Davis and Brody, 1979). At that time, however, the concern focused on sexual assault by strangers. Only in the 1990s did sexual assault by family members and paid caregivers become a widely recognized aspect of elder abuse, principally through studies in the United States, which revealed that the overwhelming majority of victims were women (Ramsey-Klawsnik, 1991 and 1993). Studies conducted in Great Britain around the same time reported that a significant number of older sexual assault victims were men (Holt, 1993). Reports of sexual assault against older people are rare (Tatara, 1996), but the resulting physical and emotional trauma can be severe and long lasting.

Abandonment occurs when dependent older people are deserted by people who are responsible for their care. Few states specifically address this form of elder abuse in protective service or abuse reporting laws (Tatara, 1995). Nonetheless, surveys by the U.S. Senate Special Committee on Aging and the American College of Emergency Physicians (Beck and Gordon, 1991) suggest that the number of older people abandoned at hospital emergency rooms has increased dramatically. This increase is attributable, at least in part, to the increasing numbers of dependent older adults and to public policies that encourage care of dependent people at home by family or other informal providers, some of whom feel ill-equipped, physically, emotionally, or financially, to assume this role.

Self-neglect and self-harm are other forms of elder abuse, but they differ from other types in that they have no perpetrator other than the older person. With self-neglect, the older person fails to meet essential needs, usually because of such factors as serious functional impairments or the desire to die. With self-abuse, the older person causes injury or pain to herself or himself, including body mutilations.

Although until recently the elder abuse literature usually did not address situations that were mutually abusive or neglectful, nurses working in home settings have long encountered situations in which two people, often a married couple, abuse each other or are both neglected. These situations may be rooted in a long-term, mutually abusive relationship, but usually, they evolve because of gradual declines in the functional abilities of both people. They also may be associated with the poor coping skills of a spouse or caregiver who is faced with increasing demands and little or no outside help. These situations are now being recognized as aspects of domestic violence.

The convergence between problems of elder abuse and domestic violence began in 1988 with the publication of a Boston prevalence survey, which found that there were more reported cases of spousal abuse (58%) among elders than cases of elder abuse by adult children (24%) (Pillemer

and Finkelhor, 1988). In that same year, the older adult population was added to the list of groups eligible for services under the Family Violence Prevention and Services Act. In the early 1990s, the American Association of Retired Persons (AARP) (1992) brought together elder abuse and domestic violence experts for a forum entitled "Abused Elders or Older Battered Women?" This forum served as the impetus for a subsequent AARP national survey of programs for older battered women and the publication of a resource guide. In the mid-1990s, the Administration on Aging awarded grants to six organizations to demonstrate domestic violence programs for older adults (Nerenberg, 1996). Also during that time, the Older Women's League selected violence against midlife and older women as the topic for their annual Mother's Day Call to Action. Since then, interest in the convergence of elder abuse and domestic violence has taken multiple forms, including research (Wolf and Pillemer, 1995; Harris, 1996), public testimony (Wolf, 1996), clinical presentations (Brandl and Raymond, 1996, 1997), and intervention programs (Seaver, 1996; Brandl, 1997). Despite this attention, there are very few viable programs addressing domestic violence and elders.

Many older people who are victims of elder abuse are aware of their situation and suffer serious psychosocial consequences from both the situation itself and their awareness of the situation (Anetzberger, 1997). The following case illustrates the awareness that some people have of their unfortunate circumstances.

When Mr. P.'s wife died, this frail man sought care in the home of a neighbor who offered both board and care in exchange for his monthly Social Security check. In reality, the neighbor provided neither, but locked Mr. P. in the basement and gave him little food. If he complained about the treatment or refused to sign over the income or property, the "caregiver" hit or kicked him. After 4 years, the situation was discovered and reported to the county protective services agency. Mr. P. later sat in the social worker's office and sadly commented, "So this is what it's like to be a protective case."

Nursing Assessment

Elder abuse is not so much assessed as it is detected, and gerontological nurses often must assume the role of detective. Because elder abuse, by its very nature, is a hidden problem, assessment begins with a suspicion about its existence. Information may be purposefully withheld, and it is rarely volunteered, except in situations in which the older person or caregiver is desperate for help. Clues to elder abuse might first be noted when an older person is seen in an emergency room or admitted to a hospital. Most often, a home visit is an essential component of the assessment process, and gaining admission to the home usually is the first assessment challenge. Many times, the situation deteriorates so gradually that it is hard to determine the onset of abuse. In borderline situations, people often choose to ignore the clues in hopes that the situation will resolve itself without intervention.

Unique Aspects of Elder Abuse Assessment

Assessment of elder abuse differs from overall nursing assessment in several respects. First, in contrast to usual health care situations in which the purpose of assessment is to plan interventions for addressing health and medical needs, one of the purposes of assessment of elder abuse is to determine whether legal interventions are appropriate or necessary. In these situations, the primary concern usually is a determination of the safety of the older person. This approach is similar to emergency room nursing, in which basic life-preserving needs are addressed immediately and other needs are considered later. Second, health care workers dealing with elder abuse often are quite limited in their goals.

They sometimes have to accept basic safety as the only goal, especially when the elder and caregiver insist on choices that are not in accordance with what the health care workers would recommend. An assessment of "safe function" is crucial, therefore, because legal interventions can be taken only in high-risk situations. Because the determination of safety often is based on medical and nursing information, the role of the nurse is especially important. In home settings, in particular, the nurse may be the only health care professional who directly assesses the situation, and the nursing assessment may be the major determinant of recommendations for legal intervention.

Third, cases of elder abuse usually involve some element of resistance from the older person or caregiver(s). It is only in rare situations that abused elders or their caregivers seek out the assistance of health care professionals. It might be impossible to establish a trusting relationship, but the nurse must try, at the very least, to establish an accepting relationship. The initial assessment, therefore, is aimed at identifying ways of gaining access and acquiring at least passive acceptance.

Fourth, in contrast to most health care situations, the nurse may be viewed as a threat rather than a help. Nurses are not accustomed to being viewed as the "bad guy," and they often must identify a way to minimize the perceived threat, even before the initial contact. This can be accomplished by identifying some person who both acknowledges that a problem exists and is willing to facilitate the introduction of a nurse. Any of the following categories of people might be helpful in gaining access and acceptance: neighbors; relatives (especially family members who do not live in the problematic home setting); staff from senior centers, offices on aging, or health care or community agencies; physicians or any other health professionals; and church-based people (e.g., clergy).

Fifth, when legal interventions are being considered, the legal rights of the person and the caregivers must be addressed. Nurses and other workers involved in elder abuse cases usually are uncomfortable making decisions that involve the rights of other adults. When legal and ethical issues are addressed in institutional settings, the decisions are guided by medical information and institutional policies, and in these settings, the role of the physician usually is the most important. In home settings, however, there are few clear guidelines and little or no physician input.

Physical Health

The nursing assessment of physical abuse and neglect focuses on the following aspects: nutrition, hydration, bruises and injuries, degree of frailty, and presence of pathologic conditions. Nutrition and hydration are important not only in determining the existence of physical neglect, but also in determining the seriousness and urgency of the situation. In community settings, a determination of nutrition and hydration status is sometimes the crucial factor as to whether emergency or involuntary measures must be taken, or whether time can be allowed for working with the person in the home setting. The guidelines discussed in Chapter 8, particularly in Table 8-1 ("Causes and Consequences of Nutrient Deficiencies"), can be applied to the detection of malnutrition and dehydration.

Skin turgor over the extremities is not necessarily a reliable indicator of hydration, especially for very old people or for people who have lost weight. Examination of the mucous membranes and an assessment of skin turgor over the sternum or abdomen provide more accurate clues to dehydration. The absence of thirst sensation does not necessarily mean the person is adequately hydrated, because older people may have a diminished thirst response. On the other hand, the presence of thirst sensation is a definite indicator of either dehydration, a physiologic disturbance, or an adverse medication effect. If a urine sample can be obtained,

a measurement of specific gravity will provide information about hydration. When a urinometer is not available, a visual examination of urine concentration will provide some clues to hydration.

When any indicators of malnutrition or dehydration are identified, the next step is to determine whether the hydration or nutritional status can be improved adequately without removing the person from the setting. The role of the nurse can be especially important in assessing not only the nutrition and hydration status, but also the measures required to alleviate deficits immediately. Sometimes, the provision of water and food is the most important intervention in neglect situations. In addition, this intervention is inexpensive and readily available, and it can be quite effective in establishing a relationship with a hungry or thirsty person!

Assessment of bruises, swelling, injuries, lacerations, pressure sores, and other indications of physical harm is an important aspect of the detection of physical neglect or abuse. In situations of physical neglect, nurses may see any of the following indicators: leg ulcers; pressure sores; dependent edema; poor wound healing; burns from stoves, cigarettes, or hot water; and bruises and injuries from falls, especially repeated falls. The presence of more than one of these indicators at the same time, or over a short period of time, should raise high levels of suspicion about physical neglect. The possibility of drug or alcohol abuse also should be considered when any of these indicators is identified, especially if the person is also depressed or socially isolated. To detect physical abuse, the nurse should look for any indication of injury caused by people who live with or visit a vulnerable older adult. Examples are marks from cuts, bites, burns, or punctures; bruises or injuries, especially of the face, head, or trunk; bruises on both upper arms, as would result from being grabbed or shaken harshly; or bruises that reflect the shape of objects, like belts or hairbrushes. If there is evidence of injuries from falls, the nurse must consider the possibility that the person was shoved or otherwise caused to fall by someone else.

Physical abuse may also be caused indirectly, as by a caregiver who gives the person excessive amounts of alcohol or drugs, especially psychoactive medications. Sometimes, caregivers who abuse drugs or alcohol will give these substances to the people for whom they care, especially if the dependent person is not able or willing to refuse. Other times, caregivers may administer excessive amounts of psychoactive medications to keep the dependent person quiet and less troublesome. If psychoactive medications are used only for the caregiver's benefit and to the detriment of the person receiving the medication, this can constitute physical or psychological abuse. Any of the following clues to substance abuse may be observed: ataxia, somnolence, clouded mentation, slurred speech, staggering gait, or extrapyramidal manifestations. If there is evidence that the caregiver of a passive and dependent older person is a substance abuser, the nurse should be particularly suspicious about the possibility that the caregiver is giving drugs or alcohol to the older person.

Other aspects of physical neglect include withholding therapeutic medications or interfering with the person's medical care. Caregivers may decide not to purchase prescriptions or provide nursing care, medical equipment, or comfort items because they do not want to spend the money. When decisions not to purchase these things are made by caregivers without the willing consent of the older adult, this may represent physical abuse. For example, a caregiver may be unwilling to spend money for nursing assistance, even though this care is necessary for the dependent older adult. If the older adult has not freely chosen to forego this available help, then this may be considered physical neglect. If the caregiver is likely to inherit the money that is being saved by the lack of paid help, this may represent financial exploitation as well.

Because physical neglect can arise from the caregiver's lack of knowledge, it is essential to assess the caregiver's understanding of the dependent person's needs. For example, caregivers may have very good intentions when they use adult briefs for the control of incontinence, but they may not understand the potential for skin breakdown. With regard to medications, caregivers may administer excessive amounts of psychoactive medications because they do not understand the correct dosing schedule. This is especially common when medications are ordered on a p.r.n. basis and the caregiver has not been given clear guidelines for determining when the medication is needed, or what the most effective dosage is. In these situations, nursing assessment of the caregiver's knowledge is especially important because educational interventions or the provision of additional services may alleviate the abuse.

Assessment of the degree of frailty of the older adult is another consideration in determining actual or potential physical abuse or neglect. For example, an older adult who is slightly obese and fully ambulatory would not have the same degree of risk for fall-related injuries as someone who weighs only 78 pounds and ambulates unsteadily with a walker. Similarly, if the 75-year-old wife of an alcoholic man can easily escape to safety when he becomes violent, and she chooses to remain in the situation, she would not necessarily be considered a protective case; however, if the woman is cognitively impaired, physically frail, or unable to move quickly, and if she is the target of his violence when he is inebriated, this situation could be defined as elder abuse.

In the presence of certain medical conditions, someone may be determined to be neglected if necessary treatments cannot be or are not being provided. For example, if the person is an insulin-dependent diabetic, it is essential to determine whether daily insulin injections can be provided. In determining whether an older adult can function safely in community settings, the nurse must consider the person's ability to follow medical regimens and the consequences of noncompliance. If a medication regimen is necessary for the control of medical conditions, such as congestive heart failure, the nurse and primary care provider must assess the person's ability to comply and the consequences of noncompliance. Assessment also should address the question of whether the medical regimen could be modified in such a way that compliance would be facilitated while still allowing the person to remain in an independent setting. In planning care for people in home settings, the ideal regimen may have to be modified to gain an increase in the level of compliance. For example, an older person who is hospitalized might be maintained on a complex medication regimen that requires some medications to be administered before meals and others after meals, and some to be administered 4 times a day and others 3 times a day. This might be the ideal way to ensure optimal medication effectiveness and minimal adverse reactions while the person is hospitalized, but such a regimen may be so complicated for the older person or the caregivers to carry out in a home setting that it might not be followed at all. In situations such as these, a thorough nursing assessment of the total medication regimen can lead to measures that simplify the regimen and result in increased compliance and alleviation of the neglect.

Activities of Daily Living

One of the purposes of assessment in elder abuse situations is to determine the necessity of legal interventions when an older adult is at risk. Therefore, a nursing assessment of the person's potential for safe performance of ADL is extremely important. For community-living older adults, an assessment of the home environment and the person's level of function in that environment is best conducted by health care workers who can directly observe the person at home. The assessment is based not only on direct observations, but also on information provided by caregivers who observe the person's daily function. Home health aides can be a valuable source of information, and they usually have a greater

degree of objectivity than family members. In some circumstances, it may be appropriate to involve occupational or physical therapists in the home assessment. When a difference of opinion exists, or when the nurse is unable to make a clear determination of the safety of the situation, a team conference may be helpful in reaching some agreement. Team conferences ideally include all the people who function in assessment or caregiving capacities and who have some degree of objectivity. In cases of suspected elder abuse, the assessment team may include many informal sources of help, such as family and neighbors, as well as formal sources of help.

Personal dress, hygiene, and grooming are among the most visible aspects of daily function, and these are assessed even in social settings. People often are viewed as neglected when they do not comply with socially defined standards of cleanliness, particularly when an unpleasant odor is noted. Although poor hygiene and grooming are important reflections of many underlying problems, these aspects of ADL do not necessarily reflect the person's safe function. When families and health care/social service workers first work with a neglected older person who is obviously in need of much personal care, they often are tempted to begin by assisting the person with bathing and grooming. Although the workers may view this as the most socially acceptable way to begin, the older person may view this approach as very threatening.

Therefore, once the nurse has assessed whether the poor hygiene is hazardous to the person's health, the nurse should assess the consequences of imposing assistance with personal care on someone who may be unwilling to accept help or to acknowledge a hygiene problem. The nurse may determine that immediate efforts to deal with personal hygiene would be detrimental to the immediate goal of establishing a relationship and the long-term goal of assisting with many aspects of daily function. When this is the case, the nurse may have to reinforce the principle that "people don't die of dirt" with caregivers and other workers. Although not ignoring the need for assistance with personal care, the nurse may need to emphasize that it is more important to address issues of nutrition, hydration, and safety first, and to avoid addressing less important issues that could interfere with the acceptance of services.

Adequate nutrition and hydration, and an ability to obtain help in an emergency, are the basic human needs that are most often called into question in cases of elder abuse. Other basic needs may also be compromised, usually in relation to specific functional impairments and environmental circumstances. For instance, for people who are bed-bound or who have very limited function, bowel and bladder elimination may be a basic need. For people with mobility limitations or serious vision impairments, safe ambulation and the ability to avoid falls are important considerations. Table 21-1 summarizes some of the specific functional and environmental conditions that present risks to basic needs.

Psychosocial Function

Assessment of psychosocial function is discussed at length in Chapter 5. In cases of elder abuse, the most important aspect of psychosocial function is assessment of the person's capacity for reasonable judgments about self-care. This is not only the most important aspect, but also the most difficult, because the determination of someone's ability to make "appropriate" judgments is based, at least in part, on subjective criteria and opinions. When judgment is impaired to the point that the person is at serious risk and does not acknowledge the risk, the person usually is considered incompetent or incapacitated. The crucial element in assessing the risk for elder abuse, therefore, is a determination not of the "goodness" or "wisdom" of decision-making abilities, but of the danger, if any, posed by the decisions. When the competence of an older adult to make safe decisions regarding self-care is in doubt, nurses may be legally bound

TABLE 21-1
Risks to Safety Associated with Functional Limitations

Functional Limitation	Risks to Safety
Any mental or physical impairment in combination with social isolation and lack of a support system	Nutrition and hydration
Mobility limitations or seriously impaired vision, especially in combination with poor judgment	Falls
Cognitive impairments in ambulatory people	Wandering, getting lost
Bed-bound status or seriously impaired ambulation	Pressure sores
Cognitive impairment, especially poor judgment	Inability to get help
Poor judgment, especially when living in an unsafe neighborhood	Basic safety and security

to make reports or consider other legal interventions. There are no federal guidelines for determining the mental capacity of abused or neglected older adults, and the legal criteria differ from state to state. The ethical and legal considerations involved in various legal interventions are discussed later in this chapter and in Chapter 22.

Support Resources

Support resources include those people, such as caregivers and friends, who influence the person's physical and psychosocial function. Some or all of the support people may directly cause the abusive situation, or they may be actively or passively contributing to the abusive situation. Therefore, the support resources used by the dependent adult are assessed in terms of both helpful and detrimental effects. In addition, support resources that are not currently being used are identified as potential sources of help.

When the support resources currently being used are the caregivers who perpetrate the abuse, the nurse must assess the potential for working with the caregivers to alleviate the negative consequences. Although it is not always easy to work with abusive caregivers, it may be even more difficult to eliminate their influence over the older adult. During the assessment, therefore, the nurse must attempt to identify any strengths of the caregiver and any willingness to change the situation voluntarily. If the caregiver has good intentions but lacks the knowledge to provide adequate care, then educational interventions and role modeling may be effective. If the caregiver is extremely stressed, then respite, along with individual or group support and counseling, may be effective interventions. In mutually abusive situations in which the designated caregiver also could be defined as abused or neglected, the nurse should attempt to identify any outside sources of support that have not been tapped. For example, in a mutually abusive situation involving a socially isolated married couple, the nurse might identify a relative or friend who is willing to assist with caregiving or decision-making responsibilities.

In situations of neglect, there usually are very few support services to assess, and the task of the nurse is to identify potential sources of help. In assessing potential support resources, the nurse also must identify the barriers that interfere with the use of these resources. The assessment of barriers to the use of resources is discussed in Chapter 5 and is summarized in Display 5-8. It is especially important to identify these barriers, because simple interventions, such as provision of information or assistance with transportation, may be effective in eliminating them. Cultural influences also must be assessed in relation to the use of support resources, as discussed in Chapter 5.

Environmental Influences

As with other aspects of elder abuse, the primary purposes of assessing the environment are to identify the factors that create risks and to determine which of these factors can be alleviated through interventions. With regard to the immediate living conditions, the nurse must assess whether minimal standards of safety and cleanliness are being maintained. When nurses assess home environments that are terribly cluttered, they must make some determination of both the meaning and the consequences of the clutter. A massive collection of clutter, like poor personal hygiene, reflects an underlying disorder and may or may not be a risk factor that needs to be addressed. Consequences of clutter range from socially unacceptable appearances to serious risks to health and safety. Therefore, the nurse must assess the person's ability to maneuver in the environment during daily activities, as well as the person's safety in emergency situations, such as a fire. When nurses and other workers are initially exposed to massive amounts of clutter, their first impulse may be to think of a way to eliminate some of the clutter. If this reaction is communicated to the resident of the cluttered home, however, it may become impossible to establish an accepting relationship, and the older adult may reject any further interventions. In assessing the home environment, therefore, nurses must be nonjudgmental, except in circumstances in which the risks are so great that immediate action must be taken.

The nurse also should assess the neighborhood environment for its impact on the safety of the person. This is especially important when the older person lives in an area of high crime or extreme isolation and is vulnerable by virtue of impaired judgment, physical frailty, or a combination of physical and psychosocial impairments. People who are only moderately forgetful may be safe in an apartment or a suburban neighborhood where neighbors watch out for them. In a high-crime neighborhood, however, forgetting to lock the doors or to take other precautions may place the person at increased risk for physical harm, financial exploitation, or other serious abuses. Likewise, in a rural environment, social isolation may increase the risks for vulnerable elderly people.

Finally, seasonal conditions can be a determinant of risk for elder abuse for those who live in climates characterized by extreme heat or cold. For example, a person who does not pay utility bills may not be in any danger as long as the weather is mild, but when the temperature turns cold, that person would be at risk for hypothermia. The same is true for people who occasionally wander outside without dressing appropriately. As long as the neighborhood is safe and the weather mild, they may be relatively safe; however, they may be at increased risk during the cold months, especially if they do not wear proper foot covering. If the person has any of the risk factors for hypothermia or heat-related illness discussed in Chapter 15, these additional risk factors also must be considered.

Threats to Life

The most immediate consideration in determining whether legal interventions are necessary is the assessment of threats to life. In home settings, it is often the nurse who assesses the urgency of the situation and whose opinion is used as the basis of legal interventions. Situations often are viewed as being of crisis proportions when they are first discovered, and the immediate reaction of the person who discovers the situation may be to remove a person from the environment. Many times, however, the person may not want to leave the home setting, or there may be no better setting in which the person can receive care immediately. In these situations, the nurse may be asked to assess the urgency and seriousness of the situation and to provide an opinion about whether or not legal interventions are justified. The nurse often is viewed as the person who can either convince the elder to accept help or convince the caregivers and social workers that the present situation is tolerable. At times, nurses are successful at convincing the person to accept help, especially if they assure the person that, with proper help, the situation can be improved.

In situations in which the caregiver is the abuser, the nurse and other team members must assess whether the caregiver presents a threat to the life of the dependent older person. If there is any evidence or history of physical violence on the part of the caregiver, and if the dependent elder does not have the ability to escape or otherwise defend himself or herself, a threat to life may exist. Threats to life also may exist if any of the following circumstances are present: (1) untreated wounds or infections; (2) inability to administer insulin correctly; (3) progressive gangrene or ulcerated conditions; (4) inability to adhere to therapeutic regimens; (5) consistent wandering in unsafe neighborhoods or in very cold weather; (6) misuse (usually unintentional) of certain medications, such as digitalis or insulin; or (7) excessive use of drugs or alcohol, either self-directed or caregiver-induced. In any of these circumstances, the nurse may be the health professional whose opinion is essential in determining the consequences of action or inaction.

When the nurse does not have firsthand knowledge of the abused or neglected older person before being notified of a "crisis" situation, the first question that should be asked, at least in the nurse's mind, is: Is this truly a crisis, or is this merely a crisis in the eyes of the person who just discovered the situation? Some of the situations that appear to be most appalling actually represent a gradual deterioration over several months or years. Therefore, the immediate assessment is aimed at determining whether there are currently any threats to the life of the abused elder, such as malnutrition, dehydration, or an untreated medical condition. Last, suicide potential must be assessed, especially in self-neglected elders who also are depressed and expressing feelings of hopelessness. All of the principles of suicide assessment, discussed in Chapter 20, can be applied to the abused and neglected elder.

Cultural Aspects

Many cultural factors can influence the perception of some aspects of elder abuse and neglect; that is, what may be defined as abusive in one culture may be acceptable in other cultures. For example, Asian Indians may consider not visiting an older family member to be a form of psychological neglect, but Anglo-Americans may consider this a way of respecting privacy and autonomy. Cultural factors also have a strong influence on caregiver roles and responsibilities. Most families have culturally influenced expectations about which family members

should provide care to dependent elders and about whether it is acceptable to enlist the aid of paid caregivers. In some families, there may be conflicts about these expectations, particularly between older and younger generations. Sometimes, these conflicts need to be identified and addressed before elder abuse or neglect can be resolved (refer to the case example at the end of this chapter).

Nurses must identify cultural factors that influence the care that is provided—or not provided—to older adults. The accompanying Culture Box lists some of the assessment questions that should be considered in identifying cultural influences. In addition to these questions, cultural assessment information on the following topics also should be considered: communication and psychosocial assessment (see Chapter 5), nutrition (see Chapter 8), sources of health

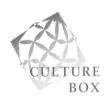

CULTURE BOX

Cultural Considerations in Assessing Elder Abuse and Neglect

- What are the family and cultural expectations concerning family caregivers? (For example, is it acceptable to employ paid caregivers, or are family members expected to provide all the care?)
- Do family members differ in their perceptions about caregiving responsibilities?
- What are the family and cultural perspectives on autonomy and independence?
- Do family members differ in their perspectives on autonomy and independence?
- How are decisions made about care of the older adult? (For example, is it a patriarchal or matriarchal family?)
- Who are the acceptable sources of social support and personal assistance?
- Who are the acceptable sources of health care (e.g., herbalists, spiritual healers, Native American practitioners)?
- What are the acceptable health care practices (e.g., herbs, homeopathy, acupuncture, faith healing, folk remedies)?
- Are there language barriers that influence the care that is provided or that limit the number of care providers?
- How does skin color affect assessment of bruises, pressure sores, and other skin changes?

care and modes of treatment (see Chapter 18), dementia (see Chapter 19), and depression (see Chapter 20). A recent article describes the use of a "Culturagram" as a screening tool to promote culturally sensitive assessment and detection of family abuse among immigrant elders (Brownell, 1997).

Nursing Diagnosis

A nursing diagnosis that would apply to many elder abuse situations is Ineffective Family Coping: Disabling. This is defined as "the state in which a family demonstrates, or is at high risk to demonstrate, destructive behavior in response to an inability to manage internal or external stressors due to inadequate resources (physical, psychological, cognitive)" (Carpenito, 1997, p. 281). Related factors include changes in family roles, unrealistic expectations about caregiving, and changes in the health status of the older adult. If the nursing assessment identifies several stressors primarily related to caregiving, the nursing diagnosis of Caregiver Role Strain might be used. This is defined as "a state in which an individual is experiencing physical, emotional, social, and/or financial burden(s) in the process of caregiving to another" (Carpenito, 1997, p. 169). Related factors involving the caregiver include ineffective coping patterns, functional or cognitive impairments, and insufficient resources (e.g., respite, financial assets, assistance with care). Related factors involving the dependent older adult include increased dependence and the presence of difficult or unsafe behaviors (e.g., paranoia, wandering, incontinence).

The nursing diagnosis of High Risk for Injury might be used for older adults who are in self-neglecting situations. The nursing diagnosis of Decisional Conflict might apply to abused or neglected older adults who live in an environment that places them at risk for harm because they are unable to make decisions about alternative environments. Related factors include fear, lack of information about alternatives, and impaired decision-making ability.

Nursing Goals

Care for older adults with the nursing diagnosis of Ineffective Family Coping is directed toward identifying and addressing the contributing factors. Goals are established according to the contributing factors. For example, if a change in the health status of the dependent older adult is a contributing factor, the nursing goal would be to assist the older adult to function at their highest possible level. Another goal would be to identify resources for assisting with the care of the dependent person. If family caregivers are experiencing multiple stressors, a goal would be to alleviate some of the caregiving burden. This would be accomplished by identifying appropriate resources and facilitating referrals for care. A related goal in many situations would be to address any barriers to accepting services. This might be accomplished through counseling and case management services provided by a nurse or social worker specializing in this kind of service.

A goal for older adults with a nursing diagnosis of Decisional Conflict would be to facilitate a decision-making process that includes the older adult as much as possible and addresses the best interest of the impaired older adult. At some point, the decision-making process may include legal issues, and at all points, the process includes ethical issues. The role of the nurse in assisting with decisions about the care of impaired older adults is discussed later in this chapter and in Chapters 19 and 22.

If abused or neglected elders or their caregivers resist voluntary interventions and are at risk of harm, then the nursing goal is to protect the older adult from harm. This is accomplished through legal interventions, such as reporting the situation to the appropriate public agency. At times, the primary goal is the protection of the rights of the person, and the role of the nurse may be that of an advocate.

Nursing Interventions

Elder abuse is a compilation of several or many nursing and social problems involving the older person, the caregivers, and the environment. Nurses identify the various underlying problems, then plan and implement appropriate interventions for each problem. Therefore, nursing interventions for elder abuse are the same interventions that are applied to whatever underlying problems have been identified. What is unique about elder abuse, however, is the inherent complexity and difficulty of most situations. From a medical perspective, abused elders would be described as the intensive care patients of the community. Like intensive care patients in hospitals, abused elders demand the highest level of skill from a variety of professionals. In cases of elder abuse, however, the team members are not specialized medical professionals, but rather are community-based workers and people who provide informal support.

A second unique aspect of interventions for elder abuse is the fact that many abused elders have some impairment in their ability to make decisions. In some cases of abuse, the decision-making abilities of the caregivers also may be impaired, as the caregiver may not be a competent decision maker or may not be acting in the best interest of the dependent elder. Most cases of elder abuse present a decision-making challenge to both professional and family caregivers. Nurses and other health care professionals generally are not prepared to deal with the underlying legal and ethical issues, or to assume the role of advocate for older adults. Even when they are prepared, most are quite uncomfortable either

making or participating in decisions for other adults.

Interventions for elder abuse are implemented in community settings, over a long period of time, by a team of formal and informal care providers. Nurses working in home and community settings have the most direct opportunities for both the prevention of and interventions for elder abuse. Nurses in institutional settings, however, have many opportunities for detecting elder abuse, working with caregivers, and facilitating referrals to appropriate community agencies. Because the role of the nurse in institutional settings is quite different from that of the nurse in community settings, each of these areas is discussed separately.

Role of the Nurse in Institutional Settings

Nurses in acute and long-term care settings can intervene in cases of elder abuse through their work with caregivers and their participation in discharge planning. When elder abuse is rooted in the caregiver's lack of information about adequate caregiving measures, the nurse can teach the caregiver about the person's care before discharge. In addition, when nurses are concerned about a caregiver's abilities, they can initiate a referral to a home care agency or a public nursing agency for follow-up. In some cases, the nurse may ascertain that the situation requires skilled nursing care, covered by Medicare, for at least a few visits. If the nurse has serious questions about a discharge plan that seems inadequate, a referral to a protective service agency may be made so that the situation can be monitored on a long-term basis.

Caregivers of dependent older adults who have been placed temporarily in institutional settings often seek advice from nurses about the management of the dependent person's care. They may be ambivalent about taking the person home, or they may be unsure or unrealistic about their own ability to provide appropriate care or to cope with the stress of the situation. In some cases, the caregivers may be seeking permission not to provide care at home, and they may seek this permission in indirect ways. In these situations, nurses often are in the best position to facilitate communication among all the decision makers, including the primary care provider, the older adult, and the various family members who are responsible for care. When nurses identify caregiver concerns, they can suggest individual counseling or support groups. One of the most effective ways to prevent elder abuse is to provide support and education for the caregivers, and the best opportunities for this may arise when the dependent older adult is in a hospital or nursing home. Nurses can encourage caregivers to use the period of institutionalization to reevaluate their own abilities to provide care at home, as well as their own need to accept additional support and assistance.

Role of the Nurse in Community Settings

Although home health aides are the health care workers most likely to observe clues to elder abuse in home settings, they often are ill-prepared to detect such clues or to deal with what they observe. Nurses in home care agencies, therefore, have a tremendous responsibility to work closely with home health aides, both in recognizing and intervening in situations of elder abuse. Home care nurses must educate home health aides about the detection of elder abuse, and they should be available if home health aides have questions or concerns about what they observe. If the home situation cannot be discussed openly during supervisory visits, the nurse may have to arrange a time for private discussion with the home health aide. In situations in which the older adult requires a significant degree of physical care or supervision, the services of a home health aide may be the most effective

means of preventing elder abuse. Often, however, the retention of a home health aide in such difficult situations depends largely on the degree of support and guidance provided by a professional nurse.

Nurses in home settings have many opportunities for teaching caregivers about adequate care through verbal and written instruction. In addition to teaching caregivers directly about the provision of physical care and the management of difficult behaviors, nurses and home health aides also can serve as role models. Some caregivers may have great difficulty managing complex medication regimens; in such cases, the nurse can simplify these regimens through the use of charts and specially designed plastic containers. Nurses also can educate caregivers about basic care needs, such as nutrition, exercise, and elimination. For example, nurses may suggest innovative ways of meeting the nutritional requirements of an elderly person who does not eat adequately. Home care nurses have the advantage of observing many creative and effective techniques used by caregivers that have never been described in any nursing texts. Thus, experienced home care nurses are continually expanding their repertoire of techniques for physical care and behavioral management, and these techniques can then be passed on to other family caregivers.

When home health aides or home care nurses detect evidence of abuse, they must decide whether or not a referral to a protective service agency is warranted. Decisions about reporting actual or suspected abuse may present an ethical dilemma for the nurse, as discussed later in this chapter. If an abuse situation is rooted in caregiver stress, the caregiver may voluntarily agree to accept help if the nurse suggests counseling resources.

Nurses in other community settings, such as clinics or senior centers, also have opportunities to intervene in elder abuse. In these settings, nurses often come in contact with spouses who have assumed a caregiving role and who need advice about resources to assist with the care of the dependent spouse. Nurses also will encounter older people who neglect themselves and need support services at home. Older adults and their caregivers may not be aware of the many community-based services that are available, and the nurse may be the only person with whom they have any contact. Community-based resources, such as group meal programs, home-delivered meals, or adult day care centers, may be an effective way of preventing or alleviating some situations of elder abuse or neglect. Nurses can facilitate referrals for whatever services are appropriate. If nurses are not familiar with specific community services, they can educate the older adult or caregiver about the general kinds of services available and the advantages of these services. Every geographic area of the United States has an area agency on aging, and nurses can suggest that older adults and caregivers use this agency as a source of information about specific programs. Information about local agencies on aging is available by calling the Eldercare Locator at (800) 677–1116.

Role of the Nurse in Multidisciplinary Teams

Because elder abuse situations usually are very complex, nursing interventions are implemented in conjunction with other interventions, using a multidisciplinary team approach. When nurses assume the role of case manager, they may have to be quite creative in finding other team members with whom to work. In community settings, the nurse is usually the health care person who can identify the need for health services and facilitate appropriate referrals. In working with homebound people, nurses may need to identify essential resources for an initial medical evaluation or for ongoing monitoring. In many areas of the country, primary care providers are resuming the old-time practice of making home visits. Nurses can determine if such a home visit

is warranted and then find an appropriate primary care provider to provide this home service. In addition, with the growing demand for home health services, there is increased availability of diagnostic tests that can be performed in the home, (e.g., radiographs, blood tests, and electrocardiograms). In many situations, these diagnostic tests are essential for determining whether involuntary care measures are justified. For instance, if the older adult refuses to go out of the home for care, home-based diagnostic measures may provide the evidence needed to convince the person or the primary care provider that hospitalization is warranted. On the other hand, results of these diagnostic tests also may be used to convince caregivers, protective services workers, and involved professionals that hospitalization is unnecessary.

Nurses can also facilitate referrals for services that will decrease the burden of caregiving responsibilities and improve the older adult's self-esteem and level of independence. For instance, speech, physical, and occupational therapy may be useful in improving the older person's ability to communicate, ambulate, and perform ADL. Referrals for skilled nursing and other skilled care services usually are made at the time of discharge from an institution, but if the person has not received institutional care, these services may not have been suggested. The nurse making a home visit may be the first health professional to suggest these resources. Sometimes, referrals may be suggested as part of a discharge plan following a stay at a health care facility, but either the older adult or the family may be reluctant to pursue those services at that time. Although an older adult or his or her family may have refused such services at one time, at another time he or she may be more receptive to accepting help. If there has been a recent change in the person's condition, the nurse may be able to obtain an order from the primary care provider to allow these services to be covered under Medicare or managed care. Nurses in home care agencies who provide skilled care usually are very happy to discuss health care services with anyone who calls for information, and they can advise the person about the possibility of having the services covered by health insurance. For example, a recent change in medications might qualify the person for skilled nursing care, and a recent fall might qualify the person for skilled physical therapy.

Nurses also can suggest medical equipment and assistive devices that would improve the person's function and relieve some of the caregiver's responsibilities. Some durable medical equipment is covered by health insurance, and medical supply companies usually are quite helpful in advising people about specific equipment. Caregivers may be unaware of disposable supplies and the many assistive devices that are available, and they may be quite responsive to suggestions from the nurse about obtaining and using these items. Any interventions that improve unsafe situations may prevent or alleviate elder abuse or neglect.

Finally, any services aimed at reducing caregiver stress or dealing with caregiver problems also may prevent or alleviate elder abuse. For example, participation in Alcoholics Anonymous may be an effective intervention in situations in which the abuse is related to the caregiver's alcoholism. Mental health counseling or support groups may be quite helpful when abuse is related to caregiver stress. Respite services can be provided through in-home care, by companions or home health aides, or through the participation of the dependent older person in an adult day care program. Sometimes, even a limited amount of respite will be sufficient to prevent or alleviate elder abuse in situations in which the caregiver is stressed and overburdened.

Range of Interventions

The range of interventions that may be needed by abused elders and their caregivers or abusers is great. These interventions can be categorized according to basic function: (1) core, or essential, integrative services; (2) emergency services, which are appropriate during crises or just before or after abuse or neglect occurs; (3) support services, or services used for managing the problem and improving the situation; (4) rehabilitative services, or services that help to diminish the likelihood of abuse or neglect by addressing the problems of either the victim or the perpetrator; and (5) preventive services, which include programs directed toward changing society in ways that diminish the likelihood of maltreatment or self-neglect.

Figure 21-1 identifies some of the specific types of services, arranged by function, that may be needed in protective situations. It should be noted that probably no community has either a full array of needed services or enough of any particular service to deal adequately with the scope of the problem locally. In recent years, however, communities throughout the country have made notable progress in understanding and addressing elder abuse and neglect. In addition, research suggests that service use may vary according to the form of abuse, and that service type may be comparable for abused elders and frail older people (Sengstock et al., 1989).

Adult Protective Services Law

Philosophically, adult protective services law provides a framework for defining the interests of society and the person. Specifically, it provides protection for the person, protection for the person offering assistance, and protection for society from possible dangers posed by the person. Each of these interests is represented in distinct legal concepts. For example, protection for the person is embodied in constitutional amendments that protect individual liberty and privacy. Protection of individual health and safety is provided for by the concept of parens patriae, which means that the state can interfere in the life of the person when interference is deemed to be in the person's best interest. Pro-

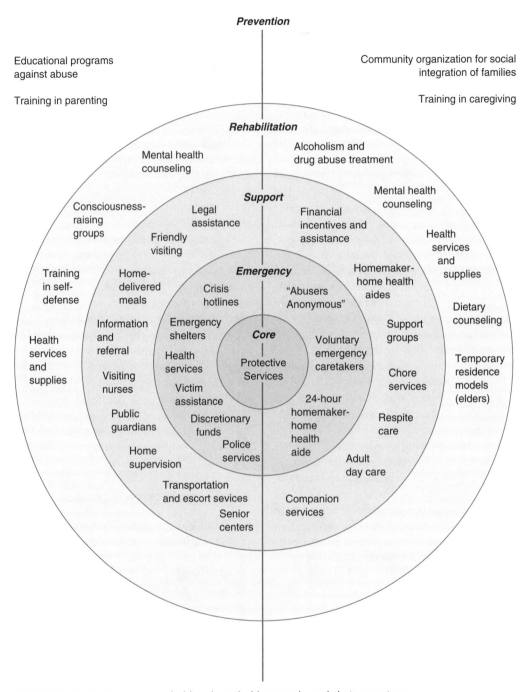

Prevention

Educational programs
against abuse

Training in parenting

Community organization for social
integration of families

Training in caregiving

Rehabilitation

Mental health
counseling

Alcoholism and
drug abuse treatment

Mental health
counseling

Support

Consciousness-
raising
groups

Legal
assistance

Friendly
visiting

Financial
incentives and
assistance

Health
services
and
supplies

Training
in self-
defense

Home-
delivered
meals

Emergency

Crisis
hotlines

"Abusers
Anonymous"

Homemaker-
home health
aides

Dietary
counseling

Health
services
and
supplies

Information
and
referral

Emergency
shelters

Core

Voluntary
emergency
caretakers

Support
groups

Health
services

Protective
Services

Chore
services

Temporary
residence
models
(elders)

Visiting
nurses

Victim
assistance

Public
guardians

Discretionary
funds

24-hour
homemaker-
home
health
aide

Respite
care

Home
supervision

Police
services

Transportation
and escort sevices

Adult
day care

Senior
centers

Companion
services

FIGURE 21-1. Services needed by abused older people and their caregivers.
Source: G. J. Anetzberger, (1982), *Report of the Elder Abuse Project: Recommenda-
tions for addressing the problem of elder abuse in Cuyahoga County,* Cleveland:
Federation for Community Planning. Used with permission.

tection for the state is covered in the police powers of the state, which authorize intervention in dangerous or unhealthy situations. Elder abuse reporting and adult protective services laws differ among the 50 states in terms of their provisions. In part, this reflects a lack of federal guidance or incentive in this area. Partly, too, it suggests the diversity of perceptions and arrangements for dealing with the complex problem of elder abuse that exists throughout the country.

Overview

Interest in state adult protective services law began in the mid-1960s and peaked during the early 1980s. Today, every state has some kind of adult protective services or elder abuse reporting law, and all but three of these were enacted or amended in the 1980s (the other three were enacted between 1973 and 1977). There are at least four reasons for this interest. First, growth in the elderly population has resulted in increased concern about all matters related to this population. As the proportion of those aged 65 years and older expanded from 8.1% of the population in 1950 to 12.5% in 1990, so did public policies related to the needs of older people. In this regard, protective services law simply represents one policy promoting the welfare of older adults. In addition, it reflects increased public awareness that older people can be disproportionately impaired and disadvantaged and, therefore disproportionately dependent on caregivers, who may or may not have the best interest of their charges at heart. Public outrage over nursing home abuse, in particular, has led to protective measures, like protective services law, encouraging safety and improved care for older people in dependent situations.

Second, as discussed earlier, adult protective services law grew out of the increased public awareness of the problem of elder abuse. With this increased awareness came the demand for state laws to address this area of family violence.

The third factor promoting interest in adult protective services law has been the belief that other laws are inadequate for protecting older people. Guardianship law often is regarded as restrictive and antiquated. Because the intent of the criminal code is to punish offenders rather than to assist victims, it fails to correct the conditions leading to or resulting from elder abuse. In addition, the criminal code typically does not address neglect and the many forms of exploitation experienced by older people. Finally, under many domestic violence laws, for example, the battered parent must charge a relative or other perpetrator with abusive behavior and seek relief from the situation in that manner. Usually, an older person is unwilling to do this for family or other reasons, and so remains at risk. None of these "protective" laws, therefore, adequately meet the safety needs of older people.

The last reason for interest in adult protective services law concerns the passage of protective laws for other populations subject to maltreatment. Very simply, protective services laws for older adults have been enacted on the coattails of similar laws for abused children and spouses. In fact, child abuse laws have served as models for legislation addressing the rights and needs of abused older adults (Wolf, 1988). In part, this is justified. If adults are impaired, then they are often in dependent situations, much as are small children. Even the most severely impaired adults, however, are not just children grown old or dependent. They are categorically different under the law by virtue of the rights and responsibilities inherent in adult status. Therefore, statutes that do not recognize this fact—and some adult protective services laws do not—reflect a bias against older people and a stereotyping of people who are disabled.

Purpose and Structure

Overall, laws protecting maltreated and self-neglected older people usually have four intents: (1) to promote the identification and referral of abuse or neglect; (2) to convey public and centralized authority for addressing protective matters; (3) to establish a system of protective services to prevent, correct, or discontinue abuse or neglect that is discovered; and (4) to permit, under certain circumstances, involuntary access for the purpose of investigation and service delivery. The structure under which these intents are fulfilled usually includes the receipt of reports by local departments of welfare or social services, although in some states, reports are received by departments of aging or prosecutors' offices.

Reports generally are accepted for neglect, exploitation, and physical, sexual, and psychological abuse; in several states, they also are accepted for abandonment and cruel punishment. In most states, reporting is mandatory for health, social service, and safety professionals and paraprofessionals. People in these categories can be penalized for failure to report, with the typical penalty being a charge of a misdemeanor, with or without specific financial penalty. In some states, however, imprisonment, civil liability for damages, or notification of the state licensing board may be the consequence of failure to report. Most state laws also protect the confidentiality of reports and the identity of all people involved in making the report.

Response to the report on the part of the public authority responsible for implementation usually is prompt; sometimes, the law mandates a response within 24 to 72 hours of receipt of a report. In this context, response means investigation of the situation, which generally includes a home visit with the alleged victim and consultation with people knowledgeable about the situation. Service intervention for endangered older people often can include health care, support services, protective placement, emergency services, or financial management. Under most state laws, intervention must be accepted voluntarily by mentally capable older adults. Less than 10% of adult protective services clients receive interventions without their consent (Duke,

1997). Likewise, most laws emphasize the principles of self-determination, use of the least restrictive interventions, and due process in their implementation.

The intent of adult protective services law is to protect the vulnerable aged. The fact that this intent has not always or everywhere been realized is a result of factors that limit the effective and appropriate implementation of these laws, such as the following:

1. Only a handful of states have enacted elder abuse reporting or adult protective services law with any accompanying appropriations. Therefore, most public authorities have had to implement the laws using already-diminished state and federal dollars.
2. Alleged perpetrators and people failing to report elder abuse or neglect rarely are prosecuted and, given the vague wording of many statutes, may not be prosecutable (Tatara, 1995).
3. The public authority is seldom accountable to anyone, including the court, with the result that it can and sometimes does assume unreasonable control over elderly clients.

Responsibilities of Nurses

Notwithstanding its limitations, adult protective services law reduces the endangerment of, and secures the help required by, thousands of abused and neglected older adults every year (Lachs et al., 1996). Although the primary role in law implementation is assumed by the protective service worker, an essential secondary role is offered by nurses. There are five dimensions to this role: reporting, assessment, consultation, court testimony, and acute and ongoing care. Only the first dimension, however, tends to be explicit in law.

Reporting

Nurses usually are identified in adult abuse and protective services laws as mandatory reporters (Stiegel, 1995; Tatara, 1995). This is because the various duties ordinarily assumed by nurses place them in a critical position for witnessing the consequences of abuse and neglect (Reynolds and Stanton, 1983; VanderMeer, 1992). Also, nurses are in a critical position to foster collaboration between health care professionals as abuse reporters and adult protective service or law enforcement officials as abuse investigators or interventionists (Capezuti et al., 1997). Mandatory reporting laws do not require reporters to *know* whether abuse or neglect has occurred, but merely to report it if they *suspect* its occurrence. The responsibility for problem verification rests with the public agency charged with law implementation, not with the reporter or referral source. Suspecting elder abuse means detecting signs of violence, such as bruises, welts, or fractures. It also means recognizing conditions resulting from the deprivation of proper shelter, food, or medical care, such as frostbite, malnutrition, oversedation, or mental changes.

Most mandatory reporting laws provide immunity for people reporting elder abuse or neglect. On this basis, nurses can report suspected cases of maltreatment or self-neglect without fear of civil or criminal liability, so long as the report is made in good faith and without malicious purpose. A few laws further offer immunity in the workplace. Accordingly, nurses cannot be fired, transferred, or demoted for making a report. The last provision of mandatory reporting that bears consideration concerns the locus of responsibility for making the report, which in all state laws rests with the individual nurse. Even if the nurse is part of a large agency or hospital, he or she cannot delegate that responsibility to someone else, be it a supervisor or an attending physician. The nurse alone has the responsibility for reporting, and for the consequences—both legal and moral—of failing to do so.

This does not mean that it may not be advantageous to establish a protocol concerning such reporting. Many agencies and hospitals have done this. Protocols and detection teams do not erode individual responsibility in this matter, however. They simply clarify roles and enhance the credibility of the report. Excellent examples of elder abuse detection protocols are available, and they should be considered for use by nurses in all health care settings involving multiple professions and levels of authority (e.g., Fulmer and O'Malley, 1987; Chelucci and Coyle, 1990; Fulmer and Anetzberger, 1995; Quinn and Tomita, 1997). A typical protocol for hospital- or agency-based nurses appears in Display 21-1.

Assessment

Protective service workers often call upon nurses to assess older people suffering from abuse or neglect. Sometimes, this request comes during an emergency, when it is believed that the client's life is endangered. More commonly, however, nurses are asked to make routine assessments of new protective clients, or of existing clients who are exhibiting changes in health status. Indeed, nurses often are the preferred health care worker for conducting such assessments owing to their holistic approach to health assessment, their availability through public health departments or visiting nurse associations, their willingness to make home visits, and the relative ease with which older people usually accept.

Because assessment was discussed earlier in this chapter, only one aspect requires further examination here. Assessment is best accomplished through the use of an established assessment instrument, which can summarize observations, facilitate the collection of vital information in a single document, prevent forgetting of multiple indicators, provide a basis for referral or action, standardize the detection and evaluation process, and offer documentation for possible court action (Lachs and Fulmer, 1993; Hwalek et al., 1996). Excellent examples of elder abuse assessment instruments based on a nursing perspective include those by Ferguson and Beck (1983), Hwalek (1985), Fulmer and

---

DISPLAY 21-1
Sample Protocol for Nurses with Regard to Elder Abuse

Performing an Initial Assessment

- Gather data on the client's clinical presentation; observe the client and interview the client, caregivers, or both.
- Analyze data that raise a suspicion of abuse, neglect, or exploitation; consider objective findings and whether these fit the explanations; consider client-caregiver interactions.

If There Is Reason for Suspicion, Use an Assessment Guide

If There Is Continued Suspicion, Consult the Abuse Detection Team

- Report pertinent findings to the primary nurse.
- Summarize findings from the assessment guide on progress notes.
- Discuss the information with the assigned primary care provider and social worker as soon as possible.

- Determine the need to report abuse or neglect to authorities charged with investigation under law.
- Document additional facts, and whether a report was made, in the progress notes.

Meeting with the Client and Caregivers to Inform Them of the Intent to Report

- Include representatives from at least two health care, social service, or other professional disciplines in the meeting.
- Document the interaction and the results of the meeting in the progress notes.

Follow-up Actions

- Provide a report to the appropriate abuse detection team member for handling and distribution.
- Identify any security measures that must be taken to protect the client.
- Implement appropriate interventions.

Source: Cleveland Metropolitan General/Highland View Hospital, (1987), Statement of policy and procedure: Abuse/neglect cases, reporting of suspected elder abuse (unpublished manuscript).

Wetle (1986), Hamilton (1989), and Fulmer and Gould (1996). Whatever instrument is adopted for this purpose, however, it should be able to assess and document the following:

1. Background data (e.g., client's name and address),
2. Signs of maltreatment or self-neglect according to type (e.g., bruises or welts in cases of suspected physical abuse),
3. Severity of signs (e.g., an immediate life threat),
4. Indicators of maltreatment intentionality (e.g., a caregiver who will not allow the nurse to be alone with the client),
5. Symptoms of acute or chronic illness or impairment (e.g., incontinence),
6. Functional incapacity (e.g., an inability to dress or toilet without assistance),

7. Aggravating social conditions (e.g., a client who lives alone and is socially isolated),
8. Source of information (e.g., agency referral), and
9. Recommended action (e.g., referral of the case to home health care service providers).

Consultation

Nurses serve as important resources for protective services workers when questions arise regarding the health status of clients. In such situations, telephone contact between the nurse and protective services worker usually provides the necessary information. Typical questions relate to medications, continence, nutrition and hydration, and disease signs. Consultation ordinarily is an informal arrangement, based on established networks among service providers in a given community. Sometimes, however, consultation is formally organized through clinical consultation teams belonging to protective services coalitions. Such a team exists in Cleveland, Ohio under the auspices of the Western Reserve Consortium for the Prevention and Treatment of Elder Abuse. There, upon request by a consortium member, the team reviews individual cases and offers the referring agencies or people guidance as to how abuse dynamics might be addressed. Because the team includes representatives from the disciplines of law, nursing, medicine, psychiatry, and social work, a variety of perspectives is offered. In addition, because consultation is voluntarily sought, recipients show little defensiveness.

The final kind of consultation in adult protective services relates to training and education. Nurses are used by protective services agencies to train workers in health assessment, disease identification and detection, recognition of endangerment, and other topics. Training usually is accomplished through in-service programs, although it is occasionally presented within the context of workshops or conferences.

Court Testimony

Nationally, very few cases involve involuntary intervention through adult protective services law. In those that do, court assistance usually is sought to gain access, either to conduct the investigation or to deliver services. When legal intervention is indicated, the older person generally is mentally impaired and unable to make decisions that would alleviate or eliminate the endangerment. Sometimes, a caregiver or other person may refuse to allow intervention on behalf of the abused or neglected elder. Other times, legal intervention is required on the basis of life-threatening circumstances. Cases requiring legal intervention involve the presentation of evidence to a judge or referee to document that the older person is abused or neglected, that he or she requires protective services, and that no other means of receiving protective services exist, except through court action. Much of this evidence is provided through the records kept by protective services workers. Additional evidence is secured through mental or physical health evaluation by psychologists or physicians. Occasionally, however, the nurse who assessed the situation or offered care might be called to offer testimony and submit records.

Testimony provides two types of evidence: direct observation and opinion. Direct observation is an eyewitness account of the health status or function of the older person. Opinion represents conclusions drawn from specific observations or from general training and experience. To be effective, opinion must never be overstated or relate to areas outside the nurse's scope of practice or expertise. Medical records are useful as evidence because they are maintained in the regular course of client care by people who understand the facts being documented. Their usefulness is further enhanced if they are timely, legible, thorough, and objective (Kapp and Bigot, 1985). In addition, corrections to the medical records must be obvious and clear, removing any doubt about the destruction of relevant evidence.

Acute and Ongoing Care

As discussed in the nursing interventions section of this chapter, nurses provide essential care and treatment for abused and neglected older people. They help correct the conditions caused by maltreatment and self-neglect, and they prevent their recurrence through such activities as treating injuries, monitoring medication, educating caregivers, obtaining assistive devices, and facilitating service referrals. In this role, as in others, nurses work cooperatively with other professionals and with paraprofessionals, applying their training and experience in an attempt to help the victims of elder abuse.

Ethical Issues

Ethical issues in adult protective services are similar to ethical issues in medicine and other fields. There are no answers, so to speak, no absolutes, and no rights and wrongs. Rather, there are only differing perspectives and different implications, depending on what course of action is taken. It is probably more important to remember this in the realm of adult protective services than in other fields. Law, community pressures, and personal concepts of professionalism sometimes lead to the erroneous assumption that a problem, such as maltreatment or self-neglect, can easily or simply be resolved. Unfortunately, protective situations involving older people are rarely easily resolved.

Abused or neglected children can be removed from their parents' home and placed elsewhere when warranted. This is not so with most older people, whose rights as adults protect them from intrusion unless they have been judged to be incompetent or incapacitated by a court of law. One aspect of the dilemma surrounding ethical issues in adult protective services is the societal fact that adults do have rights. These rights include freedom from intrusion, the right to fair treatment, freedom from unnecessary restraint, and the right to self-determination. Another aspect of the dilemma involves the characteristics of protective situations that sometimes make respecting personal rights so difficult. Some such characteristics are listed as follows:

1. In situations that are urgent or dangerous, it is hard to walk away, even when the older person says, "leave me alone."
2. Public pressure to "do something, no matter what" places pressure on care providers who are trying to resolve the situation while respecting the rights of the older person.
3. Contradictory societal values may pit individual rights against other values, such as paternalism and protectionism.
4. The goals of nurses are directed toward helping others. This fact presents difficulties for nurses when others do not accept their help, especially when the lack of help has detrimental consequences.
5. Serious decisions often have to be made with-

out an adequate base of information. Older adults may be too impaired to provide accurate information, the situation may not allow time for a good assessment, or pertinent information may be withheld by the older person or the caregivers.
6. The questionable mental status of many abused or neglected elders places decision-making responsibility in the hands of other people. One option in these situations is to seek guardianship or another form of surrogate care. Although this option may deprive the person of certain rights unnecessarily, other options might mean that basic human needs are not being met adequately, or at all.
7. The intrusive nature of legal interventions, including protective services law, robs older adults of fundamental rights. Mandatory reporting provisions, for example, by their very nature, invade privacy. Likewise, the sharing of information among agencies involved in case planning infringes on confidentiality.

Ethical dilemmas about particular situations sometimes can be resolved by applying practice guidelines (Anetzberger et al., 1997) or a hierarchy of values or principles. Display 21-2 presents the principles of adult protective services, developed from long-term experience with abused elders. These principles are arranged from the most to the least important considerations with regard to interventions for abused or neglected elders.

The bottom line is that adult protective services are steeped in ethical dilemmas. Some of these dilemmas are related to the five basic roles played by nurses, social workers, and others: reporter, investigator, service provider, administrator, and planner. Although the professional backgrounds of the people assuming these roles vary considerably, ordinarily, the "helping professions" are represented, especially nursing and social work. Each role that is assumed has a particular sphere of responsibility in addressing

DISPLAY 21-2
Principles of Adult Protective Services

I. Freedom over Safety. The client has a right to choose to live at risk of harm, providing she or he is capable of making that choice, harms no one, and commits no crime.

II. Self-Determination. The client has a right to personal choices and decisions until such time that she or he delegates, or the court grants, the responsibility to someone else.

III. Participation in Decision Making. The client has a right to receive information to make informed decisions and to participate in all decision making affecting her or his circumstances to the extent that she or he is able.

IV. Least Restrictive Alternative. The client has a right to service alternatives that maximize choice and minimize lifestyle disruption.

V. Primacy of the Adult. The worker has a responsibility to serve the client, not the community people concerned about appearances, the landlord concerned about crime, or the family concerned about finances.

VI. Confidentiality. The client has a right to privacy and secrecy.

VII. Benefit of Doubt. If there is evidence that the client is making a reasoned choice, the worker has a responsibility to see that the benefit of doubt is in her or his favor.

VIII. Do No Harm. The worker has a responsibility to take no action that places the client at greater risk of harm.

IX. Avoidance of Blame. The worker has a responsibility to understand the origins of any maltreatment and to commit no action that would antagonize the perpetrator and so reduce the chances of terminating the maltreatment.

X. Maintenance of the Family. The worker has a responsibility to deal with the maltreatment as a family problem, if the perpetrator is a family member, and to try to find the necessary family services to resolve the problem.

Source: G. J. Anetzberger, (1988, May), *Ethical issues,* paper presented at the National Conference on Elder Abuse: Linking Systems and Community Services, Milwaukee, WI. Used with permission.

elder abuse and neglect. The reporter detects the situation and describes it to someone authorized by law to deal with it. The investigator is the legal agent for assessing the situation and determining the need for protective services. The service provider offers interventions for correcting or discontinuing maltreatment or self-neglect. The administrator manages a protective services program. Finally, the planner develops policies and programs, as well as community education initiatives, aimed at preventing or treating the problem.

In each of these roles, professional workers face different ethical dilemmas. Issues of the reporter role include questions about whether to make a report and the consequences of the report. The role of the investigator involves confronting questions about privacy, openness, and confidentiality. The service provider deals with issues about the rights of the elder, the rights of the caregivers, and the degree of risk. Program planners and administrators face dilemmas about service priorities and the lack of funds, staff, and other critical resources. Nurses most often deal with ethical issues in their roles as reporters, investigators, and service providers.

TABLE 21-2
Ethical Questions and Suggested Solutions Regarding Abused Elders

Ethical Question/Implications	Suggested Solution
When do I report elder abuse? (If I report too soon, I may needlessly invade someone's privacy. If I wait, the situation may worsen.)	Report elder abuse when you believe that, without intervention, the situation will deteriorate or endanger the elder.
What if my report places the elder in more danger, or labels someone inaccurately? What if it causes the elder to shy away from me and my agency?	Report elder abuse if you believe that the protective services system can reduce the risk better than the current interventions.
How do I decide if the elder or the caregiver receives priority? (If my priority is the elder, I may alienate his or her family members, who serve as the primary sources of care. If my priority is the family, then the care plan may be contrary to the elder's wishes and may not adequately respect his or her rights.)	With certain exceptions, the elder should receive priority. These exceptions are limited to circumstances in which the elder has been judged to be incompetent by a court of law or is endangering others by his or her behavior.
Is it more important to maintain standards of confidentiality than to comply with a reporting law?	State law takes precedence over professional standards.
Does the right of an elder to refuse services extend to total self-neglect and intentional suicide? How can I know that endangered elders clearly understand the consequences of their self-neglect? How can I accept abandoning the situation?	Ethical dilemmas such as these often can be resolved through the use of a hierarchy of values or principles, such as those summarized in Display 21-2.
Can emergency services be thrust upon an elder who would have refused them under ordinary circumstances? If the elder's life is endangered, then is it not my primary responsibility to use my nursing skills in life-saving ways, no matter what the elder chooses? Even if the elder might have refused services in the past, does that mean he or she absolutely would refuse them now?	If the elder is incapable of deciding whether to accept or reject emergency services, then these services should be provided, subject to the constraints of the protective services law. This offers the elder essential protection, but recognizes his or her right to refuse ongoing services when the emergency has subsided and he or she is capable of making decisions on his or her own behalf.

Table 21-2 identifies some of the ethical problems, as well as related solutions, that nurses may encounter in their roles in adult protective services.

Additional Legal Interventions

Adult protective services law cannot address every situation of endangerment or elder abuse. In particular, it has limited application when considerable property needs protection, the maltreatment is significant and repeated, the older person's mental impairment is substantial and permanent, or there is a desire to prevent maltreatment rather than to treat the problem. Under these conditions, other legal interventions should be considered in conjunction with, or as alternatives to, adult protective services.

Determining the Need for Legal Intervention

Older people who are mentally impaired may require legal intervention. This is especially true when the impairment substantially reduces insight, judgment, memory, or cognition. All of these abilities are essential to life in a complex and ordered society. Without these abilities, the following functional consequences may occur: bills may go unpaid, personal hygiene may be ignored, prescribed medication may be forgotten, the home environment may deteriorate, and unscrupulous people may abscond with property. Although nurses are not the primary people responsible for determining the appropriateness of legal interventions, they often are called upon to assist in assessing the person's abilities. This is appropriate, because nurses often are in the best position to assess the person's abilities to meet basic human needs.

A complete assessment and home evaluation usually requires the involvement of a multidisciplinary team. These teams have been established as special units in some hospitals. Other teams are components of agencies offering protective or case management services to older people and their families. In either instance, multidisciplinary teams include the perspectives of law, nursing, medicine, psychiatry, social work, and rehabilitation therapy. Additional disciplines are included if the situation requires. When legal interventions are being considered, the multidisciplinary team must conduct a complete assessment, including assessment of the person's ability to function safely in the home environment, of the involvement of the family and significant others in meeting basic needs, and of the ability of the older person to participate in developing a safe and realistic plan of action.

Another consideration is that, whenever feasible, problems should be remedied using services other than legal intervention. For example, an impairment may improve or a risk may be decreased through the use of resources, such as counseling, telephone reassurance, adult day care, home-delivered meals, caregiver support groups, or homemaker/home health aide services. Alternatively, residence in a protected setting may be necessary. Assisted living settings and board and care settings offer full accommodations, including meals, as well as a range of services, such as social interaction and transportation, while ensuring the continuance of community living and personal freedom.

Assessment is emphasized here because knowlege of the nature of the older person's impairment, functional limitations, and personal or social resources is essential. Without this knowledge, it becomes impossible to determine appropriate interventions. Generally, legal intervention is indicated when assessment reveals all of the following conditions: (1) decisions must be made about the older person's health, living arrangements, money, or property; (2) the older person is unable to make sound decisions related to these matters because of impaired mental function; (3) there is a risk to the older person's health, safety, money, or property as a result; and (4) the risk would be reduced or eliminated if someone else made decisions on behalf of the older person in these matters.

Considerations in the Choice of Legal Interventions

Three features of legal interventions should be considered in selecting those most appropriate for addressing the older person's needs: voluntary versus involuntary nature of the action; temporary versus long-term intervention; and limited versus extensive loss of personal freedom (Bookin, 1992). Some legal interventions are voluntary and, therefore, require the consent of the older person before they are implemented. Money management, power of attorney, and various types of bank accounts, such as joint or direct deposit, are of this nature. Other legal interventions, such as guardianship or civil commitment, are either voluntary or involuntary, but they tend to be used on an involuntary basis when others in the community believe that the older person's safety or property is in jeopardy. Because these legal interventions involve a much more extensive loss of personal freedom than voluntary ones, they should be employed with extreme caution.

Some legal interventions are temporary, or can be terminated whenever the older person elects. These characteristics apply to all voluntary measures, but do not apply to most involuntary ones. Some measures, like guardianship, may be easier to initiate than to discontinue. Others, like civil commitment, may be accompanied by long-term stigma, even when the intervention is terminated. Last, domestic violence law or the criminal code may be used to deal with abusers, and they should be included in the range of legal interventions available to abused older adults.

Determining Mental Incompetence or Incapacity

Although the concepts of incompetence and incapacity tend to be broadly and loosely applied by the public, they are subject to specific legal interpretation and are of particular importance to health professionals (Sabatino, 1996). These legal interventions establish criteria for determining whether or not an older person can decide the course of treatment. According to Culver (1985), competent people understand and appreciate information about their health care, the benefits and risks of treatment, and the application of information to themselves. Similarly, Haddad (1988) suggests that competent patients are those who are able to make and express choices concerning life that are rational and have reasonable outcomes. Finally, Schimer and Kahana (1992) offer five parameters to consider in determining a person's competence: (1) ability to communicate choices to others; (2) capacity to understand information about a proposed course of treatment; (3) appreciation of the situation and personal consequences of making a specific health care decision; (4) ability to manipulate information

rationally; and (5) making of a decision that will produce a reasonable outcome.

A distinction is sometimes drawn between decisional and legal incapacity or incompetence. The characteristics of decisional incapacity are that it is medically determined by a physician, allows immediacy of action, provides no privation of rights, and does not presume legal incompetence (High, 1987). By contrast, the Uniform Guardianship and Protective Proceeding Act (1993), which is the basis for most state laws, defines an "incapacitated person" as follows: "Any person who is impaired by reason of mental illness, mental deficiency, physical illness or disability, chronic use of drugs, chronic intoxication, or other cause except minority, to the extent that he [or she] lacks sufficient understanding or capacity to make or communicate reasonable decisions concerning his [or her] person." Accordingly, the characteristics of legal incapacity are that it can be determined only through court action, requires some time to adjudicate, and results in the removal of personal rights. Neither form of incapacity or incompetence is easy to determine. Both require a review of assessment findings and consideration of the older person's requirements for surrogate decision making. Various mental status assessment instruments may facilitate this process, but they do not exclude the need to consider all aspects of the older person's situation, including personal resources, before determining incapacity.

Evaluating Nursing Care

Nursing care of abused or neglected older adults is evaluated by the extent to which nursing goals are achieved. If a nursing goal is to alleviate the contributing factor of unnecessary dependence, the care is evaluated by whether the older adult is functioning at a higher level of independence. If a nursing goal is to address caregiver stress, the nursing care might be evaluated by the caregiver accepting help with the care, attending caregiver support groups, and expressing less stress about their caregiving responsibilities. In cases in which the nursing goal is to protect an incompetent older adult from harm, nursing care might be evaluated by the extent to which the least restrictive legal interventions are implemented. In such cases, nursing care is evaluated in terms of protecting the older adult from harm while also protecting his or her rights. Evaluation of elder abuse and neglect situations often involves ethical considerations.

Chapter Summary

Elder abuse and neglect is one of the most complex issues involved in the nursing care of older adults because it involves legal and ethical considerations regarding the rights of the older person. Conclusions derived from the theories that have evolved to explain elder abuse indicate that elder abuse causation is extremely complex, with many variables associated with both the victim and the perpetrator. Also, the underlying factors vary according to the different types of elder abuse. Factors that increase the risk of elder abuse include invisibility and vulnerability of the elder and psychosocial factors affecting older adults and their caregivers. Types of elder abuse include physical or psychological abuse, physical or psychological neglect, exploitation, and violation of rights.

Nursing assessment of elder abuse begins with a suspicion of abuse or neglect, and it involves the careful detection of clues. Assessment is accomplished best through the coordinated efforts of members of a multidisciplinary team. Nurses assess many aspects of physical and psychosocial function, with emphasis on safe function and identification of threats to life. Nursing diagnoses to address elder abuse and neglect include Ineffective Family Coping, Caregiver Role Strain, and High Risk for Injury. Nursing goals include the alleviation of contributing fac-

tors and the protection of incompetent older adults.

Nurses assume many roles, particularly with regard to adult protective services laws. Responsibilities of nurses include reporting, assessment, consulting, court testimony, caregiver education, and direct nursing care. Nurses need to be familiar with the range of services (see Figure 21-1) and the legal interventions that might be used for abused or neglected older adults. Ethical considerations can be addressed by applying principles of adult protective services (see Display 21-2). Table 21-2 proposes some possible solutions that nurses might use to resolve ethical questions about the care of abused or neglected older adults.

Critical Thinking Exercises

1. In each of the following categories, identify factors that are currently contributing to elder abuse and neglect in the United States:
   a. demographic statistics
   b. changes in families
   c. health care systems
   d. health status and other characteristics of older adults
   e. social awareness
2. What is different about the nursing assessment of abused or neglected elders compared to the nursing assessment of other older adults?
3. Put yourself in the place of the visiting nurse in the case example that follows regarding Mrs. B. Identify some strategies you would use to establish a relationship with her.
4. What do you believe about family caregiving responsibilities? How would you deal with families whose values about caregiving differ significantly from yours?
5. What are your beliefs about the degree of risk a frail elder should be allowed to take? Under what circumstances should an elder be denied the right to remain in his or her own home?

Case Example

Mrs. B. is an 82-year-old divorced and widowed mother of four. She lives in a senior citizens' apartment located in the downtown area of a large city. The building is regularly serviced by subsidized transportation to grocery stores and shopping malls, and has a nutrition center on the ground floor. Mrs. B.'s eldest son died in an accident 12 years ago. Her daughter lives 65 miles away, but she comes once a week to do the grocery shopping and other errands. Two sons live within 4 miles of their mother's apartment. Mrs. B. lived in the home of one son and his wife until they argued 1 year ago. The remaining son lives alone in a small apartment. He visits his mother two or three times a week and frequently takes her to lunch or dinner. Mrs. B. has been hospitalized for major depression eight times since her eldest son's death. She also has been diagnosed as having hypertension, rheumatoid arthritis, and non-insulin-dependent diabetes.

Mrs. B. was referred to a home health agency for follow-up after her last hospital stay because her medication regimen, which she had followed for 6 years, had been changed while she was in the hospital. At the time of discharge, Mrs. B. was given a 30-day supply of unit-dose medications. She was to take DiaBeta, 2.5 mg, once a day; Inderal, 40 mg, twice a day; Paxil, 20 mg, once a day; folic acid, 1 mg, once a day; and methotrexate, 2.5 mg, four tablets each Wednesday. Scheduled medication times were 8 AM and 8 PM. The home health nurse was to instruct Mrs. B. in her medication regimen, including what medications she was to take, how she was to take them, what each medication was expected to do, and possible side effects. The nurse was also to assess Mrs. B.'s ability to follow instructions and her adherence to the medication regimen.

Because Mrs. B.'s vision was impaired from diabetes, she had difficulty reading the labels on the medication boxes. The nurse used marking pens to paint each box end a different color. The nurse then made a chart for Mrs. B., with each day of the week and the time for administration marked at the top and the name of each medicine marked in bold black on the left margin, underlined with the corresponding color from the box ends. The chart was divided into boxed sections for each day, time, and medication. If a medicine was to be taken at 8 AM, the box beside the name was colored in the corresponding color in the 8 AM column. If more than one tablet was to be taken, the number of tablets per dose was printed in bold black on the top of the box. The nurse visited twice a day for 2 days to allow Mrs. B. to use the chart with supervision until Mrs. B. was comfortable with it. On the third morning, the nurse telephoned Mrs. B. at 8:15 AM and asked if Mrs. B. had any problems taking her pills. Mrs. B. happily reported that she had taken all the pills, including the four methotrexate, without any difficulty. The nurse then scheduled Mrs. B. to be seen 3 times a week for ongoing assessment.

Mrs. B.'s pharmacist was very helpful in continuing to refill her prescriptions with unit-dose tablets, using her marked boxes to avoid any errors. Mrs. B.

successfully managed her medications for 6 months. At that time, the nurse noted a change in her mannerisms, accompanied by slurred speech and an unbalanced gait. Mrs. B. had bruises on her forehead, knees, and arms, but she insisted that she had not fallen. Her blood pressure was 210/104, and her blood glucose level was 410. A pill count revealed that Mrs. B. had not taken her medications for 2 1/2 days. After a consultation with her primary care provider, Mrs. B. was admitted to the hospital. Tests revealed that she had suffered a stroke, resulting in left-sided weakness and short-term memory loss.

Mrs. B. left the hospital against medical advice and returned to her apartment, refusing visits from the home health nurse. She insisted that her children come and administer her medications and prepare her meals because she was unable to do this for herself. Mrs. B. reasoned that she had cared for her children when they were young, so they should come when she needed them. The children tried to assist Mrs. B. for 4 days, but were unable to meet her demands and those of their jobs and families. Mrs. B. agreed to a visit from the home health nurse "to make my children do right."

Mrs. B.'s children were present for the assessment. Mrs. B. was unable to stand or transfer to the commode without help. She could not use her chart and color-coded boxes to take her pills. Mrs. B. flatly refused to consider admission to a nursing facility to receive therapy to regain her strength, and she would not consider living with her daughter or either son. The family was unable to continue to provide the care that Mrs. B. needed. The nurse explained to Mrs. B. that it was not safe for her to remain in her apartment without assistance. She suggested that Mrs. B. hire an aide until other arrangements could be made, because her children were not obligated to lose their jobs or jeopardize their family relationships to care for her. A referral was made for a social worker and a physical therapist to evaluate Mrs. B. After their visits the next day, Mrs. B. agreed to be admitted to a nursing home for therapy, and she decided to remain there and pay for her care when it was no longer covered by Medicare. Mrs. B.'s family continued to visit her often, and she no longer chided them for their inability to maintain her at home.

If Mrs. B. had insisted on remaining in her apartment, the nurse and social worker would have been obligated to make a referral to Adult Protective Services. Legal interventions, such as guardianship, might have been initiated. For further discussion of legal issues, refer to Chapter 22.

Educational Resources

Clearinghouse on Abuse and Neglect of the Elderly
College of Human Resources, University of Delaware, Newark, DE 19716
(302) 831-3525

National Center on Elder Abuse
810 First Street, NE, Suite 500, Washington, DC, 20002
(202) 682-2470
www.gwjapan.com/NCEA

National Eldercare Locator
1112 16th Street, NW, Suite 100, Washington, DC 20036
(800) 677-1116

•Information about community services for older adults in all geographic areas of the United States (written in English and Spanish)

References

American Association of Retired Persons (AARP). (1992). *Abused elders or older battered women? Report on the AARP Forum.* Washington, DC: AARP.

Anetzberger, G. J. (1987). *The etiology of elder abuse by adult offspring.* Springfield, IL: Charles C Thomas.

Anetzberger, G. J. (1990). Abuse, neglect and self-neglect: Issues of vulnerability. In Z. Hanel, P. Ehrlich, & R. Hubbard (Eds.), *The vulnerable aged: People, services, and policies* (pp. 140–148). New York: Springer.

Anetzberger, G. J. (1997). Elderly adult survivors of family violence: Implications for clinical practice. *Violence Against Women, 3*(5), 499–514.

Anetzberger, G. J., Dayton, C., & McMonagle, P. (1997). A community dialogue series on ethics and elder abuse: Guidelines for decision-making. *Journal of Elder Abuse & Neglect, 9*(1), 33–50.

Anetzberger, G. J., Korbin, J. E., & Austin, C. (1994). Alcoholism and elder abuse. *Journal of Interpersonal Violence, 9*(2), 184–193.

Anetzberger, G. J., Korbin, J. E., & Tomita, S. K. (1996). Defining elder mistreatment in four ethnic groups across two generations. *Journal of Cross-Cultural Gerontology, 11,* 187–212.

Beck, M., & Gordon, J. (1991, December 23). A dumping ground for granny: Weary families drop her in the emergency room. *Newsweek,* 64.

Bendik, M. (1992). Reaching the breaking point: Dangers of mistreatment in elder caregiving situations. *Journal of Elder Abuse & Neglect, 4*(3), 39–59.

Block, M. R., & Sinnott, J. D. (Eds.). (1979). *The battered elder syndrome: An exploratory study.* College Park, MD: University of Maryland, Center on Aging.

Bookin, D. (Ed.). (1992). *Working with impaired elders in the community: A guide to the decision-making process and legal interventions.* Cleveland, OH: Federation for Community Planning.

Boydston, L. S., & McNairn, J. A. (1981). Elder abuse by adult caretakers: An exploratory study. In U.S. House Select Committee on Aging, *Physical and financial abuse of the elderly* (Committee Publication No. 97-297). Washington, DC: U.S. Government Printing Office.

Brandl, B. (1997). *Developing services for older abused women: A guide for domestic abuse programs.* Madison, WI: Wisconsin Coalition Against Domestic Violence.

Brandl, B., & Raymond, J. (1996). Older abused and battered women: An invisible population. *Wisconsin Medical Journal, 95*(5), 298–300.

Brandl, B., & Raymond, J. (1997). Unrecognized elder abuse victims: Older abused women. *Journal of Case Management, 6*(2), 62–68.

Bristowe, E. (July, 1987). Family mediated abuse of noninstitutionalized frail elderly men and women living in British Columbia. Paper presented at the Third National Conference of Family Violence Researchers, University of New Hampshire, Durham, NH.

Brownell, P. (1997). The application of the Culturagram in cross-cultural practice with elder abuse victims. *Journal of Elder Abuse & Neglect, 9*(2), 19–33.

Burston, G. R. (1975). Granny-battering. *British Medical Journal, 3,* 592.

Butler, R. N. (1975). *Why survive? Being old in America.* New York: Harper & Row.

Byers, B., & Lamanna, R. A. (1993). Adult protective services and elder self-endangering. In B. Byers & J. E. Hendricks (Eds.), *Adult protectice services: Research and practice* (pp. 61–85). Springfield, IL: Charles C. Thomas.

Capezuti, E., Brush, B. L., & Lawson, W. T. (1997). Reporting elder mistreatment. *Journal of Gerontological Nursing, 23*(7), 24–32.

Carpenito, L. J. (1997). *Nursing diagnosis: Application to clinical practice* (7th ed.). Philadelphia: J. B. Lippincott.

Chelucci, K., & Coyle, J. (1990). *Elder abuse: Acute care and resource manual.* Toledo, OH: Authors.

Chen, P. N., Bell, S., Dolinsky, D., Doyle, J., & Dunn, M. (1981). Elderly abuse in domestic settings: A pilot study. *Journal of Gerontological Social Work, 4,* 3–17.

Coyne, A. C., Reichman, W. E., & Berbig, L. J. (1993). The relationship between dementia and elder abuse. *American Journal of Psychiatry, 150,* 643–646.

Crouse, J. S., Cobb, D. C., & Harris, B. B. (1981). *Abuse and neglect of the elderly in Illinois: Incidence and characteristics, legislation and policy recommendations.* Springfield, IL: State of Illinois, Department of Aging.

Culver, C. M. (1985). The clinical determination of competence. In M. Kapp, H. E. Pies, & A. E. Doudera (Eds.), *Legal and ethical aspects of health care for the elderly.* Ann Arbor, MI: Health Administration Press.

Davis, L. J., & Brody, E. M. (1979). *Rape and older women: A guide to prevention and protection.* Rockville, MD: U.S. Department of Health, Education, and Welfare.

Douglass, R. L., & Hickey, T. (1983). Domestic neglect and abuse of the elderly: Research findings and systems perspectives for service delivery planning. In J. I. Kosberg (Ed.), *Abuse and maltreatment of the elderly: Causes and interventions* (pp. 115–133). Littleton, MA: John Wright.

Douglass, R. L., Hickey, T., & Noel, C. (1980). *A study of maltreatment of the elderly and other vulnerable adults.* Ann Arbor, MI: University of Michigan, Institute of Gerontology.

Duke, J. (1997). A national study of involuntary protective services to adult protective services clients. *Journal of Elder Abuse & Neglect, 9*(1), 51–68.

Ferguson, D., & Beck, C. M. (1983). H.A.L.F.: A tool to assess elder abuse within the family. *Geriatric Nursing, 4,* 301–304.

Fulmer, T., & Anetzberger, G. J. (September, 1995). Knowledge about family violence interventions in the field of elder abuse. Background paper for the Committee on the Assessment of Family Violence Interventions of the

National Research Council and Institute of Medicine, Washington, DC.

Fulmer, T. T., & Gould, E. S. (1996). Assessing neglect. In L. A. Baumhover & S. C. Beall (Eds.), *Abuse, neglect, and exploitation of older persons: Strategies for assessment and intervention* (pp. 89–103). Baltimore: Health Professions Press.

Fulmer, T. T., & O'Malley, T. A. (1987). *Inadequate care of the elderly: A health care perspective on abuse and neglect.* New York: Springer.

Fulmer, T., & Wetle, T. (1986). Elder abuse screening and intervention. *Nurse Practitioner, 11*(5), 33–38.

Galbraith, M., & Zdorkowski, R. (1986). Systematizing the elder abuse literature. In M. Galbraith (Ed.), *Elder abuse: Perspectives on an emerging crisis* (pp. 168–176). Kansas City, KS: Mid-American Congress on Aging.

Gioglio, G. R., & Blakemore, P. (1983). *Elder abuse in New Jersey: The knowledge and experience of abuse among New Jerseyans.* Trenton, NJ: New Jersey Department of Human Services.

Greenberg, J. R., McKibben, M., & Raymond, J. A. (1990). Dependent adult children and elder abuse. *Journal of Elder Abuse & Neglect, 2*(1/2), 73–86.

Griffin, L. W. (1994). Elder maltreatment among rural African-Americans. *Journal of Elder Abuse & Neglect, 6*(1), 1–27.

Haddad, A. M. (1988). Determining competency. *Journal of Gerontological Nursing, 14*(6), 19–22.

Hamilton, G. P. (1989). Prevent elder abuse: Using a family systems approach. *Journal of Gerontological Nursing, 15*(3), 21–26.

Harris, S. B. (1996). For better or for worse: Spouse abuse grown old. *Journal of Elder Abuse & Neglect, 8*(1), 1–33.

High, D. M. (1987). Planning for decisional incapacity: A neglected area in ethics and aging. *Journal of the American Geriatrics Society, 35*, 814–820.

Holt, M. G. (1993). Elder sexual abuse in Britain: Preliminary findings. *Journal of Elder Abuse & Neglect, 5*(2), 64–71.

Homer, A. C., & Gilleard, C. (1990). Abuse of elderly people by their carers. *British Medical Journal, 301*, 1359–1362.

Hudson, M. F. (1991). Elder mistreatment: A taxonomy with definitions by Delphi. *Journal of Elder Abuse & Neglect, 3*(2), 1–20.

Hudson, M. F. (1994). Elder abuse: Its meaning to middle-aged and older adults—Part II: Pilot results. *Journal of Elder Abuse & Neglect, 6*(1), 55–82.

Hwalek, M. (1985). *Sengstock-Hwalek comprehensive index of elder abuse.* Detroit: Wayne State University.

Hwalek, M., Goodrich, C. S., & Quinn, K. (1996). The role of risk factors in health care and adult protective services. In L. A. Baumhover & S. C. Beall (Eds.), *Abuse, neglect, and exploitation of older persons: Strategies for assessment and intervention* (pp. 123–141). Baltimore: Health Professionals Press.

Kapp, M. B., & Bigot, A. (1985). *Geriatrics and the law: Patient rights and professional responsibilities.* New York: Springer.

Kivela, S. (1995). Elder abuse in Finland. In J. I. Kosberg & J. L. Garcia (Eds.), *Elder abuse: International and cross-cultural perspectives* (pp. 31–44). New York: Haworth Press.

Kosberg, J. I., & Nahmiash, D. (1996). Characteristics of victims and perpetrators and milieus of abuse and neglect. In L. A. Baumhover and S. C. Beall (Eds.), *Abuse, neglect, and exploitation of older persons: Strategies for assessment and intervention* (pp. 31–49). Baltimore: Health Professionals Press.

Krassen Maxwell, E., & Maxwell, R. J. (1992). Insults to the body civil: Mistreatment of elderly in two Plain Indian tribes. *Journal of Cross-Cultural Gerontology, 7*, 3–23.

Lachs, M. S., & Fulmer, T. (1993). Recognizing elder abuse and neglect. *Clinics in Geriatric Medicine, 9*(3), 665–681.

Lachs, M. S., & Pillemer, K. (1995). Abuse and neglect of elderly persons. *The New England Journal of Medicine, 332*(7), 437–443.

Lachs, M. S., Williams, C., O'Brien, S., Hurst, L., & Horwitz, R. (1996). Older adults: An 11-year longitudinal study of adult protective service use. *Archives of Internal Medicine, 156*, 449–453.

Lachs, M. S., Williams, C., O'Brien, S., Hurst, L., & Horwitz, R. (1997). Risk factors for reported elder abuse and neglect: A nine-year observational cohort study. *The Gerontologist, 37*, 469–474.

Lau, E., & Kosberg, J. (1979). Abuse of the elderly by informal care providers. *Aging, 299–300*, 10–15.

Longres, J. F. (1995). Self-neglect among the elderly. *Journal of Elder Abuse & Neglect, 7*(1), 69–86.

Luppens, J., & Lau, E. (1983). The mentally and physically impaired elderly relative: Consequences for family care. In J. I. Kosberg (Ed.), *Abuse and maltreatment of the elderly: Causes and interventions* (pp. 204–219). Boston: John Wright-PSG.

Lustbader, W. (1996). Self-neglect: A practitioner's view. *Aging, 367*, 51–60.

McLaughlin, J. S., Nickell, J. P., & Gill, L. (1980). An epidemiological investigation of elderly abuse in southern Maine and New Hampshire. In U. S. House Select Committee on Aging, *Elder abuse* (Committee Publication No. 68-463). Washington DC: U.S. Government Printing Office.

Montoya, V. (1997). Understanding and combating elder abuse in Hispanic communities. *Journal of Elder Abuse & Neglect, 9*(2), 5–17.

Moon, A., & Williams, O. (1993). Perceptions of elder abuse and help-seeking patterns among African-American, Caucasian American, and Korean-American elderly women. *The Gerontologist, 33*, 386–395.

Nagpaul, K. (1997). Elder abuse among Asian Indians: Traditional versus modern perspectives. *Journal of Elder Abuse & Neglect, 9*(2), 77–92.

Nerenberg, L. (1996). *Older battered women: Integrating aging and domestic violence services.* Washington, DC: National Center on Elder Abuse.

Oakar, M. R., & Miller, C. A. (1983). Federal legislation to protect the elderly. In J. I. Kosberg, (Ed.), *Abuse and maltreatment of the elderly: Causes and interventions* (pp. 422–435). Boston: John Wright-PSG.

Ogg, J., & Bennett, G. (1992). Elder abuse in Britain. *British Medical Journal, 305,* 988–989.

O'Malley, J., Segars, J., Perez, R., Mitchell, V., & Knuepfel, G. M. (1979). *Elder abuse in Massachusetts: A survey of professionals and para-professionals.* Boston: Legal Research and Services for the Elderly.

Paveza, G. J., Cohen, D., Eisdorfer, C., Freels, S., Semla, T., Ashford, J. W., et al. (1992). Severe family violence and Alzheimer's disease: Prevalence and risk factors. *The Gerontologist, 32,* 493–497.

Phillips, L. R. (1986). Theoretical explanations of elder abuse: Competing hypotheses and unresolved issues. In K. A. Pillemer and R. S. Wolf (Eds.), *Elder abuse: Conflict in the family* (pp. 197–217). Dover, MA: Auburn House.

Pillemer, K. A. (1986). Risk factors in elder abuse: Results from a case-control study. In K. A. Pillemer & R. W. Wolf (Eds.), *Elder abuse: Conflict in the family* (pp. 239–263). Dover, MA: Auburn House.

Pillemer, K. A., & Finkelhor, D. (1988). The prevalence of elder abuse: A random sample survey. *The Gerontologist, 28,* 51–57.

Pillemer, K. A., & Suitor, J. J. (1992). Violence and violent feelings: What causes them among family caregivers? *Journal of Gerontology, 47*(4), S165–S172.

Podnieks, E. (1992). National survey on abuse of the elderly in Canada. *Journal of Elder Abuse & Neglect, 4*(1/2), 5–58.

Poertner, J. (1986). Estimating the incidence of abused older persons. *Journal of Gerontological Social Work, 9*(3), 3–15.

Quinn, M. J., & Tomita, S. K. (1986). *Elder abuse and neglect: Causes, diagnosis, and intervention strategies.* New York: Springer.

Quinn, M. J., & Tomita, S. K. (1997). *Elder abuse and neglect: Causes, diagnosis, and intervention strategies* (2nd ed.). New York: Springer.

Ramsey-Klawsnik, H. (1991). Elder sexual abuse: Preliminary findings. *Journal of Elder Abuse & Neglect, 3*(3), 73–90.

Ramsey-Klawsnik, H. (1993). Interviewing elders for suspected sexual abuse: Guidelines and techniques. *Journal of Elder Abuse & Neglect, 5*(1), 5–18.

Rathbone-McCuan, E., & Bricker-Jenkins, M. (1992). A general framework for elder self-neglect. In E. Rathbone-McCuan & D. R. Fabian (Eds.), *Self-neglecting elders: A clinical dilemma* (pp. 13–24). New York: Auburn House.

Reynolds, E., & Stanton, S. (1983). Elderly abuse in a hospital: A nursing perspective. In J. I. Kosberg (Ed.), *Abuse and maltreatment of the elderly: Causes and interventions* (pp. 391–403). Boston, MA: John Wright.

Sabatino, C. P. (1996). Competency: Refining our legal fictions. In M. Smyer, K. W. Schaie, & M. B. Kapp (Eds.), *Older adults' decision-making and the law* (pp. 1–28). New York: Springer.

Schimer, M. R., & Kahana, J. S. (1992). *Legal issues in the care of older adults: "The magic of legal labels."*

Cleveland, OH: Western Reserve Geriatric Education Center.

Seaver, C. (1996). Muted lives: Older battered women. *Journal of Elder Abuse & Neglect, 8*(2), 3–21.

Sengstock, M. C., Hwalek, M. H., & Petrone, S. (1989). Services for aged abuse victims: Service types and related factors. *Journal of Elder Abuse & Neglect, 1*(4), 37–56.

Sengstock, M. C., & Liang, J. (1982). *Identifying and characterizing elder abuse.* Detroit: Wayne State University, Institute of Gerontology.

Stearns, P. J. (1986). Old age family conflict: The perspective of the past. In K. A. Pillemer & R. S. Wolf (Eds.), *Elder abuse: Conflict in the family* (pp. 3–24). Dover, MA: Auburn House.

Stein, K. F. (1991). *Working with abused and neglected elders in minority populations: A synthesis of research.* Washington, DC: National Aging Resource Center on Elder Abuse.

Steinmetz, S. K. (1981). Elder abuse. *Aging, 315–316,* 6–10.

Steinmetz, S. K. (1988). *Duty bound: Elder abuse and family care.* Newbury Park, CA: Sage.

Stiegel, L. A. (1995). *Recommended guidelines for state courts handling cases involving elder abuse.* Washington, DC: American Bar Association.

Tatara, T. (1995). *An analysis of state laws addressing elder abuse, neglect, and exploitation.* Washington, DC: National Center on Elder Abuse.

Tatara, T. (1996). *Elder abuse: Questions and answers—An information guide for professionals and concerned citizens.* Washington, DC: National Center on Elder Abuse.

Tatara, T. (1997, November). Attitudes toward elder mistreatment and reporting: A multicultural study. Paper presented at the Annual Scientific Meeting of the Gerontological Society of America, Cincinnati, OH.

Texas Department of Human Services, Region 09. (1985, November). *Self neglect study.* Paper presented at the Adult Protective Services Conference, San Antonio, TX.

Uniform Guardianship and Protective Proceedings Act. (1993). References and annotations: Table of jurisdictions wherein Act has been adopted.

U.S. House Select Committee on Aging. (1981). *Elder abuse: An examination of a hidden problem* (Committee Publication No. 97-277). Washington, DC: U.S. Government Printing Office.

U.S. House Select Committee on Aging. (1990). *Elder abuse: A decade of shame and inaction.* Washington, DC: U.S. Government Printing Office.

VanderMeer, J. L. (1992). Elder abuse and the community health nurse. *Journal of Elder Abuse & Neglect, 4*(4), 37–45.

Vinton, L. (1991). An exploratory study of self-neglectful elderly. *Journal of Gerontological Social Work, 18*(1/2), 55–68.

Wolf, R. S. (1988). The evaluation of policy: A 10-year retrospective. *Public Welfare, 46,* 7–13.

Wolf, R. S. (1996). Elder abuse and family violence: Testimony presented before the U.S. Senate Special Committee on Aging. *Journal of Elder Abuse & Neglect, 8*(1), 81–96.

Wolf, R. S., Godkin, M. A., & Pillemer, K. A. (1984). *Elder abuse and neglect: Final report from three model projects.* Worchester, MA: University of Massachusetts Medical Center, University Center on Aging.

Wolf, R. S., Godkin, M. A., & Pillemer, K. A. (1986). Maltreatment of the elderly: A comparative analysis. *Pride Institute Journal of Long-Term Home Health Care, 5*(4), 10–17.

Wolf, R. S., & Pillemer, K. A. (1995, November). The older battered woman: Wives and mothers compared. Paper presented at the Annual Scientific Meeting of the Gerontological Society of America, Los Angeles, CA.

Health Care for Older Adults

Chapter

22

**Learning
Objectives**

1. *Discuss the benefits and limitations of the most common health insurance programs in relation to the planning of care for older adults.*

2. *Provide examples of various health care settings that are designed to address the unique needs of older adults in the United States.*

3. *Discuss various aspects of legal and ethical issues affecting older adults.*

4. *Discuss cultural considerations of legal and ethical aspects of care of older adults.*

The 1965 Medicare and Medicaid amendments of the Social Security Act marked the beginning of a revolution in health care for older adults in the United States. Gerontological nursing and other areas of health care specialization evolved as part of this revolution. In Chapter 1, gerontological nursing was discussed in relation to the broad social changes that have influenced the older adult population in the United States. This chapter addresses the ways in which the health care system influences gerontological nursing practice. The specific topics discussed are health insurance for older adults, gerontological health care settings, and legal and ethical considerations.

Health Insurance for Older Adults

In the United States, older people have not always used as many formal health care services as they do today. Before Medicare and Medicaid, only a minute proportion of the federal budget was appropriated for health care for older people, and little attention was paid to their health and medical needs. Now the pendulum has swung in the other direction. Older people constitute the largest group of health care

consumers, and costs of retirement and health care benefits constitute an increasingly larger proportion of the federal budget. Now, most discussions of the federal budget include references to the need to cut the cost of Medicare and Medicaid and to provide for the stability of Social Security. In the past few years, major changes have occurred in health insurance with the advent of managed care programs. The next sections review trends in health care and health insurance for older adults.

Relevance to Gerontological Nurses

At a minimum, gerontological nurses must be knowledgeable enough about current health care policies relating to older people to be able to understand some of the barriers and challenges of implementing nursing care plans and discharge plans. For example, knowing the Medicare criteria for skilled home care services enables the nurse to make referrals for this type of nursing care when appropriate. Also, nurses need to keep up-to-date on recent changes, not only so they can guide older adults in the many choices of health care delivery systems that are now available, but also so they can identify opportunities for new roles for gerontological nurses. As discussed in Chapter 1, roles of gerontological nurses are expanding rapidly. Much of this expansion is directly related to changes in health insurance and health delivery systems. For example, after several decades of anticipation, opportunities for Medicare reimbursement for advance practice nurses have finally become a reality. Also, a recent nursing article emphasized the need to identify and develop the skills that are necessary for gerontological nurses to function knowledgeably and expertly in managed care environments. The "managed care skill set" includes a sound business orientation, advance practice clinical skills, and a firm grasp of the organization, financing, delivery, and policy implications of managed care (Malloy, 1997).

Nurses are encouraged to supplement information in this chapter by consulting current nursing and gerontology journals and the references and Internet sites listed in the Educational Resources section of this chapter. Also, the article by Melillo (1996), in the reference section, provides an excellent review of the Medicare and Medicaid programs as they relate to older adults.

Medicare

Medicare is a program of health insurance available to people who are eligible for benefits under Social Security. Medicare covers primarily hospital and physician services and some skilled care services in homes and nursing homes. It does not cover medications, dental care, most vision care, most routine or preventive services, or nonskilled long-term care. There are two parts to Medicare. Part A is funded through Social Security payroll taxes, whereas Part B is financed through monthly premiums and general revenues. Medicare, therefore, is part of the national budget and is subject to the same political processes that affect other budget items.

Hospital insurance (Part A) covers medical or psychiatric inpatient care in a hospital and in a skilled nursing facility after a hospital stay. It also covers part of the approved costs of durable medical equipment, and it covers skilled home care services and hospice care for those patients meeting the criteria. Beneficiaries have a co-pay amount for hospital services, which increases every year and is the equivalent of the average cost of 1 day of hospital care. Costs of hospital and skilled nursing facility care are paid on the basis of benefit periods. A benefit period begins on the first day of hospital admission and ends 60 days after any payments are made for hospital or skilled nursing facility care. Strict criteria must be met for coverage of services in a skilled nursing facility, and there is a limit to the number of days that are covered. The Medicare home care benefit is intended to provide medically oriented, acute or restorative, skilled nursing care on an intermittent, short-term basis to homebound patients who are under the care of a physician. These services are described in the section entitled Home Care Services. Supplemental medical insurance (Part B) covers all or part of the cost of approved physician's services and other outpatient services, such as diagnostic imaging and laboratory services. Additional services covered under Part B include certain ambulance services, mammograms and Papanicolaou (Pap) smears, durable medical equipment used at home, and services of certain specially qualified, nonphysician, health care practitioners (e.g., nurse practitioners).

When Medicare was first established, there was a limit on the types of services covered, but little regulation of the amount of reimbursement for these services. During the first 10 years of Medicare, health care costs increased more than 1000%, or an average of 141% per year, compared to 11.4% for the gross national product. This does not mean that older people were the primary beneficiaries of these federal expenditures. From 1967 to 1975, Medicare expenditures quadrupled, but only 25% of this increase was accounted for by increased use of services. In fact, older people began to pay more out-of-pocket expenses for their health care. Today, older people spend a larger percentage of their income on their health care needs than they did in the 1960s. Older adults who are disabled or have lower incomes spend even higher percentages of their income on their health care needs (Liu et al., 1993; Rubin and Koelin, 1993). Currently, at least 30% of personal health care bills are paid by older people themselves or by their families. Thus, although older people are receiving more health care than in the past, they are paying more money for their care.

The explanation for these trends may be found in the unprecedented rise in health care costs that occurred in the late 1960s. One cause of these escalating costs was the high rate of inflation in the general economy and the even higher rate in the health care industry. Contributing factors included malpractice concerns, expensive technology, duplication of equipment and services, lack of less costly alternatives to institutional care, and the legal and ethical constraints that encourage the use of high technology to prolong life. By the early 1990s, the Medicare system was rewarding physicians for performing more services (e.g., expensive diagnostic tests) rather than spending time explaining why services would not be necessary. With the trend toward careful scrutiny of Medicare-covered services and the concomitant trend toward managed care, these practices are changing, as discussed in the section on New Models of Health Insurance.

When Medicare was enacted in 1965, the federal government had not anticipated the dramatic rise in health care costs. This was evident from their grossly underestimated projections for the 1970s and 1980s. In 1972, Congress amended Medicare in an attempt to control the rapidly growing costs of this federal program. These amendments established Professional Standard Review Organizations to review use of services. These same amendments extended

Medicare coverage to include adults of any age who had end-stage renal disease or were disabled for 2 years or more as a result of any disease. Although these amendments provided some control over the use of services, the costs of the program continued to escalate far beyond the cost estimates.

In the early 1980s, the federal government took a serious look at health care expenditures and began to deal with the problem of cost containment. In addition to cost containment issues, goals of the federal government during this period included increasing expenditures for defense and diminishing the role of the government in health and social programs. One way of accomplishing these goals was to target for revision the large part of the federal budget that went toward Medicare, Medicaid, Social Security, and other programs for older people. The three-pronged approach that was adopted to cut health care costs included an increase in the amount paid by individual participants, restriction of the amount of Medicare payment for services, and promotion of voluntary reductions in costs of health care services.

In 1982, a system of prospective payment was instituted in place of the system that provided reimbursement for services provided. With this system, payment was based on the expected cost of treating a patient with a specific diagnosis, classified according to a diagnosis-related group (DRG). Payment was provided at a predetermined rate based on whatever DRG the patient was assigned. This system of reimbursement initially was applied to those patients covered by Medicare insurance, but it has been used as a model by private insurance companies as well. Thus, hospitals are no longer guaranteed payment for actual services rendered. Rather, they are financially rewarded when the cost of patient care is less than that associated with a specific DRG, and they are penalized when the cost of patient care is more than that allowed for that particular DRG. This system promotes the early discharge of hospitalized patients, who tend to be relatively sicker at the time of discharge, and shifts the burden of care from hospitals to families, nursing homes, and other community-based care providers. This approach has given rise to the phrase, "quicker and sicker," which became the theme of discharge planning in the 1980s. Other results of the change to a prospective system of payment are a dramatic increase in the number of outpatient procedures and the development of postacute and subacute care programs.

One of the major limitations of Medicare is the lack of coverage for preventive services. This is of particular concern because these are the very services that are most important in delaying the onset of chronic illnesses and improving the health and function of older adults. During the 1990s, Medicare began covering mammograms, influenza immunizations, and a few other preventive services. One of the benefits of the movement toward managed care organizations (MCOs) is the provision of, and even encouragement of, preventive services.

Medicaid

Medicaid legislation was passed at the same time as Medicare, and its intent was to provide health insurance for poor people. Although Medicare falls entirely under the jurisdiction of the federal government, Medicaid is a state-run program that receives partial funding from federal sources and is subject to certain federal guidelines. To qualify for Medicaid, people must have very limited income and assets, or they must have limited assets and be spending a high proportion of their income on medical expenses. Each state determines the specific income and asset limits, and state and federal regulations restrict the transfer of assets from one family member to another to qualify for Medicaid.

Although initially intended to meet the health care needs primarily of poor people, Medicaid has become an important program for older people who require long-term care. Since the late 1960s, Medicaid has paid for skilled nursing care and for care received in intermediate care facilities. In 1973, Medicaid was extended to all adults meeting the criteria for Supplemental Security Income, including those requiring long-term care. Although states have some discretion with regard to eligibility criteria for Medicaid, the federal government has mandated that they pay for nursing home care for all eligible adults. Thus, Medicaid has become increasingly important as a source of payment for long-term care, and it pays about 50% of the costs associated with nursing home care. Traditionally, Medicaid has been biased toward institutional care rather than community-based long-term care, but this is changing. States can apply to the Health Care Financing Administration for approval of Medicaid-waiver programs that provide community-based services to people who would otherwise need nursing home care. These programs are discussed in the section on New Models of Health Insurance.

Private Insurance

Because of the many limitations of Medicare as a health insurance program, about 75% of older adults purchase additional insurance coverage from private companies. Private health insurance policies include all of the following types: medigap policies, MCOs, hospital indemnity policies, specific disease policies, long-term care policies, and continuation of employer-provided policy. Medigap, MCOs, and long-term care policies are discussed in detail; the other policies are described briefly.

Employer-provided policies generally provide the best supplemental insurance, but they are available only to retired people (or their spouses) who continue a health insurance policy from their employer. These policies are likely to cover prescription medications, and they may cover some long-term care services that are not covered by Medicare. Hospital indemnity policies pay cash amounts for each day of inpatient hospital care; they may also include benefits for surgical procedures or days spent in a skilled nursing facility. Specific disease policies are limited to paying for services related to a specific disease, and they are likely to duplicate benefits covered under Medicare or other primary insurance policies.

Medigap policies are designed to supplement Medicare benefits, and they are now regulated by federal and state laws. The National Association of Insurance Commissioners has developed 10 standard plans that insurance companies must follow in the provision of medigap policies. Plan A contains basic benefits, such as coverage for coinsurance payments and additional payments for hospital days. Other plans (B through J) cover Part A deductible and additional services, such as preventive medical care, skilled nursing coinsurance, and medical care in foreign countries. The most comprehensive policies cover the cost of medications. Limits are applied to the drug benefit and some of the other benefits. A relatively new type of supplemental policy is the Medicare Select policy, which is the same as the medigap policies but with coverage only when services are provided by a designated, preferred provider. This option is still being evaluated by Congress and has been extended at least until 1998.

Long-term care insurance is a recent development in the health insurance industry. When these policies were introduced in the late 1980s, they were unregulated, and many of the policies contained large loopholes and significant barriers to receiving benefits. During the 1990s, many states enacted laws mandating certain standards suggested by the National Association of Insurance Commissioners. Suggested requirements for long-term care insurance policies include inflation protection and caps on rates. A good long-term care policy will provide payment for a range of options, including home care services and assisted living facilities. Policies also should include additional options that may be available in the future. A major drawback of this type of insurance for older people is that the premiums are based on the age of the person when he or she initially signs up for the policy. For many older adults, the cost of the policy will outweigh the benefits. These policies will likely become increasingly important, particularly for young-old and middle-aged people, because one of the major trends of the late 1990s is to shift responsibility for long-term care financing from the federal government to states, individuals, and families (Cohen, 1998). Nurses can obtain information about long-term care policies from several of the agencies listed in the Educational Resources section.

New Models of Health Insurance

Persistent increases in health care costs for Medicare and Medicaid programs have provided incentive for the development of new models of health insurance and health care delivery. Since the early 1980s, the federal government has allowed Medicare beneficiaries to enroll in approved MCOs, such as health maintenance organizations (HMOs). This move marked the first time that Medicare payments were based on criteria other than a fee-for-service basis. By the mid-1990s, older adults in every state could choose from a variety of MCOs, as alternatives to Medicare, for their primary health care insurance. People who enrolled in a Medicare MCO or HMO continued to pay Part B premiums to Medicare, but they did not pay Medicare deductibles or coinsurance amounts. MCOs and HMOs receive capitation payments of 95% of the average amount paid to fee-for-service providers in the same geographic area. The intent is to reduce the cost of federal health insurance costs and to provide choices for Medicare beneficiaries. The major advantage to participants is that these plans generally cover the costs of medications, vision care, and preventive services. Some plans even place a heavy emphasis on preventive services. Also, there is decreased emphasis on hospitalization and increased emphasis on the use of subacute care, home health care, and skilled nursing care. The major disadvantage for some participants is that the choice of health care providers is limited by the MCO or HMO, and permission is needed from a primary care provider before services can be obtained. Many issues are being raised about the clinical, ethical, and financial aspects of MCOs. For example, a recent nursing article discussed the importance of nurses advocating for standards of clinical practice that can be used to address conflicts of interest regarding payment incentives (Haack, 1997). A recent review of quality measures found that, with a few exceptions, Medicare recipients fare as well or better in MCOs compared to fee-for-service plans (Colenda and Sherman, 1998).

Innovative programs have recently been implemented and are still being developed to extend the MCO concept by covering a limited amount of long-term care services for people with chronic conditions. The On Lok program in the Chinatown area of San Francisco, which opened in 1983, was the first Medicare-waiver Social Health Maintenance Organization (SHMO) model established. The success of this model prompted the development of similar programs, called Programs of All-inclusive Care for the Elderly (PACE), in the late 1980s. Federal legislation in 1990 allowed additional replication sites, and these are still being developed in the late 1990s. The distinguishing features of these programs are: (1) the provision of community-based, long-term care services to nursing-home-eligible clients, (2) integrated funding through Medicare and Medicaid, (3) integrated service delivery through adult day health centers, and (4) case management through multidisciplinary teams (Branch et al., 1995). Other models of integrated care, such as the home hospital program, are currently being

planned, implemented, and evaluated (Leff et al., 1997; Cohen, 1998). For a review of cultural considerations relating to health insurance and long-term care, see the Culture Box on page 661.

Gerontological Health Care Settings

An outgrowth of the establishment of geriatrics and gerontology as areas of health care specialization has been the recent development of innovative programs—both institutional and noninstitutional—designed to address the unique needs of the older population. Although some of these programs have arisen from an increased concern about health expenditures, many are the result of an increased awareness of the importance of meeting chronic care needs of older adults in a way that addresses both financial concerns and quality-of-life issues. As the number and variety of settings have increased, so have the opportunities for gerontological nurses. Indeed, just as older adults now have a broader selection of places where they can receive care, nurses now have a wider array of practice settings for providing care to older adults. Some of the recent developments in both institutional and noninstitutional gerontological care are discussed in the following sections. Nurses can obtain additional information about services provided in these settings by contacting the organizations listed in the Educational Resources section of this chapter. Nurses and families also can obtain specific information about services that are available in their communities by contacting local offices on aging, community information services, and their local Alzheimer's Association.

Acute Care Settings

Although most health care services for older adults are provided in nonacute settings, most nurses who care for older adults provide the

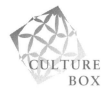

CULTURE
BOX

Cultural Considerations Relating to Health Insurance and Long-Term Care

Health Insurance

- Older Hispanics and African Americans are more likely than White Americans to have no health insurance, or to have no insurance except Medicare.
- Almost half of older Korean Americans have no health insurance (Kim and Kim, 1992).
- Native Americans receive health services, including home care services, from the Indian Health Service.

Long-Term Care

- The following are rates of nursing home utilization by people aged 65 years and older according to different cultural groups in the United States: 5% of White elderly, 4% of African Americans, 3% of Hispanic Americans, 3% of American Indian and Alaska Natives, and 2% of Asian and Pacific Americans (American Association of Retired Persons, 1987).
- The following are rates of nursing home utilization by people aged 85 years and older according to different cultural groups in the United States: 26% of White elderly, 17% of African Americans, 12% of Asian Americans, and 11% of Hispanic Americans (Damron-Rodriguez et al., 1994).
- Older Hispanics who enter a nursing home have greater degrees of disability than do non-Hispanic Whites (Bassford, 1995).
- Korean Americans generally prefer independent or assisted living residences over living with family members or in a nursing home setting (Kim, 1997).
- The lower rate of nursing home use by older African Americans may be related to a higher use of paid home care, informal-only care, and no care (Wallace et al., 1998).

care in hospital settings. As with other aspects of health care, however, hospital care of older adults is rapidly changing. As discussed in the section on health insurance for older adults, there have been major shifts in health care services because of changes in health insurance. Increasingly, even acute care services are being provided more frequently in outpatient settings. The terms transitional care and subacute care are now being used in reference to services that continue the work of the hospital after discharge (Kane and Kane, 1997). Inpatient hospital stays now are part of a continuum of care that necessitates careful preadmission and postdischarge planning and coordination of services.

In the 2 decades since establishment of the Medicare program, hospital admissions for older adults have increased at a rate 5 times faster than that of the population in general. In the past 15 years, the average length of stay and the number of hospital admissions for older people have been decreasing gradually. This trend has led to frustration on the part of hospital nurses who have less time to prepare the older patient for discharge. In addition, it has become increasingly important for nurses to include family caregivers in discharge planning and to facilitate referrals for postdischarge care.

As in other health care settings, acute care settings are developing new ways of delivering care to older adults in an effort to improve both the quality and efficiency of care. Some hospitals are establishing geriatric units, staffed by specially trained health care workers who work together as an interdisciplinary team (e.g., Inouye et al., 1993a). In addition to nurses, the team typically includes a geriatrician, pharmacist, social worker, various rehabilitation therapists (e.g., speech, physical, and occupational therapists), and mental health professionals (e.g., psychologists or psychiatrists). The focus of these programs is to assist older adults with complex problems to remain at their highest level of function. This is an important focus for geriatric care, because the prevention of functional decline during hospitalization may decrease the need for nursing home care (Rudberg et al., 1996). Key elements of one such program include a specially adapted environment; an emphasis on independence, rehabilitation, and prevention of disability; intensive review of care to minimize the adverse effects of medications and procedures; and discharge planning with the goal of returning the patient to his or her home (Landefeld et al., 1995). Gerontological clinical nurse specialists often have a strong role in these programs (e.g., Inouye et al., 1993b). Geropsychiatric and geriatric rehabilitation programs are other new models of hospital-based geriatric care that are evolving to address the unique and complex needs of older people.

Long-Term Care

Although "institutional care" and "long-term care" have been used interchangeably in reference to nursing home care, neither term is synonymous with nursing home care. The close association between nursing home care and long-term care arises from the fact that, before the late 1970s, nursing homes were the primary resource, and usually the only formal resource, for people who needed long-term care that could not be provided by their families. Institutional

care accurately refers to care that is provided in acute care, subacute, rehabilitative, or chronic care settings, such as nursing homes. Long-term care accurately refers to a continuum of services that holistically address comprehensive needs in a variety of settings. During the 1990s, distinctions between sites and types of health care became blurred, as almost any type of care could be delivered in any setting (Kane and Kane, 1997). Long-term care services include all those services designed to provide care for people at different stages of dependence for an extended period of time. As their functional abilities change, older people use different services according to their level of dependence and the availability of social supports.

The phrase "aging in place" refers to the concept of older adults being able to remain in one setting even though their needs change. This same concept, under the name "in-place progression," has been applied to a model of care for people with Alzheimer's disease who remain in the same bedroom and on the same nursing care unit from the mid-stages of the disorder until their death (Weaverdyck et al., 1998). Conceptualizations of future long-term care programs describe a service delivery system that integrates the entire range of health, community-based, and in-home services. These long-term care programs will be characterized by the following: client-driven services, a single point of access, assessment and coordination of all services, payment based on a capitation system, and mandatory accountability and quality of service (Beck and Chumbler, 1997). The range of long-term care services, including institutional services and community-based services, is discussed in the following sections.

Cost of care is a major determinant of the services that are used by older adults. Nurses need to keep in mind that Medicare has very strict requirements for coverage of skilled services in home or nursing home settings. The type of long-term care services that are most commonly needed by chronically ill people who require assistance with their activities of daily living (ADL) is rarely covered by Medicare or private health insurance. Medicaid may cover some services, but strict financial criteria must be met before a person is eligible for services. Older adults must rely on family members for their care and pay out-of-pocket for the care that is not available from family members. In the late 1990s, the average monthly cost of nursing home care ranged from $3000 to $4000 nationwide. The monthly cost of assisted living facilities is usually between $1000 and $3000. Costs and insurance coverage of other long-term services are briefly discussed in the appropriate following sections. Gerontological nurses need to keep cost factors in mind when discussing the various options for long-term care with older adults and their families.

Nursing Home Care

Since the 1970s, about 5% of people older than 65 years of age have received care in nursing homes at any point in time. Although the proportion of older people receiving care in nursing homes has remained stable and is expected to increase only slightly in the next decades, the characteristics of people in nursing homes have changed. Indeed, the characteristics of typical nursing home residents in 1985 have been described as follows: the average age is 82 years; 90% have no living spouse; women outnumber men by a ratio of 3 to 1; 50% have a progressive dementing condition; 50% have arthritis, cardiovascular disease, or both; one third have impaired vision and one third have impaired hearing; help is required in several or all ADL; only 20% return home, and 70% stay for longer than 1 year (U.S. House Select Committee on Aging, 1986, pp. 5–6).

This picture of the very old woman who needs help in performing ADL and who has no one who can provide the care at home must be viewed with caution, however. The recent and dramatic changes in the delivery of health care for older adults have resulted in increasing numbers of people being admitted to nursing homes from hospitals for short-term nursing care. A longitudinal study of people admitted to nursing homes in 1976 showed that 34% were discharged within the first month, and an additional 18% were discharged within the next 2 months. Less than 50% of the cohort remained in the nursing home after 3 months, and only 14% remained for more than 3 years (Liu and Manton, 1984). Therefore, even before DRGs, only about 50% of the residents in nursing homes were there for long-term care. As a consequence of the trend toward earlier discharges from hospitals, it is expected that more older people will be admitted to nursing homes for short-term care than for long-term care. In fact, one gerontologist concluded that people aged 65 or older have a 50/50 chance of being in a nursing home at some point in their life (McConnel, 1984). Thus, the characteristics presented earlier might accurately describe those older people who are in nursing homes for long-term stays, but they are not applicable to the many older people who stay in nursing homes for short-term care.

The chance of being admitted to a nursing home is determined not only by the characteristics of the person who needs the care, but also by the availability and characteristics of caregivers. It has long been recognized that, for many dependent people, the reason for moving to a nursing home is not a change in that person's condition but rather a change in the availability or abilities of the caregiver. Nursing home residents are generally more disabled than community-living older people, but for each person living in a nursing home, there are two to three equally disabled older people living in the community with family or paid caregivers (Kane and Kane, 1997). A study of community-based people with dementia found that the best predictors of institutionalization were factors associated with the type of caregiver arrangement and how much distress was reported by the caregiver (Lieberman and Kramer, 1991). Place of residence is another factor that is currently being examined as a factor in relative risk of receiving institutional long-term care. Recent data from the Longitudinal Study on Aging found that older adults who lived in less urbanized and thinly populated nonmetropolitan areas had the highest likelihood of admission for short- or long-term nursing home stays, and that older people from large metropolitan areas had the lowest rate of admission (Coward et al., 1996).

Characteristics of the dependent person that are likely to increase the risk of institutionalization include White race, living alone, advanced age, and functional and/or cognitive impairments (Wolinsky et al., 1993; Nielsen et al., 1996; Chenier, 1997; Scott et al., 1997). Married people have about half the risk for nursing home admission of unmarried people, and people who have at least one daughter or sibling reduce their risk by one fourth (Freedman, 1996). Caregiver factors that are associated with the decision to seek institutional placement of people with dementia include use of services, length of caregiving, enjoyment of caregiving, caregiver health and burden, and caregiver reactions to behaviors (Cohen et al., 1993; Nielsen et al., 1996). Caregiver factors that have been found to increase the need for institutional care of people without cognitive impairments are increasing age and caregiver burden, which includes the number of tasks performed, restricted social contact, deteriorating physical or mental health, and perceived stress due to caregiving (Chenier, 1997). It is the combination of dependence in performing ADL and lack of caregiver resources that brings older people to nursing homes for long-term care. Therefore, an accurate assessment of so-

cial supports and resources for help in the community is at least as important as an accurate assessment of the person's functional abilities.

Family Caregiving and Care Management Services

Services provided to older adults in their own homes constitute one of the most rapidly growing components of health care services. Although 85% of all in-home care is provided by family and other unpaid workers, the remaining 15% is provided by informal and formal paid caregivers. The family members most likely to become primary caregivers are adult daughters (29%), wives (23%), husbands (13%), and sons (9%) (Whitlatch and Noelker, 1996). Family caregiving has become more complex and difficult as more and more family members have moved away from their hometowns. Also, the entry of more women into the paid workforce has significantly diminished the availability of traditional family caregivers. These trends, along with the significant increase in the number of people aged 85 years and older, have led to the need for professional geriatric care management services. These services are most often provided by a nurse or social worker who assesses the needs for in-home and other long-term care services and then plans, coordinates, and oversees the services. For many older adults, the geriatric care manager serves as the primary care coordinator who is responsible for implementing a long-term care plan in the absence of family members who have the ability to do so. Professional geriatric care management services are provided by individual professionals and by non-profit and for-profit organizations. By the late 1990s, more than two dozen organizations (including the American Nurses' Credentialing Center) were addressing the need for credentialing of this rapidly evolving profession. Nurses can keep up-to-date on developments in care management services by contacting the organizations listed in the Educational Resources section at the end of this chapter.

Home Care Services

Although older people and other dependent populations have always received much of their health care at home, they have not always had formal home care services. Proprietary home care agencies were virtually nonexistent before Medicare, but their growth has spiraled in the past 2 decades. In 1975, the federal government's Health Services Program was established, making grants available for the establishment, operation, or expansion of programs providing health care at home. In the same year, federal funds were made available for home-based services through the Older Americans Act and Title XX Social Services Act. The primary target groups for home care services are the 15% of the community-living older people who are unable to perform major activities, and those older people who have been discharged "quicker and sicker" to home from acute care hospitals.

Basic services that are provided by home care agencies and covered by Medicare, MCOs, and other health insurance (when qualifying criteria are met) include skilled nursing care, social work services, speech-language therapy, physical therapy, occupational therapy, nutritional counseling, home health aide services, and medical supplies and equipment. All of the following eligibility criteria must be met for Medicare coverage: the person must be homebound (i.e., leaving the home requires considerable and taxing effort); the services must be ordered by a primary care provider; there must be a need for skilled nursing or rehabilitative services; and the person must require intermittent, but not full-time, care. There are two kinds of typical home care recipients who qualify for skilled home care services: (1) those who are homebound but able to manage most of their daily care at some level of independence; and (2) those who, although

homebound and dependent in many functional areas, have assistance from families or have paid help to supplement the skilled care services. Care is provided by or under the direction of a licensed professional nurse. Some of the care, such as bathing, linen changes, range of motion exercises, and assistance with transfers and ambulation, can be given by home health aides. Geropsychiatric nursing services are also covered if the person qualifies, and clinical practice guidelines have been published in the nursing literature for psychiatric home health nurses (Freed and Rice, 1997).

For people who do not meet the Medicare criteria, these same services are available, but must be paid for out-of-pocket; likewise, they also are available to the small percentage of people who qualify under public programs or through private health insurance plans. In addition, home care services that are not defined as skilled are widely used by people who can pay for such services. These services may include companionship, homemaker, and home health aide services and typically provide assistance with ADL, such as personal care and meal preparation.

Formal home care agencies generally have a registered nurse perform the initial assessment and supervise the home health aide. Some agencies, however, are little more than registry services, and do not provide nursing assessments or supervision. Companionship, homemaker, and home health aide services also are available informally on a word-of-mouth basis or through informal registries kept by church groups, community agencies, or offices on aging. In the late 1990s, the cost of this kind of service averaged about $8 to $12 per hour on an informal basis, and about $14 to $20 per hour through a formal agency. Some agencies set a minimum number of hours per day or per week for which payment must be received. Rates usually are higher if more than one person in the household needs assistance.

Adult Day Care Centers

A more recent development in community-based care for older people is the adult day care center. The goals of these programs are to maintain or improve the functional abilities of impaired older people who can benefit from structured activities; to provide relief for caregivers of dependent older adults; to improve the quality of life for impaired older adults; and to delay or prevent the need for institutional care. Participants in adult day care programs usually are impaired to the point that they need supervision or assistance in several functional areas. Most participants have a caregiver who assists with their needs when they are not at the day care center. Although some participants primarily suffer from depression or functional impairments, most suffer from a dementing illness and are cognitively impaired. With regard to functional abilities, many participants are as dependent in their care as people in institutional settings. The major difference between day care participants and residents of nursing homes or assisted living facilities is that day care participants return to their home setting and are cared for by family members when they are not at the adult day care center.

Only a few health insurance policies cover adult day health care programs, and most costs are paid by families. Exceptions to this include the PACE model (discussed in the section on New Models of Health Insurance), in which adult day health centers are the central place of service provision (Branch et al., 1995). Some adult day care programs may have a sliding fee scale, and a few programs may receive subsidies to reduce the cost to families. In some states, public funds are available to pay for these services, especially if the person would otherwise be admitted to a nursing home where the care would be covered by Medicaid. It is likely that additional public funds for adult day care will become available as the long-term care needs of older adults are addressed through public policy.

Day Hospitals

Day hospitals are less common in the United States than adult day care centers, and when they are established, it is often in conjunction with hospitals, nursing homes, or rehabilitation centers. People needing day hospital care usually are quite impaired physically and need substantial amounts of assistance or supervision. The primary reasons people participate in a day hospital program are that they can benefit from therapy programs, and their primary caregivers can obtain relief from responsibilities, perhaps enabling them to be employed in a daytime job. Day hospices are now being developed for people with terminal illnesses, and there may soon be a joint effort to care for physically dependent older people and terminally ill adults in day hospital settings. In the near future, oncology nurses and gerontological nurses might be working together to develop and implement models of day nursing care to meet the needs of impaired adults who want to remain at home.

Respite Services

Despite the increased availability of home care services, most care for dependent older people is still provided by family members. The term "respite" first appeared in the gerontological literature in the late 1970s as the needs of family caregivers were being recognized. Respite services can be provided in the home or in a community or institutional setting, but they are provided for people who are living in a home setting and are being cared for by family members or other unpaid help. The primary goal of respite services is to address the needs of caregivers by allowing them to be relieved periodically from the usual stress and burden of their caregiving responsibilities. Various types of respite services exist: day care, day hospitals, overnight nursing home care, short-term nursing home care, or provision of in-home companions or home health aides.

Health Promotion Programs

In addition to the programs that address the needs of frail older adults, there are numerous settings in which the health care needs of able older adults are addressed. It is becoming increasingly common for nurses to provide health services and perform periodic health screening activities in senior centers and other places where able older adults gather, such as continuing care retirement communities (e.g., Petit, 1994). Because of the availability of portable equipment for measuring blood glucose levels, cholesterol levels, and other indicators of health status, screening programs have become commonplace. By assuming dominant roles in these programs, nurses can make them health promotion programs rather than simply screening or monitoring programs.

With the growing interest in health promotion activities in the United States, older adults are joining the ranks of people who are concerned about their own health and fitness. Organized group activities, such as senior wellness programs, are becoming increasingly common. Among the health promotion activities offered by these programs are blood pressure checks; safe driving courses; smoking cessation classes; flu shots and other immunizations; health screenings, such as for vision and hearing; various types of exercise, such as walking, aerobics, aquatics, or t'ai chi; classes on topics such as nutrition, stress reduction, and general health care; education about and screenings for the early detection of cancer, such as skin or breast cancer; and classes about seasonal health issues, such as hypothermia, heat-related illnesses, and colds and flu.

Many of these senior wellness activities take place in or are sponsored by community-based senior centers that exist in almost every community. Hospitals are becoming more involved in providing this kind of program, and they are employing nurses to address the needs of older adults in the community. In addition, there is a widening array of assisted living and other housing options for older people, and many of these programs sponsor health promotion activities. The development of so-called life-care communities, where older people receive different types of care as their needs change, also has spurred an interest in health promotion activities. With all of these options, the opportunities for nurse-provided health promotion activities also are expanding.

Housing Options and Community-Based Services

Since the 1980s, a wide range of housing options has evolved to address the needs of the growing number of older adults who require assistance with their daily needs but who do not need full-time care. In recent years, environmental psychologists have studied and emphasized how older people adapt to environments that have been designed and built to address their needs. These studies have found that carefully designed environments can assist older people who would have difficulty in conventional housing settings (Kendig and Pynoos, 1996). One result of this emphasis is that a wide variety of housing options is now available for older adults. As of the 1990s, 5% of people aged 65 years or older and 25% of people aged 85 years or older were living in a form of congregate housing (Kendig and Pynoos, 1996). Nurses need to be aware of these options so they can suggest appropriate settings for older adults. Display 22-1 describes various housing options for older adults that are available in most parts of the United States. It is important to keep in mind that this is one of the most rapidly evolving areas of program development for older adults. For example, in the late 1990s, studies were conducted to evaluate attitudes of caregivers and professionals toward a new housing alternative for dependent older adults, called the Homecare Suite, described in Display 22-1 (Altus et al., 1997). Increasing at-

DISPLAY 22-1
Housing Options for Older Adults

Family Residence or Apartment. The older person may own, rent, or live with a family member who owns or rents. He or she lives alone, with a spouse or significant other, or with other, often younger, family members. If assistance is needed, the family provides it, or services are provided by outsiders.

Homecare Suite. A fully accessible, modular apartment is installed in the attached garage of a caregiver's home. The unit is fully insulated and contains its own water, heating, and air conditioning systems. It can be purchased, rented, or leased for whatever length of time it is needed.

Foster-Care or Board-and-Care Home. The older person lives with unrelated people in a private home. Each resident has a private or shared bedroom and shared use of common space, such as a living room and dining room. The foster family or board-and-care operator usually provides meals, housekeeping, and supervision of or assistance with basic and instrumental activities of daily living.

Shared Housing. The older person shares a house or apartment with one or more unrelated people. Each occupant has a private or semiprivate bedroom and shares the rest of the dwelling, expenses, and chores. Offices on aging may coordinate these programs and provide some services.

Congregate Housing. Older persons occupy individual apartments within a specially designed, multi-unit dwelling. Supportive services, such as meals, housekeeping, transportation, and social and recreational activities, are provided.

Retirement Community. Self-sufficient older people live in a specially designed residential development with owned or rented units. Recreational programs and support services (e.g., transportation, laundry, and housekeeping) are usually available.

Life-Care or Continuing-Care Retirement Community. Older adults reside in a residential complex that has been designed to provide a full range of services and accommodations to meet each resident's needs as they change. The development includes independent housing, congregate housing, assisted living, and nursing home care. Each resident usually pays a significant fee and enters into a contract with the organization. This legal agreement guarantees lodging, nursing services, and other health-related services for a specified term or for the remainder of the resident's life. Strict admission criteria may apply.

Assisted Living Facility. Older adults live in their own apartment (usually one or two rooms and a bathroom), and they share common areas for meals and social activities. One to three meals a day are provided. Assistance with laundry, housekeeping, transportation, personal care, and medication administration usually is available, as is some degree of protective supervision and 24-hour emergency services. Fees vary depending on the number of services used, and service agreements may be adjusted as the needs of the resident change. Some assisted living facilities are being designed specifically for people with dementia.

tention is being paid to designing environments that can address the changing needs of older adults so that they can age in place. Nurses can keep up-to-date on such developments by consulting the Educational Resources listed at the end of this chapter.

Many older people are unaware of the types of community-based services for which they may be eligible. Additionally, if community-based services are not culturally relevant, they may not be used by older adults or their families, even when they are aware of their existence.

DISPLAY 22-2
Community Resources for Older Adults

National Eldercare Locator (800-677-1116). This program provides free information about state or local resources in any part of the United States according to the zip code of the location where services are desired. This is a collaborative project of the U.S. Administration on Aging, the National Association of Area Agencies on Aging, and the National Association of State Units on Aging.

Senior Information and Referral Service. This service is often listed in the front of telephone directories under the heading "Community Services," and is sometimes referred to as "Infoline." Callers are given the names of agencies that might address their needs.

Area Agency on Aging. Funded through state, county, and local resources, these agencies provide a range of services. Some area agencies on aging employ social workers and registered nurses to make assessments and provide supportive services (e.g., referrals, case management, assistance with daily living needs). Eligibility for these services is based on economic need and the ability to address the safety and quality-of-life needs of older people living in their home environment.

Senior Centers. Sometimes the sites for hot meals, these community centers provide social, educational, and recreational programs for older adults.

Home-Delivered Meals. This program provides daily home delivery of hot meals to homebound people. Fees generally are based on a sliding scale. Special dietary needs can sometimes be addressed.

Companions and Friendly Visitors. Volunteers visit homebound older adults in their homes. Some also do errands or provide escort service to community activities.

Telephone Reassurance. Volunteers make scheduled, usually daily (sometimes more frequent) telephone calls to older people to provide support and reality orientation.

Personal Emergency Response Systems. This type of program is a home emergency response system that initiates a phone call to designated people when it is activated by a remote control device. Public funding is available in some areas to assist low-income older adults in acquiring such a system.

Energy Assistance Programs. State and local programs offer financial assistance for utility bills for qualifying people. Older adults should check with local utility companies or the local office on aging.

Home Weatherization and Home Repair Service. Home repairs and maintenance (e.g., insulation, window caulking, and installation) are provided for low-income people by contractors paid by government agencies.

Because the use of these resources may improve the quality of life for the older adult and their family caregivers, nurses need to address any lack of information about these services. Also, nurses need to assess barriers to the use of community services, as discussed in Chapter 5. Nurses in all settings have many opportunities to suggest the use of the community-based services that are described in Display 22-2.

Legal and Ethical Aspects of Care

In the past decade, legislative efforts have attempted to address legal and ethical issues related to older adults. For example, in the 1980s, state and federal governments addressed elder abuse through legislation and policy (discussed in Chapter 21). Beginning in the mid-1980s, state and federal governments began to focus on legal and ethical issues relating to patients' rights, residents' rights, end-of-life decisions, and the quality of care provided under Medicaid and Medicare programs. Many of these legislative and policy changes affect dependent older adults to a greater extent than other populations. The next sections review some of the pertinent legal and ethical issues that are relevant to nursing care of older adults. This review focuses on the role of the nurse in addressing these issues. Additional legal and ethical considerations are reviewed in Chapter 21 in relation to vulnerable elders.

Legislation Affecting Nursing Homes

As the regulator of Medicare and Medicaid programs, Congress has the responsibility to ensure that dollars expended for health care are well spent. In response to cited examples of poor quality of care in nursing homes dating back to the 1960s, Congress mandated an Institute of Medicine study that was published in 1986. Recommendations of the study included the increased use of registered nurses, the use of standardized resident assessments, and the implementation of nurse's aide training and certification. Subsequently, the Omnibus Budget Reconciliation Act (OBRA) was passed in 1987 and began to be implemented in 1990. This legislation was the outcome of joint efforts of the Health Care Financing Administration, the National Citizens Coalition for Nursing Home Reform, the American Association for Retired Persons, representatives from the long-term care industry, and health care professionals.

The OBRA states that each resident in a long-term care facility is to be at his or his highest practicable level of physical, mental, and psychosocial well-being, and that the long-term care facility is to accomplish this in an atmosphere that emphasizes residents' rights. To assist facilities in accomplishing this goal, OBRA mandates that all Medicaid- and Medicare-funded facili-

ties use a standardized form, known as the Minimum Data Set (MDS) for Resident Assessment and Care Planning. This form includes a Resident Assessment Instrument (RAI), which is a structured, multidimensional, resident assessment and problem identification system (discussed in Chapter 17). OBRA requires that, within 14 days of admission and at least annually thereafter, nursing facility staff perform a comprehensive, interdisciplinary assessment of every resident. Also, a care plan must be developed from that assessment, with the goal of continually evaluating the resident's highest functional level and preventing any deterioration of that status unless it is assessed and clearly documented that the deterioration was unavoidable. A primary responsibility of nurses is to ensure that the comprehensive assessment is done at the appropriate times. Also, the nurse must ensure that the assessment tool is used as a basis for planning care that addresses the changing needs of the resident. By October of 1991, the RAI was being used in all Medicaid- and Medicare-funded nursing homes; in 1995, a second version of the MDS was developed to replace the first version.

Advance Directives

The Patient Self-Determination Act (PSDA) was enacted by Congress in 1990 as a part of OBRA, and became effective December 1, 1991. This legislation is designed to protect the health care consumer by requiring that all providers of Medicare and Medicaid services (1) inform patients of their right to refuse treatments, (2) provide information about their state's provisions for implementing advance directives, and (3) include documentation of patients' advance directives in their medical records. The PSDA, which also directs participants to provide education for their staff and the community on advance directives, is binding for hospices, hospitals, home health agencies, extended care facilities, and health maintenance organizations. An advance directives protocol for geriatric nursing has recently been published (refer to Mezey et al., 1996). The nursing literature is also addressing such issues as implementing information programs about the PSDA (e.g., Drugay and Gallagher, 1993) and facilitating communication about advance directives and end-of-life care (e.g., Dunlap, 1997; Perrin, 1997).

Advance directives are legally binding documents that allow competent people to document what medical care should be rendered should they become incompetent to make such decisions. There are two types of advance directives: (1) living wills and medical directives, and (2) health care proxy or durable power of attorney for health care. All states and the District of Columbia have laws addressing advance directives, but only about 20% of people in the United States have advance directive documents. State laws vary regarding the scope and other details of advance directives, and nurses need to have up-to-date information about their own state laws. Most states require a periodic update of the advance directives (e.g., every 5 to 7 years). Information about legal requirements for advance directives is widely available in health care institutions. Nursing organizations, such as the National League for Nursing and the American Nurses' Association, also are developing guidelines and recommendations for nursing roles in end-of-life decision making. Information can be obtained from the organizations listed in the Educational Resource section of this chapter.

Most older people are willing to discuss end-of-life issues, but they expect health care professionals to initiate the topic. Also, older adults generally prefer that family members, rather than health care providers, be surrogate decision makers, and they trust that family members will make appropriate choices. In light of this, nurses have an obligation to older adults and their surrogate decision makers to assist them in the decision-making process by providing accurate in-

formation on rights and statutes, answering questions concerning their care, listening to patient and family needs, and acting as liaisons with primary care providers when necessary. Nurses can encourage older people to talk to their families and relay their wishes before a crisis occurs, even if they are reluctant to execute a legal document.

When an advance directive does exist, it is the nurse's responsibility to inform other members of the health care team and to make certain that it is readily accessible in the chart. Each caregiver should read the directive and know what it covers. The nurse also should make certain that the older person's family, especially the designated surrogate, is aware of the document and its contents. An interdisciplinary team, composed of a social worker, minister, therapists, nurses, and primary care provider, can provide information and support, and may benefit surrogate decision makers by relieving them of guilt they may experience when making and implementing difficult decisions.

Living Wills and Medical Directives

Living wills evolved as a component of right-to-die statutes, and many changes have been instituted since the first legislation was enacted in 1976 in California. Living wills are now recognized in every state and in the District of Columbia. Living wills are legal documents whose purpose is to allow people to specify what type of medical treatment they would want if they became incapacitated and terminally ill. People must be competent to initiate a living will, and they can revoke it after they have written it. Living wills should not be misunderstood as the equivalent of a "do not resuscitate" order. Although living wills do affirm the right of the person to refuse treatment, the precise treatments are not always specified. Also, the living will applies only to situations in which the person is considered "terminally ill," and there may be disagreement about whether this criterion is met. Some states require that the living will document the authorization of certain procedures, such as the withholding or withdrawal of artificially or technologically supplied hydration or nutrition.

Advance medical directives are similar to living wills, but they are broader. In addition to focusing on the right to refuse treatments, medical directives address the person's desires for medical treatment that should be provided. These directives can provide instructions about specific interventions, such as antibiotics, cardiopulmonary resuscitation, and food and nutrition. They can also address circumstances (e.g., irreversible brain damage) that might not be defined as a terminal illness. These documents can provide reassurance to people who fear that medical treatments will be withheld. Although they do guarantee that the person's preferences will be considered, they do not guarantee that a medical intervention will be provided regardless of the circumstances. Because of the inability to predict medical advances that might become available, and because of the changing health condition of the person executing the document, medical directives should be reviewed periodically. Given the restrictions of living wills and the complexity of medical directives, older people who wish to use them should be encouraged to consult their attorneys and to fill out a durable power of attorney for health care as well. In this way, the person will have legally recognized advance directives that facilitate decision making about end-of-life issues.

Durable Power of Attorney for Health Care

A durable power of attorney for health care is an advance directive that takes effect whenever an adult cannot, for any reason, provide informed consent for health care treatment decisions. It allows a surrogate health care decision maker, also called a health care proxy, to be named by the person before he or she becomes incapable of directing his or her own care. The document usually provides the surrogate with

written guidelines stating the person's wishes, such as with regard to termination of life support. It is imperative that the health care proxy have a copy of the living will and any medical directives. The health care proxy also should discuss end-of-life treatment issues with the person. Like other powers of attorney, the durable power of attorney for health care must be initiated when the person is competent. The durable power of attorney for health care can go into effect immediately, and the person does not have to be diagnosed as terminally ill. Because language can sometimes be vague, it is advisable to encourage older people to discuss their wishes with their primary care provider, other health care workers, and their designated surrogate before a crisis develops. As stated earlier, it is advisable to offer the support of an interdisciplinary team to the surrogate decision maker, particularly when difficult end-of-life decisions are being discussed.

Competency, Capacity, and Autonomy

Competency is a legal term that refers to the ability to fulfill one's role and handle one's affairs in an adequate manner. If a person has been designated as incompetent, a guardianship or conservatorship is established to manage and assume responsibility for all personal and financial decisions. Adults are presumed to be competent to make decisions concerning their own treatment, but the patient's family or other caregivers may seek to have the person declared incompetent. Before a guardian can be appointed, a competency hearing is held in a probate court. Nurses may be called on to participate in these hearings. If the person is declared by the court to be incompetent, the judge may assign either a partial or a full guardianship. With a partial guardianship, the incompetent person is permitted to make limited decisions. When a full guardianship is assigned, the person loses all of his or her rights to make such decisions. The role of the nurse in determining competency is discussed in Chapters 5 and 21, and models for assessment can be found in the nursing literature (e.g., Weisensee et al., 1994).

Capacity and incapacity are terms that refer to the ability of a person to consent to or refuse a specific medical treatment or procedure. There are no legal guidelines for determining decision-making capacity, but health care institutions may have procedures, usually involving an interdisciplinary team process, for assessing someone's decision-making capacity. It is widely agreed that capacity is based on the following characteristics: (1) appreciation of the right to make a choice, (2) understanding of the risks and benefits of the medical intervention and lack of intervention, (3) ability to communicate about the decision, (4) stability over time, and (5) consistency with the person's usual beliefs and values. Determination of decision-making capacity should not be based on a particular diagnosis, nor should it be decided on the basis of advanced age. Rather, determination of decision-making capacity should be based on a careful evaluation of the person's ability to understand the issues involved in one specific decision-making situation and to communicate about these issues. For example, a person with dementia may be able to participate in a decision about a health care proxy but not be able to participate in a complex decision about medical interventions for prostate cancer that may or may not progress. In this situation, it might be reasonable for the person to designate his wife or one of his children to make the treatment decision for him. An article by Mezey et al. (1997) provides an excellent overview of issues and nursing responsibilities related to assessment of decision-making capacity.

Autonomy is the personal freedom to direct one's own life as long as it does not impinge on the rights of others. An autonomous person is capable of rational thought and is able to recognize the need for problem solving. The person can identify the problem, search for alternatives, and select a solution that allows their continued personal freedom, as long as it does not cause any harm to another's rights or property. Loss of autonomy and, therefore, loss of independence, is a very real fear among the elderly. Nurses have a responsibility to older people and to their families to assist them, often as impartial mediators, when issues concerning personal autonomy arise. However, nurses must refer older people to the appropriate community agencies for further evaluation when patient safety becomes an issue. For a case example and further discussion of autonomy and other legal issues, refer to Chapter 21.

Cultural Considerations

Health care providers need to be aware of the strong Anglo-centric bias of certain laws, such as the PSDA. There are many significant cultural differences with regard to patterns of decision making about medical interventions and health care services. For example, some families may believe it is a sign of respect to protect an elder from the burdens of receiving information about their health status and making decisions about medical interventions and long-term care plans. This may present a conflict for health care professionals who believe that all competent adults are entitled to information about their own health. It is imperative that health care providers determine culturally influenced patterns of decision making with such questions as "Whom do you talk to about your health care decisions?" or "Who will help you decide about where you are going to live?" In some situations, it may be appropriate to ask a family member about decision-making patterns. It is especially important to be sensitive to cultural differences when discussing advance directives and end-of-life issues. The Culture Box on page 674 summarizes some cultural variations in decision-making patterns and in perspectives regarding advance directives. Practical information about consent forms, decision-making patterns, and end-of-life

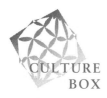

Cultural Considerations Relating to Legal and Ethical Aspects of Care

Decision-Making Patterns

- In many cultures, decisions regarding elder care and health care are based on the good of the family.
- In many cultures, it is a sign of respect to protect elders from the burden and responsibility of making decisions about their own health care.
- Families in some cultures expect that medical information will be given to the designated family authority figure, who then will decide what to do with the information.
- In many cultures, the opinions of all adult family members are acknowledged, but there is a designated authority figure who ultimately makes the final decision.
- In many cultures, the primary health care provider is seen as the authority figure who should make decisions based on his or her knowledge. In such instances, it is not considered necessary or even desirable to discuss options with patients or their surrogates.
- In a study of frail older people, the following percentages of participants expressed their own health care wishes, in contrast to having an alternative decision-maker: 91% of Whites, 85% of Hispanics, 83% of Asians, and 67% of Blacks (Hornung et al., 1998).

Legal and Ethical Aspects of Care

- Autonomy and informed consent are Anglo-centric concepts that are not a part of many cultures.
- People should have the right to refuse to be informed of their medical conditions and to request that health care decisions be discussed with the designated family authority figure, even when the person is competent (Cheng, 1997).
- Because Native Americans tend to see the cycle of birth, life, and death as natural, they may see no need for advance directives.
- Because some people may be suspicious of written documents, health care providers may need to rely on discussions with designated surrogates for communication of the authentic wishes of the patient (Hepburn and Reed, 1995).

End-of-Life Issues

- In some cultures, it is taboo to discuss impending death with the person who is terminally ill or to discuss end-of-life issues in advance of need.
- Although it might be taboo for Asians to discuss end-of-life treatment issues, it may be acceptable and common to discuss funeral arrangements and preferences for burial (Cheng, 1997).
- Because of the complexity of end-of-life issues and culturally influenced styles of communicating about these issues, health care providers may need to involve cultural interpreters in discussions about these decisions (Hepburn and Reed, 1995).

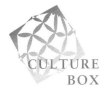

CULTURE
BOX

Cultural Considerations Relating to Legal and Ethical Aspects of Care (Continued)

- Health care providers need to determine the expectations of family members and other caregivers during terminal stages of illness.
- Health care providers need to assess whether there are culturally based rituals that are done at the time of death that need to be addressed in a health care setting.

issues as viewed from many cultural perspectives is described in an excellent pocket guide, written by nurses, entitled *Culture and Nursing Care* (Lipson et al., 1996).

Chapter Summary

Medicare and Medicaid programs were enacted in 1965 to provide medical and long-term care services to older adults and poor people. Before the 1980s, there were very few major changes in these programs, and very few options available for older adults. During the 1990s, health insurance for older adults became one of the most rapidly evolving areas of health care. Long-term care and other health services for older adults are now undergoing major changes, and these changes are likely to continue well into the 21st century. Older adults now have several options for health insurance and many options for health care services in a variety of settings. Nurses, too, have many opportunities for providing numerous types of health care services to older adults in a variety of settings.

During the 1990s, nurses and other health care professionals have been affected by laws, such as the PSDA and the OBRA. As a result of these laws, health care professionals must be prepared to discuss advance directives, and nursing homes must meet certain requirements with regard to the care of residents. Also, nurses must be familiar with issues related to competency, capacity, and autonomy. Concepts asso-

ciated with the PSDA are strongly rooted in the Anglo-centric perspective, and they may be difficult to apply to people of non-Anglo cultures. Nurses need to be culturally sensitive in identifying and addressing these issues.

Critical Thinking Exercises

1. You are working at a senior center and several of the people there ask you whether they should sign up for the new managed care program that is being advertised in various brochures. What approach would you use in providing information to assist them with decision making?

2. Mrs. F., who is 82 years old, is a resident in the skilled care section of the nursing home where you work. She had been living alone in her own home before being admitted to the hospital with a fractured hip 4 weeks ago. She has regained much of her independence and walks with a walker and one-person assist. She expects to ambulate independently using a walker within 2 weeks, at which time she expects to return to her own home. She tells you she is thinking about moving from her home, but that she doesn't need a nursing home. She asks you what kind of services would be available in her own home and what kind of housing options are available. What additional information would you want before you answered her questions? What information would you share with her? What suggestions would you make?

3. A Mexican American woman, aged 78 years old, is being admitted to the hospital with hemiplegia following a stroke. There are no advance directives on her chart. What information would you want to know before you approached her about a living will and durable power of attorney for health care? How would you explain these documents to her?

Educational Resources

American Association of Retired Persons
601 E Street, NW, Washington, DC 20049
(202) 434–2277
www.aarp.org

American Bar Association, Senior Lawyers Division
750 North Lake Shore Drive, Chicago, IL 60611
(312) 988–5000
www.abanet.org/srlawyers/home.html

American Nurses Association (ANA)
600 Maryland Ave., #100 West, Washington, DC 20024
(800) 274–4262
www.nursingworld.org

Black Elderly Legal Assistance Support Project
National Bar Association, 1225 11th Street, NW, Washington, DC 20001
(202) 842–3900

Health Care Financing Administration
U.S. Department of Health and Human Services, 7500 Security Boulevard, Baltimore, MD 21244–1850
Medicare Hotline (800) 638–6833; TDD (800) 820–1202
www.hcfa.gov

Health Insurance Association of America
555 13th Street, NW, Washington, DC 20004
(202) 824–1600

National Association of Professional Geriatric Care Managers
1604 North Country Club Road, Tucson, AZ 85716–3102
(602) 881–8008

National Gerontological Nursing Association (NGNA)
7250 Parkway Drive, #510, Hangover, MD 21076
(800) 723–0560
www.nursingcenter.com/people/nrsorgs/ngna

National Senior Citizens Law Center
1101 14th Street, NW, Suite 400, Washington, DC 20005
(202) 289–6976
www.nsclc.org

References

Altus, D. E., Mathews, R. M., & Kosloski, K. D. (1997). Examining attitudes toward the Homecare Suite: A new housing alternative for elders. *Journal of Applied Gerontology, 16*, 459–476.

American Association of Retired Persons (AARP), Minority Affairs Initiative. (1987). *A portrait of older minorities: Minority elderly in California*. Washington, DC: AARP.

Bassford, T. L. (1995). Health status of Hispanic elders. *Clinics in Geriatric Medicine, 11*(1), 25–38.

Beck, C., & Chumbler, N. (1997). Planning for the future of long-term care: Consumers, providers, and purchasers. *Journal of Gerontological Nursing, 23*(8), 6–13.

Branch, L. G., Coulam, R. F., & Zimmerman, Y. A. (1995). The PACE evaluation: Initial findings. *The Gerontologist, 35*, 349–359.

Cheng, B. K. (1997). Cultural clash between providers of majority culture and patients of Chinese culture. *Journal of Long-Term Home Health Care, 16*(2), 39–43.

Chenier, M. C. (1997). Review and analysis of caregiver burden and nursing home placement. *Geriatric Nursing, 18*, 121–126.

Cohen, C. A., Gold, D. P., Shulman, K. I., Wortley, J. T., McDonald, G., & Wargon, M. (1993). Factors determining the decision to institutionalize dementing individuals: A prospective study. *The Gerontologist, 33*, 714–720.

Cohen, M. A. (1998). Emerging trends in the finance and delivery of long-term care: Public and private opportunities and challenges. *The Gerontologist, 38*(1), 80–89.

Colenda, C. C., & Sherman, F. T. (1998). Managed Medicare: An overview for the primary care physician. *Geriatrics, 53*(1), 57–63.

Coward, R. T., Netzer, J. K., & Mullens, R. A. (1996). Residential differences in the incidence of nursing home admissions across a six-year period. *Journal of Gerontology: Social Sciences, 51B*, S258–S267.

Damron-Rodriguez, J., Wallace, S. P., & Kingston, R. (1994). Service utilization and minority elderly: Appropriateness, accessibility and acceptability. *Gerontology and Geriatrics Education, 15*(1), 45–64.

Drugay, M., & Gallagher, G. (1993). Patient self-determination act: Implementing an information program in a nursing facility. *Journal of Gerontological Nursing, 19*(12), 29–34.

Dunlap, R. K. (1997). Teaching advance directives: The why, when, and how. *Journal of Gerontological Nursing, 23*(12), 11–16.

Freed, P., & Rice, R. (1997). Managing mental illness at home—Part II: Clinical guidelines for psychiatric home health nurses. *Geriatric Nursing, 18*, 178–179, 181.

Freedman, V. A. (1996). Family structure and the risk of nursing home admission. *Journal of Gerontology: Social Sciences, 51B*, S61–S69.

Haack, M. R. (1997). Payment incentives and conflicts of interest within a managed care environment. *Journal of Gerontological Nursing, 23*(8), 22–25.

Hepburn, K., & Reed, R. (1995). Ethical and clinical issues with Native-American elders. *Clinics in Geriatric Medicine, 11*(1), 97–111.

Hornung, C. A., Eleazer, G. P., Strothers, H. S., Wieland, G. D., Eng, C., McCann, R., & Sapir, M. (1998). Ethnicity and decision-makers in a group of frail older people. *Journal of the American Geriatrics Society, 46*, 280–286.

Inouye, S. K., Acampora, D., Miller, R. L., Fulmer, T., Hurst, L. D., & Cooney, L. M. (1993a). The Yale geriatric care program: A model of care to prevent functional decline in hospitalized elderly patients. *Journal of the American Geriatrics Society, 41*, 1345–1352.

Inouye, S. K., Wagner, D. R., Acampora, D., Horwitz, R. I., Cooney, L. M., & Tinetti, M. E. (1993b). A controlled trial of a nursing-centered intervention in hospitalized elderly medical patients: The Yale geriatric care program. *Journal of the American Geriatrics Society, 41*, 1353–1360.

Kane, R. L., & Kane, R. A. (1997). Long-term care. In C. K. Cassel, H. J. Cohen, E. B. Larson, D. E. Meier, N. M. Resnick, L. Z. Rubenstein, & L. B. Sorenson (Eds.), *Geriatric medicine* (3rd ed., pp. 81–96). New York: Springer.

Kendig, H., & Pynoos, J. (1996). Housing. In J. E. Birren (Ed.), *Encyclopedia of gerontology: Age, aging, and the aged* (Vol. 1, pp. 703–713). San Diego: Academic Press.

Kim, K. S. (1997). Long-term care for the Korean American elderly: An exploration for a better way of services. *Journal of Long-Term Home Health Care, 16*(20), 35–38.

Kim, P. K., & Kim. J-S. (1992). Korean elderly: Policy, program, and practice implications. In S. M. Furoto, R. Biswas, D. K. Chung, K. Murase, & F. Ross-Sheriff (Eds.), *Social work practice with Asian Americans* (pp. 227–239). Newbury Park, CA: Sage.

Landefeld, C. S., Palmer, R. M., Kresevic, D. M., Fortinsky, R. H., & Kowal, J. (1995). A randomized trial of care in a hospital medical unit especially designed to improve the functional outcomes of acutely ill older patients. *The New England Journal of Medicine, 332*, 1338–1344.

Leff, B., Burton, L., Bynum, J. W., Harper, M., Greenough, W. B., Steinwachs, D., & Burton, J. R. (1997). Prospective evaluation of clinical criteria to select older persons with acute medical illness for care in a hypothetical home hospital. *Journal of the American Geriatrics Society, 45*, 1066–1073.

Lieberman, M. A., & Kramer, J. H. (1991). Factors affecting decisions to institutionalize demented elderly. *The Gerontologist, 31*, 371–374.

Lipson, J. G., Dibble, S. L., & Minarik, P. A. (1996). *Culture & nursing care: A pocket guide.* San Francisco: UCSF Nursing Press.

Liu, K., & Manton, K. G. (1984). The characteristics and utilization pattern of an admission cohort of nursing home patients (II). *The Gerontologist, 24*, 70–76.

Liu, K., Perozek, M., & Manton, K. (1993). Catastrophic acute and long-term care costs: Risks faced by disabled elderly persons. *The Gerontologist, 33*, 299–307.

Malloy, C. (1997). Managed care: What is its impact on nursing education and practice? *Journal of Gerontological Nursing, 23*(8), 26–31.

McConnel, C. E. (1984). A note on the lifetime risk of nursing home residency. *The Gerontologist, 24*, 193–198.

Melillo, K. D. (1996). Medicare and Medicaid: Similarities and differences. *Journal of Gerontological Nursing, 22*(7), 12–21.

Mezey, M., Bottrell, M. M., Ramsey, G., & The NICHE Faculty. (1996). Advance directives protocol: Nurses helping to protect patient's rights. *Geriatric Nursing, 17*, 204–210.

Mezey, M., Mitty, E., & Ramsey, G. (1997). Assessment of decision-making capacity: Nursing's role. *Journal of Gerontological Nursing, 23*(3), 28–35.

Nielsen, J., Henderson, C., Cox, M., Williams, S., & Green, P. (1996). Characteristics of caregivers and factors contributing to institutionalization. *Geriatric Nursing, 17*, 124–127.

Perrin, K. O. (1997). Giving voice to the wishes of elders for end-of-life care. *Journal of Gerontological Nursing, 23*(3), 18–27.

Petit, J. M. (1994). Continuing care retirement communities and the role of the wellness nurse. *Geriatric Nursing, 15*(1), 28–31.

Rousseau, P. (1995). Native-American elders: Health care status. *Clinics in Geriatric Medicine, 11*(1), 83–95.

Rubin, R. M., & Koelin, K. (1993). Out-of-pocket health expenditure differentials between elderly and non-elderly households. *The Gerontologist, 33*, 595–602.

Rudberg, M. A., Sager, M. A., & Zhang, J. (1996). Risk factors for nursing home use after hospitalization for medical illness. *Journal of Gerontology: Medical Sciences, 51A*, M189–M194.

Scott, W. K., Edwards, K. B., Davis, D. R., Cornman, C. B., & Macera, C. A. (1997). Risk of institutionalization among community long-term care clients with dementia. *The Gerontologist, 37*, 46–51.

U.S. House Select Committee on Aging. (1986). *The rights of America's institutionalized aged: Lost in confinement.* (Committee Publication No. 99-543). Washington, DC: U.S. Government Printing Office.

Wallace, S. P., Levy-Storms, L., Kington, R. S., & Andersen, R. M. (1998). The persistence of race and ethnicity in the use of long-term care. *Journal of Gerontology: Social Sciences, 53B,* S104–S112.

Weaverdyck, S. E., Wittle, A., & Delaski-Smith, D. (1998). In-place progression: Lessons learned from the Huron Woods' Staff. *Journal of Gerontological Nursing, 24*(1), 31–39.

Weisensee, M. G., Kjervik, D. K., & Anderson, J. B. (1994). Impairment of short-term memory as a criterion for de-termination of incompetency. *Geriatric Nursing, 15,* 35–40.

Whitlatch, C. J., & Noelker, L. S. (1996). Caregiving and caring. In J. E. Birren (Ed.), *Encyclopedia of gerontology: Age, aging, and the aged* (Vol. 1, pp. 253–268). San Diego: Academic Press.

Wolinsky, F. D., Callahan, C. M., Fitzgerald, J. F., & John-son, R. J. (1993). Changes in functional status and the risks of subsequent nursing home placement and death. *Journal of Gerontology: Social Sciences, 48,* S93–S101.

Appendix

Review of Physiologic Aspects of Function

This material, which is divided into 11 sections, reviews the aspects of physiologic function that were discussed in Parts III and IV of this text. The purpose of this review is to provide an outline summary of the most important considerations regarding various aspects of physiologic function. The numbers in parentheses refer to the tables and displays that provide more detailed summaries of the topic. This outline can be used in conjunction with the tables and displays in the chapters as a guide to applying the functional consequences theory to specific aspects of physiologic function.

I. Hearing

Age-Related Changes (Table 6-1)
- External ear: thicker hair, thinner skin, increased keratin
- Middle ear: less resilient tympanic membrane, calcified ossicles, stiffer muscles and ligaments
- Inner Ear: Fewer neurons and hair cells, diminished blood supply, degeneration of spiral ganglion

Risk Factors
- Prolonged exposure to noise
- Genetic predisposition to otosclerosis
- Past or present use of ototoxic medications (Display 6-1)
- Systemic diseases (e.g., diabetes, Paget's disease)
- Auditory diseases (e.g., Ménière's disease)
- Background noise

Negative Functional Consequences (Table 6-1)
- Presbycusis (diminished ability to hear high-pitched sounds, especially in the presence of background noise)
- Predisposition to impacted cerumen
- Diminished sensory input, impaired social interaction

Nursing Assessment: Interview Questions (Display 6-2)
- Past and present risk factors (e.g., use of ototoxic medications, noise exposure, family history of otosclerosis)
- Attitudes about hearing aids if impairment is present
- Impact of hearing impairment on communication and quality of life

Nursing Assessment: Observations
- Behavioral cues to impaired hearing (Display 6-3)
- Otoscopic examination for impacted cerumen (Display 6-4)
- Tuning fork tests for hearing (Display 6-4)

Nursing Interventions
- Use of techniques to enhance communication with individuals who have a hearing impairment (Display 6-6)
- Removal of impacted cerumen
- Medical evaluation of underlying diseases and ototoxic medications
- Education about the use and care of a hearing aid (Display 6-5)
- Evaluation at a speech and hearing center for aural rehabilitation and hearing aids (Table 6-2, Display 6-5)

- Use of assistive hearing devices by nurses for people who are hearing impaired

Positive Functional Consequences
- Improved communication
- Improved social interactions
- Safer functional level

II. Vision

Age-Related Changes (Table 7-1)
- Corneal yellowing and opacity; changes in curvature
- Increase in lens size and density
- Decreased pupillary size; atrophy of ciliary muscle
- Fewer photoreceptor cells and a diminished blood supply in the retina

Risk Factors
- Environmental factors (e.g., glare, poor lighting)
- Diseases affecting vision (e.g., cataracts, glaucoma, macular degeneration, diabetes)

Negative Functional Consequences (Table 7-1)
- Presbyopia (diminished ability to focus on near objects)
- Need for 3 to 5 times more light than previously
- Increased sensitivity to glare
- Slowed response to changes in illumination
- Altered color perception
- Difficulty with night driving
- Increased risk for unsafe mobility
- Increased difficulty in performing activities of daily living (ADL)

Nursing Assessment: Interview Questions
(Display 7-1)
- Past and present risk factors and diseases that affect vision
- Influence of vision changes on performance of ADL
- Source of and attitudes about ophthalmologic evaluation
- Attitudes regarding use of low-vision aids

Nursing Assessment: Observations
- Behavioral cues to visual function (Display 7-2)
- Vision screening tests (Display 7-3)

Nursing Interventions
- Referrals for further evaluation (Display 7-4)
- Aids for improving visual performance (Displays 7-5 and 7-6)
- Provision of optimal illumination (Display 7-7)
- Environmental modifications (Display 7-8)

Positive Functional Consequences
- Improved visual performance
- Increased safety and improved overall ability to perform ADL
- Improved quality of life

III. Digestion and Nutrition

Age-Related Changes
- Less efficient chewing, diminished taste sensation
- Loss of elasticity in intestinal wall
- Slower motility throughout gastrointestinal tract
- Need for fewer calories but same amount of nutrients

Risk Factors
- Absence of teeth
- Conditions that may lead to nutritional deficiencies (Table 8-1)
- Medication-food interactions (Table 8-2)
- Adverse medication effects that can influence nutrition (Table 8-3)
- Any functional impairment interfering with the ability to obtain, prepare, consume, or enjoy food
- Psychosocial and environmental factors (e.g., depression, isolation)
- Cultural factors (Culture Box page 239)

Negative Functional Consequences
- Decreased absorption of iron, folic acid, vitamin B_{12}
- Malnutrition and dehydration with subsequent cognitive impairments
- Tendency to develop constipation as a result of risk factors

Nursing Assessment: Interview Questions
(Display 8-1)
- Usual nutrient intake and eating pattern
- Risks that interfere with any aspect of eating
- Symptoms of gastrointestinal dysfunction

Nursing Assessment: Observations
- All aspects of obtaining, preparing, eating, and enjoying food (Display 8-2)
- Behavioral cues to nutrition and digestion (Display 8-2)
- Physical examination and laboratory data regarding nutritional status (Display 8-3)

Nursing Interventions
- Education regarding nutrition and digestion (Display 8-4)
- Daily food guide for older adults (Display 8-5)
- Environmental modifications in institutional settings
- Referrals to community resources (e.g., home-delivered meals, group meal programs)

Positive Functional Consequences
- Optimal nutrition
- Prevention of constipation
- Improved overall functional level, including mental performance and psychosocial function
- Improved quality of life

IV. Urinary Elimination

Age-Related Changes (Table 9-2)
- Kidney: Diminished blood flow, decreased number of nephrons, changes in tubules
- Urinary muscles: Hypertrophy of bladder muscle, replacement of smooth muscle with connective tissue, relaxation of pelvic floor
- Neurologic control: Degenerative changes in cerebral cortex

Risk Factors
- Genitourinary disorders (e.g., prostatic hyperplasia)
- Systemic diseases, functional impairments
- Any factor that interferes with socially appropriate urinary elimination
- Environmental factors (Display 9-1)
- Medications (Table 9-1)

Negative Functional Consequences (Table 9-2)
- Decreased glomerular filtration rate, decreased efficiency of homeostatic mechanisms
- Delayed excretion of water-soluble medications

- Diminished bladder capacity, urinary urgency and frequency
- Decrease in interval between the signal of the need to void and the actual emptying of the bladder
- Chronic residual urine and consequent predisposition to bacteriuria
- Urinary incontinence (Table 9-3)

Nursing Assessment: Interview Questions
(Display 9-2)
- Risk factors that increase the potential for incontinence
- Risk factors that influence renal function and the maintenance of homeostasis
- Symptoms of impaired urinary elimination
- Misunderstandings about urinary elimination; attitudes about incontinence
- Psychosocial consequences of incontinence

Nursing Assessment: Observations
- Barriers that interfere with socially appropriate urinary elimination (Display 9-1)
- Signs of impaired urinary elimination (Display 9-3)

Nursing Interventions
- Education related to urinary elimination (Display 9-4)
- Environmental modifications to prevent incontinence (Display 9-5)
- Medications to control incontinence (Table 9-4)
- Pelvic floor exercises (Display 9-6)
- Continence training programs (Displays 9-7 and 9-8)
- Incontinence aids and equipment (Display 9-9)

Positive Functional Consequences
- Prevention or alleviation of incontinence
- Improved psychosocial function and quality of life

V. Cardiovascular Function

Age-Related Changes (Table 10-1)
- Arterial stiffening
- Hypertrophy of the left ventricular wall
- Alterated conduction mechanism
- Thicker, less elastic, more dilated veins

- Increased peripheral resistance
- Altered baroreflex mechanism

Risk Factors
- Obesity
- Cigarette smoking
- Dietary habits that contribute to hyperlipidemia
- Inactivity
- Advanced age
- Conditions that predispose the person to postural hypotension (Display 10-1)

Negative Functional Consequences (Table 10-1)
- Atherosclerosis
- Increased blood pressure (Table 10-2)
- Diminished adaptive response to intense exercise
- Increased susceptibility to cardiac arrhythmias
- Increased susceptibility to postural hypotension
- Decreased cerebral blood flow
- Varicosities, increased susceptibility to venous stasis

Nursing Assessment: Interview Questions
- Detection of postural hypotension and cardiovascular disease (Display 10-2)
- Risks for cardiovascular disease (Displays 10-2 and 10-4)

Nursing Assessment: Observations
- Heart rate and rhythm
- Lying and standing blood pressure measurements (Display 10-3)

Nursing Interventions
- Nursing decisions regarding management of hypertension (Display 10-5)
- Education regarding risks for cardiovascular disease (Display 10-6)
- Education regarding postural hypotension (Display 10-7)

Positive Functional Consequences
- Improved cardiovascular performance
- Optimal oxygen perfusion of all body organs and tissues
- Diminished risk for falls
- Improved quality of life

VI. RESPIRATORY FUNCTION

Age-Related Changes (Table 11-2)
- Upper airway changes: calcification of cartilage, altered neuromuscular function and reflexes
- Increased anteroposterior chest diameter
- Chest wall stiffness, weakened muscles
- Enlarged alveoli; thinner alveolar walls
- Alterations in lung volumes and airflow (Table 11-1)

Risk Factors
- Tobacco smoking
- Occupational hazards (Display 11-1)

Negative Functional Consequences (Table 11-2)
- Mouth breathing, diminished coughing, decreased efficiency of gag reflex
- Increased use of accessory muscles, increase in the energy expended for respiratory function
- Diminished efficiency of gas exchange, decreased arterial PO_2 levels
- Decreased vital capacity, slight decrease in overall efficiency
- Increased susceptibility to lower respiratory infections

Nursing Assessment: Interview Questions (Display 11-2)
- Overall respiratory function
- Smoking, attitudes regarding smoking

Nursing Assessment: Observations
- Physical assessment findings similar to those for an adult of any age
- Pneumonia or tuberculosis that may not be accompanied by usual signs and symptoms

Nursing Interventions
- Education about pneumonia and influenza (Display 11-3)
- Education about cigarette smoking (Display 11-4)

Positive Functional Consequences
- Decreased susceptibility to upper respiratory infections (a functional consequence of age-related changes, even without interventions)
- Prevention of lower respiratory infections, and early detection if infections do occur

VII. Mobility and Safety

Age-Related Changes (Table 12-2)
- Diminished muscle mass
- Degenerative changes in joints
- Osteoporosis (Display 12-1, Table 12-1)
- Changes in central nervous system

Risk Factors for Osteoporosis (Display 12-2)
- Female, White, thin, small bones
- Inadequate calcium intake
- Immobility
- Advanced age

Risk Factors for Falls and Fractures
(Display 12-3)
- Age-related changes in gait, sensory function, and central nervous system
- Medical conditions and psychosocial impairments
- Medications
- Environmental influences

Negative Functional Consequences (Table 12-2)
- Diminished muscle strength, endurance, and coordination
- Increased difficulty in performing ADL
- Increased susceptibility to falls
- Increased susceptibility to fractures

Nursing Assessment: Interview Questions
(Display 12-4)
- Overall musculoskeletal performance
- Risks for osteoporosis (Display 12-2)
- Risks for falls (Display 12-3)

Nursing Assessment: Observations
- Environmental influences (Display 12-5)
- ADL and IADL (Displays 17-1 and 17-2)

Nursing Interventions
- Interventions for postmenopausal osteoporosis: medications, calcium and vitamin D supplementation, lifestyle interventions
- Education regarding interventions for osteoporosis (Alternative box page 366)
- Prevention of falls (Display 12-6)

Positive Functional Consequences
- Prevention of falls
- Prevention of fractures
- Improved quality of life
- Decreased health care expenditures

VIII. Skin and Its Appendages

Age-Related Changes (Table 13-1)
- Decreased rate of epidermal proliferation
- Thinner dermis, flattened dermal-epidermal junction
- Diminished moisture content
- Decreased dermal blood supply
- Decreased number of sweat and sebaceous glands
- Decreased number of melanocytes and Langerhans' cells

Risk Factors
- Exposure to ultraviolet rays (sunlight)
- Adverse medication effects
- Personal hygiene practices
- Immobility

Negative Functional Consequences (Table 13-1)
- Dry skin, discomfort
- Irregular pigmentation
- Increased susceptibility to injury, bruising, mechanical stress, ultraviolet radiation effects, blister formation
- Delayed wound healing, increased susceptibility to infection
- Decreased tactile sensitivity, increased susceptibility to burns
- Decreased sweating and shivering, increased susceptibility to hypothermia and hyperthermia
- Increased susceptibility to skin cancer

Nursing Assessment: Interview Questions
(Display 13-1)
- Risk factors and abnormal conditions
- Personal care practices

Nursing Assessment: Observations
(Display 13-2)
- Examination of the skin
- Examination of hair and nails
- Personal care practices
- Skin lesions common in older adults (Table 13-2)

Nursing Interventions (Display 13-3)
- Maintenance of healthy skin
- Personal care practices
- Avoidance of risks

Positive Functional Consequences
- Improved comfort level
- Prevention of burns and injuries

IX. Sleep and Rest

Age-Related Changes (Table 14-1)
- Alterations in sleep stages
- Decreased time spent in deep sleep and dream stages

Risk Factors
- Behaviors based on myths and misunderstandings
- Psychosocial influences (e.g., dementia, depression)
- Environmental influences
- Sleep apnea
- Lack of daytime activity or stimulation
- Physiologic disturbances (Table 14-2)
- Adverse medication effects (Table 14-3)

Negative Functional Consequences (Table 14-1)
- Longer time needed to fall asleep
- Aroused more easily
- Different quality of sleep
- Same quantity of sleep during 24 hours
- More time spent in bed

Nursing Assessment: Interview Questions
(Display 14-1)
- Perception of quality and quantity of sleep
- Pre-bedtime activities
- Sleep pattern and habits

Nursing Assessment: Observations
- Pre-bedtime activities
- Actual sleep pattern (observed in institutional settings)

Nursing Interventions
- Education about age-related changes affecting sleep
- Measures to promote healthy sleep (Display 14-2)
- Chemical agents (L-tryptophan and melatonin)
- Considerations regarding hypnotics (Display 14-3, Table 14-4)
- Relaxation and mental techniques to promote sleep (Display 14-4)
- Environmental modifications

Positive Functional Consequences
- Diminished daytime drowsiness
- Improved quality of life and overall functional level

X. Thermoregulation

Age-Related Changes
- Diminished subcutaneous tissue
- Decreased efficiency of vasoconstriction
- Delayed and diminished shivering
- Decreased peripheral circulation
- Decreased efficiency of sweating
- Diminished ability to acclimatize to heat

Risk Factors (Table 15-1)
- Dehydration, electrolyte imbalance
- Aged 75 years or older
- Systemic diseases or physiologic disturbances
- Inactivity, immobility
- Alcohol consumption
- Adverse medication effects

Negative Functional Consequences
- Lower normal range of body temperature
- Increased susceptibility to hypothermia and heat-related illnesses
- Diminished febrile response to infection

Nursing Assessment: Interview Questions
(Display 15-1)
- Risks for hypothermia and hyperthermia (Table 15-1)

Nursing Assessment: Observations
(Display 15-1)
- Baseline body temperature and normal diurnal fluctuation
- Altered febrile response to illness

Nursing Interventions
- Eliminating risk factors
- Maintaining normal body temperature
- Education regarding prevention of hypothermia and heat-related illnesses (Display 15-2)

Positive Functional Consequences
- Prevention of hypothermia and heat-related illnesses
- Awareness of normal temperature, and improved ability to detect an altered febrile response

XI. Sexual Function

Age-Related Changes in Women (Table 16-2)
- Absence of ovulation
- Atrophy of reproductive organs
- Thinner and drier vaginal wall
- Diminished length and width of vagina
- Diminished lubrication during sexual activity

Age-Related Changes in Men (Table 16-2)
- Degenerative changes affecting reproductive organs

Risk Factors
- Attitudes, stereotypes, misunderstandings, lack of knowledge
- Social circumstances (e.g., lack of partner)
- Pathologic conditions
- Functional impairments
- Environmental constraints
- Adverse medication and chemical effects (Table 16-1)

Negative Functional Consequences
- Loss of reproductive ability in women
- More prolonged and less intense response to sexual stimulation (Table 16-2)
- Diminished sexual activity as a result of risks and social circumstances (*not* age-related changes)

Nursing Assessment
- Assessment of personal attitudes toward sexuality and aging (Display 16-1)
- Cultural aspects of sexual function (Culture Box page 459)
- Interview atmosphere and format (Display 16-2)
- Interview questions for older men and women (Display 16-2)

Nursing Interventions
- Education regarding sexual function in older adults (Display 16-3)
- Interventions in long-term care facilities
- Education regarding sexual function in people with arthritis or cardiac disease (Displays 16-4 and 16-5)
- Considerations regarding hormonal replacement therapy (Display 16-6)
- Education regarding medical therapies for erectile dysfunction (Display 16-7)

Positive Functional Consequences
- Improved and prolonged enjoyment of sexual activity
- Improved attitudes of staff toward expressions of sexuality by residents in long-term care facilities
- Improved quality of life

Index

The letter *f* following a page number indicates a figure; the letter *t* following a page number indicates a table, display, Culture Box, or Alternative and Preventive Health Care Practices box.

Feel-age, 19–20
Feminist nursing paradigm, 52
Fever. *See* Febrile response
Fiber, dietary
    cardiovascular function and,
        306*t*, 315*t*, 316*t*
    constipation and, 253*t*
    deficiency of, 235*t*
    effect on medications, 503*t*
    requirements for, 234, 255*t*
    soluble and insoluble, 234
Financial resources. *See* Eco-
        nomic resources
Floaters, 205
Fluid imbalance
    cognitive impairment and,
        506*t*, 545*t*
    depression and, 588*t*
    psychosocial consequences of,
        247
    thermoregulation and, 424
Fluid intake, 241, 249*t*, 250*t*,
        253*t*, 255*t*, 266, 268,
        272, 278–280, 279*t*,
        286*t*, 289–290, 392*t*,
        424, 603*t*
    water requirement, 236–237
Fluid intelligence, 104–106
Folate, 111, 247
    deficiency of, 160*t*, 235*t*
Folk healers, 136
Folk treatments, 136, 512*t*
Food
    enjoyment of, 243–246, 251–
        252, 254
        alleviating factors interfer-
            ing with, 252–254
    preparation of. *See* Meal *en-
        tries*
    procurement of. *See* Grocery
        shopping
Food additives, 254
Food and Drug Administration,
        258
Food and Nutrition Information
        Center, 258
Food selection, 230
Forced expiratory volume, 327*t*
Forearm fracture, 349
Foster-care home, 668*t*
Fovea, 205
Fractures, 351. *See also* Osteopo-
        rosis; *specific fracture
        sites*

cultural variations in, 357*t*
economic impact of, 359
gender differences in, 357
increased susceptibility to,
        356–357
postural hypotension and,
        298–299, 311, 317,
        317*t*
prevention of, 349, 367–370,
        369*t*
racial differences in, 357
visual impairment and, 207
Fracture threshold, 357
Frail elderly, 5–6
Frailty, of older adults, 625
Freckles, senile, 390*t*
Free radical theories of aging, 39
Friendly visitors, 669*t*
Frontotemporal dementia, 536,
        542
Functional age, 20–21
Functional assessment, 41, 43,
        57
    in acute care setting, 481
    criteria for activities of daily
        living, 485–486*t*, 487
    criteria for instrumental activi-
        ties of daily living, 487,
        487–488*t*
    current trends in, 480–484
    format for, 484–487,
        485–486*t*
    goals of, 484
    history of, 480–484
    instruments for, 481, 484
Functional assessment indices,
        484
Functional consequences. *See
        also specific area of
        functioning*
    definition of, 55–56, 56*t*
    negative, 55–56, 56*t*
    positive, 55–56, 56*t*
    theoretical underpinning, 57
Functional consequences theory,
        43, 51–62, 54*f*
    concepts underlying, 54–62,
        56*t*
Functional health theories,
        40–41
Functional impairment
    cognitive impairment and,
        555*t*
    coping strategies for, 88*t*

depression and, 588–589,
        598
mental illness and, 84
psychosocial changes and, 72
safety and, 627*t*
self-esteem and, 90, 153
sexual function and, 449
urinary incontinence and,
        268–269
Functional incontinence, 272*t*
Functional status, 17, 26, 43
    age-related changes in, 41
    health and, 17
Furniture, assessment of safety
        of, 363*t*

Gag reflex, 325–326, 330*t*, 331*f*
Gait
    age-related changes in, 348
    postfall syndrome, 358
    psychosocial function and,
        138
    training, 367–368
Gas exchange, age-related
        changes in, 327, 330*t*,
        331*f*
Gastric emptying, 231–232, 494
Gastric juice, 231–232, 494,
        496*t*
Gastrointestinal disturbances
    medication-related, 243*t*
    sleep and, 405*t*
Gastrointestinal tract. *See also* Di-
        gestion
    changes in and medication,
        494–495, 496*t*
Gay men, 446, 457, *See also* Ho-
        mosexuality
GDS/FAST (Global Deterioration
        Scale/Functional Assess-
        ment Staging), 547–
        549, 548*t*
GDS (Geriatric Depression
        Scale), 594
Gender
    medication effects and, 496
    osteoporosis and, 349
    sleep patterns and, 401–402
    susceptibility to fractures and,
        357
Gender-sensitive nursing para-
        digm, 52